METHODS IN MOLECULAR BIOLOGY™

Series Editor
John M. Walker
School of Life Sciences
University of Hertfordshire
Hatfield, Hertfordshire, AL10 9AB, UK

For further volumes:
http://www.springer.com/series/7651

Ovarian Cancer

Methods and Protocols

Edited by

Anastasia Malek

Laboratory of Oncoendocrinology,
N.N. Petrov Institute of Oncology, St. Petersburg, Russia

Oleg Tchernitsa

Labs of Molecular Tumor Pathology and Functional Gemonics,
Charité-Universitatsmedizin Berlin, Berlin, Germany

Humana Press

Editors
Anastasia Malek
Laboratory of Oncoendocrinology
N.N. Petrov Institute of Oncology
St. Petersburg, Russia

Oleg Tchernitsa
Labs of Molecular Tumor Pathology
and Functional Gemonics
Charité-Universitatsmedizin Berlin
Berlin, Germany

ISSN 1064-3745 ISSN 1940-6029 (electronic)
ISBN 978-1-4939-5962-4 ISBN 978-1-62703-547-7 (eBook)
DOI 10.1007/978-1-62703-547-7
Springer New York Heidelberg Dordrecht London

Printed on acid-free paper

Humana Press is a brand of Springer
Springer is part of Springer Science+Business Media (www.springer.com)

Preface

Ovarian cancer (OC) is the most lethal malignancy of the female reproductive system and is also the fifth leading cause of cancer death in women. The etiology of OC is poorly understood, and there are no reliable predictive factors or preceding chronic diseases. As OC is mostly asymptomatic in its initial stages, early detection is difficult. By the time OC is diagnosed, the tumor has often progressed to an advanced stage. Despite aggressive primary therapy and a sufficient initial response rate, advanced OC has a strong tendency to relapse and develop drug resistance. In order to improve this dismal situation, a better understanding of the biology of OC at the molecular, cellular and histological levels is essential. Molecular and cell biology methods are clearly applicable to the field of ovarian cancer research. However, proper study design and interpretation of the results from these types of experiments requires careful consideration of the specific features associated with OC.

In more then 90 % of cases, ovarian cancer has an epithelial origin. It is assumed to develop from cells belonging to the simple monolayer ovarian surface epithelium, a tissue similar to the remainder of the mesothelium that overlays the peritoneal cavity. However, in contrast to the mesothelium, the ovarian surface epithelium undergoes cyclic hormonal influence and local destruction associated with ovulation. Repair of the ovarian surface after ovulation can result in the development of ovarian cysts lined with epithelial tissue. This portion of the ovarian surface epithelium can become isolated and may be constantly exposed to hormones and growth factors. Together, these observations provide grounds for the hypothesis that the epithelium associated with cysts represents a primary source of ovarian cancer. An alternative theory is based on the morphological similarity between ovarian cancer and tumors within the Mullerian system (fallopian tubes, cervix, uterus), suggesting that ovarian cancer may develop from Mullerian-type epithelia. In addition, other mechanisms have also been suggested regarding the origin of ovarian cancer. Thus, the unclear etiology of this cancer should reinforce the importance of focusing on the proper choice of normal reference tissues for structural and functional genetic studies.

After development of an ovarian tumor, single cancer cells or cell clusters are released into the peritoneal cavity. Each cluster drifts until it encounters the lining of the cavity. It then attaches to the visceral or parietal peritoneum, spreads out, and launches an invasion into the mesothelium. There are two factors that can trigger this process. The first is anoikis, a specific type of apoptotic death of single floating cells that is induced by loss of contact with the epithelial basal membrane. The second factor is the peritoneal lymph drainage route, which can draw cancer cells into the lymphatic system. OC cells avoid anoikis and lymphatic clearance via attachment to the mesothelium. Further successful metastatic spread requires concerted regulation of critical cellular processes, including apoptosis, proliferation, cell–cell and cell–matrix adhesion, migration, and breakdown of the extracellular matrix. Due to their intra-peritoneal localization, gene expression and structural and metabolic properties of ovarian cancer cells may differ from that of tumours that spread via the lymphatic or blood vasculature, requiring the use of specific techniques for investigation.

A detailed understanding of the mechanisms associated with ovarian cancer onset and progression requires the development of appropriate experimental models for in vitro and in vivo studies. Ovarian cancer cell lines derived from ascites or primary ovarian tumour have been used extensively and can very effective for studying the processing growth regulation. There are many in vitro approaches aimed at recapitulating specific aspects of OC progression such as cell motility, invasiveness, adhesive properties, development of multicellular spheroids. Animal models of OC have been created to mimic this cancer in the context of a whole organism. Thus, syngenic models help to study initiating event of ovarian cancerogenesis while transplantation of human tumours into athymic mice is providing with useful tools for therapeutics development.

The primarily goal of this book is to provide readers with methods that have been created or adapted to study various aspects of ovarian cancer. Thus, Part I contains chapters describing methods used to study structural genetic alterations present in ovarian cancer. It is essential to note that these chapters do not contain laboratory protocols, but instead focus on statistical approaches needed for evaluation of complex results and integration of this data with epi-genetic, expression, and clinical data. Part II presents descriptions of basic techniques used to investigate gene methylation status, with an emphasis on the differences between these methods and on their specific applications. Methods used to analyze genome expression activity and some specific classes of RNAs are combined in Part III. The last chapter of Part III presents a mathematical approach for gathering data associated with structural and regulatory gene expression profiling in order to better understand coordinated regulation of these genes. Next, Part IV describes the methods used to study structural features of ovarian cancer cells in terms of proteins, lipids and glycosides content. Techniques used to culture ovarian cancer cells and to assay malignant properties of ovarian cancer in vitro are included in Part V. In vitro and in vivo models that recapitulate ovarian cancer development are described in Part VI. The last part of this book relates to ovarian cancer-oriented drug delivery research. Each section of the book is introduced with a short review describing the current state of the field. These introductory passages are intended to provide a comparative overview of all of the methods presented in the section and to note any missing approaches.

The secondary goal of this book is to demonstrate the broad applicability of well-known molecular biology techniques to ovarian cancer research and to encourage readers to adopt other general methods for use in their studies, while taking into account the specifics of ovarian cancer biology.

The editors believe that this book will be helpful for beginning, as well as experienced investigators, to optimize study designs, to correctly select the most applicable methods, and to produce interesting and novel results.

St. Petersburg, Russia *Anastasia Malek*
Berlin, Germany *Oleg Tchernitsa*

Contents

Contributors

ACHIM AIGNER • *Rudolf-Boehm-Institute for Pharmacology and Toxicology, Clinical Pharmacology University of Leipzig, Leipzig, Germany*
PETER ALTEVOGT • *D015, Tumorimmunology, German Cancer Research Centre (DKFZ), Heidelberg, Germany*
MARINA BAGNOLI • *Department of Experimental Oncology and Molecular Medicine, Unit of Molecular Therapies, Fondazione IRCCS, Istituto Nazionale dei Tumori, Milan, Italy*
JIRI BARTEK • *Genome Integrity Unit, Danish Cancer Society Research Center, Copenhagen, Denmark; Laboratory of Genomic Integrity and Institute of Molecular and Translational Medicine, Palacky University, Olomouc, Czech Republic*
CHRISTOPHER F. BASSIL • *Division of Gynecologic Oncology, Duke University Medical Center, Durham, NC, USA*
KARL-FRIEDRICH BECKER • *Department of Pathology, Technische Universität München, Munich, Germany*
DAVID D.L. BOWTELL • *Cancer Genetics and Genomics Laboratory, Peter MacCallum Cancer Centre, East Melbourne, VIC, Australia*
SILVANA CANEVARI • *Department of Experimental Oncology and Molecular Medicine, Unit of Molecular Therapies, Fondazione IRCCS, Istituto Nazionale dei Tumori, Milan, Italy*
JEREMY CHIEN • *Mayo Clinic College of Medicine, Rochester, MN, USA*
MINE S. CICEK • *Department of Health Sciences Research, Mayo Clinic College of Medicine, Rochester, MN, USA*
IAN R. CORBIN • *Advanced Imaging Research Center, University of Texas Southwestern Medical Center at Dallas, Dallas, TX, USA*
JÚLIA COSTA • *Instituto de Tecnologia Química e Biológica, Universidade Nova de Lisboa, Lisbon, Portugal*
CARLO M. CROCE • *Department of Molecular Virology, Immunology and Medical Genetics and Comprehensive Cancer Center, Ohio State University, Columbus, OH, USA*
JUAN CUI • *Department of Biochemistry and Molecular Biology, University of Georgia, Athens, GA, USA*
NEVENKA DIMITROVA • *Philips Research North America, Briarcliff Manor, NY, USA*
MAURO FERRARI • *The Methodist Hospital Research Institute, Houston, TX, USA*
MIRANDA Y. FONG • *Department of Physiology and Biophysics, University of Louisville, Louisville, KY, USA*
JOSHY GEORGE • *Cancer Genetics and Genomics Laboratory, Peter MacCallum Cancer Centre, East Melbourne, VIC, Australia*
ELLEN L. GOODE • *Department of Health Sciences Research, Mayo Clinic College of Medicine, Rochester, MN, USA*
KYLIE L. GORRINGE • *Peter MacCallum Cancer Centre, East Melbourne, VIC, Australia*
JAMES B. GREENAWAY • *Department of Biomedical Sciences, University of Guelph, Guelph, ON, Canada*

DANIELA GUTSCH • *Faculty of Medicine, Biochemical-Pharmacological Center, Institute of Pharmacology, Philipps-University Marburg, Marburg, Germany*
NAFIS HASAN • *Thomas Jefferson University, Philadelphia, PA, USA*
XIAOPING HE • *Mayo Clinic College of Medicine, Rochester, MN, USA*
SABRINA HÖBEL • *Rudolf-Boehm-Institute for Pharmacology and Toxicology, Clinical Pharmacology University of Leipzig, Leipzig, Germany*
BINGDING HUANG • *Collaborative Innovation Center for Diagnosis and Treatment of Infectious Diseases, Zhejiang University, Hangzhou, Zhejiang Province, P. R. China*
ZHIQING HUANG • *Division of Gynecologic Oncology, Duke University Medical Center, Durham, NC, USA*
EVGENY N. IMYANITOV • *Laboratory of Molecular Oncology, N.N. Petrov Institute of Oncology, St.-Petersburg, Russia*
EGIDIO IORIO • *Department of Cell Biology and Neurosciences, Istituto Superiore di Sanità, Rome, Italy*
MARILENA V. IORIO • *Department of Experimental Oncology, Fondazione IRCCS, Istituto Nazionale Tumori, Milan, Italy*
SHAM S. KAKAR • *Department of Physiology and Biophysics, University of Louisville, Louisville, KY, USA*
SITHARTHAN KAMALAKARAN • *Philips Research North America, Briarcliff Manor, NY, USA*
SEBASTIAN KANDZIA • *Oligosaccharide Analytics, GlycoThera, Hannover, Germany*
DONGMEI LAI • *The International peace maternity and child health hospital, School of medicine, Shanghai Jiaotong University, Shanghai, China*
DOUGLAS A. LEVINE • *Department of Surgery, Gynecology Service, Memorial Sloan-Kettering Cancer Center, New York, NY, USA*
LISHA LI • *Collaborative Innovation Center for Diagnosis and Treatment of Infectious Diseases, Zhejiang University, Hangzhou, Zhejiang Province, P. R. China*
ANDRÉ LIEBER • *Division of Medical Genetics, University of Washington, Washington, DC, USA; Department of Pathology, University of Washington, Washington, DC, USA*
BIAOYANG LIN • *Collaborative Innovation Center for Diagnosis and Treatment of Infectious Diseases, Zhejiang University, Hangzhou, Zhejiang Province, P. R. China*
QIONG LIN • *Institute for Biomedical Engineering-Cell Biology, RWTH Aachen University Medical School, Aachen, Germany*
JIE LIU • *Collaborative Innovation Center for Diagnosis and Treatment of Infectious Diseases, Zhejiang University, Hangzhou, Zhejiang Province, P. R. China*
JINSONG LIU • *Department of Pathology, University of Texas M. D. Anderson Cancer Center, Houston, TX, USA*
XIAOYAN LOU • *Collaborative Innovation Center for Diagnosis and Treatment of Infectious Diseases, Zhejiang University, Hangzhou, Zhejiang Province, P. R. China*
ROBERT LUCITO • *Hofstra North Shore-LIJ School of Medicine, Hofstra University, Hempstead, NY, USA*
ANASTASIA MALEK • *Laboratory of Oncoendocrinology, N.N. Petrov Institute of Oncology, St. Petersburg, Russia*
KATHARINA MALINOWSKY • *Department of Pathology, Technische Universität München, Munich, Germany*
AMAN MANN • *Sanford-Burnham Medical Research Institute, La Jolla, CA, USA*
MATTHEW J. MAURER • *Department of Health Sciences Research, Mayo Clinic College of Medicine, Rochester, MN, USA*
JONATHAN MCDUNN • *Metabolon, Inc., Durham, NC, USA*

ANNE-MARIE MES-MASSON • *Department of Medicine, University of Montréal, Montréal, QC, Canada*
SUSAN K. MURPHY • *Division of Gynecologic Oncology, Duke University Medical Center, Durham, NC, USA*
MARK W. NACHTIGAL • *Department of Biochemistry and Medical Genetics, University of Manitoba, Winnipeg, MB, Canada; Department of Obstetrics Gynecology and Reproductive Sciences, University of Manitoba, Winnipeg, MB, Canada; Manitoba Institute of Cell Biology, CancerCare Manitoba, Winnipeg, MB, Canada*
SARA NAPOLI • *Laboratory of Experimental Oncology, Institute of Oncology Research, Bellinzona, Switzerland*
IRINA NAZARENKO • *Department of Environmental Health Sciences, Freiburg University Medical Centre, Freiburg, Germany*
SELENE NUNEZ-CRUZ • *Department of Obstetrics and Gynecology, Penn Ovarian Cancer Research Center, University of Pennsylvania, Philadelphia, PA, USA*
JIM J. PETRIK • *Department of Biomedical Sciences, University of Guelph, Guelph, ON, Canada*
MARIA ELENA PISANU • *Department of Cell Biology and Neurosciences, Istituto Superiore di Sanità, Rome, Italy*
FRANCA PODO • *Department of Cell Biology and Neurosciences, Istituto Superiore di Sanità, Rome, Italy*
LISE PORTELANCE • *University of Montréal Hospital Research Centre, Montréal Cancer Institute, Montréal, QC, Canada*
DAVID PUETT • *Department of Biochemistry and Molecular Biology, University of Georgia, Athens, GA, USA*
ALESSANDRO RICCI • *Department of Cell Biology and Neurosciences, Istituto Superiore di Sanità, Rome, Italy*
PAUL C. ROBERTS • *Department of Biomedical Sciences and Pathobiology, Virginia Polytechnic Institute and State University, Blacksburg, VA, USA*
ANNE-KATHLEEN RUPP • *D015, Tumorimmunology, German Cancer Research Centre (DKFZ), Heidelberg, Germany*
EVA M. SCHMELZ • *Department of Human Nutrition, Foods and Exercise, Virginia Tech, Blacksburg, VA, USA*
NATHALIE SCHOLLER • *Department of Obstetrics and Gynecology, Penn Ovarian Cancer Research Center, University of Pennsylvania, Philadelphia, PA, USA*
CHRISTINA SCHOTT • *Department of Pathology, Technische Universität München, Munich, Germany*
WEIWEI SHAN • *Department of Obstetrics and Gynecology, Baylor College of Medicine, Houston, TX, USA*
VIJI SHRIDHAR • *Mayo Clinic College of Medicine, Rochester, MN, USA*
JOHN SINCLAIR • *Cell Communication Team, The Institute of Cancer Research, London, UK*
GORDON K. SMYTH • *Bioinformatics Division, Walter and Eliza Hall Institute of Medical Research, Parkville, VIC, Australia*
ROBERT STRAUSS • *Genome Integrity Unit, Danish Cancer Society Research Center, Copenhagen, Denmark*
TAKEMI TANAKA • *Thomas Jefferson University, Philadelphia, PA, USA*
BRIGITTE L. THÉRIAULT • *Campbell Family Cancer Research Institute, Ontario Cancer Institute, University Health Network, Toronto, ON, Canada*

JOHN F. TIMMS • *Cancer Proteomics Laboratory, EGA Institute for Women's Health, University College London, London, UK*
VINAY VARADAN • *Philips Research North America, Briarcliff Manor, NY, USA*
ILEABETT M. ECHEVARRIA VARGAS • *Department of Biochemistry, School of Medicine, University of Puerto Rico, San Juan, PR, USA*
PABLO E. VIVAS-MEJÍA • *Department of Biochemistry and Cancer Center, School of Medicine, University of Puerto Rico, San Juan, PR, USA*
WOLFGANG WAGNER • *Helmholtz Institute for Biomedical Engineering, Aachen, Germany*
ULRIKE WEIRAUCH • *Rudolf-Boehm-Institute for Pharmacology and Toxicology, Clinical Pharmacology University of Leipzig, Leipzig, Germany*
CLAUDIA WOLFF • *Department of Pathology, Technische Universität München, Munich, Germany*
KAZIMIERZ O. WRZESZCZYNSKI • *Bioinformatics and Genomics, Cold Spring Harbor Laboratory, Cold Spring Harbor, NY, USA*
YING XU • *Department of Biochemistry and Molecular Biology, University of Georgia, Athens, GA, USA*
LIJUAN YANG • *The International peace maternity and child health hospital, School of medicine, Shanghai Jiaotong University, Shanghai, China*
WEI YU • *Collaborative Innovation Center for Diagnosis and Treatment of Infectious Diseases, Zhejiang University, Hangzhou, Zhejiang Province, P. R. China*
MARTIN ZENKE • *Institute for Biomedical Engineering-Cell Biology, RWTH Aachen University Medical School, Aachen, Germany*
SHIHUA ZHANG • *Institute of Applied Mathematics, Academy of Mathematics and Systems Science, Chinese Academy of Science, Beijing, China*

Part I

Evaluation of Genomic Alteration

Chapter 1

Ovarian Cancer Genome

Evgeny N. Imyanitov

Abstract

Ovarian cancer (OC) is a relatively frequent malignant disease with a lifetime risk approaching to approximately 1 in 70. As many as 15–25 % OC arise due to known heterozygous germ-line mutations in DNA repair genes, such as BRCA1, BRCA2, RAD51C, NBN (NBS1), BRIP, and PALB2. Sporadic ovarian cancers often phenocopy the features of BRCA1-related hereditary disease (so-called BRCAness), i.e., show biallelic somatic inactivation of the BRCA1 gene. Tumor-specific BRCA1 deficiency renders selective sensitivity of transformed cells to platinating compounds and several other anticancer drugs, which explains high response rates of OC to systemic therapies. High-throughput molecular profiling of OC is instrumental for further progress in identification of novel OC diagnostic markers as well as for the development of new OC-specific treatments. However, interpretation of the huge bulk of incoming data may present a challenge. There is a critical need in the development of bioinformatic tools capable to integrate the multiplicity of available data sets into biologically and medically meaningful pieces of knowledge.

Key words Ovarian cancer genome, Mutations, Gene polymorphisms, High-throughput methods, BRCA1

Ovarian cancer (OC) is a relatively frequent malignant disease with a lifetime risk approaching to approximately 1 in 70. As compared to other common tumor types, OC is characterized by a number of unique bioclinical features. Ovarian neoplasms are usually asymptomatic or produce only nonspecific symptoms at early stages of the disease, so the majority of OC cases are diagnosed only at the time of distant metastatic spread. While localized ovarian tumors have excellent cure rates (80–95 %), even the advanced disease appears to be relatively well manageable at least in some patients. In contrast to other cancer entities, thorough cytoreductive surgery is highly effective for the treatment of women affected by late-stage OC. Furthermore, the majority of ovarian carcinomas demonstrate a pronounced response to conventional cytotoxic therapy, especially to platinum-containing regimens. Up to 20 % of stage IV OC patients treated by surgical tumor debulking and standard chemotherapy enjoy long-term survival that is apparently the best statistics among advanced epithelial malignant tumors [1, 2].

Anastasia Malek and Oleg Tchernitsa (eds.), *Ovarian Cancer: Methods and Protocols*, Methods in Molecular Biology, vol. 1049, DOI 10.1007/978-1-62703-547-7_1, © Springer Science+Business Media New York 2013

Contribution of inherited mutated genes in the incidence of ovarian cancer is noticeably higher than for other common malignancies. Indeed, as many as 15–25 % OC arise due to known heterozygous germ-line mutations in DNA repair genes. Recent studies show that the lists of predisposing genes for breast and ovarian cancers may have nearly complete overlap. In addition to the well-established significance of the BRCA1 and BRCA2, there is evidence for contribution of mutations in NBN (NBS1), BRIP, RAD51C, PALB2, and some other genes [3, 4]. Interestingly, sporadic ovarian cancers often phenocopy the features of BRCA1-related hereditary disease (so-called BRCAness), i.e., show biallelic somatic inactivation of the BRCA1 gene. Tumor-specific BRCA1-deficiency renders selective sensitivity of transformed cells to platinating compounds and several other anticancer drugs, which explains the high response rate of OC to the systemic treatment [5].

It is frequently underestimated that the majority of information gained by ovarian cancer research concerns its most frequent histological type, i.e., serous carcinomas. Unlike some other epithelial tumors, various histological categories of OC preserve relatively high level of differentiation, rarely demonstrate mixed histology, and appear to have entirely distinct molecular pathogenesis and clinical behavior. It is sometimes stated that serous, mucinous, endometrioid, and clear-cell types of OC deserve to be considered as four distinct diseases and need to be subjected to separate epidemiological, clinical, and biological investigations [6].

While formulating the priorities for ovarian cancer research, most of the experts outline the utmost significance of timely recognition of the disease. Indeed, early-stage ovarian cancer is more or less curable by the already available means; however, the sensitivity and specificity of existing diagnostic tools remain insufficient. Gene-based identification of those women at-risk, who need tighter surveillance than average population, is one of the possible solutions. Another approach includes the development of specific molecular markers, which would be accessible to the laboratory detection even when the growing tumor mass is still tiny [1, 6].

Search for novel drug targets is also a primary focus for genomic OC research. Although the initial sensitivity of OC to conventional cytotoxic agents is widely acknowledged, most of the tumors inevitably develop the multidrug resistance during the therapy. Furthermore, the platinating drugs, taxanes, and other compounds demonstrate evident effect only towards serous ovarian carcinomas, while the treatment of other histological types of OC is significantly more complicated. In addition, most of the routinely used cytotoxic drugs have pronounced adverse effects; for example, patients receiving platinum-containing regimens often suffer from severe neurological and renal complications that call for the development of drugs with improved safety profile [1, 6].

While approximately two dozens of targeted drugs have been approved for the treatment of several common cancer types in the past, there are no novel breakthrough agents for the management of ovarian cancer. It is hoped that advances in molecular portraying of OC will provide new therapeutic leads [7].

As mentioned above, the significant portion of ovarian carcinomas are attributed to rare highly or moderately penetrant inactivating gene defects [4, 6]. It was believed until recently that the rest of ovarian cancer incidence can be explained by unfavorable combination of common low-penetrance gene polymorphisms. Recent genome-wide association studies (GWAS) succeeded to identify a number of OC-predisposing alleles [8–11]. Although the statistical significance of these data sets seems convincing and therefore allows to exclude the possibility of chance variations, the difference of odds ratios (OR) from 1 (i.e., the degree of the additional risk carried by an unfavorable allele) is uniformly low. Therefore, low-penetrance gene scanning is unlikely to enter predictive genetic testing for OC in the near future.

An array profiling has identified a number of recurrent abnormalities in ovarian cancer. Comprehensive catalogs of OC molecular karyotypes have become available since recently. A number of studies provided systematic description of DNA methylation patterns in ovarian tumors. These data have been successfully integrated with the results of transcriptome studies. Molecular portraying of ovarian tumors has allowed to identify new determinants of malignant growth, describe novel bioclinical subtypes of OC, reveal previously unknown causes of drug resistance, etc [12–18]. At the time of writing of this manuscript, there was still no publications on the whole-genome sequencing of ovarian tumors, but it is beyond the doubt that the massive information on new OC-specific mutations will appear very soon.

As high-throughput methods become increasingly accessible to the biomedical researchers, it is getting more and more difficult to manage the huge bulk of incoming data. First, development of principles for discrimination between biologically meaningful and "noise" molecular events presents a great challenge. Second, it is instrumental to develop bioinformatic tools, which would allow to reveal relationships between pathogenically linked abnormalities, i.e., to identify pathways leading to malignant transformation and tumor maintenance. Third, while all currently available technologies, i.e., genomics, transcriptomics, methylomics, proteomics, metabolomics, and massive parallel sequencing, are technically capable to describe only a certain aspect of cancer disease, true biological picture can be obtained only by integrating these data strata into a single module. Papers presented in this issue provide excellent examples of the progress in the gathering, analysis, and interpretation of the data on ovarian cancer genome.

References

1. Cannistra SA (2004) Cancer of the ovary. N Engl J Med 351:2519–2529
2. Tropé CG, Elstrand MB, Sandstad B, Davidson B, Oksefjell H (2012) Neoadjuvant chemotherapy, interval debulking surgery or primary surgery in ovarian carcinoma FIGO stage IV? Eur J Cancer 48(14):2146–2154
3. Meindl A, Hellebrand H, Wiek C, Erven V, Wappenschmidt B, Niederacher D, Freund M, Lichtner P, Hartmann L, Schaal H, Ramser J, Honisch E, Kubisch C, Wichmann HE, Kast K, Deissler H, Engel C, Müller-Myhsok B, Neveling K, Kiechle M, Mathew CG, Schindler D, Schmutzler RK, Hanenberg H (2010) Germline mutations in breast and ovarian cancer pedigrees establish RAD51C as a human cancer susceptibility gene. Nat Genet 42: 410–414
4. Walsh T, Casadei S, Lee MK, Pennil CC, Nord AS, Thornton AM, Roeb W, Agnew KJ, Stray SM, Wickramanayake A, Norquist B, Pennington KP, Garcia RL, King MC, Swisher EM (2012) Mutations in 12 genes for inherited ovarian, fallopian tube, and peritoneal carcinoma identified by massively parallel sequencing. Proc Natl Acad Sci U S A 108:18032–18037
5. Turner N, Tutt A, Ashworth A (2012) Hallmarks of 'BRCAness' in sporadic cancers. Nat Rev Cancer 4:814–819
6. Bast RC Jr, Hennessy B, Mills GB (2009) The biology of ovarian cancer: new opportunities for translation. Nat Rev Cancer 9:415–428
7. Cheung HW, Cowley GS, Weir BA, Boehm JS, Rusin S, Scott JA, East A, Ali LD, Lizotte PH, Wong TC, Jiang G, Hsiao J, Mermel CH, Getz G, Barretina J, Gopal S, Tamayo P, Gould J, Tsherniak A, Stransky N, Luo B, Ren Y, Drapkin R, Bhatia SN, Mesirov JP, Garraway LA, Meyerson M, Lander ES, Root DE, Hahn WC (2011) Systematic investigation of genetic vulnerabilities across cancer cell lines reveals lineage-specific dependencies in ovarian cancer. Proc Natl Acad Sci U S A 108:12372–12377
8. Bolton KL, Tyrer J, Song H, Ramus SJ, Notaridou M, Jones C, Sher T, Gentry-Maharaj A, Wozniak E, Tsai YY, Weidhaas J, Paik D, Van Den Berg DJ, Stram DO, Pearce CL, Wu AH, Brewster W, Anton-Culver H, Ziogas A, Narod SA, Levine DA, Kaye SB, Brown R, Paul J, Flanagan J, Sieh W, McGuire V, Whittemore AS, Campbell I, Gore ME, Lissowska J, Yang HP, Medrek K, Gronwald J, Lubinski J, Jakubowska A, Le ND, Cook LS, Kelemen LE, Brook-Wilson A, Massuger LF, Kiemeney LA, Aben KK, van Altena AM, Houlston R, Tomlinson I, Palmieri RT, Moorman PG, Schildkraut J, Iversen ES, Phelan C, Vierkant RA, Cunningham JM, Goode EL, Fridley BL, Kruger-Kjaer S, Blaeker J, Hogdall E, Hogdall C, Gross J, Karlan BY, Ness RB, Edwards RP, Odunsi K, Moyisch KB, Baker JA, Modugno F, Heikkinenen T, Butzow R, Nevanlinna H, Leminen A, Bogdanova N, Antonenkova N, Doerk T, Hillemanns P, Dürst M, Runnebaum I, Thompson PJ, Carney ME, Goodman MT, Lurie G, Wang-Gohrke S, Hein R, Chang-Claude J, Rossing MA, Cushing-Haugen KL, Doherty J, Chen C, Rafnar T, Besenbacher S, Sulem P, Stefansson K, Birrer MJ, Terry KL, Hernandez D, Cramer DW, Vergote I, Amant F, Lambrechts D, Despierre E, Fasching PA, Beckmann MW, Thiel FC, Ekici AB, Chen X; Australian Ovarian Cancer Study Group; Australian Cancer Study (Ovarian Cancer); Ovarian Cancer Association Consortium, Johnatty SE, Webb PM, Beesley J, Chanock S, Garcia-Closas M, Sellers T, Easton DF, Berchuck A, Chenevix-Trench G, Pharoah PD, Gayther SA (2010) Common variants at 19p13 are associated with susceptibility to ovarian cancer. Nat Genet 42:880–884
9. Bolton KL, Ganda C, Berchuck A, Pharaoh PD, Gayther SA (2012) Role of common genetic variants in ovarian cancer susceptibility and outcome: progress to date from the Ovarian Cancer Association Consortium (OCAC). J Intern Med 271:366–378
10. Goode EL, Chenevix-Trench G, Song H, Ramus SJ, Notaridou M, Lawrenson K, Widschwendter M, Vierkant RA, Larson MC, Kjaer SK, Birrer MJ, Berchuck A, Schildkraut J, Tomlinson I, Kiemeney LA, Cook LS, Gronwald J, Garcia-Closas M, Gore ME, Campbell I, Whittemore AS, Sutphen R, Phelan C, Anton-Culver H, Pearce CL, Lambrechts D, Rossing MA, Chang-Claude J, Moysich KB, Goodman MT, Dörk T, Nevanlinna H, Ness RB, Rafnar T, Hogdall C, Hogdall E, Fridley BL, Cunningham JM, Sieh W, McGuire V, Godwin AK, Cramer DW, Hernandez D, Levine D, Lu K, Iversen ES, Palmieri RT, Houlston R, van Altena AM, Aben KK, Massuger LF, Brooks-Wilson A, Kelemen LE, Le ND, Jakubowska A, Lubinski J, Medrek K, Stafford A, Easton DF, Tyrer J, Bolton KL, Harrington P, Eccles D, Chen A, Molina AN, Davila BN, Arango H, Tsai YY, Chen Z, Risch HA, McLaughlin J, Narod SA, Ziogas A, Brewster W, Gentry-Maharaj A, Menon U, Wu AH, Stram DO, Pike MC; Wellcome Trust Case-Control Consortium, Beesley J, Webb PM; Australian Cancer Study (Ovarian Cancer); Australian Ovarian Cancer Study Group; Ovarian

Cancer Association Consortium (OCAC), Chen X, Ekici AB, Thiel FC, Beckmann MW, Yang H, Wentzensen N, Lissowska J, Fasching PA, Despierre E, Amant F, Vergote I, Doherty J, Hein R, Wang-Gohrke S, Lurie G, Carney ME, Thompson PJ, Runnebaum I, Hillemanns P, Dürst M, Antonenkova N, Bogdanova N, Leminen A, Butzow R, Heikkinen T, Stefansson K, Sulem P, Besenbacher S, Sellers TA, Gayther SA, Pharoah PD; Ovarian Cancer Association Consortium (OCAC) (2010) A genome-wide association study identifies susceptibility loci for ovarian cancer at 2q31 and 8q24. Nat Genet 42:874–879

11. Song H, Ramus SJ, Tyrer J, Bolton KL, Gentry-Maharaj A, Wozniak E, Anton-Culver H, Chang-Claude J, Cramer DW, DiCioccio R, Dörk T, Goode EL, Goodman MT, Schildkraut JM, Sellers T, Baglietto L, Beckmann MW, Beesley J, Blaakaer J, Carney ME, Chanock S, Chen Z, Cunningham JM, Dicks E, Doherty JA, Dürst M, Ekici AB, Fenstermacher D, Fridley BL, Giles G, Gore ME, De Vivo I, Hillemanns P, Hogdall C, Hogdall E, Iversen ES, Jacobs IJ, Jakubowska A, Li D, Lissowska J, Lubiński J, Lurie G, McGuire V, McLaughlin J, Medrek K, Moorman PG, Moysich K, Narod S, Phelan C, Pye C, Risch H, Runnebaum IB, Severi G, Southey M, Stram DO, Thiel FC, Terry KL, Tsai YY, Tworoger SS, Van Den Berg DJ, Vierkant RA, Wang-Gohrke S, Webb PM, Wilkens LR, Wu AH, Yang H, Brewster W, Ziogas A; Australian Cancer (Ovarian) Study; Australian Ovarian Cancer Study Group; Ovarian Cancer Association Consortium, Houlston R, Tomlinson I, Whittemore AS, Rossing MA, Ponder BA, Pearce CL, Ness RB, Menon U, Kjaer SK, Gronwald J, Garcia-Closas M, Fasching PA, Easton DF, Chenevix-Trench G, Berchuck A, Pharoah PD, Gayther SA (2009) A genome-wide association study identifies a new ovarian cancer susceptibility locus on 9p22.2. Nat Genet 41:996–1000

12. Gorringe KL, Ramakrishna M, Williams LH, Sridhar A, Boyle SE, Bearfoot JL, Li J, Anglesio MS, Campbell IG (2009) Are there any more ovarian tumor suppressor genes? A new perspective using ultra high-resolution copy number and loss of heterozygosity analysis. Genes Chromosomes Cancer 48:931–942

13. Gorringe KL, Campbell IG (2009) Large-scale genomic analysis of ovarian carcinomas. Mol Oncol 3:157–164

14. Gorringe KL, George J, Anglesio MS, Ramakrishna M, Etemadmoghadam D, Cowin P, Sridhar A, Williams LH, Boyle SE, Yanaihara N, Okamoto A, Urashima M, Smyth GK, Campbell IG, Bowtell DD, Australian Ovarian Cancer Study (2010) Copy number analysis identifies novel interactions between genomic loci in ovarian cancer. PLoS One 5:e11408

15. Kennedy BA, Deatherage DE, Gu F, Tang B, Chan MW, Nephew KP, Huang TH, Jin VX (2011) ChIP-seq defined genome-wide map of TGFβ/SMAD4 targets: implications with clinical outcome of ovarian cancer. PLoS One 6:e22606

16. Yu W, Jin C, Lou X, Han X, Li L, He Y, Zhang H, Ma K, Zhu J, Cheng L, Lin B (2011) Global analysis of DNA methylation by Methyl-Capture sequencing reveals epigenetic control of cisplatin resistance in ovarian cancer cell. PLoS One 6:e29450

17. Wrzeszczynski KO, Varadan V, Byrnes J, Lum E, Kamalakaran S, Levine DA, Dimitrova N, Zhang MQ, Lucito R (2011) Identification of tumor suppressors and oncogenes from genomic and epigenetic features in ovarian cancer. PLoS One 6:e28503

18. Fekete T, Rásó E, Pete I, Tegze B, Liko I, Munkácsy G, Sipos N, Rigó J Jr, Györffy B (2012) Meta-analysis of gene expression profiles associated with histological classification and survival in 829 ovarian cancer samples. Int J Cancer 131:95–105

Chapter 2

Identifying Associations Between Genomic Alterations in Tumors

Joshy George, Kylie L. Gorringe, Gordon K. Smyth, and David D.L. Bowtell

Abstract

Single-nucleotide polymorphism (SNP) mapping arrays are a reliable method for identifying somatic copy number alterations in cancer samples. Though this is immensely useful to identify potential driver genes, it is not sufficient to identify genes acting in a concerted manner. In cancer cells, co-amplified genes have been shown to provide synergistic effects, and genomic alterations targeting a pathway have been shown to occur in a mutually exclusive manner. We therefore developed a bioinformatic method for detecting such gene pairs using an integrated analysis of genomic copy number and gene expression data. This approach allowed us to identify a gene pair that is co-amplified and co-expressed in high-grade serous ovarian cancer. This finding provided information about the interaction of specific genetic events that contribute to the development and progression of this disease.

Key words Amplicon, Deletion, Oncogene, Bioinformatics, CGH, Copy number

1 Introduction

Genetic co-alteration and cancer. When cancer is viewed as an evolutionary system where the unit of selection is the cancer cell, genomic alterations are one of the means by which cells obtain their selective advantage. These alterations provide a survival advantage to the cancer cell by deregulating biochemical pathways that enable the cell to acquire the necessary traits to undergo malignant transformation [1]. If a biological pathway can be activated by a number of distinct molecular aberrations, then after the occurrence of any one of the alterations, the cell is unlikely to obtain an additional survival advantage from the occurrence of the remaining alterations. Thus it is reasonable to assume that such events will occur in a mutually exclusive fashion—for example, mutations in *BRAF* and *KRAS* are generally mutually exclusive in borderline ovarian cancer [2]. Conversely, biochemical pathways that have synergistic effects

Joshy George and Kylie L. Gorringe have contributed equally to this chapter.

Anastasia Malek and Oleg Tchernitsa (eds.), *Ovarian Cancer: Methods and Protocols*, Methods in Molecular Biology, vol. 1049, DOI 10.1007/978-1-62703-547-7_2, © Springer Science+Business Media New York 2013

may be expected to co-occur. Co-amplified genes are thought to cooperatively drive breast cancer [3] and glioblastoma [4] and, using the technique described herein, we identified a cooperative interaction between *CCNE1* and *TPX2* via gene amplification (and overexpression) [5, 6]. Thus, identifying the relationships between regions of aberrations can throw light on the biological pathways targeted by genomic alterations.

Methodological approach. We developed a method to identify the relationship between distinct genomic events in tumor samples using SNP mapping array data and to correlate this relationship with gene expression data. The method uses the following steps to compute the association between any two genomic events: First, a contingency table of the counts of each combination of the genomic alterations across the samples is constructed. Then a Poisson log-linear model is fitted to the contingency table describing the aberration status. The statistical significance of the association is then computed using a score test that yields a standard normal z-statistic [7]. This method is applied to all possible pairs of genomic alterations to identify the association between genomic alterations in an unbiased manner. The number of possible pairs (and the number of hypothesis tested) increases quadratically with the number of genomic events considered. In order to limit the number of events, we only test the relationship between significantly altered genomic regions, such as those that are frequently targeted by copy number gain or loss. The statistical test assumes a parametric distribution for the events and may not be satisfied in all the cases. Hence we also developed a permutation test to compute the association between all the events.

Outcome and interpretation. We have used the above methods to identify co-occurring and mutually exclusive genomic copy number aberrations using high-resolution SNP array data. The method requires a large number of samples but has the advantage over other methods of not requiring any prior knowledge of pathways or assumption of gene function. Pair-wise correlation of the expression levels of genes within the regions can be used to further identify interacting events, which assists in identifying the most relevant genes given that copy number alterations frequently affect large genomic regions containing many genes. This chapter describes the method in detail, along with a reference implementation in R[1] (*see* **Note 1**). Even though we have only used this method to identify the association between genomic regions significantly altered by copy number, it can readily be extended to identify associations between other genomic events such as point mutations or regions of DNA methylation. Through such a comprehensive analysis, a cooperative pathway could be identified that indicates a critical nexus for a subset of tumors. Mutually exclusive events may

[1] http://www.R-project.org

identify different genomic lesions leading to disruption of a common pathway (e.g., *KRAS/BRAF*). Using the genomic events as prognostic markers for such pathways may stratify patients that could benefit from a targeted therapy. Coexisting events may also indicate possible mechanisms for resistance to targeted therapies, such as deletion of *PTEN* in *BRAF* mutant tumors that are resistant to BRAF inhibitors [8], and suggest potential combination therapies.

2 Materials

2.1 Input Data

1. Affymetrix SNP 6.0 Human Genome Mapping arrays
   Copy number profiles were estimated from the SNP6 CEL files downloaded from the TCGA data portal [9].
2. Affymetrix hthgu133a microarray
   Gene expression profiles corresponding to the same samples for which copy number was obtained were estimated using the CEL files downloaded from the TCGA data portal.

2.2 Bioinformatics Toolboxes

The following R-packages are used in this analysis: Biobase, hthgu133a.db, aroma.affymetrix, and DNAcopy. In addition significant regions of gains and losses were computed using GISTIC available from the Broad Institute [10].

3 Methods

The first step involves the identification of significantly altered genomic regions using genomic data of all tumor samples. In this document we demonstrate the steps using tumor DNA copy number values obtained using Affymetrix SNP 6.0 Human Genome Mapping arrays. Alternate technologies to identify genomic copy number changes in tumor samples can be used without affecting the remaining steps. The method described below assumes standard wet-lab processing and scanning of Affymetrix SNP 6.0 Human Genome Mapping arrays (*see* **Note 2**).

3.1 Data Preprocessing and Segmentation

The steps below summarize detailed code provided in the Supplementary File (*see* **Note 1**). Unless otherwise stated, all steps are performed in R.

1. Normalize arrays using the R-package "aroma.affymetrix" [11] to remove systematic biases introduced due to allelic cross talk, PCR fragment length bias, and differences in GC content.
2. The log ratio of the genomic copy number data is computed at every SNP marker by subtracting the log-transformed normalized signal of a tumor sample from the data of normal

lymphocyte DNA from the same patient, if available, generating log_2 ratio values. On tumor samples for which matched normal tissue was not available, the average signal from all the normals generated in the same laboratory can be used as reference (*see* **Note 2**).

3. Segment tumor samples using DNAcopy [12] (*see* **Note 3**).
4. Identify frequent regions of amplification or deletion by Genomic Identification of Significant Targets in Cancer (GISTIC) [10] using the web-based interface (http://genepattern.broadinstitute.org) with CNA thresholds of ±0.3, a minimum of ten markers and a q-value threshold of 0.25 (*see* **Note 4**).

3.2 Association Between Regions of Aberrations (Score Test)

The basic idea is depicted as a schematic in Fig. 1. We evaluated two methods of calculating associations between regions of aberration, termed the "score test" and the "permutation test." The procedure for the score test is given below and the permutation described in **Note 5**.

1. Create matrix. The input required for the association analysis is a matrix of recurrently altered regions. This matrix is of dimension $N \times M$, where N is the number of samples and M is the number of recurrently altered regions identified by GISTIC. Samples are thus represented as rows and recurrent regions are represented as columns of this matrix. The matrix entry at any location is 1 or 0 depending on the presence or absence of the aberration in that sample. This matrix can be created in R from a GISTIC output file as detailed in **Note 4**. The relationship between any two pairs of aberrations can then be identified using the following steps.
2. Construct a contingency table of the counts at each combination of aberration status.
3. A Poisson log-linear model is fit to the contingency table.
4. Statistical significance of association between aberrations can be tested using a score test that yields a standard normal z-statistic. If the genomic alterations that occur at any locus are unique, the contingency table becomes 2×2, and the statistical significance can be tested by comparing two binomial proportions.
5. Statistical significance of association between all possible pairs of alterations is computed, and the false discovery rate estimated using the Benjamini and Hochberg method.

The following R code computes the association between all possible pairs of alterations in the matrix names "aberration.matrix". The columns in this matrix represent the genomic events and rows represent the samples. The number of pairs tested is equal to $n(n-1)/2$, where n is the number of genomic events under

Sample	1q gain	8q gain	16p loss	TP53 mutation
1	1	1	0	1
2	1	0	0	1
3	1	1	0	1
4	1	0	0	0
5	1	0	0	1
6	1	0	1	1
7	0	0	1	0
8	0	1	1	0
9	0	0	1	0
10	0	1	1	0
11	0	0	1	0
12	0	1	1	0

Construct contingency table

P=0.015	TP53 mutated	TP53 wild type
1q gain +	5	1
1q gain -	0	6

Test for significance

Repeat for all pairs and correct for multiple testing

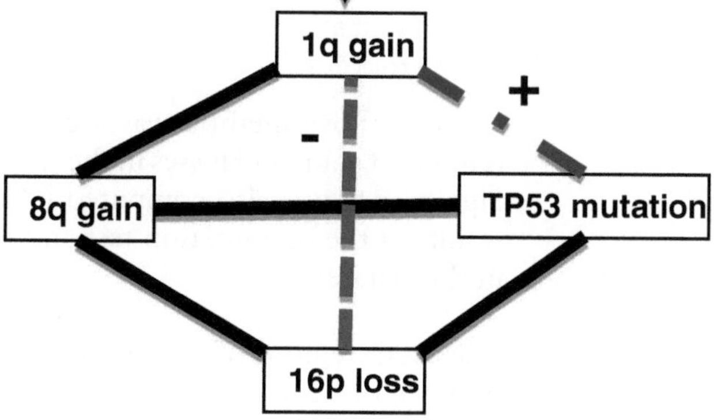

Fig. 1 Schematic presentation of analytic approach

consideration. The code below uses the standard z-statistic for comparing two binomial proportions.

```
num.regions <- ncol(aberration.matrix)
num.entries  <- (num.regions*(num.regions-1))/2
```

```
reg1 <- character(length = num.entries)
reg2 <- character(length = num.entries)
direction <- character(length = num.entries)
pvals <- numeric(length = num.entries)
row.num = num.regions - 1
cnt <- 1
for(i in 1: row.num)
{
   k <- i+1
   for(j in k:num.regions)
   {
      reg1[cnt] <- colnames(aberration.matrix)[i]
      re3g2[cnt] <- colnames(aberration.matrix)[j]
      tab     <-
table(aberration.matrix[,i],aberration.
matrix[,j])
      n0 <- tab[1,1] + tab[1,2]
      n1 <- tab[2,1] + tab[2,2]
      p01 <- tab[1,1]/n0
      p11 <- tab[2,1]/n1
      p1 <- (tab[1,2] + tab[2,2])/(n0 + n1)
      se <- sqrt(p1*(1-p1)*(1/n0 + 1/n1))
      z <- (p11 - p01)/se
      pvals[cnt] <- 2*pnorm(abs(z),lower.tail=FALSE)
      if( z < 0 ) direction[cnt] <- "Co-occur"
      if( z > 0 ) direction[cnt] <- "Mutually exclusive"
      cnt <- cnt + 1
   }
}
pvals.adj <- p.adjust(pvals,"fdr")
res.stats <- data.frame(reg1, reg2, pvals, pvals.adj,
direction)
```

The above method was used to identify associations between regions of gains and losses in the genome of ovarian cancer patients. Significance was also computed using a permutation test, but the results of the permutation test and the score test were concordant in this dataset [5].

3.3 Analysis of Expression Correlations Between Associated Copy Number Aberrations

Recurrent regions of copy number change typically contain a large number of genes, and consequently it is difficult to identify the target gene of the alterations. The same difficulty translates to identifying the genes cooperatively involved in disease pathogenesis. Here we describe how the transcriptional profiles of the genes can be used to identify interacting genes associated with regions of significantly correlated copy number change. We assume that the gene expression profiles of the same samples used for DNA copy number are also available.

3.3.1 Creation of the Expression Profile Matrix

Gene expressions of all the samples in the cohort were profiled using the Affymetrix hthgu133a microarray (*see* **Note 6**). Typically microarray platforms had multiple probe sets mapping to several regions of each gene. In this case the probe set with the maximum gene expression is taken as the representative value. The reference implementation given below organizes the expression profile for all the genes for all the samples. It is assumed that the normalized data is available as a matrix "exp" (the output of expression array files from R) with columns representing the samples and rows representing the probe set.

```
library(Biobase)
library(hthgu133plusa.db)
r.m = rowMeans(exp)
o = order(r.m,decreasing=T)
exp.ord <- exp[o,]
geneSymbol
as.character(mget(rownames(exp.
ord),hthgu133plusaSYMBOL))
idx <- duplicated(geneSymbol)
exp.sel <- exp.ord[!idx,]
rownames(exp.sel) = mget(rownames(exp.
   sel),hthgu133aSYMBOL)
```

3.3.2 Creation of Copy Number Profiles

The following code creates the copy number profile of all the genes within all the samples. The segmented log ratio at the midpoint of the gene is used as the copy number level of the gene.

```
cn.profile <- NULL
for (i in 1:nrow(gene.anns))
{
   idx <- seg$chrom == chr & seg$loc.start < pos
      & seg$loc.end >
pos
   profile <- seg[idx,]
   rownames(profile) <- profile$ID
   profile.ord <- profile[rownames(exp.sel),]
   rbind(cn.profile,profile.ord$seg.mean)
}
```

3.3.3 Identify Potentially Interacting Genes Through the Integration of Expression (Subheading 3.3.1) and Copy Number (Subheading 3.3.2) Data

Once the copy number profiles and expression profiles of all the genes are created, this data can be used to identify the potentially interacting pair of genes within the regions identified in earlier section. The expression profile of a gene is correlated with its own copy number profile to check for the evidence for copy number-related expression changes. The correlation between the expression profiles of genes in different regions is then used to rank gene pairs for potential interaction. This method was used to identify the

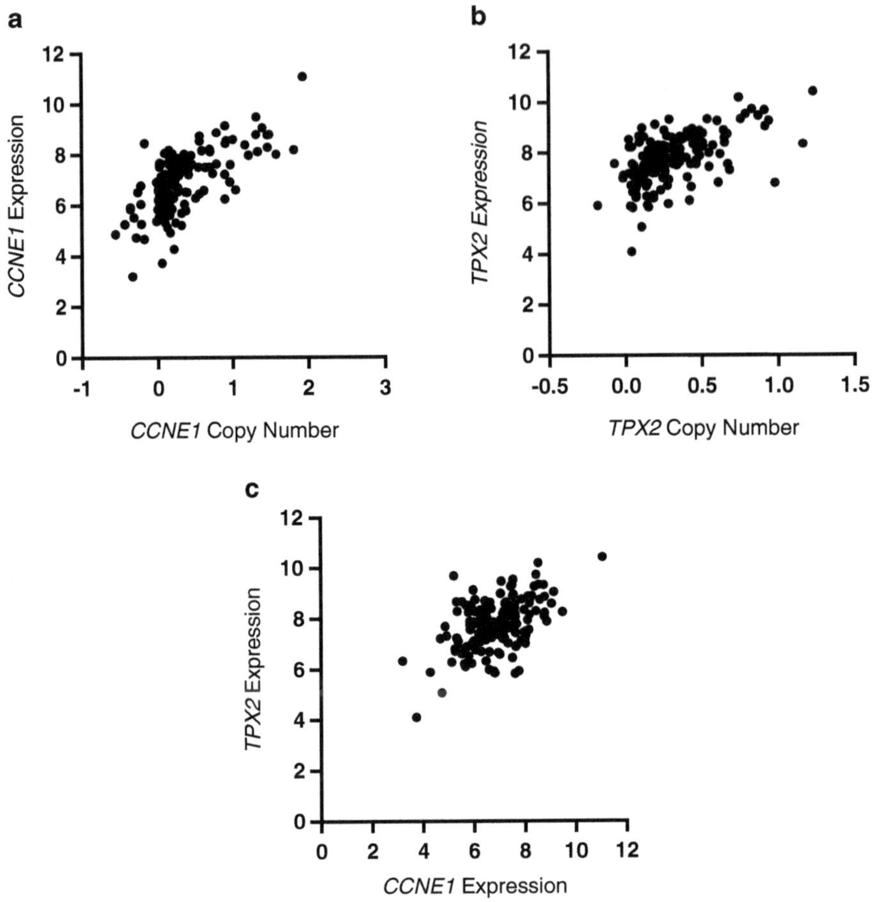

Fig. 2 Integrated analysis of copy number and gene expression. (**a**) Perform steps 1 and 2 for all genes in Regions 1 and 2. (**b**) For all genes that show a significant correlation between expression and copy number, perform step 3 for all gene pairs between Regions 1 and 2. (**c**) Rank gene pairs by the significance of the expression correlation in step 3

interaction between *CCNE1* and *TPX2* in ovarian cancer [6]. Analysis of significantly altered regions in high-grade serous ovarian cancer identified co-amplification of 19q12 and 20q11. Integrated analysis of copy number and gene expression identified the interaction between *CCNE1* and *TPX2* (Fig. 2).

The reference implementation below assumes the list of genes in the two regions to be altered in a correlated manner is available in character vectors named Region1.genes and Region2.genes.

```
num.pairs <- length(Region1.genes)*length(Region2.genes)

Gene1 <- character(length = num.pairs)
Gene2 <- character(length = num.pairs)
G1.cn.exp <- numeric(length = num.pairs)
G2.cn.exp <- numeric(length = num.pairs)
G1.G2.exp <- numeric(length = num.pairs)
```

```
cnt <- 1
for(i in 1: length(Region1.genes))
{
   gene1 <- Region1.genes[i]
   Gene1[cnt] <- gene1
   gene1.cn <- cn.profile[gene1,]
   gene1.exp <- exp.sel[gene1,]
   G1.cn.exp[cnt] <- cor.test(gene1.cn,gene1.exp)$p.value
   for(j in 1: length(Region2.genes))
   {
      gene2 <- Region2.genes[j]
      Gene2[cnt] <- gene2
      gene2.cn <- cn.profile[gene2,]
      gene2.exp <- exp.sel[gene2,]
      Gene1[cnt] <- gene1
      Gene2[cnt] <- gene2
      G2.cn.exp[cnt]  <-  cor.test(gene1.cn,
         gene1.exp)$p.value
      G1.G2.exp[cnt]            <-
cor.test(gene1.exp,gene2.exp)$p.value
      cnt <- cnt + 1
   }
}
res <- data.frame(Gene1, Gene2, G1.cn.exp,G2.
 cn.exp,G1.G2.exp)
colnames(res) <- c("Gene A","Gene B","Gene A CN-mRNA
  correlation","Gene B CN-mRNA correlation","Gene A
  Gene-B mRNA correlation")
write.csv(res,"correation_results_for_iden-
tifying_interacting_genes.csv")
```

4 Notes

1. R is an open-source programming language and environment for statistical computing and is freely available for almost all operating systems under the GNU general public license. The open-source nature of this environment makes the algorithms transparent and enables the extension of this environment via user-developed packages, making it a very popular platform for statistical software development. A document containing reference implementations can be downloaded from http://bioinformatics.petermac.org/supplements/George_et_al_2013_SupplementaryFile.pdf.
2. We used a dataset comprising CEL files from tumor samples and matching normal data (from lymphocytes), when available. We found that using matched normal samples reduced

the incidence of copy number polymorphisms in the data (but not completely excluding them, *see* ref. 13). In most cases data has better quality when normalized against matching normals (since they were run in the same batch), but in some cases using a baseline of multiple normal samples improved the quality of data (we used all available normal samples that passed QC).

3. The signal from the tumor sample and its corresponding normal sample can be used to compute the log ratio signal and identify regions of gains and losses in the tumor sample. If the genomic copy number at any locus is normal, the log ratio signal of markers within that region should be close to zero. A positive log ratio value suggests a gain in the region, whereas a negative value suggests a loss. However, gains and calls based on individual markers can result in false positives and negatives, and the situation can be improved by taking into consideration the physical constraints of copy number alterations. Copy number alterations are discrete events affecting contiguous regions of the genome. This fact can be used to improve the signal to noise ratio by combining information from neighboring markers. DNAcopy is an R-package that implements a circular binary segmentation (CBS) that can be used to improve the signal to noise ratio of the signal. This method identifies change point boundaries, and the mean value of the log ratios within a segment is reported as the copy number value within that segment.

4. GISTIC is a convenient method for this analysis; however, any list of significant regions (or mutations) can be used, for example, one generated through a frequency alone approach. GISTIC has the advantage, however, of not only identifying significant regions of aberrations but also scoring the presence or absence of these events in all the samples used to detect these aberrations in a matrix suitable for the next steps.

5. A permutation test is a statistical significance test in which the distribution of the test statistic under the null hypothesis is obtained by calculating all possible values of the test statistic under rearrangements of the labels on the observed data points. If the labels are exchangeable under the null hypothesis, then the resulting test will yield exact significance levels. To use this method, every column in the alteration matrix was permuted independently. The permutations did not change the number of nonzero entries in any column. The null hypothesis under test is that there is no association between the two genomic alterations and the *P*-value can be computed by taking the ratio $\frac{M+1}{N+1}$, where M is the number of times a test statistic greater than or above the original test statistic observed during the N permutations [14]. The average rank obtained for every pair of

regions from a large number of permutations can be used to estimate the false discovery rate.

6. There are no specific constraints on the platforms used to assess either the copy number profiles or the gene expression profiles of the tumor samples, so long as the expression probes can be mapped to their genomic location using the same genome build as the copy number probes.

References

1. Hanahan D, Weinberg RA (2011) Hallmarks of cancer: the next generation. Cell 144:646–674
2. Anglesio MS, Arnold JM, George J, Tinker AV, Tothill R et al (2008) Mutation of ERBB2 provides a novel alternative mechanism for the ubiquitous activation of RAS-MAPK in ovarian serous low malignant potential tumors. Mol Cancer Res 6:1678–1690
3. Kwek SS, Roy R, Zhou H, Climent J, Martinez-Climent JA et al (2009) Co-amplified genes at 8p12 and 11q13 in breast tumors cooperate with two major pathways in oncogenesis. Oncogene 28(17):1892–1903
4. Bredel M, Scholtens DM, Harsh GR, Bredel C, Chandler JP et al (2009) A network model of a cooperative genetic landscape in brain tumors. JAMA 302:261–275
5. Gorringe KL, George J, Anglesio MS, Ramakrishna M, Etemadmoghadam D, et al (2010) Copy number analysis identifies novel interactions between genomic loci in ovarian cancer. PLoS One 5(9): e11408
6. Etemadmoghadam D, George J, Cowin PA, Cullinane C, Kansara M et al (2010) Amplicon-dependent CCNE1 expression is critical for clonogenic survival after cisplatin treatment and is correlated with 20q11 gain in ovarian cancer. PLoS One 5:e15498
7. Smyth GK (2003) Pearson's goodness of fit statistic as a score test statistic. Statistics and science: a festschrift for Terry Speed. Institute of Mathematical Statistics, Ann Arbor, MI, pp 115–126
8. Villanueva J, Vultur A, Herlyn M (2011) Resistance to BRAF inhibitors: unraveling mechanisms and future treatment options. Cancer Res 71:7137–7140
9. TCGA (2011) Integrated genomic analyses of ovarian carcinoma. Nature 474:609–615
10. Beroukhim R, Getz G, Nghiemphu L, Barretina J, Hsueh T et al (2007) Assessing the significance of chromosomal aberrations in cancer: methodology and application to glioma. Proc Natl Acad Sci U S A 104: 20007–20012
11. Bengtsson H, Irizarry R, Carvalho B, Speed TP (2008) Estimation and assessment of raw copy numbers at the single locus level. Bioinformatics 24:759–767
12. Venkatraman ES, Olshen AB (2007) A faster circular binary segmentation algorithm for the analysis of array CGH data. Bioinformatics 23:657–663
13. Gorringe KL, Campbell IG (2008) High-resolution copy number arrays in cancer and the problem of normal genome copy number variation. Genes Chromosomes Cancer 47:933–938
14. Phipson B, Smyth GK (2010) Permutation P-values should never be zero: calculating exact P-values when permutations are randomly drawn. Stat Appl Genet Mol Biol 9:Article39

Chapter 3

Analysis of Genome-Wide DNA Methylation Profiles by BeadChip Technology

Qiong Lin, Wolfgang Wagner, and Martin Zenke

Abstract

This chapter covers the genome-wide DNA methylation analysis using microarray platforms, such as Illumina Infinium HumanMethylation27 BeadChips or HumanMethylation450 BeadChips. Using our previously published ovarian cancer dataset (Bauerschlag et al., Oncology 80:12–20, 2011), we introduce the underlying design principles of these methylation array platforms and describe common yet effective bioinformatic strategies for data analysis, including data preprocessing, clustering methods, and differential methylation tests. We also describe the downstream analytic techniques for the results derived from the methylation array, i.e., gene set enrichment analysis and sequence-based motif analysis, which can be utilized for generating biological hypotheses.

Key words HumanMethylation27 BeadChip, HumanMethylation450 BeadChip, Methylation, Microarray analysis, Clustering, Differential gene expression, Ovarian cancer

1 Introduction

DNA methylation is crucial for myriad cellular processes, such as differentiation, aging, and malignant transformation, and represents one of the most widely studied epigenetic modifications in human [1–7]. Cytosine DNA methylation typically occurs in the sequence context of CpG dinucleotides (CpGs; CpG sites). Throughout the genome CpG sites are rare, whereas short regions with an exceptionally high frequency of CpGs (i.e., >0.6) exist, referred to as CpG islands (CGIs). In human, CGIs associate with approximately 60 % of gene promoter regions and most of them are in an unmethylated state [8]. Changes in the methylation level of the promoter-associated CpGs or CGIs can result in either gene silencing or activation. Frequently, DNA methylation in promoter regions is associated with downregulation of gene expression. In cancer cells, tumor-suppressor genes are often hypermethylated in their promoter regions and the gene expression is switched off

Anastasia Malek and Oleg Tchernitsa (eds.), *Ovarian Cancer: Methods and Protocols*, Methods in Molecular Biology, vol. 1049, DOI 10.1007/978-1-62703-547-7_3,

[9, 10]. Recent studies indicate that DNA methylation is also involved in regulation of RNA splicing [11].

Microarray and next-generation sequencing-based technologies allow analysis of DNA methylation at single-base resolution or enrichment of methylated DNA regions (reviewed in ref. [12, 13]). The gold-standard technique for assessing DNA methylation is based on sodium bisulfite conversion. In the presence of bisulfite, unmethylated cytosines of genomic DNA are chemically deaminated to uracil, while methylated cytosines are resistant to bisulfite treatment and remain cytosine. Applying the same principle, Illumina Infinium HumanMethylation27 BeadChip detects the DNA methylation status of 27,578 CpG sites throughout the genome. The interrogated CpG sites cover the promote regions of 14,475 genes, including nearly 13,000 well-annotated genes in the NCBI CCDS Database (Genome Build 36) and over 1,000 cancer-related genes or targets. In addition, 110 CpG sites located within miRNA promote regions are presented on the array. For individual CpG sites, a pair of bead-bound probes is used to detect the presence of T (unmethylated state) or C (methylated state). The beta value, which is a quantitative measurement of the methylation level of single CpG site, is subsequently determined by calculating the ratio of the fluorescent intensities of the methylated probe (*M*) and unmethylated probe (*U*) according to the following formula:

$$\text{Beta} = \frac{\text{Max}(M,0)}{\text{Max}(M,0) + \text{Max}(U,0) + 100}$$

Here, Max(*M*, 0) and Max(*U*, 0) indicate the maximum value between *M* and 0 and *U* and 0, respectively. The number 100 in the denominator is a constant offset to standardize beta values when both methylated and unmethylated probe intensities are low. The beta value, ranging from 0 (completely unmethylated) to 1 (completely methylated), relates to the percentage of methylation for a given CpG site.

A major limitation of HumanMethlyation27 BeadChip is that most interrogated CpG sites are located in the gene promoter region. However, methylation across the gene and the role of the CpG sites in the intragenic or gene body regions have attracted considerable interest recently [10]. Therefore, HumanMethylation450 BeadChip was developed, allowing the measurement of over 450,000 CpG sites distributed across the gene promoters, 5′ untranslated regions (UTR), first exon, gene body, and 3′ UTR.

In general, the pipeline of DNA methylation microarray data analysis includes the following steps:

1. Data preprocessing: collect sample information, assess array quality, and normalize or format the raw data.
2. Global comparisons and clustering analysis: perform pair-wise comparison by scatter plots to observe the global methylation changes between two samples or groups; employ principal

component analysis (PCA) and hierarchical clustering (HC) to investigate the class composition of the samples and identify outliers or low-quality samples.

3. Differential methylation analysis: identify the differentially methylated CpG sites using statistic methods, such as *t*-test for two groups and ANOVA for multiple groups (at least three groups). It is crucial to perform multiple testing correction for *p*-value, as the test is repeatedly applied.
4. Downstream bioinformatics analysis: integrate genome methylation profiles with various kinds of biological information. For example, perform sequence-based analysis to identify common motifs of differentially methylated genes; perform functional analysis such as gene set enrichment analysis, to evaluate a list of differentially methylated genes by using predefined gene sets or pathways. These analyses allow us to organize the methylation array results in biological context and help us to design biological hypotheses.
5. Validation of the microarray data: select representative or interesting CpG sites, and subject them to more precise measurements (e.g., pyrosequencing) for verification.

In our previous study [14], we performed a global DNA methylation analysis of ovarian cancer patients by using HumanMethylation27 BeadChip. The bioinformatics analyses showed that differential DNA methylation of various cytosines correlated with progression-free interval (PFI) after therapy. However, this becomes only significant by classification according to PFI with a cutoff of 28 months. Gene ontology analysis revealed that differentially methylated genes were significantly overrepresented in the categories telomere organization, mesoderm development, and immune regulation. In this chapter, we will introduce the basic analytical pipeline of HumanMethylation27 BeadChip by this dataset. Please note that most of these analyses can also be applied to HumanMethlyation450 BeadChips or gene expression microarrays [15]. The validation step in the pipeline is beyond the scope of this introduction and therefore will not be covered here. However, we emphasize that obtaining a biological validation by more precise or alternative measurements is inevitably important for microarray-based bioinformatic results.

2 Materials

2.1 Input Data

Illumina HumanMethylation27 BeadChip data can be either obtained from GenomeStudio Methylation module or retrieved from NCBI Gene Expression Omnibus (GEO) [16] and ArrayExpress Archive [17], which are two widely used data repositories (*see* **Note 1**).

2.2 Bioinformatics Toolbox

Most of the tools, which are designed and used for microarray data gene expression analysis, are also well suited for DNA methylation arrays. The data analysis described here is mainly done by MultiExperiment Viewer (MEV) [18], DAVID bioinformatics resources [19], and Multiple EM for Motif Elicitation (MEME) [20] more tools are introduced in **Note 2**.

1. MEV (http://www.tm4.org/), an open-source application, provides a rich toolbox for analyzing microarray data, such as clustering, classification, visualization, and statistic analysis. All functions are accessible in a graphical user interface.
2. DAVID (http://david.abcc.ncifcrf.gov/home.jsp) bioinformatics resources include several web-accessible programs, which provide a comprehensive set of functional annotation tools, aiming at extracting biological meaning from large gene lists. One key module is gene set enrichment analysis.
3. MEME (http://meme.sdsc.edu/meme/cgi-bin/meme.cgi) detects sequence patterns called motifs from a group of DNA sequences by evaluating their similarities.

3 Methods

3.1 Data Preprocessing

1. Obtain the raw data of HumanMethylation27 BeadChips from the GenomeStudio Methylation (M) module. The raw data usually reports the beta values, Cy3 and Cy5 intensities, detective *p*-values, and additional measurements for each probe. To keep the essential information for data analysis, the raw data are imported into Excel, and unique probe ID column (termed as TargetID) and beta value columns (termed as AVG_Beta) are extracted. As a result a table, in which each row represents a single probe and each column represents an array or a sample, can be structured and subsequently exported in tab-delimited file format (Table 1). Please note that a TargetID serves as a unique identifier of each probe, used for mapping probe to genes. Alternative data source and data submission are discussed in **Notes 3** and **4**.
2. Control correct probe and sample annotation. The probe annotation table is readily obtained from web link mentioned in **Note 3**, if it is not provided in the raw data. The table contains comprehensive probe information, including its sequence, chromosome location, NCBI Entrez Gene ID, and distance to the transcription start site. The first column of the table is the unique probe ID, which represents the key for linking the annotation file and raw data. The sample annotation table is related to the experiment design. The vital information, such as array names, conditions, and treatments, should be included to facilitate the data interpretation.

Table 1
Structured methylation data

TargetID	Gene symbol	More gene annotations	Sample 1 beta value	Sample 2 beta value	Sample 3 beta value
cg00000292	ATP2A1	–	0.213	0.147	0.207
cg00002426	SLMAP	–	0.063	0.081	0.047
cg00003994	MEOX2	–	0.007	0.019	0.007
cg00005847	HOXD3	–	0.553	0.791	0.703
cg00006414	ZNF398	–	0.016	0.007	0.011

The first column of the data table contains the unique identifier of each probe (i.e., TargetID), which is followed by gene annotation columns (e.g., official gene symbol, NCBI Entrez Gene ID, and chromosome location). The next columns are beta values of each probe in different samples

3.2 Loading Data

1. Launch MEV program, go to *File> Load Data*, and select a prepared methylation file. In the file loader preview table, click the upper-leftmost beta value, and click *Load*. Data will be displayed as a heatmap, in which columns are the samples/conditions and rows are the probes. By default, the cells are color-coded using a continuous spectrum from green (low beta value) to red (high) via black (medium). By clicking any spots in the heatmap, we can explore *Spot Information* of individual probe, including the beta value, gene annotations, and sample information.
2. Go to *Display> Set Color Scale Limits.* As beta values range from 0 to 1, we need to change upper and lower limits accordingly. Click *Update Limits* button and set midpoint value as suggested by MEV.
3. Go to *Utilities> Append Gene Annotation* and select a gene annotation file (*see* Subheading 3.1, **step 2**). For both the loaded methylation data and the annotation file, choose "TargetID" as *Gene Identifier* and then click *OK.* Go to *Display> Gene/Row Labels* and select *Label by Gene_ID.* You will find that the row names of the heatmap are changed to the NCBI Entrez Gene ID.

3.3 Clustering Analysis

Principal component analysis (PCA) and hierarchical clustering (HC) are often used for investigating sample relations, for instance, to assess similarities and differences between samples or to determine clusters among them (*see* **Note 5**).

3.3.1 Principal Component Analysis

PCA represents a classical statistical method that reduces the dimensionality of the data while retaining most of the variation in the dataset [21]. The HumanMethylation27 BeadChip contains more than 27,000 highly informative CpG sites per sample. PCA achieves the data reduction by reducing 27,000 variables into a smaller number of artificial variables, called principal components, which will capture most of the variance within the data. Thus, samples can be represented and visualized by the first few components, such as first two or three components [3, 22].

1. Go to *Analysis> Data Reduction > PCA*.
2. Select *Cluster sample*, as we are interested in sample relations, and then press *OK*.
3. Navigate to the PCA results on the left side of the main interface. Click *2D view> 1, 2*. The samples will be shown as dots in a two-dimensional space according to the first and second principal components (Fig. 1a).
4. Go to *3D view*, right-click, and select *show spheres* and *show text*; the data will be projected into a 3D space.

3.3.2 Hierarchical Clustering

HC is a commonly used method for class discovery. In the context of cancer research, it often helps us to identify the subtypes of a particular cancer. Distance metric and linkage methods are two important parameters for HC. The selection of them will severely influence the composition of the clusters. We prefer to use Pearson correlation and average linkage method, which usually generate robust and biological relevant clustering results.

1. Go to *Analysis> Clustering> HCL*.
2. Click *Sample Tree*, *Pearson Correlation* distance metric, and *Average linkage clustering* method.
3. Navigate to the HCL results on the left side of the main interface and click *HCL tree*. A tree diagram, referred to as dendrogram, will be shown on top of the heatmap.
4. You can cut the dendrogram along branches at desired height to obtain a desired number of clusters. By right-clicking the subtree and *Store Cluster*, you can color-code the clusters and save them for further analysis (Fig. 1b).

3.4 Differential Methylation

Statistical methods can address the question on which genes are differentially methylated between two (or more) investigated groups, such as cancer patients versus healthy individuals. In general, statistical models are either parametric or nonparametric. The parametric tests, such as *t*-test and ANOVA, assume that the data follow a particular distribution (e.g., normal distribution), whereas the nonparametric tests make less stringent assumptions on the data distribution. MEV offers many statistic functions. Here we used *t*-test to demonstrate the basic approach to identify the differential methylation (*see* **Note 6**).

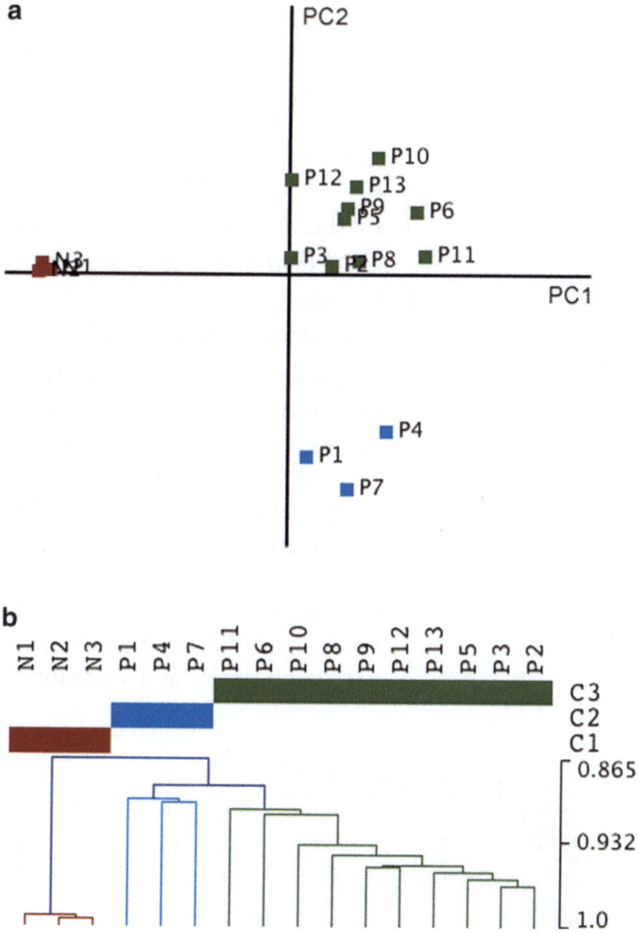

Fig. 1 Clustering analysis. (**a**) Normal tissue (N) and ovarian cancer patient samples (P) are separated into three clusters by PCA and color-coded accordingly. Each dot represents one methylation array/sample. The spatial distribution of samples indicates their biological relations. (**b**) HC of the same samples investigated by PCA in (**a**). Pearson correlation distance metric and average linkage were applied. The PCA and HC indicate that epigenetic profiles of ovarian cancer patient samples with a progression-free interval (PFI) <28 months (*green* cluster) are related and different from those with a PFI >28 months (*blue* cluster), while all ovarian cancer patient samples are distinct from healthy individuals (*red* cluster)

1. Go to *Analysis*> *Statistics*> TTEST.
2. To perform unpaired *t*-test, select the *Between subjects* panel and assign samples to group A, group B, or neither group. If samples are dependent, paired *t*-test should be utilized in the *Paired* panel.
3. In the *P-value Parameters* panel, by default (*p-value based on t-distribution*), classic parametric *t*-test will be performed. In this

case, the p-value of a gene is taken directly from the theoretical t-distribution on the basis of the calculated t-value. Alternatively, select *p-value based on permutation*, and nonparametric tests will be applied, which obtain the p-value from the sample-specific permutation distribution. For *Overall alpha (critical p-value)*, set 0.05 as a threshold.

4. In the *P-value/False Discovery Corrections* panel, select *standard Bonferroni correction* for multiple testing correction.
5. In the *Hierarchical Clustering* panel, check *Construct Hierarchical Trees for: Significant genes only.*
6. Navigate to the t-test results on the left side of the main interface and click *Cluster Information.* It shows the number of significant genes that are detected by t-test. Click *Hierarchical Tree*, the significant genes are shown in a heatmap with both gene and sample clustering. This allows to visually inspect the methylation patterns between different groups. The interesting gene clusters are readily identified according to the gene dendrogram located on the left side of the heatmap (Fig. 2a). Click *Table Views> Significant Genes*, it shows a tabular display with each probe as a separate row, and each column a different

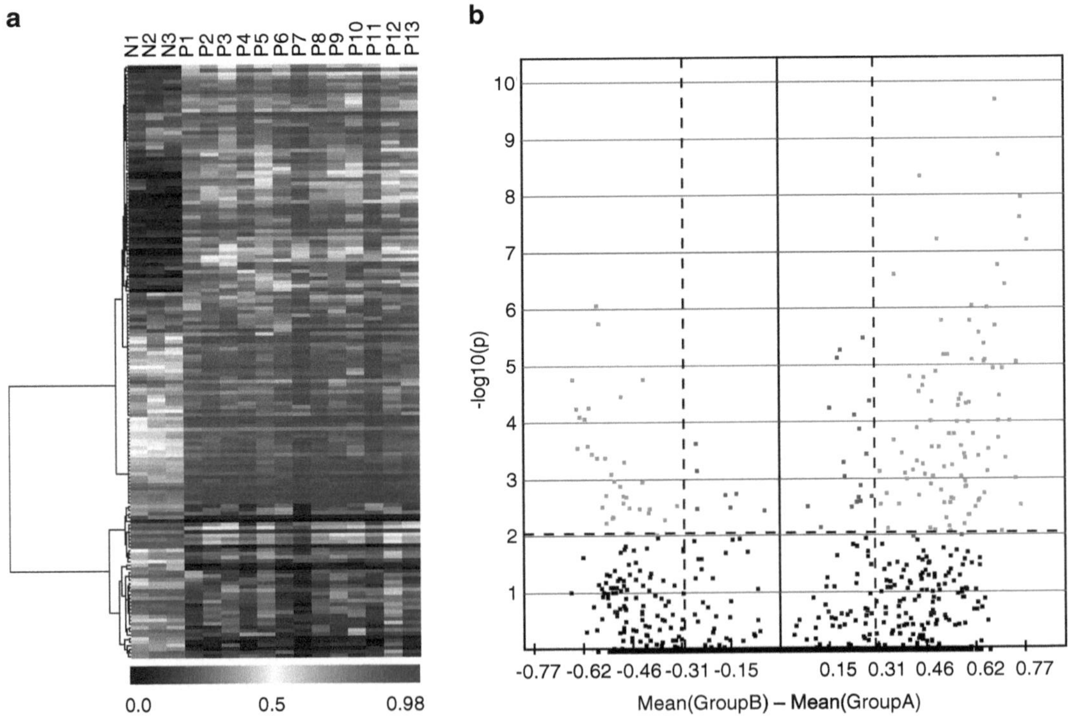

Fig. 2 Differential methylation analysis. (**a**) The heatmap of differentially methylated genes detected by t-test. The beta values of the CpG sites that were significantly differentially methylated (p-value < 0.05) between normal and patient samples are depicted in heatmap format. The cells are color-coded using a continuous spectrum from *blue* (low beta value) to *red* (high) via *white* (medium). (**b**) The volcano plots show, for each CpG site, the change of methylation levels on the x-axis versus a measure of statistic significance (p-value) on the y-axis

attribute of that probe. By clicking the column named *Adj p value*, you can sort the probes by their statistic significance in the *t*-test.

7. If we want to perform further gene filtering, first click *Volcano Plot*, then right-click in the plot, and select *Use gene selection sliders*. A new *p*-value threshold and fold change cutoff can be defined (Fig. 2b).

3.5 Gene Set Enrichment Analysis via DAVID

Gene set enrichment analysis is a common strategy to analyze gene lists derived from microarray experiment. It will highlight the most relevant biological annotations (e.g., gene ontology terms, KEGG pathways) associated with a given gene list. To demonstrate how to perform enrichment analysis, we will subject the differentially methylated genes generated from previous *t*-test to DAVID.

1. Prepare the gene list. In MEV, navigate to the *t*-test results (*see* Subheading 3.4) and copy NCBI Entrez Gene IDs of differentially methylated genes from the table under *Table Views> Significant Genes.*
2. Prepare the gene population background. This background refers to the complete set of the genes tested on the microarray. In MEV, navigate to the *Original Data* on the left side of main interface, click *Gene Table View*, and copy the NCBI Entrez Gene IDs of all CpG sites.
3. Launch your preferred web browser and access DAVID tools. Click *Start Analysis.*
4. Paste the list of differentially methylated genes, select *ENTREZ GENE ID* as the identifier, and select *Gene List* as list type. Do the same for the background, except to select *Background* as list type.
5. Perform enrichment analysis of GO biological process terms. Select *Gene_Ontology> GOTERM_BP_ALL*, and click *Functional Annotation Chart*. The significance of enrichment will be examined by a modified Fisher's exact test (EASE score). The GO terms with low EASE score (e.g., <0.05) will be listed in the resulting page.

3.6 Motif Discovery via MEME

The identification of regulatory motifs from DNA sequences is of pivotal importance in the analysis of gene regulation. A motif is a short sequence pattern that recurs in a group of related DNA sequences. Such a motif is often presumed to have a biological function relating to protein-DNA binding, mRNA processing, and transcription [23]. In the context of methylation analysis, we assume that a group of co-methylated or co-demethylated genes may share common motifs in their DNA sequences. Here we will describe how to detect motifs by an online web tool called MEME.

For demonstration, we selected top 10 co-methylated probes from the previously described *t*-test results (*see* Subheading 3.4).

1. Prepare DNA sequences. For each of 10 probes, the upstream and downstream DNA sequences of its CpG site (i.e., 124 bp) are extracted from a column named TopGenomicSeq in the probe annotation table (*see* Subheading 3.1, **step 2**). Please note that the sequence input of the MEME program should be in FASTA format.
2. Launch your preferred web browser and access to MEME. Enter your email address, as the results will be sent to your mailbox.
3. You can either upload a file containing the sequences or paste them in the input box.
4. MEME allows us to tune some key parameters of the motif discovery algorithm. We select *One per sequence* to define the frequency of the occurrence of a motif in the input sequences. We can also restrict the length of the motif; for example, set the minimum length of 6 and maximum of 10 nucleotides.
5. The MEME will report the discovered motifs and display them as sequence logos.

4 Notes

1. To obtain statistically significant results, the biological triplicate microarray experiments are strongly recommended.
2. dChip (http://www.hsph.harvard.edu/cli/complab/dchip/) and gene pattern (http://www.broadinstitute.org/cancer/software/genepattern/) represent two tools further to MEV, which are developed for microarray data analysis. They can also be applied for methylation array analysis. For advanced users, R/Bioconductor (http://www.bioconductor.org/) is recommended. Employing R environment, Bioconductor provides tools/packages designed specifically for the analysis and comprehension of high-throughput genomic data [24]. R/Bioconductor can easily cope with high-density microarrays, such as HumanMethlyation450 BeadChip.

   Gene Set Enrichment Analysis (GSEA; http://www.broadinstitute.org/gsea/index.jsp) is a statistical method to determine whether a pathway or a gene set shows significant, concordant differences between two biological states [25]. Associated with GSEA, the Molecular Signatures Database provides an enriched collection of predefined gene sets, which can be utilized for analyzing gene lists derived from microarray experiments.

3. If one wants to search and retrieve previously published microarray data, NCBI Gene Expression Omnibus (GEO) [16] and ArrayExpress Archive [17] are two widely used data repositories. Taking NCBI GEO as example, one could browse all public available Illumina HumanMethylation27 BeadChip data (http://www.ncbi.nlm.nih.gov/geo/query/acc.cgi?acc=GPL8490) as well as

   Illumina HumanMethylation450 BeadChip (http://www.ncbi.nlm.nih.gov/geo/query/acc.cgi?acc=GPL13534).

   After downloading the data, beta value columns can be extracted accordingly. In this chapter, we used our previously published ovarian cancer dataset (GSE25033) [14].

4. There are a number of benefits for submitting microarray data to a public repository. First and foremost, many journals require mandatory deposit of your data to NCBI GEO or ArrayExpress. Moreover, the submitted data receive long-term archiving at a centralized repository, which increases the usability and visibility of your data and your research. In addition, these data can be further utilized and explored by both academic and industrial researchers.

   Both above-mentioned databases provide straightforward deposit procedures.

   We recommend that you submit the Illumina methylation data to NCBI GEO via the GEOarchive spreadsheet-based submission method. You need to prepare the three following excel worksheets for the GEOarchive:

   (a) A metadata worksheet containing descriptive information and protocols for the overall experiment and individual samples
   (b) A matrix worksheet consisting of the final processed/normalized data used to draw the conclusions from your study
   (c) A matrix worksheet including non-normalized data

5. To reduce the impact of gender-associated effects on sample clustering, one should consider excluding CpG sites on sex chromosomes when performing PCA or HC.

6. In addition to the differential methylation test, Pavlidis template matching (PTM) identifies the CpG sites of which methylation levels are highly correlated with a given template (i.e., sample phenotypes) [14, 26, 27]. For example, the template can be specified according to the cancer subtypes of patients. This method ranks CpG sites by the correlation coefficient between beta values and the corresponding patient phenotypes.

Acknowledgements

This work was supported by the state North Rhine Westphalia within the BioNRW2 project "StemCellFactory" (M.Z., W.W.) and the Stem Cell Network NRW (W.W.). Q.L. and M.Z. were supported by DFG Priority Program SPP1356.

References

1. Suzuki MM, Bird A (2008) DNA methylation landscapes: provocative insights from epigenomics. Nat Rev Genet 9:465–476
2. Koch CM, Joussen S, Schellenberg A, Lin Q, Zenke M et al (2011) Monitoring of cellular senescence by DNA-methylation at specific CpG sites. Aging Cell 11(2):366–369
3. Koch CM, Suschek CV, Lin Q, Bork S, Goergens M et al (2011) Specific age-associated DNA methylation changes in human dermal fibroblasts. PLoS One 6:e16679
4. Schellenberg A, Lin Q, Schuler H, Koch CM, Joussen S et al (2011) Replicative senescence of mesenchymal stem cells causes DNA-methylation changes which correlate with repressive histone marks. Aging 3:873–888
5. Jones A, Lechner M, Fourkala EO, Kristeleit R, Widschwendter M (2010) Emerging promise of epigenetics and DNA methylation for the diagnosis and management of women's cancers. Epigenomics 2:9–38
6. Teschendorff AE, Menon U, Gentry-Maharaj A, Ramus SJ, Gayther SA et al (2009) An epigenetic signature in peripheral blood predicts active ovarian cancer. PLoS One 4:e8274
7. Teschendorff AE, Menon U, Gentry-Maharaj A, Ramus SJ, Weisenberger DJ et al (2010) Age-dependent DNA methylation of genes that are suppressed in stem cells is a hallmark of cancer. Genome Res 20:440–446
8. Portela A, Esteller M (2010) Epigenetic modifications and human disease. Nat Biotechnol 28:1057–1068
9. Ushijima T (2005) Detection and interpretation of altered methylation patterns in cancer cells. Nat Rev Cancer 5:223–231
10. Shenker N, Flanagan JM (2012) Intragenic DNA methylation: implications of this epigenetic mechanism for cancer research. Br J Cancer 106:248–253
11. Shukla S, Kavak E, Gregory M, Imashimizu M, Shutinoski B et al (2011) CTCF-promoted RNA polymerase II pausing links DNA methylation to splicing. Nature 479:74–79
12. Laird PW (2010) Principles and challenges of genomewide DNA methylation analysis. Nat Rev Genet 11:191–203
13. Beck S (2010) Taking the measure of the methylome. Nat Biotechnol 28:1026–1028
14. Bauerschlag DO, Ammerpohl O, Brautigam K, Schem C, Lin Q et al (2011) Progression-free survival in ovarian cancer is reflected in epigenetic DNA methylation profiles. Oncology 80:12–20
15. Schuldt B, Lin Q, Muller FJ, Loring J (2011) Basic approaches to gene expression analysis of stem cells by microarrays. Methods Mol Biol 767:269–282
16. Barrett T, Troup DB, Wilhite SE, Ledoux P, Evangelista C et al (2011) NCBI GEO: archive for functional genomics data sets—10 years on. Nucleic Acids Res 39:D1005–D1010
17. Parkinson H, Sarkans U, Kolesnikov N, Abeygunawardena N, Burdett T et al (2011) ArrayExpress update—an archive of microarray and high-throughput sequencing-based functional genomics experiments. Nucleic Acids Res 39:D1002–D1004
18. Saeed AI, Sharov V, White J, Li J, Liang W et al (2003) TM4: a free, open-source system for microarray data management and analysis. Biotechniques 34:374–378
19. da Huang W, Sherman BT, Lempicki RA (2009) Systematic and integrative analysis of large gene lists using DAVID bioinformatics resources. Nat Protoc 4:44–57
20. Bailey TL, Boden M, Buske FA, Frith M, Grant CE et al (2009) MEME SUITE: tools for motif discovery and searching. Nucleic Acids Res 37:W202–W208
21. Ringner M (2008) What is principal component analysis? Nat Biotechnol 26:303–304
22. Felker P, Sere K, Lin Q, Becker C, Hristov M et al (2010) TGF-beta1 accelerates dendritic cell differentiation from common dendritic cell progenitors and directs subset specification toward conventional dendritic cells. J Immunol 185:5326–5335

23. D'Haeseleer P (2006) What are DNA sequence motifs? Nat Biotechnol 24:423–425
24. Gentleman RC, Carey VJ, Bates DM, Bolstad B, Dettling M et al (2004) Bioconductor: open software development for computational biology and bioinformatics. Genome Biol 5(10):R80
25. Subramanian A, Tamayo P, Mootha VK, Mukherjee S, Ebert BL et al (2005) Gene set enrichment analysis: a knowledge-based approach for interpreting genome-wide expression profiles. Proc Natl Acad Sci U S A 102:15545–15550
26. Pavlidis P, Noble WS (2001) Analysis of strain and regional variation in gene expression in mouse brain. Genome Biol 2: RESEARCH0042.
27. Koch CM, Wagner W (2011) Epigenetic-aging-signature to determine age in different tissues. Aging 3:1018–1027

Chapter 4

Integrative Prediction of Gene Function and Platinum-Free Survival from Genomic and Epigenetic Features in Ovarian Cancer

Kazimierz O. Wrzeszczynski, Vinay Varadan, Sitharthan Kamalakaran, Douglas A. Levine, Nevenka Dimitrova, and Robert Lucito

Abstract

The identification of genetic and epigenetic alterations from primary tumor cells has become a common method to discover genes critical to the development, progression, and therapeutic resistance of cancer. We seek to identify those genetic and epigenetic aberrations that have the most impact on gene function within the tumor. First, we perform a bioinformatics analysis of copy number variation (CNV) and DNA methylation covering the genetic landscape of ovarian cancer tumor cells. We were specifically interested in copy number variation as our base genomic property in the prediction of tumor suppressors and oncogenes in the altered ovarian tumor. We identify changes in DNA methylation and expression specifically for all amplified and deleted genes. We statistically define tumor suppressor and oncogenic gene function from integrative analysis of three modalities: copy number variation, DNA methylation, and gene expression. Our method (1) calculates the extent of genomic and epigenetic alterations of defined tumor suppressor and oncogenic features for the functional prediction of significant ovarian cancer gene candidates and (2) identifies the functional activity or inactivity of known tumor suppressors and oncogenes in ovarian cancer. We applied our protocol on 42 primary serous ovarian cancer samples using MOMA-ROMA representational array assays. Additionally, we provide the basis for incorporating epigenetic profiles of ovarian tumors for the purposes of platinum-free survival prediction in the context of TCGA data.

Key words Serous ovarian cancer, Copy number variation, DNA methylation, Representational oligonucleotide microarray analysis, Methylation detection representational oligonucleotide microarray analysis, Platinum-free survival

1 Introduction

The American Cancer Society projects there will be approximately 22,240 new cases of ovarian cancer in the United States in 2013. Of those, an estimated 14,030 will succumb to the disease. In order to better treat these women and improve survival, our goal is to determine the genetic changes that have occurred in the patients' tumors and to be able to interpret the significance these changes

Anastasia Malek and Oleg Tchernitsa (eds.), *Ovarian Cancer: Methods and Protocols*, Methods in Molecular Biology, vol. 1049, DOI 10.1007/978-1-62703-547-7_4,

have on the growth and development of ovarian tumors. This aberrant growth is a result of chromosomal abnormalities and epigenetic variations [1–3]. In addition, generally low rates of somatic nucleotide mutation in ovarian cancer as compared to other solid tumors suggest an increase in the significance of copy number and epigenetic aberrations in regulating gene function. This type of regulation has been shown to affect different functional classes of genes (e.g., membrane receptors, tumor suppressors, oncogenes, and other cancer-related genes) pertaining to ovarian cancer [4].

Copy number variations (CNV) are a common occurrence in all forms of cancer [2, 5–8]. Distinct patterns of DNA instability as evident by gene copy number amplification and deletion have been observed within patient samples [2, 9–11]. A typical cancer sample exhibits an average of 17 % amplifications and 16 % deletions within an entire genome. Somatic copy number alterations have been shown to significantly affect pathways involving kinase function, cell cycle regulation, the Myc and NF-κB networks and apoptosis [2]. Detection of these alterations and identification of the specific genes responsible for cancer proliferation can help to molecularly subtype cancers and lead toward more individualized cancer-type specific therapies [9, 10, 12–16]. Epigenetic properties of the cancer genome correlate with the development and function of the cancer cell [17–21], and DNA methylation profiles have been identified in ovarian cancer [22, 23]. Specifically, DNA methylation at gene promoter regions can regulate the gene expression of various oncogenes and tumor suppressors [24–27]. Loss of function or transcriptional silencing via hypermethylation has been identified for tumor suppressor genes, while hypomethylation has been attributed to oncogenesis and the loss of imprinting properties of certain cancer-related alleles [1, 28].

These genomic and epigenetic aberrations present significant problems in both the clinical and scientific analysis of ovarian cancer especially with respect to diagnosis, the understanding of tumor progression, survival analysis, and treatment and therapeutic resistance [12, 29]. The development of successful cancer treatment protocols is reliant on the understanding of the underlying biology driving tumor progression. The magnitude of individual gene function within cancer pathways is often highly variable among tumor samples. A certain tumor suppressor or oncogene function may be gained or silenced at different frequencies by varying genomic conditions (aberrant DNA) within a tumor sample population. Epigenetic diversity and nucleotide mutations can also contribute to these varying rates of gene activity. Genome-wide copy number variation and changes in DNA methylation distribution integrated with RNA expression provide more detailed evidence for determining gene function. It is therefore essential to first accurately determine a gene's individual functional state within its cancer environment prior to understanding its cellular contribution within a cancer pathway or functional network.

Here, we provide a bioinformatics framework for the prediction of functionally relevant genes in ovarian cancer from genomic and epigenetic data. Single modality methods often capture all significant aberrations for one particular feature class of the tumor. The complexity of cancer progression and the subtle regulation of cancer genes within a continuum model of cancer function will only be accurately explained through the analysis of multiple modes of experimental data [30]. Examination of multiple cancer epigenetic and genomic modalities will help segregate cancer-specific genes from randomly altered cancer genes and can possibly elucidate the genetic mediators of ovarian tumorigenesis and predict progression of the disease [3, 31, 32]. Therefore, integrative methods that rely on a multimodal view of tumor suppressors and oncogenes are critical and necessary for a more detailed study of cancer. Here, we explain our proposed statistical methodology that predicts tumor suppressor and oncogenic functional gene candidates.

Additionally, one of the critical steps for treatment of ovarian cancer is identifying those patients who are at most risk for disease progression. Platinum-free interval is an important clinical end point used to measure ovarian tumor aggressiveness. The frontline treatment of ovarian cancer involves cytoreduction surgery followed by administration of platinum- and taxane-based chemotherapy. Approximately 25 % of patients with advanced stage cancers (stages III/IV) that initially respond to primary treatment with surgery and chemotherapy typically suffer recurrence with a drug-resistant phenotype within 6 months [3]. Consequently, there is a clinical need for both clinical and molecular features or biomarkers that can be associated with survival and disease recurrence in ovarian cancer. While significant progress has been made in measurement technologies that can simultaneously measure thousands of molecular features in a given patient sample, statistical methods to analyze this flood of data need to be carefully chosen in order to identify biomarkers that are more likely to validate and thus achieve clinical utility. We therefore propose a methodology to incorporate epigenetic features for the analysis of platinum-free survival for the purposes of identifying such clinically relevant genomic loci.

2 Material

2.1 Patient-Obtained Material and Data

1. Tumor tissue DNA samples (N.42) were collected from patients with newly diagnosed, untreated, advanced stage, serous ovarian carcinomas in Memorial Sloan-Kettering Cancer Center (*see* **Note 1**).
2. Normal ovarian tissue DNA samples (N.7) were obtained from the Cooperative Human Tissue Network (*see* **Note 2**).

3. Copy number variation, DNA methylation, and gene expression data for primary serous ovarian tumor samples (N.379) and associated platinum-free survival data (N.176) were downloaded from TCGA (http://tcga.cancer.gov/) [3].

2.2 Input Data for Statistical Analysis

1. Copy number variation data is derived from representational oligonucleotide microarray analysis (ROMA). All ROMA data is MIAME compliant and can be found in the GEO database (http://www.ncbi.nlm.nih.gov/geo/) for the subseries accession number GSE28013.
2. Genome expression profiling data was performed using the Affymetrix Human Genome U133A array: GEO platform identifier GPL96. All array data is MIAME compliant and corresponding CEL files can be found in the GEO database (http://www.ncbi.nlm.nih.gov/geo/) for the subseries accession number GSE27943.
3. DNA methylation data is derived from methylation detection representational oligonucleotide microarray analysis (MOMA). All MOMA data is MIAME compliant and can be found in the GEO database (http://www.ncbi.nlm.nih.gov/geo/) for the subseries accession number GSE27940.
4. Platinum-free survival data is calculated per ovarian tumor sample from both the publicly available and all (protected—by request) clinical data platforms downloaded from the data portal at The Cancer Genome Atlas (http://cancergenome.nih.gov/).

2.3 Bioinformatics Toolbox

All bioinformatics analysis was performed using a combination of Perl, Python, MATLAB, R (http://www.r-project.org/), and Bioconductor (http://bioconductor.org/) programming and statistical tools. R packages include "mclust," "survival," "qvalue," and "multtest." The KEGG pathway database and analysis was obtained and performed via Bioconductor (http://bioconductor.org/packages/2.6/data/annotation/html/KEGG.db.html).

3 Methods

3.1 Representational Arrays for Genomic and Epigenetic Analysis

3.1.1 Copy Number Detection via Representational Oligonucleotide Microarray (ROMA)

1. Apply the protocol for obtaining accurate DNA segmentation patterns using comparative genomic hybridization arrays including DNA extraction, restriction digestion of DNA, adaptor ligation, and PCR amplification followed by hybridization to custom-designed arrays [33] as previously outlined in a past volume [34] and extensively in varying studies [5, 35–37].
2. Use the CBS (circular binary segmentation) algorithm to segment the normalized log ratios from the array experiment. CNV segments are defined as regions of statistically combined probe (marker) intensities calculated by the CBS algorithm [36, 37].

3.1.2 Methylation Detection via Representational Oligonucleotide Microarray (MOMA)

1. Apply a similar representation array approach for DNA methylation detection. Calculate data from the MOMA experiment into a single methylation ratio (from the McrBc restriction enzyme-treated samples and control samples) for each array probe [38]. The method captures genome-wide methylation through a series of array probes intended to tile all predicted CpG islands in the genome (*see* **Note 3**).
2. Normalize probe GeoMeanRatios of all samples using the quantile normalization method [39].

3.1.3 Gene Expression Data

1. Produce gene expression data using the Affymetrix Human Genome U133A array.
2. Final signal intensities are processed using the RMA normalization method in the affy package of R Bioconductor 2.5.

3.2 Integrative Analysis of MSKCC Copy Number (ROMA), DNA Methylation (MOMA), and Expression Data

Our method is to examine the epigenetic and genomic features for possible tumor suppressors and oncogenes in primary ovarian tumors. With the base modality being copy number variation, we examine methylation and expression data for each gene under amplified or deleted copy number conditions. Therefore, an oncogene is classified as an amplified gene having low methylation and elevated expression (Fig. 1). This same amplified oncogene may be epigenetically regulated through hypermethylation in the context

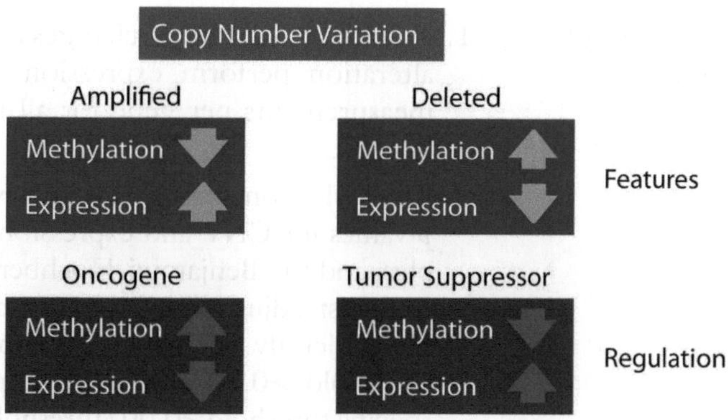

Fig. 1 Genomic and epigenetic features of tumor suppressors and oncogenes. A biological based annotation for regulated gene function by genomic and epigenetic features is shown to identify potential sample-specific functioning genes. Copy number variation is the base genomic feature for our identification of tumor suppressor and oncogenic gene properties in ovarian cancer. An oncogene can be overexpressed under amplified copy number and low methylation, while hypermethylation can be used for regulating expression in a gene-amplified state. Similarly, decreased tumor suppressor expression can be the result of partial copy number loss with hypermethylation. Tumor suppressors may also possibly be regulated via hypomethylation in a copy number deleted state. Our analysis is modeled for such properties and first examines the CNV per gene and then attributes epigenetic alteration for each copy number aberration with gene expression

of the ovarian tumor resulting in a decreased expression even if copy number is amplified. Conversely, a tumor suppressor is classified as having lowered copy number variation and hypermethylation resulting in decreased expression or is regulated through hypomethylation allowing for its expression under lowered CNV conditions (Fig. 1). This approach allows for (1) the use of predefined genomic and epigenetic features to predict functional gene candidates in ovarian tumors and (2) to reveal the functional activity of known tumor suppressors and oncogenes in ovarian cancer.

3.2.1 Copy Number Gene Assignment from ROMA

1. Identify genes contained in each ROMA loci using the UCSC Genome Browser hg17 assembly (*see* **Note 4**).
2. Determine through sample comparison between the TCGA platform and the ROMA platform (for which seven samples were in common) a ROMA platform-specific amplification and deletion threshold that captures a maximum percentage of deleted genes while maintaining a minimum false-positive percentage of amplified or neutral copy genes (*see* **Note 5**).

3.2.2 Genome-Wide Methylation Assignment from MOMA

1. MOMA probes represent single genomic loci and several contiguous fragments represent whole genes. Assign the final gene methylation value by using the maximum probe value for each MOMA fragment and attribute the maximum MOMA fragment value to the closest gene.

3.2.3 Integration of CNV and Expression Data

1. To identify significant changes in expression with copy number alteration perform expression to CNV Pearson correlation measurements per gene for all tumor samples in the ROMA data set.
2. The Wilcoxon signed-rank test is used to calculate enrichment *p*-values for CNV and expression data among tumor-only samples, and the Benjamini-Hochberg (BH) method is used for the multitest adjustment and false discovery rate (FDR) control. First, identify per gene all samples with a high copy number threshold ≥ 0.50 and a low copy number ROMA platform-specific threshold <0.00 (threshold identification was performed as stated above). Perform the Wilcoxon signed-rank test for each individual gene using the expression values obtained per sample in the amplified and deleted pools (*see* **Note 6**).

3.3 Integration of Copy Number Variation, DNA Methylation, and Expression Data

It is of interest to integrate all forms of the data when possible to determine which gene candidates are affected by CNV and methylation and have a concomitant change in gene expression. Epigenetic significance can be identified when both expression and methylation data types are examined at amplified and deleted CNV changes. Here, we combined methylation and expression data with CNV information from the MSKCC data set to isolate genes with potential oncogenic and tumor suppressor features (*see* **Note 7**).

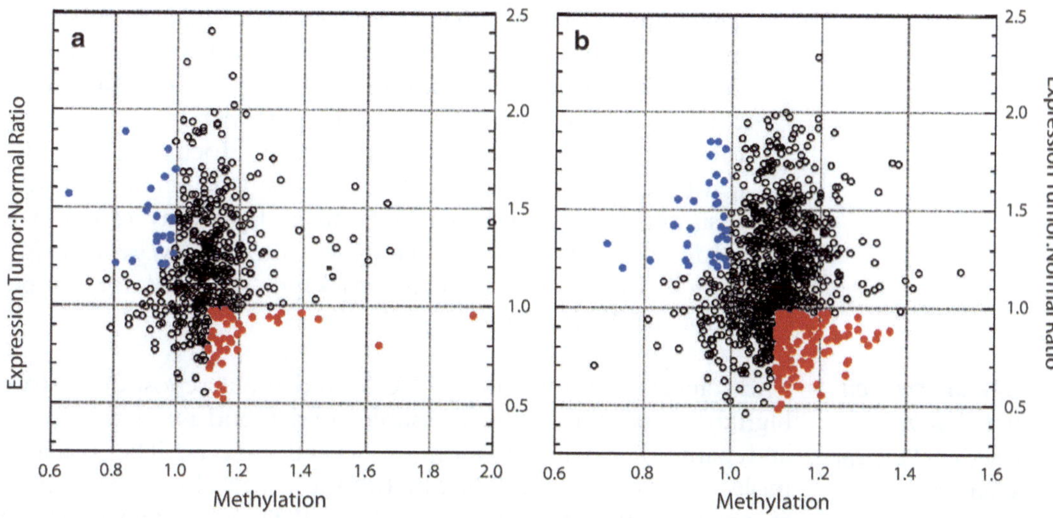

Fig. 2 Oncogenic and tumor suppressor features in ovarian cancer. We isolated genes (all points) with extreme copy number variation from the MSKCC data set. Methylation and tumor to normal expression ratio was then compared for genes at high CNV (**a**) and low CNV (**b**). Genes with oncogenic features (*blue ovals*; high expression and low methylation) and tumor suppressor features (*red ovals*; low expression and high methylation) were identified

1. Filter genes per sample with low CNV or high CNV and calculate the mean methylation and expression values for each copy number variation (Fig. 2). Determine expression thresholds for tumor to normal ratios by using a cutoff for the top 25 % and bottom 25 % of the entire expression ratio distribution, respectively (*see* **Note 8**).
2. Calculate Euclidean distances between normal and tumor samples for methylation and expression data points for all genes. If sufficient normal sample expression data is not available, a 50× bootstrap sampling was performed using the TCGA (The Cancer Genome Atlas) normal samples expression data per gene. Perform single variate and Hotelling multivariate *t*-tests on these distances to calculate all *p*-values when performing the methylation and expression analysis at varying copy number values, with statistical multiple test FDR adjustments as previously described (*see* **Note 9**).

3.4 Gene Pathway Overlay

Finally, in order to identify likely pathway changes captured by our feature-based gene analysis, test the membership of predicted genes for each defined tumor suppressor and oncogenic feature class (Fig. 1) within KEGG biological pathways.

1. In order to identify likely functional and pathway changes captured by feature-based gene analysis, test whether the membership of predicted genes in each feature class within a KEGG biological pathways is proportional to their size.

This translates to identifying pathways whose gene membership in each feature class deviates significantly from the null, as defined by a hypergeometric distribution ("phyper" R function). Choose the final list of significant pathways by controlling the false discovery rate using Benjamini-Hochberg multiple-testing correction. This analysis can easily be performed with a simple R script using KEGG.db and pathway id's downloaded from the KEGG database (http://www.genome.jp/kegg/) or the Bioconductor package; see [32] for sample script (*see* **Note 10**).

3.5 DNA Methylation Associated with Platinum-Free Survival in Ovarian Tumors

The Cancer Genome Atlas (TCGA) and other repositories store high throughout molecular measurement data and associated clinical and pathological information on several cancers. The available molecular data include DNA methylation, gene locus expression, sequencing data, and clinical data. These data sets contain a mixture of continuous and discrete/categorical variables, and any integrative analysis applying this information necessitates a careful selection of methodologies. Typically, measurements of time to metastasis, platinum-free interval (PFI) are given as continuous variables, and associated clinical data can take either discrete (hormone receptor status, grade, etc.) or continuous values such as locus expression and DNA methylation data. Deriving markers associated with prognosis from data that include both discrete and continuous measurements is a difficult challenge and frequently necessitates transformation of the data (e.g., binning), which can lead to loss of information available for analysis. Identification of CpG sites where DNA methylation state is indicative of PFI is valuable in understanding epigenetic regulation in ovarian cancer and its relationship with clinical outcome. Using the TCGA ovarian cancer clinical and genomic data, we developed a statistical methodology to infer loci whose methylation levels are associated with platinum-free survival. Biologically, DNA methylation state is discrete (i.e., any given CpG is either methylated or unmethylated). However, a tumor sample from which methylation is assessed is typically a heterogeneous mixture of cells. Therefore, a given CpG locus in each cell could be methylated or unmethylated (a discrete value), whereas the beta value that is estimated for a given CpG is a continuous value. With respect to these two possible definitions of CpG methylation, we provide two different modeling strategies to identify associations with platinum-free survival. An outline of these two strategies is depicted below and in Fig. 4.

3.5.1 Platinum-Free Survival

1. Platinum-free survival is defined as the period in months from the end of platinum-based chemotherapy until cancer progression or recurrence. Calculate platinum-free survival (PFS) data by using the clinical tables of the TCGA ovarian cancer data set and counting the number of days from end of platinum-based

chemotherapy until the patient suffered a recurrence or progression or left the study. The platinum-free survival times are right censored due to differing follow-up times for individual patients in the study, and we therefore used a Cox proportional hazards and Kaplan-Meier survival analysis to model associations between locus methylation levels and PFS.

3.5.2 Strategy to Discretize DNA Methylation and Find Associations with Platinum-Free Survival

1. The methylation values for each locus across all samples are discretized using a model-based clustering algorithm, and these discrete methylation levels are tested for correlation with survival (Fig. 4). Apply a standard expectation maximization model to discretize the continuous molecular profiling data where applicable (e.g., transform DNA methylation into high methylation or low methylation state). The beta values are therefore discretized to "0" indicating low levels of methylation or "1" indicating high methylation (*see* **Note 11**).
2. Use the "mclust" package in R to identify all CpG loci that fit a bimodal distribution of beta values across all samples. Exclude loci with non-bimodal distributions from further analysis. Use the Kaplan-Meier estimator of survival as the underlying statistical model to evaluate the association of methylation states with PFI. Individual survival curves are estimated for all samples with a given methylation state ("0" or "1") at a given locus.
3. Apply the logrank (Mantel-Haenszel) test to determine whether the two survival curves were significantly different from each other. Implement the "survfit" and "survdiff" functions in the "survival" package in R (*see* **Note 12**).

3.5.3 Strategy to Find Association Between Continuous Methylation Values and Platinum-Free Survival

The second strategy uses the continuous methylation values for each locus and performs univariate Cox regression analysis for each locus against the platinum-free survival data obtained from patient samples (Fig. 4).

1. Filter loci excluding those with very low variance (s.d. <0.2).
2. Estimate Cox coefficient for a given locus using the "coxph" function in the "survival" R package.
3. Evaluate the null hypothesis that a particular locus is not associated with survival, using the Wald test. The Wald test determines the likelihood that the estimated Cox coefficient is significantly different from zero returning a p-value for each locus.
4. Use the determined p-values to derive q-values [40] for loci within each modeling strategy by correcting for multiple testing with a false discovery rate of 5 % (*see* **Note 13**).
5. Perform multivariate Cox regression analysis on each of the selected loci along with other clinical factors such as tumor stage, age, and estrogen receptor status (*see* **Note 14**).

3.5.4 Clustering Survival Analysis

1. Pool the loci that are called as significant in either of the two strategies (Subheadings 3.5.2 and 3.5.3) as this provides the most complete set of CpG loci likely to be associated with platinum-free survival.
2. Perform hierarchical clustering on tumor samples using pooled loci with continuous methylation values.
3. Identify the major clusters and estimate Kaplan-Meier survival curves of the patients within each of the clusters (*see* **Note 15**).

4 Notes

1. Tumor DNA from 42 patients with newly diagnosed, untreated, advanced stage, serous ovarian carcinomas seen at the Memorial Sloan-Kettering Cancer Center between the period May 1992 and February 2003 was included in this study. The samples were collected under research protocols approved by the Memorial Sloan-Kettering Cancer Center IRB. Patients individually provided written informed consent to use their specimens for research purposes [32].
2. Seven ovarian tissue normal samples obtained from the Cooperative Human Tissue Network, a repository of tissue and tumor material run by the National Institutes of Health and funded by the National Institute of Cancer. Other investigators may have received specimens from the same samples. We refer to this patient and normal sample set as the MSKCC data set [32].
3. Approximately 26,000 CpG islands were obtained from the UCSC Genome Browser human genome build 17 in the range of 200–2,000 bp, and 50-mer sequence probes were constructed to overlap these regions. Using a combination of restriction enzymes where one of the enzymes is specific to methylated CpG sites (McrBc), an eventual hybridization comparison is made for each probe in the designed oligonucleotide array, and a level for DNA methylation is calculated [41].
4. The methods for obtaining accurate DNA segmentation patterns using comparative genomic hybridization arrays have been previously reviewed in a past volume [34] and extensively in varying studies [5, 35–37]. When calculating significant copy number aberrations in tumor samples from segmentation profiles, a careful examination for all germ line variations should be first performed. This can be performed by accounting for all normal loci variations found in the HapMap database (http://hapmap.ncbi.nlm.nih.gov/) [42]. In addition different strategies can be used to account for focal and arm-level variations. The Gistic method provides an excellent review and strategy for handling these variations and for the specific determination of somatic copy number variations [35].

5. Copy number variation for serous ovarian tumors and normal tissue was downloaded from TCGA (http://tcga.cancer.gov/). TCGA data was used to assess copy number variation threshold determination in ROMA [3]. When using multiple data modes, it is beneficial to examine overlapping samples for experimental consistency and data standardization.
6. In examining expression changes with copy number variation, greater gene expression differences between normal and tumor samples are not observed until we rely only on those samples containing genes with extreme amplifications and deletions. Therefore, our approach to identify genes with altered copy number variation correlated to expression was to examine the expression values of genes within high and low copy number seg.mean values. Furthermore, a small data set of expression values for normal samples may not accurately capture a true baseline for normal gene expression. By performing tumor sample specific expression analysis, we may not fully eliminate these variations but hope to limit their magnitude. Applying this to our ROMA data, the Wilcoxon signed-rank test based on CNV and gene expression captured 62 genes at a false discovery rate ≤0.05 (Table 1). We therefore integrated the

Table 1
Selected ovarian cancer genes captured by Wilcoxon signed-rank test based on copy number variation and expression data[a]

Gene name	*p*-Value	Chr.	Position	Gene function
POP4	*4.16e–04*	*19*	*34789009*	*Component of ribonuclease P*
CCNE1	*1.97e–03*	*19*	*34995400*	*Cyclin E1, ovarian cancer marker*
FOXJ3	5.88*e*–03	1	42414796	Forkhead box protein
CEBPG	1.03*e*–02	19	38556448	CCAAT-enhancer-binding protein
C19orf2	*2.29e–02*	*19*	*35125264*	*RPB5 binding protein*
UQCRB	*2.42e–02*	*8*	*97398479*	*Ubiquinol-cytochrome c reductase binding protein*
MYCBP	2.73*e*–02	1	39101222	c-MYC binding protein
MLL4	2.82*e*–02	19	40900760	Histone-lysine *N*-methyltransferase
STK3	3.33*e*–02	8	99536036	Serine/threonine-protein kinase 3
PHF20L1	*3.57e–02*	*8*	*133856785*	*PHD finger protein 20-like 1*
EBAG9	4.73*e*–02	8	110621104	Estrogen receptor-binding fragment-cancer-associated protein
OXR1	4.76*e*–02	8	107739211	Oxidation resistance protein

[a]Results of Wilcoxon signed-rank test with BH correction of selected genes in ovarian cancer tumor samples. Italics indicate genes also captured from the TCGA data set. All full results can be obtained in [32]

expression data with CNV to determine the genes that are more likely to be candidates as functioning cancer genes with potential tumor suppressor and oncogenic CNV-expression features. This makes the number of genes in further studies more approachable for functional validation of genes affected by genetic aberrations (see ref. 32 for complete results).

7. Identification of tumor active and inactive genes is a rational strategy for the better understanding of cancer progression in each individual sample. Here, we propose a gene function analysis strategy based on three modalities, copy number variation, DNA methylation, and RNA expression data. Though a reasonable assumption, other cellular factors such as genetic mutation, biophysical regulation, or normal cellular pathway disturbances can lead to the activation or inactivation of gene function. Furthermore, one modality such as copy number variation may have a more dominant effect on the expression of a gene, especially if the other modality (in this case DNA methylation) remains unchanged.

8. The heterogeneous tissue complexity of the ovarian cancer tumor sample must be considered throughout the analysis. By using conservative thresholds of extreme copy number deletions and amplifications and a 25 % distribution range for high and low methylation capture, we seek to capture mainly aberrations that are specific to the tumor cell in the sample.

9. We isolated 126 genes with tumor suppressor properties of low CNV, low tumor to normal expression ratios and were hypermethylated (Fig. 2b). When compared to both the methylation and expression values among the normal data samples, 114 out of these 126 genes had p-values below 5×10^{-2} (all results from this analysis can be obtained from [32]). The classic tumor suppressor RB1 (retinoblastoma protein, p-value 2×10^{-16}), the tumor suppressor BIK (Bcl-2-interacting

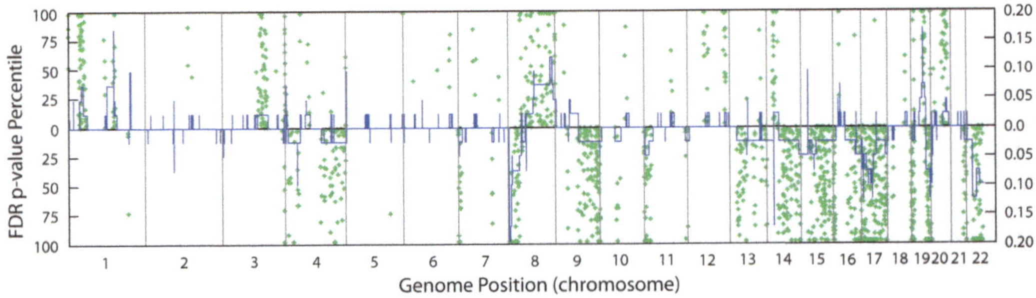

Fig. 3 Ranking of significantly expressed and methylated genes with copy number variation. Predicted MSKCC data set genes (*green circle*) with changes in methylation and expression are overlayed by a genome-wide stair plot of ROMA probe sample frequencies per deletion and amplification (*blue line*). Each predicted gene is percentile ranked according to its FDR p-values (<0.05) between normal and tumor samples

killer, apoptosis-inducing protein, p-value 1×10^{-13}), and the transcriptional repressor CTCF (p-value 4.5×10^{-5}) are among this feature class of gene. Examining genes with oncogenic properties such as high tumor to normal expression ratios, high CNV, and low methylation, we find 33 genes (Fig. 2a). A total of 238 genes were identified using tumor suppressor and oncogenic gene features. In addition, we show all predicted genes (ranked by percentile by their FDR p-value <0.05) per chromosome with relation to the ROMA probe copy number variation sample frequency (Fig. 3). Regions of amplification and deletion are shown along with the number of genes with significant expression and methylation differences from normal. A total of 941 genes were identified with significant changes from normal (based on Euclidean distance measurements) in both DNA methylation and expression in amplified and deleted copy number loci, 25 % (238) of which were also discovered using the tumor suppressor and oncogene gene features protocol. Therefore, we illustrate how loci with minor CNV frequency among tumor samples can still contain significantly altered expression and methylation gene features such as seen in chromosomes 2, 6, 10, and 12 (Fig. 3). These specific gene identifications within less frequent aberrant loci can potentially lead to a better understanding of direct functional gene contributions in ovarian subtype cancer networks.

10. When analyzing for significant pathways or gene set enrichment, the total number and accuracy of contents in each pathway will significantly affect any statistical analysis for relevance. Many times pathway significance is not revealed since all the genes in a large functional pathway annotation are not captured. A simpler strategy is to first determine the number of genes in the pathway annotation that have been covered (sensitivity) by experimental data and then examine only the captured genes for significant variance. Performing a KEGG pathway enrichment analysis on the predicted genes for each feature class identifies KEGG pathways associated with cancer: endometrial cancer (hsa05213), ErbB signaling pathway (hsa04012), amino acid metabolism (hsa00340), epithelial cell signaling in *h. pylori* infection (hsa0512), and regulation of actin cytoskeleton (hsa4810).
11. When discretizing beta values into high and low methylation states, it is important to assess the true distribution of the beta values across all samples and eliminate from considerations all CpG sites with unimodal distributions. The estimation of the number of underlying distributions that gave rise to the observed beta values can be evaluated by the use of the Bayesian Information Criterion (BIC). In our own work, we eliminated

loci which BIC indicated poorer fit to bimodal distributions over other unimodal or multimodal (>2 modes) distributions.

12. In the scenario of testing for survival association of discrete molecular features, the power of the Mantel-Haenszel test for differences between survival curves may be compromised if the relative size of the two subgroups of patients is highly skewed. It is therefore important to filter out loci that have uneven distribution of high and low methylation states. One needs to remove, from tests of association, any loci that do not have a minimum number of patients in each subgroup prior to checking for association with platinum-free survival.
13. The survival analysis is carried out using the "survival," "multtest," and "qvalue" packages in R. Additionally, in order to ensure that the selected loci stratified patients independent of other clinical factors, loci whose Cox regression coefficient remained statistically significant and did not change by more than 20 % when included with the above pathophysiological variables were chosen as being independent indicators of platinum-free survival.
14. In the scenario of the continuous molecular feature, the Cox regression framework makes the assumption that the values of the molecular features being tested for association with platinum-free survival are multiplicatively related to the hazard. For example, when Kaplan-Meier plots of patient subgroups show intersecting survival curves, the proportional hazards assumption is violated. In such cases, the Cox regression framework will not accurately estimate the average relative risk of a molecular feature, resulting in reduced power of the test of association. Performing multiple-testing correction after associating a list of molecular features with survival outcome is particularly important. There are many statistical methodologies that can be chosen for multiple-testing correction, and the choice depends on assumptions of the prevalence of such prognostic markers in the population of the molecular features being tested. It is important for end users of these statistical tools to review a good summary of the trade-offs and assumptions underlying different multiple-testing correction algorithms [43].
15. These 300 loci with continuous methylation values were then pooled together and used to cluster (using hierarchical clustering) the tumor samples. Loci information is available upon request. The major clusters are identified, and Kaplan-Meier survival curves of the patients within each of the clusters are estimated (Fig. 4). Our strategy has led to the identification of patient groups with significantly different platinum-free survival outcomes using methylation data. The utility of these 300 genes would, however, need to be validated on an independent data set.

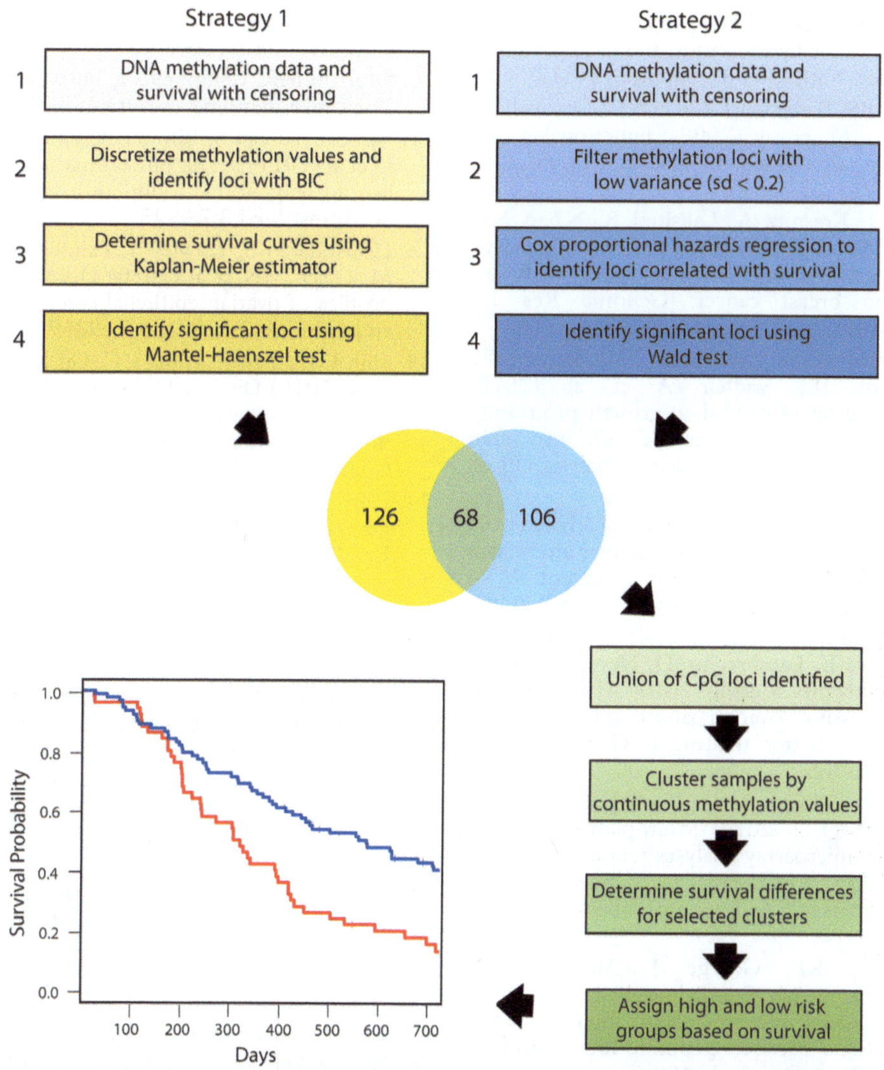

Fig. 4 Modeling strategies for an epigenetic-based ovarian cancer platinum-free survival analysis. Two different modeling strategies reliant on continuous or discrete epigenetic and clinical information are used to identify loci for which methylation levels are correlated with platinum-free survival. Patient survival curves are estimated from predicted and integrated epigenetic significant loci

References

1. Ting AH, McGarvey KM, Baylin SB (2006) The cancer epigenome-components and functional correlates. Genes Dev 20: 3215–3231
2. Beroukhim R, Mermel CH, Porter D, Wei G, Raychaudhuri S et al (2010) The landscape of somatic copy-number alteration across human cancers. Nature 463:899–905
3. Bell D, Berchuck A, Birrer M, Chien J, Cramer DW et al (2011) Integrated genomic analyses of ovarian carcinoma. Nature 474:609–615
4. Bast RC Jr, Hennessy B, Mills GB (2009) The biology of ovarian cancer: new opportunities for translation. Nat Rev Cancer 9:415–428
5. Degenhardt YY, Wooster R, McCombie RW, Lucito R, Powers S (2008) High-content analysis of cancer genome DNA alterations. Curr Opin Genet Dev 18:68–72
6. Santarius T, Shipley J, Brewer D, Stratton MR, Cooper CS (2010) A census of amplified and overexpressed human cancer genes. Nat Rev Cancer 10:59–64

7. Pinkel D, Albertson DG (2005) Array comparative genomic hybridization and its applications in cancer. Nat Genet 37(Suppl):S11–S17
8. Taylor BS, Barretina J, Socci ND, Decarolis P, Ladanyi M et al (2008) Functional copy-number alterations in cancer. PLoS One 3:e3179
9. Hicks J, Krasnitz A, Lakshmi B, Navin NE, Riggs M et al (2006) Novel patterns of genome rearrangement and their association with survival in breast cancer. Genome Res 16: 1465–1479
10. Ramakrishna M, Williams LH, Boyle SE, Bearfoot JL, Sridhar A et al (2010) Identification of candidate growth promoting genes in ovarian cancer through integrated copy number and expression analysis. PLoS One 5:e9983
11. Chen S, Auletta T, Dovirak O, Hutter C, Kuntz K et al (2008) Copy number alterations in pancreatic cancer identify recurrent PAK4 amplification. Cancer Biol Ther 7(11): 1793–1802
12. Despierre E, Lambrechts D, Neven P, Amant F, Lambrechts S et al (2010) The molecular genetic basis of ovarian cancer and its roadmap towards a better treatment. Gynecol Oncol 117:358–365
13. Andrews J, Kennette W, Pilon J, Hodgson A, Tuck AB et al (2010) Multi-platform whole-genome microarray analyses refine the epigenetic signature of breast cancer metastasis with gene expression and copy number. PLoS One 5:e8665
14. Gorringe KL, George J, Anglesio MS, Ramakrishna M, Etemadmoghadam D et al. (2010) Copy number analysis identifies novel interactions between genomic loci in ovarian cancer. PLoS One 5:e11408
15. Etemadmoghadam D, deFazio A, Beroukhim R, Mermel C, George J et al (2009) Integrated genome-wide DNA copy number and expression analysis identifies distinct mechanisms of primary chemoresistance in ovarian carcinomas. Clin Cancer Res 15:1417–1427
16. Malek JA, Mery E, Mahmoud YA, Al-Azwani EK, Roger L et al (2011) Copy number variation analysis of matched ovarian primary tumors and peritoneal metastasis. PLoS One 6:e28561
17. Delcuve GP, Rastegar M, Davie JR (2009) Epigenetic control. J Cell Physiol 219:243–250
18. Feinberg AP, Tycko B (2004) The history of cancer epigenetics. Nat Rev Cancer 4: 143–153
19. Sadikovic B, Al-Romaih K, Squire JA, Zielenska M (2008) Cause and consequences of genetic and epigenetic alterations in human cancer. Curr Genomics 9:394–408
20. Stratton MR, Campbell PJ, Futreal PA (2009) The cancer genome. Nature 458:719–724
21. Fang F, Turcan S, Rimner A, Kaufman A, Giri D et al (2011) Breast cancer methylomes establish an epigenomic foundation for metastasis. Sci Transl Med 3:75ra25
22. Houshdaran S, Hawley S, Palmer C, Campan M, Olsen MN et al (2010) DNA methylation profiles of ovarian epithelial carcinoma tumors and cell lines. PLoS One 5:e9359
23. Shih IM, Chen L, Wang CC, Gu J, Davidson B et al (2010) Distinct DNA methylation profiles in ovarian serous neoplasms and their implications in ovarian carcinogenesis. Am J Obstet Gynecol 203(6):584.e1–584.e22
24. Laird PW (2010) Principles and challenges of genome-wide DNA methylation analysis. Nat Rev Genet 11:191–203
25. Veeck J, Esteller M (2010) Breast cancer epigenetics: from DNA methylation to microRNAs. J Mammary Gland Biol Neoplasia 15:5–17
26. Iacobuzio-Donahue CA (2009) Epigenetic changes in cancer. Annu Rev Pathol 4:229–249
27. Campan M, Moffitt M, Houshdaran S, Shen H, Widschwendter M et al (2011) Genome-scale screen for DNA methylation-based detection markers for ovarian cancer. PLoS One 6:e28141
28. Ehrlich M (2002) DNA methylation in cancer: too much, but also too little. Oncogene 21: 5400–5413
29. Yap TA, Carden CP, Kaye SB (2009) Beyond chemotherapy: targeted therapies in ovarian cancer. Nat Rev Cancer 9:167–181
30. Berger AH, Knudson AG, Pandolfi PP (2011) A continuum model for tumour suppression. Nature 476:163–169
31. Mankoo PK, Shen R, Schultz N, Levine DA, Sander C (2011) Time to recurrence and survival in serous ovarian tumors predicted from integrated genomic profiles. PLoS One 6:e24709
32. Wrzeszczynski KO, Varadan V, Byrnes J, Lum E, Kamalakaran S et al (2011) Identification of tumor suppressors and oncogenes from genomic and epigenetic features in ovarian cancer. PLoS One 6:e28503
33. Lucito R, Healy J, Alexander J, Reiner A, Esposito D et al (2003) Representational oligonucleotide microarray analysis: a high-resolution method to detect genome copy number variation. Genome Res 13:2291–2305
34. Lucito R, Byrnes J (2009) Comparative genomic hybridization by representational oli-

gonucleotide microarray analysis. Methods Mol Biol 556:33–46

35. Mermel CH, Schumacher SE, Hill B, Meyerson ML, Beroukhim R et al (2011) GISTIC2.0 facilitates sensitive and confident localization of the targets of focal somatic copy-number alteration in human cancers. Genome Biol 12:R41
36. Olshen AB, Venkatraman ES, Lucito R, Wigler M (2004) Circular binary segmentation for the analysis of array-based DNA copy number data. Biostatistics 5:557–572
37. Venkatraman ES, Olshen AB (2007) A faster circular binary segmentation algorithm for the analysis of array CGH data. Bioinformatics 23:657–663
38. Kamalakaran S, Kendall J, Zhao X, Tang C, Khan S et al (2009) Methylation detection oligonucleotide microarray analysis: a high-resolution method for detection of CpG island methylation. Nucleic Acids Res 37:e89
39. Bolstad BM, Irizarry RA, Astrand M, Speed TP (2003) A comparison of normalization methods for high density oligonucleotide array data based on variance and bias. Bioinformatics 19:185–193
40. Storey JD, Tibshirani R (2003) Statistical significance for genomewide studies. Proc Natl Acad Sci U S A 100:9440–9445
41. Kamalakaran S, Varadan V, Giercksky Russnes HE, Levy D, Kendall J et al (2010) DNA methylation patterns in luminal breast cancers differ from non-luminal subtypes and can identify relapse risk independent of other clinical variables. Mol Oncol 5:77–92
42. Consortium TIH (2003) The International HapMap Project. Nature 426:789–796
43. Benjamini Y, Hochberg Y (1995) Controlling the false discovery rate: a practical and powerful approach to multiple testing. J R Stat Soc Ser B 57:289–300

Chapter 5

Survival Prediction Based on Inherited Gene Variation Analysis

Mine S. Cicek, Matthew J. Maurer, and Ellen L. Goode

Abstract

There is a significant variation of outcome among ovarian cases. Clinical features such as age, stage, comorbidities, or degree of debulking are known prognostic factors for the disease. However, additional variation remains unexplained, some of which may be due to inherited factors. Here, we describe identification of survival-associated inherited variants in ovarian cancer that can enhance our current prognostic capabilities.

Key words Survival prediction, Inherited variation, tagSNP, Candidate genes, Pathway analysis, Ovarian cancer-related pathways

1 Introduction

Ovarian cancer is the most lethal of gynecologic malignancies in the United States [1], yet much remains unknown about reasons for the observed differences in outcome across patients. Paclitaxel (Taxol)- and platinum-based chemotherapy (either cisplatin or carboplatin) represent standard therapy after surgical debulking [2]. Unfortunately, even with modern chemotherapy, most patients with advanced disease relapse and die of ovarian cancer; 10-year overall survival remains around 30 % [3–5]. Clinical features such as age, stage, comorbidities, or degree of debulking are known prognostic factors [6]. However, additional variation in outcome among patients remains unexplained, some of which may be due to inherited factors (germline, as opposed to tumor or somatic changes) that vary among patients. Inherited variation may influence outcome through differential metabolism of chemotherapeutic agents (e.g., variants in *ERCC1* and *ABCB1* modifying chemo-response), variable immune response, or through a variety of other host-related factors. For example, inherited *BRCA1* and *BRCA2* mutations are known to correlate with ovarian cancer survival [7].

Anastasia Malek and Oleg Tchernitsa (eds.), *Ovarian Cancer: Methods and Protocols*, Methods in Molecular Biology, vol. 1049, DOI 10.1007/978-1-62703-547-7_5, © Springer Science+Business Media New York 2013

To identify survival-associated variants, one can examine genome-wide or candidate genes. As an example of a candidate pathway approach, we hypothesized that inherited variants in mechanistic ovarian cancer-related pathways may contribute to genetically determined differences in ovarian cancer outcome. In particular, variants related to tumor angiogenesis may influence outcome as a major contributor to pathogenesis; anti-angiogenic therapy with bevacizumab represents the most successful application of a biologically targeted ovarian cancer therapy [8]. Aberrant inflammatory processes can impact multiple tumorigenic pathways [9]. Detoxifying molecules are key in response to oxidative stress [10] and the processing of chemotherapeutic agents. Alterations of cell cycle regulators cooperate in ovarian tumor development, and tumor molecular analyses show frequent mutation of these regulators [11]. Host defense mechanisms that eliminate mutated cells through permanent growth arrest (cellular senescence) are considered crucial tumor suppressive mechanisms [12]. Apoptotic pathways have been shown to be frequently altered in both tumor progression and drug resistance [13]. Glycosylation [14–16], one-carbon transfer [17], and other processes may also be susceptible to inherited changes which lead to differential ovarian cancer outcome.

A unique aspect of our approach was the clinical, demographic, and treatment homogeneity of the patients studied which, when combined with high data completeness, allowed us to assess the role of inherited variants above and beyond known clinical factors. The use of a clinic-based population provided the ability to account for detailed clinical data, which are not routinely available in population-based studies, while restriction to patients living within a defined surrounding geographic region minimized the potential for the referral bias sometimes seen in clinic-based studies. Centralized pathology review, high-quality genotyping, covariate adjustment, and conservative interpretation of results are also strengths of this study. The downside of an observational study is that compared to a randomized controlled trial, follow-up (e.g., measurement of toxicities) is less standardized. Our comprehensive efforts in selecting ovarian cancer-related polymorphisms, genes, and pathways were critical in this work. We used bioinformatics tools to help us choose genes included in this study in a systematic way.

Identifying survival-associated inherited variants can help to elucidate the most important drivers of ovarian cancer, representing ideal targets for tailored therapeutics, and may also enhance our current prognostic capabilities. Causality is not necessarily established by a correlation between a set of genes and clinical endpoints. In addition, a variety of mechanisms regulate gene expression including DNA methylation, histone deacetylation, copy-number changes, and targeting by micro-RNAs. Therefore, an integration procedure that incorporates this biologically useful knowledge is highly desirable.

2 Materials

2.1 Input Data

Analytic approach is designed to integrate extended collection of patient-relevant information and dataset characterizing SNPs of ovarian cancer—implicated genes and pathways.

2.1.1 Patients' Material and Data

1. Blood samples from 325 patients with pathologically confirmed primary invasive epithelial ovarian cancer (*see* **Note 1**).
2. Full collection of clinical data (histology, surgery outcome, chemotherapy, etc.) (*see* **Note 2**).
3. Illumina GoldenGate™ BeadArray assay genotype data.

2.1.2 Candidate Genes and Pathways Selection Sources

1. Cancer Genome Anatomy Project database.
2. Biokarta database.
3. KEGG PATHWAY databases.
4. Results of comparative (Affymetrix U95Av2 microarrays-based) advanced- versus early-stage ovarian cancer analysis [18].

2.1.3 Relevant tagSNPs Identification

1. HapMap Consortium's release 21a (genome build 34) [19].
2. Perlegen Sciences (genome build 34) [20].
3. SeattleSNPs (http://pga.mbt.washington.edu, genome build 35).
4. Panel 2 of the National Institute for Environmental Health Science SNPs (www.egp.gs.washington.edu, genome build 35).

2.2 Bioinformatics Toolbox

Statistical approaches are commonly used association testing methods which take advantage of multiple free and open-source softwares.

2.2.1 Statistical Approaches

1. Cox proportional regression model.
2. Confidence interval estimation algorithm.
3. Association testing method.

2.2.2 Available Software

1. R is an open-source statistical computing environment with a wide range of statistical analysis and graphical techniques (http://www.r-project.org/).
2. PLINK is a free genotype analysis toolset that has a wide array of relevant QC and analysis techniques available (http://pngu.mgh.harvard.edu/purcell/plink/).
3. Haploview is an open-source software package that can determine haplotypes as well as generate LD plots (http://www.broadinstitute.org/scientific-community/science/programs/medical-and-population-genetics/haploview/haploview) [21].

3 Methods

3.1 Gene Selection

1. Select relevant pathways and genes using available databases. With the goal of comprehensiveness, key genes within the pathways of angiogenesis (N = 18 genes), apoptosis (N = 18), cell cycle (N = 39), cellular senescence (N = 33), detoxification (N = 15), glycosylation (N = 26), inflammation (N = 26), and one-carbon transfer (N = 21) were identified using a number of sources including peer-reviewed published literature, the Cancer Genome Anatomy Project, Biokarta, and KEGG PATHWAY databases.
2. Add candidate genes significantly overexpressed in ovarian cancer as it was shown in previous expression profiling studies. Twenty-five genes previously shown to have a 50 % or more reduction in expression in ovarian tumor versus normal tissue using the Affymetrix U133A GeneChip array were included [18].
3. Include in the list any other interesting candidate genes. In our study we included a small number of genes related to NF-κB (*NFKBIA*, *NFKBIB*) and hormone metabolism (*CYP19A1*, *SULT1E1*) as well as the granulin-epithelin precursor (*GRN*) [22], and transcription elongation factor A (SII)-like 7 (*TCEAL7*) [23] based on unpublished data and recent reports.
4. The complete list of 227 included genes is provided in Table 1 (*see* **Note 3**).

3.2 Single Nucleotide Polymorphism (SNP) Selection

3.2.1 Select tagSNPs.

1. Identify tagSNPs via analysis of unrelated Caucasian genotypes from the HapMap Consortium's release 21a (genome build 34) [19], Perlegen Sciences (genome build 34) [20], SeattleSNPs (http://pga.mbt.washington.edu, genome build 35), and Panel 2 of the National Institute for Environmental Health Science SNPs (www.egp.gs.washington.edu, genome build 35).
2. Choose SNPs from each source from the region within 5 kb of the most 5′ and 3′ exons of each gene.
3. Identify tagSNPs by applying the ldSelect algorithm [24] to group (i.e., bin) SNPs with minor allele frequency (MAF) ≥ 0.05 and pair-wise linkage disequilibrium (LD) threshold of $r^2 \geq 0.8$.
4. Following binning, select tagSNPs for analysis from the source with the greatest number of SNPs with MAF ≥ 0.05 and the greatest number of LD bins that also met criteria for predicted likelihood of successful genotyping using the Illumina GoldenGate Assay™ quality score metrics.

Table 1
List of investigated genes (*N* = 227) and number of SNPs analyzed by pathway

Pathway	Genes	*N* SNPs analyzed (*N* attempted)
Angiogenesis	*EIF2B5, ELAVL1, HIF1A, KDR, MMP1, MMP2, MMP26, MMP3, MMP9, NOS3, PDGFD, PDGFRA, TIMP1, TIMP2, TIMP3, VEGFA, VEGFC, VHL*	130 (147)
Apoptosis	*APAF1, ATM, BAD, BAX, BCL2L1, BID, CASP10, CASP3, CASP6, CASP7, CASP8, CASP9, CYC1, EIF2S1, PARP1, PTK2, STAT1, TLN1*	118 (122)
Cell cycle	*ABL1, CCNA1, CCNA2, CCNB1, CCNB2, CCND1, CCND2, CCND3, CCNE1, CCNE2, CCNG1, CCNG2, CDC2, CDC25A, CDC25B, CDK2, CDK4, CDK6, CDK7, CDKN1A, CDKN1B, CDKN2A, CDKN2B, CDKN2C, CDKN2D, CUL1, E2F1, E2F2, E2F3, E2F4, E2F5, E2F6, PLK1, RB1, RBL1, RBL2, SKP2, TFDP1, TFDP2*	222 (244)
Cellular senescence	*ACTB, AKT1, ARID1A, BCL2, EGFR, ERCC3, FHIT, HRAS, IGF1, IGF1R, IGF2, KRAS, MYC, NF1, NR3C1, PIK3CB, POLR2A, PRKCA, SHC1, SMARCA2, SMARCA4, SMARCB1, SMARCC1, SMARCC2, SMARCE1, SOS1, SRC, TBP, TEP1, TERT, TNKS, TP53, XRCC5*	211 (223)
Detoxification	*ADH1A, ADH1B, ADH1C, ADH4, ADH5, ADH6, CYP1A1, CYP1A2, EPHX1, GSTM1, GSTP1, NAT1, NAT2, NQO1, NQO2*	108 (114)
Glycosylation	*FUT10, FUT3, FUT5, FUT6, FUT7, FUT8, FUT9, GALNT1, GALNT14, GALNT2, GALNT3, GALNT5, GALNT6, GALNT7, MGAT2, MGAT3, MGAT5, POFUT1, ST3GAL1, ST3GAL3, ST3GAL4, ST3GAL5, ST6GAL1, ST6GALNAC5, ST8SIA2, ST8SIA5*	95 (101)
Inflammation	*ALOX12, ALOX15, ALOX5, CCL11, CCL2, CCL3, CCR3, CRP, CXCL16, IL10, IL15RA, IL18, IL1A, IL1B, IL1RN, IL4R, IL6, IL6R, IL7R, IL8RA, IL8RB, IL9, PTGS1, PTGS2, TLR2, TNF*	154 (163)
One-carbon transfer	*AHCYL1, ALDH1L1, DHFR, DNMT1, DNMT3A, DNMT3B, DPYD, FOLR1, MAT2B, MBD4, MGMT, MTHFD1, MTHFD1L, MTHFD2, MTHFR, MTHFS, MTR, MTRR, SHMT1, SLC19A1, TYMS*	179 (187)
Under-expressed	*ABCB1, ACTG1, ARPC4, COL8A1, DKK3, DUSP1, EHD2, ELOVL4, F3, FGF2, FGF5, FOXD1, GALK1, HNT, KCNG1, LAMA4, MAPRE2, NRP2, P2RX5, PAPPA, PPP1R3A, PPP3CC, TBX3, TPM1, ULBP2*	120 (154)
Miscellaneous	*CYP19A1, GRN, NFKBIA, NFKBIB, SULT1E1, TCEAL7*	79 (81)
		1,416 (1,536)

Under-expressed genes from Dressman et al., J Clin Oncol. 25: 517–525, 2007 [34] and Lancaster et al., Int J Gynecol Cancer 16: 1733–1745, 2006 [18]; N analyzed SNPs excludes 50 (3 %) which failed genotyping and 70 (5 %) with incorrect genomic coordinates or low MAF

3.2.2 Putative functional SNPs. SNPs (within 1 kb upstream, 5′ UTR, 3′ UTR or non-synonymous) with MAF ≥ 0.05 identified in Ensembl version 34.

3.2.3 Select SNPs, tagging at least one other SNP using pair-wise binning in Tagger for SNPs in HapMap with Caucasian MAF ≥ 0.05, $r^2 \geq 0.8$, within 10 kb of genes (*CDC25B*, *CUL1*, *E2F3*, and *SMARCA2*) [25].

3.2.4 Select all non-intronic SNPs within 10 kb of each gene with a MAF > 0.05 (glycosylation genes).

3.2.5 Select SNPs within 10 kb of each gene with MAF > 0.05 among the CEU samples of HapMap Consortium's release 21a (genome build 34) [19] were binned if r2 ≥ 0.8, and include all non-synonymous SNPs.

3.2.6 Alternative SNP selections (non-intronic, non-synonymous, etc.) (see Note 4).

3.2.7 Finally, evaluate each SNP for compatibility with Illumina GoldenGate™ BeadArray assay ensuring all designability scores ≥ 0.6 and no SNP pairs within 60 bp.

3.3 Genotyping

1. Extract genomic DNA from 10 to 15 mL fresh peripheral blood using the Gentra AutoPure LS Puregene salting out methodology.
2. Perform Illumina GoldenGate™ BeadArray assay (*see* **Note 5**).

3.4 Statistical Analysis

3.4.1 Genotype QC and Dataset Creation

1. Exclude samples based on QC. This includes duplicate samples, identical samples based on pair-wise concordance, samples that failed genotyping, samples with low call rates (e.g., <97 %), and samples that are missing or ineligible based on clinical or phenotype criteria.
2. Exclude SNPs based on QC. This includes SNPs with low-quality calling (i.e., poor clustering), SNPs with low call rates (e.g., <95 %), SNPs with large deviation from HWE (e.g., $p < 0.0001$), and SNPs with high Mendelian or concordance errors in duplicates.
3. Perform SNP imputation if desired to fill in missing SNPs and create a complete-case SNP dataset [26] (*see* **Note 6**).
4. Determine what the phenotype endpoint will be (overall survival, progression-free survival, etc.) and relevant inclusion and exclusion criteria. Determine if models will be adjusted for relevant prognostic factors; if so, select variables and incorporate into models. Determine what the primary analysis will be (i.e., overall survival adjusted for age, stage, and tumor grade). The power from a survival analysis is based on the number of events, not the total N. Thus, event rate and number of events need to be considered when identifying the number of prognostic factors to include (*see* **Note 7**).

5. Create analysis dataset, merging SNP data with phenotype data. Incorporate SNP annotation, including gene, location, and function as appropriate.

3.4.2 Models and Analysis

1. *SNP level effects.* Run a Cox proportional hazards model with desired phenotype as the outcome and SNP as the predictor; adjust for prognostic factors as determined above. The SNP is generally modeled as a 0, 1, 2 variable, where the number is the count of minor alleles. This model has a good power to detect a variety of SNP effects (recessive, dominant, etc.). This model is repeated for each SNP in the study, with the hazard ratio, 95 % CI, and *p*-value reported. This is generally performed on complete cases for each SNP and not using imputation SNPs, unless confidence in imputation is high. Significant SNPs may be examined graphically using Kaplan-Meier plots; however, these would be a representation of unadjusted SNP effects.
2. *Gene-level effects.* Run principal components analysis on the collection of SNPs from a gene or region of interest and extract the first n principal components that account for 90 % of the total variation in the SNPs. Include these in a multivariable Cox regression analysis and generate global *p*-value using multiple degree-of-freedom likelihood ratio tests. SNP imputation is recommended to avoid loss of cases due to missing data (*see* **Note 8**).
3. *Haplotypes.* Haplotype analyses may be performed if SNPs are selected for haplotypes; this may be less relevant if SNPs are chosen based on a tagging approach. If desired, determine the haplotypes on the SNPs of interest and then include the haplotypes in a multivariable Cox model as shown above for gene-level tests. Low-frequency haplotypes may need to be combined to limit the number of predictors in the tables and for adequate model fitting.
4. *Pathway-level effects.* Determine the pathways or biological gene groupings a priori to analysis [27].
5. *Multiple comparisons.* Multiple comparison testing may be performed as appropriate. There is generally a large number of SNP level tests performed; these tests are not all independent as there is correlation between selected SNPs within a gene, even after tagging. See LD plots below for a visualization of this. Therefore, Bonferroni-type corrections will be conservative, and we generally prefer to report the raw (uncorrected) *p*-values and let the reader interpret the significance of results. Gene-level and pathway-level analyses greatly reduce the number of tests. Thus, we usually use gene-level tests to identify

genes or regions of interest and then examine individual SNPs within those genes. We may also report any highly significant SNPs that are not in significant genes.

6. *Linkage disequilibrium.* Examination of linkage disequilibrium (LD) between SNPs within a gene or region of interest is suggested. We prefer to use r^2 to measure LD as it represents the power of one SNP to predict the genotype of another.
7. *Software.* A number of open-source software packages are available for the described analyses. R (http://www.r-project.org/) is an open-source statistical computing environment with a wide range of statistical analysis and graphical techniques. PLINK (http://pngu.mgh.harvard.edu/purcell/plink/) is a free genotype analysis toolset that has a wide array of relevant QC and analysis techniques available. However, it does not handle survival models at the time of this writing, so those analyses, as well as the PCA for gene-level testing, would need to be performed using general statistics software, such as R. Haploview (http://www.broadinstitute.org/scientific-community/science/programs/medical-and-population-genetics/haploview/haploview) is an open-source software package that can determine haplotypes as well as generate LD plots. Both R and Haploview have plug-ins with PLINK.
8. *Tables and figures.* Presentation of results is often based on user preference. We suggest the generation of the following tables and figures at a minimum:
   (a) *Patient characteristics table.* Summary of patients in study, relevant phenotype, and adjustment and inclusion/exclusion variables. This is generally Table 1 in the manuscript.
   (b) *QC summary tables.* Summary of QC checks performed, including call rates, excluded samples, and SNPs. This is generally used internally with the results summarized in text format for the manuscript.
   (c) *Results tables.* Single SNP models are reported as a table of hazard ratio, 95 % CI, and p-value for each SNP, along with relevant annotation. Depending on the size of the genotyping study, all SNPs may be reported in the manuscript or only significant SNPs with the remaining SNPs in a supplementary table. Gene-level PCA results are reported as a table of the p-value and number of principal components required for each gene.
   (d) *LD plots.* LD plot for each gene or region of interest. This is generally used internally, though significant genes may be presented in the manuscript.
   (e) *KM curves.* KM curves for significant SNPs may be presented in the manuscript.

4 Notes

1. Recruitment of patients from Mayo Clinic's gynecologic surgery and medical oncology departments, including administration of questionnaires and venipuncture, used established protocols [28]. The protocol was approved by the Institutional Review Board, and all participants gave written informed consent. Eligible patients were women aged 20 years or older living in MN, IA, WI, IL, ND, or SD (the upper Midwest, USA) and ascertained within 1 year of a diagnosis of pathologically confirmed primary invasive epithelial ovarian cancer. Three hundred and twenty-five invasive patients recruited between December 14, 1999 and March 19, 2006 and diagnosed within the preceding year were studied.
2. Data on clinical features of disease including histology, surgical outcomes, and chemotherapy were abstracted by an experienced research nurse with review by gynecologic and medical oncology clinicians. Epidemiologic risk factor data including family history, reproductive factors, and exposure to known and suspected ovarian cancer risk factors were obtained through administration of a 16-page written questionnaire. Data on vital status was obtained from several sources including the Mayo Clinic computerized medical record, the Mayo Clinic Tumor Registry, which follows patients annually for overall survival who were diagnosed or received initial treatment at Mayo Clinic, and the National Death Index. Follow-up data was obtained through July 31, 2008.
3. A total of 1,536 SNPs on 227 genes were selected. There are not an optimal number of SNPs/genes that should be included in the analysis. This approach is widely used for small number of targeted genes as well as for GWAS.
4. For glycosylation genes, a tagSNP approach was not used; rather, all non-intronic SNPs within 10 kb of each gene with a MAF >0.05 were attempted. For inflammation genes, SNPs within 10 kb of each gene with MAF >0.05 among the CEU samples of HapMap Consortium's release 21a (genome build 34) [19] were binned if $r^2 \geq 0.8$, and all non-synonymous SNPs were included. For *CYP1A1*, variants were selected using resequencing data among 60 Caucasian-American subjects [29] via both the tagSNP method (MAF ≥ 0.05, $r^2 \geq 0.8$) [24] and a haplotype-tagging method (MAF ≥ 0.02, haplotype frequency ≥ 0.01, $r^2 \geq 0.9$).
5. Extract Genomic DNA from 10 to 15 mL fresh peripheral blood using the Gentra AutoPure LS Purgene salting out methodology (Gentra, Minneapolis, MN) and stored at 4 °C. Samples were bar-coded to ensure accurate and reliable

processing and plated with duplicates and lab standards. Following DNA activation, incubation, amplification, and automated genotype calling, quality control exclusions were performed based on poor clustering, low call rates (<95 %), and duplicate samples with unusually high number of discrepancies. No samples were excluded from cases eligible for the current analysis. Of the 1,536 attempted SNPs, we excluded SNPs which failed completely (or nearly completely), had low call rates (<95 %), and were monomorphic among all samples. Of the remaining 1,479 SNPs, prior to the analysis, additional review excluded tagSNPs found to be incorrect due to a chromosome 7 misalignment (*ABCB1*, *CDK6*, *PPP1R3A*, *NOS3*), SNPs found to be >10 kb from the gene of interest in current genome build 36.3 (*GSTM1* rs366631; *TIMP1* rs2283736; *MGAT5* rs1257189, rs1257187; *AKT1* rs4983559; *TFDP2* rs733996, rs7644383, rs11720300), and SNPs with observed MAF <0.01 in the current sample subset (*ADH4* rs13112924, *RBL1* rs1780703, *TCEAL7* rs17340307, *ERCC3* rs1803541, *CUL1* rs6958001, *IL4R* rs1801275, *SHMT1* rs2168781, *BCL2* rs4987792, *FUT6* rs364637, and *TIMP3* rs1962223). Thus, 1,416 SNPs are included in the analyses.

6. We also employed a simulation-based approach to examine whether the genes among varied biological-based pathway showed greater significance than expected due to chance. These gene set approaches can help a researcher further identify meaningful associations within biological or other predefined gene groupings. See Fridley and Biernacka for an expanded discussion of these analysis approaches [27].

7. Survival (or more generally time-to-event) genotyping studies present different sets of challenges than etiology studies. Power is limited by the number of events in the dataset, whether the event is death or a measure of disease progression. Covariates are also different in a time to event model, as you hope to account for heterogeneity in case outcome, rather than potential confounders of case versus control status. Researchers need to decide whether to examine the association of SNPs alone or after adjustment for known clinical factors that influence outcome heterogeneity in their population. Factors such as stage, morphology, tumor grade, residual disease from primary debulking surgery, and others are associated with overall survival in patients with ovarian cancer, and we chose to adjust for these factors in our study. The final adjustment list would require approximately 20 degrees of freedom to include in the survival model, which was not desirable given the sample size of the study. These clinical factors have been established in other studies and precise estimation of their effect size and direction was not as important as examining the SNP effect in

the models. Thus, we developed a single degree of freedom risk score with the clinical factors. This single degree of freedom risk score was then used as the lone adjustment variable in our SNP Cox models. We have used this approach with success on other studies [30–32], and our unpublished simulation studies have shown this approach yields similar results as including all the clinical variables in the model, with the 1 degree-of-freedom risk score tending to results in tighter estimates of the SNP effects.

8. Gene-level tests provide some benefits over single SNP approaches [33]. Our additional internal simulations have shown that principal components analysis (PCA)-based gene tests have good power to detect effects under a wide range of genetic models while greatly reducing the number of discovery tests performed, thus reducing the multiple testing concerns. PCA tests do not provide information about the nature of the association (protective or deleterious) but further investigation of SNPs within a significant gene can help further identify the nature of associations with outcome.

Acknowledgement

This work was supported by the National Cancer Institute (R01-CA86888, R01-CA122443, P50-CA136393-01A1), the Fred C. and Katherine B. Andersen Foundation, and the Mayo Foundation.

References

1. Siegel R, Naishadham D, Jemal A (2012) Cancer statistics, 2012. Cancer J Clin 62:10–29
2. Cannistra SA (2004) Cancer of the ovary. N Engl J Med 351:2519–2529
3. Hoskins WJ, Bundy BN, Thigpen JT, Omura GA (1992) The influence of cytoreductive surgery on recurrence-free interval and survival in small-volume stage III epithelial ovarian cancer: a Gynecologic Oncology Group study. Gynecol Oncol 47:159–166
4. McGuire V, Jesser CA, Whittemore AS (2002) Survival among U.S. women with invasive epithelial ovarian cancer. Gynecol Oncol 84:399–403
5. Barnholtz-Sloan JS, Schwartz AG, Qureshi F, Jacques S, Malone J et al (2003) Ovarian cancer: changes in patterns at diagnosis and relative survival over the last three decades. Am J Obstet Gynecol 189:1120–1127
6. Aletti GD, Gallenberg MM, Cliby WA, Jatoi A, Hartmann LC (2007) Current management strategies for ovarian cancer. Mayo Clin Proc 82:751–770
7. Bolton KL, Chenevix-Trench G, Goh C, Sadetzki S, Ramus SJ et al (2012) Association between BRCA1 and BRCA2 mutations and survival in women with invasive epithelial ovarian cancer. JAMA 307:382–389
8. Nimeiri HS, Oza AM, Morgan RJ, Friberg G, Kasza K et al (2008) Efficacy and safety of bevacizumab plus erlotinib for patients with recurrent ovarian, primary peritoneal, and fallopian tube cancer: a trial of the Chicago, PMH, and California Phase II Consortia. Gynecol Oncol 110:49–55
9. Inoue J, Gohda J, Akiyama T, Semba K (2007) NF-kappaB activation in development and progression of cancer. Cancer Sci 98:268–274

10. Storz P (2005) Reactive oxygen species in tumor progression. Front Biosci 10:1881–1896
11. D'Andrilli G, Giordano A, Bovicelli A (2008) Epithelial ovarian cancer: the role of cell cycle genes in the different histotypes. Open Clin Cancer J 2:7–12
12. Chiantore MV, Vannucchi S, Mangino G, Percario ZA, Affabris E et al (2009) Senescence and cell death pathways and their role in cancer therapeutic outcome. Curr Med Chem 16:287–300
13. Hajra KM, Tan L, Liu JR (2008) Defective apoptosis underlies chemoresistance in ovarian cancer. Adv Exp Med Biol 622:197–208
14. Ho SB, Niehans GA, Lyftogt C, Yan PS, Cherwitz DL et al (1993) Heterogeneity of mucin gene expression in normal and neoplastic tissues. Cancer Res 53:641–651
15. Baldus SE, Engelmann K, Hanisch FG (2004) MUC1 and the MUCs: a family of human mucins with impact in cancer biology. Crit Rev Clin Lab Sci 41:189–231
16. Saldova R, Wormald MR, Dwek RA, Rudd PM (2008) Glycosylation changes on serum glycoproteins in ovarian cancer may contribute to disease pathogenesis. Dis Markers 25:219–232
17. Yap TA, Carden CP, Kaye SB (2009) Beyond chemotherapy: targeted therapies in ovarian cancer. Nat Rev Cancer 9:167–181
18. Lancaster JM, Dressman HK, Clarke JP, Sayer RA, Martino MA et al (2006) Identification of genes associated with ovarian cancer metastasis using microarray expression analysis. Int J Gynecol Cancer 16:1733–1745
19. Frazer KA, Ballinger DG, Cox DR, Hinds DA, Stuve LL et al (2007) A second generation human haplotype map of over 3.1 million SNPs. Nature 449:851–861
20. Hinds DA, Stuve LL, Nilsen GB, Halperin E, Eskin E et al (2005) Whole-genome patterns of common DNA variation in three human populations. Science 307:1072–1079
21. Barrett JC, Fry B, Maller J, Daly MJ (2005) Haploview: analysis and visualization of LD and haplotype maps. Bioinformatics 21:263–265
22. Jones MB, Michener CM, Blanchette JO, Kuznetsov VA, Raffeld M et al (2003) The granulin-epithelin precursor/PC-cell-derived growth factor is a growth factor for epithelial ovarian cancer. Clin Cancer Res 9:44–51
23. Chien J, Staub J, Avula R, Zhang H, Liu W et al (2005) Epigenetic silencing of TCEAL7 (Bex4) in ovarian cancer. Oncogene 24:5089–5100
24. Carlson CS, Eberle MA, Kruglyak L, Nickerson DA (2004) Mapping complex disease loci in whole-genome association studies. Nature 429:446–452
25. de Bakker PI, Yelensky R, Pe'er I, Gabriel SB, Daly MJ et al (2005) Efficiency and power in genetic association studies. Nat Genet 37:1217–1223
26. Li Y, Willer C, Sanna S, Abecasis G (2009) Genotype imputation. Ann Rev Genomics Hum Genet 10:387–406
27. Fridley BL, Biernacka JM (2011) Gene set analysis of SNP data: benefits, challenges, and future directions. Eur J Hum Genet 19:837–843
28. Sellers TA, Schildkraut JM, Pankratz VS, Vierkant RA, Fredericksen ZS et al (2005) Estrogen bioactivation, genetic polymorphisms, and ovarian cancer. Cancer Epidemiol Biomarkers Prev 14:2536–2543
29. Olson JE, Ingle JN, Ma CX, Pelleymounter LL, Schaid DJ et al (2007) A comprehensive examination of CYP19 variation and risk of breast cancer using two haplotype-tagging approaches. Breast Cancer Res Treat 102:237–247
30. Cerhan JR, Wang S, Maurer MJ, Ansell SM, Geyer SM et al (2007) Prognostic significance of host immune gene polymorphisms in follicular lymphoma survival. Blood 109:5439–5446
31. Habermann TM, Wang SS, Maurer MJ, Morton LM, Lynch CF et al (2008) Host immune gene polymorphisms in combination with clinical and demographic factors predict late survival in diffuse large B-cell lymphoma patients in the pre-rituximab era. Blood 112:2694–2702
32. Wang SS, Maurer MJ, Morton LM, Habermann TM, Davis S et al (2008) Polymorphisms in DNA repair and one-carbon metabolism genes and overall survival in diffuse large B-cell lymphoma and follicular lymphoma. Leukemia 23(3):596–602
33. Gauderman WJ, Murcray C, Gilliland F, Conti DV (2007) Testing association between disease and multiple SNPs in a candidate gene. Genet Epidemiol 31:383–395
34. Dressman HK, Berchuck A, Chan G, Zhai J, Bild A et al (2007) An integrated genomic-based approach to individualized treatment of patients with advanced-stage ovarian cancer. J Clin Oncol 25:517–525

Part II

Targeted Analysis of DNA Methylation

Chapter 6

Main Principles and Outcomes of DNA Methylation Analysis

Susan K. Murphy, Christopher F. Bassil, and Zhiqing Huang

Abstract

Epigenetic modifications, including DNA methylation, are critically important mediators of normal cell function over the course of our lives. These modifications therefore also can play prominent roles in the development of disorders and diseases, including ovarian cancer. Genome-wide studies are now beginning to comprehensively decipher the methylome in normal and diseased tissues and cells, providing new insights into the distribution, specificity, and magnitude of modifications that occur and raising questions about these changes at specific loci. Further study of these alterations in specific tissues usually involves targeted approaches, of which there are a number available, all with distinct advantages and disadvantages. Here we provide a brief overview of DNA methylation and some of the methylation alterations that have been identified in ovarian cancer, as well as some of the technical approaches used to study these modifications.

Key words DNA methylation, Ovarian cancer, Bisulfite conversion, Methylation-specific PCR, Bisulfite sequencing, Pyrosequencing

1 DNA Methylation as a Biological Phenomenon

There are several major forms of epigenetic gene regulation that can become deregulated and contribute to the initiation and progression of a number of human diseases, including noncoding RNAs, histone modifications, and DNA methylation, which together interact to remodel chromatin. DNA methylation is a powerful form of gene regulation that plays a crucial role in normal mammalian development [1, 2]. The ability to methylate DNA extends to bacteria and plants, and this modification is involved in many gene regulatory systems. Cross-species comparative epigenomic analyses have revealed intriguing trends for both conserved and divergent features of DNA methylation in eukaryotic evolution. In mammals, DNA methylation is critical for the proper function of the genome, including genomic imprinting, X-chromosome inactivation, and transposon silencing and for controlling the expression of endogenous genes.

Anastasia Malek and Oleg Tchernitsa (eds.), *Ovarian Cancer: Methods and Protocols*, Methods in Molecular Biology, vol. 1049, DOI 10.1007/978-1-62703-547-7_6,

Patterns of methylation are stably maintained through somatic cell division and may even be inherited across generations. These patterns are sometimes perturbed in important human diseases, such as those associated with imprinting disorders and cancer [3–5].

Genome-wide studies are beginning to elucidate complex methylation profiles present within the human genome, and how changes in these profiles are associated with disease. DNA methylation occurs primarily at cytosine-guanine (CG) dinucleotide pairs, at the 5-carbon position of the cytosine base. About 70–80 % of the CG dinucleotides throughout the genome are methylated. DNA methyltransferase enzymes are responsible for the covalent transfer of a methyl group to cytosine using S-adenosylmethionine as the methyl group donor. CG dinucleotides are overall depleted throughout the genome, thought to be due to endogenous deamination of methylated cytosines to thymines over the course of evolution [6]. In spite of this relative depletion of CG dinucleotides, there are regions of the genome where dense clusters of CGs exist; these are often unmethylated and associated with the transcription start sites of genes [7]. Within gene bodies, CG methylation appears to be favored in exons over introns. Although the biological function of gene body methylation or mechanisms by which gene bodies are targeted by the methylation machinery are not well-understood, the preferential methylation of exons in plant and animal species appears to be an evolutionarily conserved phenomenon [8].

2 Alteration of DNA Methylation and Ovarian Carcinogenesis

In many types of cancer, DNA methylation is altered such that regions of the genome that normally exhibit methylation, such as repetitive elements, become hypomethylated [9] while other regions of the genome that are normally unmethylated, including promoter regions of tumor suppressor genes, acquire methylation [10]. The stability and somatic heritability of DNA methylation make it an attractive molecular biomarker for risk assessment, early disease detection, prognosis, and prediction of response to therapy. DNA methylation may also be useful for disease monitoring and for the identification of new therapeutic targets in cancer.

A preliminary study of DNA methylation in specimens from 50 women with ovarian cancer analyzed matched preoperative serum, tumor tissue, and ascites/peritoneal washings and reported that one or more of the tumor suppressor genes analyzed (breast cancer 1, early onset (*BRCA1*), RAS association domain family member 1, isoform A (*RASSF1A*), adenomatous polyposis coli (*APC*), $p14^{ARF}$, $p16^{INK4a}$, and death associated protein-kinase (*DAPK*)) showed methylation in all 50 of the tumors, regardless of histology, stage, or grade of the tumor [11]. Serum from 41 of the patients showed an identical pattern of hypermethylation as that detected in the tumors. The peritoneal fluid from 27 of 29 women also showed the same methylation profiles as the matched tumor. These findings suggest the ability to noninvasively detect alterations in methylation that are associated with the disease. Furthermore, the serum methylation profiles from all eight women with stage I disease matched that of the tumor. None of the tissues examined from 40 control women (serum, non-neoplastic tissues, or peritoneal fluid) showed hypermethylation of these genes. This study therefore indicates that, at least for this subset of genes, methylation changes occur early in the disease process. This study supports the utility of using DNA methylation profiles for early detection of epithelial ovarian cancer using specimens obtained through relatively noninvasive means.

3 Assessment of DNA Methylation Status in Ovarian Cancer Diagnostics and Therapy

Discovery and quantitation of methylation changes offer great potential for disease detection and prognosis and may also impact individualization of therapies used to treat the disease [12]. The fast-paced development of technologies for assessing DNA methylation has provided powerful means to also monitor changes in these profiles. Abnormal DNA methylation of CpG islands in the promoter region of tumor suppressor genes in ovarian cancer is well established as a common mechanism of gene silencing and serves as an alternative to genetic mutation to abrogate gene function. Classic tumor suppressor genes, including *BRCA1*, $p16^{INK4a}$, mutL, *E. coli* homolog of, 1 (*MLH1*), and *RASSF1A*, and many more have been identified as hypermethylated with associated loss of expression in ovarian cancers [13–18]. Thus far, only limited numbers of genes have been shown as specifically aberrantly methylated in tumor cells based on histologic origin or other common features. For example, *BRCA1* methylation is believed to be restricted to ovarian and breast cancers [19]. However, DNA methylation biomarkers that are specific to epithelial ovarian cancer remain to be discovered.

The methylation status of individual genes has been investigated for potential prognostic use in ovarian cancer. Studies have shown an association between DNA methylation of insulin-like growth factor-binding protein 3 (*IGFBP-3*), cyclin-dependent kinase inhibitor 2A (*CDKN2A*), *BRCA1*, and *MLH1* and increased risk of ovarian cancer progression [20–23]. Determining a methylation signature that can predict time to relapse and/or overall survival would greatly impact individualized care regimens. Understanding and overcoming resistance to chemotherapy is central to improving survival of ovarian cancer patients.

Several studies in breast and ovarian cancers have shown that *BRCA1* is hypermethylated in 10–15 % of sporadic ovarian tumors and that hypermethylation is associated with the loss of RNA and protein expression. Ovarian cancer patients with *BRCA1* hypermethylation have better survival [24], which may be due to reduced ability to repair DNA damage induced by chemotherapy, thereby improving clinical response to treatment [25]. However, the low frequency of *BRCA1* methylation in epithelial ovarian cancers suggests that genome-wide screening for additional informative DNA methylation targets will be required.

4 Bisulfite Modification as an Essential Step for DNA Methylation Analysis

Sodium bisulfite has differential effects on unmethylated and methylated cytosines that lead to deamination of unmethylated cytosines with conversion to uracils under acidic conditions. Methylated cytosines are not affected, enabling discrimination of methylated from unmethylated cytosines throughout the converted DNA. Bisulfite treatment has played a pivotal role in the analysis of DNA methylation. Successful bisulfite modification is essential for ensuring accuracy in assessing DNA methylation. Incomplete bisulfite conversion is the single largest confounder of bisulfite-based methods of DNA methylation analysis [26]. To achieve high bisulfite conversion, it is important that the DNA is of good purity and that appropriate reagents and procedures are used for bisulfite modification. We have found excellent performance, ease of use, and consistently high conversion rates using commercially available kits, such as those offered by Zymo Research or Qiagen. We typically treat 500–800 ng of DNA with sodium bisulfite, which can provide sufficient template for up to 40 PCR reactions (25 μl reaction volume) in our hands.

There are several important considerations regarding the treatment of genomic DNA with sodium bisulfite. Incubation of genomic DNA with sodium bisulfite is a harsh chemical treatment and leads to DNA fragmentation. Depending on the intended application, this fragmentation may hinder the downstream assays being performed. This may be alleviated in part by adjusting the time of the incubation step of the DNA with the sodium bisulfite. Several companies have recently developed kits for sodium bisulfite modification that substantially reduce this incubation time, which should lead to decreased DNA fragmentation. Use of shorter incubation times should be accompanied by methods to confirm the conversion efficiency. DNA extracted from formalin fixed, paraffin-embedded (FFPE) tissues presents an even greater challenge since the formalin fixation also leads to fragmentation of the DNA before the bisulfite treatment. Reversal of the DNA-protein cross-links followed by ligation of the DNA fragments has been successfully used to generate data from FFPE specimens on the Illumina

Infinium platform [27]. This platform utilizes technology requiring a single-base extension of the bisulfite-modified DNA so the mosaicism generated by performing ligation of DNA fragments from the entirety of the genome is not an issue, but it does require DNA fragments of at least 1 kb to work effectively. Another consideration is that DNA extracted from buccal swabs or saliva is often contaminated with substantial amounts of bacterial DNA. It is therefore important to determine that there is sufficient human DNA present in the specimen to ensure an adequate quantity for bisulfite treatment and your intended application.

5 Methods of DNA Methylation Analysis

Three PCR-based techniques for targeted analysis of DNA methylation that utilize bisulfite-modified DNA are described in the following chapters.

The first technique we describe is methylation-specific (MS) PCR, which is a relatively fast and inexpensive method for generation of qualitative (methylation present or absent) data for the region analyzed. We then describe a protocol for bisulfite sequencing of cloned alleles, which is useful for capturing the methylation status of each individual CG dinucleotide within the region studied. This method can also provide semiquantitative information about the number of alleles showing a given methylation profile and allow for detection of methylation patterns across alleles. Lastly, we describe bisulfite pyrosequencing, a quantitative method of determining the actual percent methylation of each CG within the sequence analyzed for the DNA specimen under study. There are many variations of these protocols that are beyond the scope of this chapter. We describe our preferred methodologies.

In traditional MS-PCR, two sets of primers are designed for the amplification of methylated or unmethylated DNA followed by gel electrophoresis. MS-PCR is a simple, fast, sensitive, and specific method for determining the methylation status of virtually any CG-rich region [28]. The use of PCR as the step to distinguish methylated from unmethylated DNA in MS-PCR allows for a significant increase in the sensitivity of methylation detection and thus can be used with limiting amounts of DNA. In addition, MS-PCR is suitable for the analysis of large numbers of samples as it can be carried out in a 96-well plate format. Although many newer methods have been developed, MS-PCR is still a popular technique used for analysis of DNA methylation. However, disadvantages of MS-PCR include the low quantitative accuracy and the increased risk for false positives. MS-PCR can indeed be performed in a more quantitative fashion by incorporating use of fluorescent hydrolysis probes (MethyLight) or fluorescent dyes (such as SYBR) that enable real-time detection of the MS-PCR amplification products. The tremendous amplification of the starting template during

PCR can also lead to inaccuracies in estimations of the level of methylated or unmethylated DNA present, especially when the reactions are allowed to plateau due to exhaustion of reagents or primers. Use of fewer PCR cycles may help prevent this type of discrepancy but also decreases the analytical sensitivity of the assay. Use of appropriately designed primers and a higher annealing temperature may also help prevent false-positive events.

Bisulfite sequencing of cloned alleles offers a more quantitative approach to methylation analysis as compared to MS-PCR. Sequencing of individual cloned alleles provides the methylation status for individual molecules and provides a measure of the proportion of alleles showing methylation at each CG cytosine when sufficient numbers of clones are sequenced. However, sequencing of single alleles can be time-consuming because it requires the selection and analysis of multiple clones, independent PCR, and sequencing reactions for each and can be costly when used as routine methodology.

Another quantitative approach that is more amenable to high-throughput analysis is bisulfite pyrosequencing, which utilizes pyrophosphate, released after each nucleotide is incorporated, to drive an enzymatic cascade that results in the luciferase-catalyzed conversion of luciferin to oxyluciferin and production of light. The light produced as the end result of this reaction is directly proportional to the number of nucleotides incorporated and hence the number of template molecules present in the reaction mix. Bisulfite pyrosequencing therefore yields quantitative information regarding the methylation status of single CG sites. Pyrosequencing requires careful primer design since the reaction is carried out at relatively low temperature, and the assays should be tested to insure that there is not substantial bias in the amplification efficiency of methylated versus unmethylated template DNA for the primer pair used. As with any bisulfite-based method of DNA methylation analysis, pyrosequencing also requires complete bisulfite conversion, which in part depends on high purity DNA. Unlike the other methods of analysis, bisulfite pyrosequencing incorporates bisulfite conversion controls into every sequence run, thus providing an internal control for each template to check the efficiency of the conversion. This method can be performed using a small amount of DNA (we use 40 ng of template DNA per pyrosequencing reaction, assuming complete recovery of the bisulfite-modified DNA). The main disadvantages of this method are the requirement for specialized instrumentation and the limitation of the DNA length analyzed (~115 bp maximum) so that only a limited number of CG sites are included within the sequence analyzed. However, because of the highly quantitative nature of this method coupled with the precision it affords and the reliability of the data, pyrosequencing is widely used by many research laboratories.

References

1. Li E, Bestor TH, Jaenisch R (1992) Targeted mutation of the DNA methyltransferase gene results in embryonic lethality. Cell 69:915–926
2. Okano M, Bell DW, Haber DA, Li E (1999) DNA methyltransferases Dnmt3a and Dnmt3b are essential for de novo methylation and mammalian development. Cell 99:247–257
3. Robertson KD (2005) DNA methylation and human disease. Nat Rev Genet 6:597–610
4. Doi A, Park IH, Wen B, Murakami P, Aryee MJ et al (2009) Differential methylation of tissue- and cancer-specific CpG island shores distinguishes human induced pluripotent stem cells, embryonic stem cells and fibroblasts. Nat Genet 41(12):1350–1353
5. Esteller M (2008) Epigenetics in cancer. N Engl J Med 358:1148–1159
6. Duncan BK, Miller JH (1980) Mutagenic deamination of cytosine residues in DNA. Nature 287:560–561
7. Glass JL, Thompson RF, Khulan B, Figueroa ME, Olivier EN et al (2007) CG dinucleotide clustering is a species-specific property of the genome. Nucleic Acids Res 35:6798–6807
8. Feng S, Cokus SJ, Zhang X, Chen PY, Bostick M et al (2010) Conservation and divergence of methylation patterning in plants and animals. Proc Natl Acad Sci U S A 107:8689–8694
9. Ross JP, Rand KN, Molloy PL (2010) Hypomethylation of repeated DNA sequences in cancer. Epigenomics 2:245–269
10. Sharma S, Kelly TK, Jones PA (2010) Epigenetics in cancer. Carcinogenesis 31: 27–36
11. Ibanez de Caceres I, Battagli C, Esteller M, Herman JG, Dulaimi E et al (2004) Tumor cell-specific *BRCA1* and *RASSF1A* hypermethylation in serum, plasma, and peritoneal fluid from ovarian cancer patients. Cancer Res 64:6476–6481
12. Murphy SK (2012) Targeting the epigenome in ovarian cancer. Future Oncol 8:151–164
13. Bondurant AE, Huang Z, Whitaker RS, Simel LR, Berchuck A et al (2011) Quantitative detection of *RASSF1A* DNA promoter methylation in tumors and serum of patients with serous epithelial ovarian cancer. Gynecol Oncol 123:581–587
14. Baldwin RL, Nemeth E, Tran H, Shvartsman H, Cass I et al (2000) *BRCA1* promoter region hypermethylation in ovarian carcinoma: a population-based study. Cancer Res 60: 5329–5333
15. Catteau A, Harris WH, Xu CF, Solomon E (1999) Methylation of the *BRCA1* promoter region in sporadic breast and ovarian cancer: correlation with disease characteristics. Oncogene 18:1957–1965
16. McCluskey LL, Chen C, Delgadillo E, Felix JC, Muderspach LI et al (1999) Differences in *p16* gene methylation and expression in benign and malignant ovarian tumors. Gynecol Oncol 72:87–92
17. Strathdee G, Appleton K, Illand M, Millan DW, Sargent J et al (2001) Primary ovarian carcinomas display multiple methylator phenotypes involving known tumor suppressor genes. Am J Pathol 158:1121–1127
18. Rathi A, Virmani AK, Schorge JO, Elias KJ, Maruyama R et al (2002) Methylation profiles of sporadic ovarian tumors and nonmalignant ovaries from high-risk women. Clin Cancer Res 8:3324–3331
19. Bianco T, Chenevix-Trench G, Walsh DC, Cooper JE, Dobrovic A (2000) Tumour-specific distribution of *BRCA1* promoter region methylation supports a pathogenetic role in breast and ovarian cancer. Carcinogenesis 21:147–151
20. Wiley A, Katsaros D, Fracchioli S, Yu H (2006) Methylation of the insulin-like growth factor binding protein-3 gene and prognosis of epithelial ovarian cancer. Int J Gynecol Cancer 16:210–218
21. Katsaros D, Cho W, Singal R, Fracchioli S, Rigault De La Longrais IA et al (2004) Methylation of tumor suppressor gene *p16* and prognosis of epithelial ovarian cancer. Gynecol Oncol 94:685–692
22. Wiley A, Katsaros D, Chen H, Rigault de la Longrais IA, Beeghly A et al (2006) Aberrant promoter methylation of multiple genes in malignant ovarian tumors and in ovarian tumors with low malignant potential. Cancer 107:299–308
23. Gifford G, Paul J, Vasey PA, Kaye SB, Brown R (2004) The acquisition of *hMLH1* methylation in plasma DNA after chemotherapy predicts poor survival for ovarian cancer patients. Clin Cancer Res 10:4420–4426
24. Turner N, Tutt A, Ashworth A (2004) Hallmarks of "BRCAness" in sporadic cancers. Nat Rev Cancer 4:814–819
25. Chaudhry P, Srinivasan R, Patel FD (2009) Utility of gene promoter methylation in prediction of response to platinum-based chemotherapy

in epithelial ovarian cancer (EOC). Cancer Invest 27:877–884

26. Warnecke PM, Stirzaker C, Song J, Grunau C, Melki JR et al (2002) Identification and resolution of artifacts in bisulfite sequencing. Methods 27:101–107
27. Thirlwell C, Eymard M, Feber A, Teschendorff A, Pearce K et al (2010) Genome-wide DNA methylation analysis of archival formalin-fixed paraffin-embedded tissue using the Illumina Infinium HumanMethylation27 BeadChip. Methods 52:248–254
28. Herman JG, Graff JR, Myohanen S, Nelkin BD, Baylin SB (1996) Methylation-specific PCR: a novel PCR assay for methylation status of CpG islands. Proc Natl Acad Sci U S A 93:9821–9826

Chapter 7

Methylation-Specific PCR

Zhiqing Huang, Christopher F. Bassil, and Susan K. Murphy

Abstract

Defining DNA methylation patterns in the genome has become essential for understanding diverse biological processes including the regulation of gene expression, imprinted genes, and X chromosome inactivation and how these patterns are deregulated in human diseases. Methylation-specific (MS)-PCR is a useful tool for qualitative DNA methylation analysis with multiple advantages, including ease of design and execution, sensitivity in the ability to detect small quantities of methylated DNA, and the ability to rapidly screen a large number of samples without the need for purchase of expensive laboratory equipment. This assay requires modification of the genomic DNA by sodium bisulfite and two independent primer sets for PCR amplification, one pair designed to recognize the methylated and the other pair the unmethylated versions of the bisulfite-modified sequence. The amplicons are visualized using ethidium bromide staining following agarose gel electrophoresis. Amplicons of the expected size produced from either primer pair are indicative of the presence of DNA in the original sample with the respective methylation status.

Key words DNA methylation, Polymerase chain reaction, Primer design, Annealing temperature, Gel electrophoresis

1 Introduction

Methylation-specific PCR (MS-PCR) as described herein is a qualitative technique used for detecting the presence of methylation in bisulfite-converted DNA [1]. The procedure relies on a standard PCR protocol modified to include two sets of methylation-specific primer pairs, which are designed to anneal to sequences containing CpG dinucleotides in the region to be analyzed (Fig. 1). Primers designed to detect methylated DNA (M primers) are designed under the assumption that the region will be fully methylated, and thus will contain cytosines in the sequence at CG dinucleotides. Conversely, the primers designed to detect unmethylated DNA (U primers) are designed assuming the region is unmethylated, and therefore will contain thymines rather than cytosines at CG dinucleotides. The annealing temperature for M primers will be higher than that for U primers, given their correspondence to the same genomic DNA sequence. This is due to the presence of

Anastasia Malek and Oleg Tchernitsa (eds.), *Ovarian Cancer: Methods and Protocols*, Methods in Molecular Biology, vol. 1049, DOI 10.1007/978-1-62703-547-7_7, © Springer Science+Business Media New York 2013

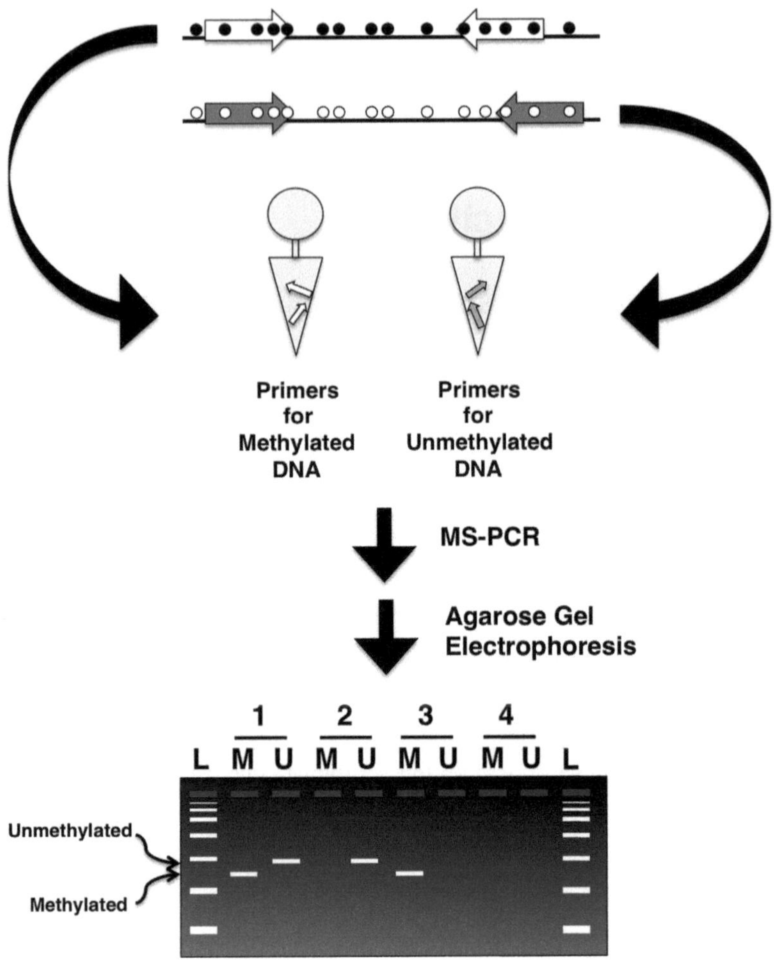

Fig. 1 Methylation-specific PCR. Methylation-specific PCR involves use of two sets of primer pairs that are designed to the methylated (methylated cytosines are represented by the *filled circles*) and unmethylated (*unfilled circles*) versions of the bisulfite-modified genomic DNA. It is helpful if the primers are designed such that there is a distinguishable size difference in the amplicons produced. Following PCR amplification, the amplicons are resolved by agarose gel electrophoresis. Hypothetical results are presented in the figure. Sample 1 shows amplicons for both the methylated (M) and unmethylated (U) primers sets; sample 2 contains only unmethylated DNA; sample 3 contains only methylated DNA; and sample 4 is a negative control. *L* DNA ladder

cytosines in the M primer sequence versus thymines in the U primer sequence for the same CG positions and the higher temperature required to melt C-G hydrogen bonds versus T-A hydrogen bonds in the DNA. The annealing temperature can usually be increased for the U primers to a level similar to that of the M primers by simply extending the number of bases at the 5′ end of the U primers.

The two primer sets are generally used to amplify template DNA in separate reactions, although with careful design and optimization, multiplexing the two primer sets in MS-PCR reactions is possible [2]. In this case, design the M and U primer pairs such that the amplicons produced are sufficiently divergent in size to enable clear separation upon agarose gel electrophoresis. This has the added benefit of enabling amplification from the same template and reaction mix. There are limitations to this approach, including that the sequences to which the primers anneal will be in different locations, which may not be homogeneous in methylation status, and there may be bias in amplification efficiency for one or the other amplification product (e.g., the shorter amplification product may be produced faster and thus will be at higher molarity than the longer product, all else being equal). PCR is followed by gel electrophoresis in which the presence of bands under UV transillumination following ethidium bromide staining qualitatively suggests either the presence or absence of methylation in the template DNA. Because MS-PCR as described here is nonquantitative, these results provide a "present-or-absent" insight into methylation.

Primer design for methylation analysis can be challenging because the sequence to be analyzed is often CG-dense and has reduced complexity after bisulfite modification due to conversion of non-CG cytosines to uracils. MethPrimer is a free online primer design tool specifically for methylation studies (available at http://www.urogene.org/methprimer) [3]. This software provides suggestions for design of primers for both MS-PCR and bisulfite sequencing. The selected genomic sequence can be input using a simple copy and paste function; the software then performs an in silico bisulfite conversion and provides suggestions for primer sequences and positioning. Parameter settings include the target size, regions to exclude, number of primer pairs to be output, the product size, primer Tm, primer length, number of CGs to include in the primers, and number of non-CG cytosines to include in the primers as well as the maximum Tm difference for MS-PCR primers.

MS-PCR is a simple, sensitive, and specific method for detecting the methylation status of virtually any genomic region. Although numerous techniques for study of DNA methylation have been developed, MS-PCR remains a useful approach widely used for DNA methylation analysis. In addition to the ability of MS-PCR to detect aberrant methylation of genes in cancer, MS-PCR is also used to assess DNA methylation relevant to other biological processes, such as genomic imprinting and X chromosome inactivation. However, the nonquantitative "methylation-present-or-absent" results obtained from MS-PCR reactions can be a disadvantage, as can the potential for false positive results. Appropriately designed primers, optimization of PCR reactions, and inclusion of appropriate control reactions can improve the quality of the analysis.

This chapter describing the MS-PCR technique is divided into subsections that explain preparing and running the PCR reactions, agarose gel electrophoresis and interpreting results.

2 Materials

2.1 Kits

1. EpiTect Unmethylated and Methylated Bisulfite-Converted Controls (Qiagen, Valencia, USA).
2. HotStarTaq Polymerase Kit (Qiagen, Valencia, USA): DNA polymerase, 10× PCR buffer, 25 mM $MgCl_2$.

2.2 Reagents and Supplies

Prepare all solutions using nuclease-free water. Unless otherwise indicated, store reagents at room temperature.

1. Bisulfite-converted DNA (20 ng/μl). The bisulfite-converted DNA is stable for up to 6 months at −80°C, up to 3 months at −20 °C, and for 1–2 weeks at 4°C. Avoid freeze-thaws.
2. Primers specific to bisulfite-modified, methylated DNA.
3. Primers specific to bisulfite-modified, unmethylated DNA.
4. 100 mM dNTP set, PCR grade (Invitrogen, Carlsbad, USA). dNTPs should be stored at −20 °C in 10–20 μl aliquots. Dilute to 10 mM with nuclease-free water before use.
5. Tris–Borate–EDTA buffer (TBE): 0.089 M Tris-base, 0.089 M boric acid, 0.002 M EDTA, pH 8.3.
6. Parafilm® M Barrier Film (SPI Supplies, West Chester, USA).
7. Ethidium bromide in dropper bottle (0.625 mg/ml) (Genesee Scientific, Research Triangle Park, USA).
8. 10× Orange G gel loading buffer. Dissolve 15 ml of glycerol and 100 mg of Orange G powder in water up to final volume 50 ml, vortex to mix. Store at 4 °C.
9. 50 bp DNA Ladder, 1,000 μg/ml (New England Biolabs, Ipswich, USA). Prior to use, dilute 20 μl DNA Ladder into 160 μl nuclease-free water. Add 20 μl Orange G Gel Loading Buffer. Store at 4 °C.
10. GenePure LE Quick Dissolve Agarose (ISC BioExpress, Kaysville, USA).

2.3 Equipment

1. Thermocycler.
2. Gel casting tray and running box.
3. Power supply.
4. UV Transilluminator.

3 Methods

3.1 Polymerase Chain Reaction

1. Prepare the PCR Master Mix with the primer sets specific to the methylated and unmethylated bisulfite-modified DNAs. An example for a 25 μl PCR reaction using the Qiagen HotStarTaq PCR kit is shown below (*see* **Notes 1** and **2**):

Stock	Reaction mix volumes (μl)	Final concentration
10× PCR buffer	2.5	1×
25 mM $MgCl_2$	1.5	1.5 mM
dNTP mix (10 mM each)	0.5	0.2 mM each
M forward primer	1	100–500 nM
M reverse primer	1	100–500 nM
U forward primer	1	100–500 nM
U reverse primer	1	100–500 nM
HotStarTaq DNA polymerase	0.2	2.0–2.5 U
DNA (to be added last)	1	10–50 ng
Nuclease-free water	17.3	
Total volume	25	

2. Thoroughly mix the PCR Master Mix by vortexing for several seconds. Spin down briefly to insure liquid is collected at the bottom of the tube.
3. Transfer the appropriate amount of PCR Master Mix (25 μl minus the volume of DNA to be added) to reaction wells (*see* **Note 3**).
4. Add template DNA to Master Mix in reaction wells.
5. Seal the reaction wells. Mix the PCR mixture by vortexing for several seconds. Spin down briefly.
6. Transfer reaction wells containing PCR mixture to a thermocycler. Perform PCR as follows: initialization step 95 °C/15′, then cycling by denaturation step 94 °C/30″, annealing step *X*°C/30″ (*see* **Note 1**), and extension step 72 °C/30″, for 25–35 cycles followed by extension at 72 °C for 10′. The samples can be analyzed immediately or can be stored at −20 °C prior to use.

3.2 Gel Electrophoresis

1. For an 8 × 10 cm, 2 % agarose gel, add 50 ml of 1× TBE Buffer to 1.0 g of agarose in a glass beaker (*see* **Note 4**). Swirl gently to mix.

2. Microwave the buffer/gel mixture until the agarose is fully dissolved (usually 1–2 min). Watch closely, as it may be necessary to pause the microwave occasionally for a few seconds to avoid having the mixture boil over.
3. In a fume hood, add one drop of ethidium bromide solution (*see* **Note 5**) to the molten agarose mixture (final concentration 0.5 μg/ml) and swirl gently until fully mixed.
4. Still in the fume hood, carefully pour molten agarose into a gel casting tray with barrier ends and comb(s) in place. Let solidify for 15–20 min.
5. Remove the end barriers from the gel. Fill the gel box with 1× TBE buffer so that the surface of the gel is just submerged in the buffer solution. Carefully remove the comb(s) using a very gentle rocking motion while constantly applying slight upward pressure.
6. Add 10 μl of prepared 50 bp DNA ladder to the desired marker lane(s) for each row of samples to be run.
7. For each of the samples that will be run on the gel, pipet 1 μl of Orange G Gel Loading Buffer onto a short strip of Parafilm® M Barrier Film. The liquid will bead up on the film, making it easy to pipet. Carefully pipet 10 μl of the PCR product onto one of the Orange G drops, pipet up and down to mix, and then slowly load the sample into the corresponding well of the gel, making sure to keep the pipet tip within the well while slowly dispensing the sample so that any runover of sample into adjacent wells is prevented. Repeat for the remaining samples.
8. Run gel at an appropriate voltage for the desired time (*see* **Note 6**).

3.3 Interpreting Results

1. After the gel has finished its run, and using gloved hands, pour the 1× TBE gel running buffer into the sink.
2. Carefully remove the gel from the gel box and place onto the UV transilluminator (*see* **Note 7**).
3. Turn on the UV light. PCR amplicons are visible on the gel due to intercalation of the ethidium bromide into the double-stranded DNA, which causes fluorescence. There should not be any visible bands in the no template controls. If there are bands present in these lanes of the anticipated size, then there is contamination and the reactions must be redone to determine the source of the contamination. The positive control methylated DNA should show an appropriately sized amplicon for the M primer set only, while the positive control unmethylated DNA should show an appropriately sized amplicon for only the U primer set (*see* **Notes 8** and **9**).
4. Dispose of the gel, which contains ethidium bromide, according to relevant guidelines.

4 Notes

1. Optimal reaction conditions (incubation times and temperatures, concentrations of primers, $MgCl_2$, and template DNA) vary and need to be optimized. The primer annealing temperatures are a good point at which to start when optimizing the PCR reactions, using the lowest annealing temperature for the primer sets. Every effort should be made to try and choose primers with similar annealing temperatures to avoid bias in performance during the PCR reactions.
2. High-performance liquid chromatography (HPLC) purification of the primers helps to assure that the primers are full length, thus improving the specificity of the primers for the intended target sequence.
3. The template DNA required varies and should be optimized. We typically elute 800 ng of bisulfite-converted DNA with 40 μl of elution buffer (with the concentration of bisulfite-converted DNA at about 20 ng/μl, assuming that all DNA was recovered after the bisulfite modification process) and use 1–3 μl (20–60 ng of input DNA) in each 25 μl PCR reaction.
4. The concentration of TBE used to prepare the gel must match that used as running buffer. If the gel is prepared with 1× TBE, it must be run in 1× TBE running buffer.
5. Ethidium bromide intercalates double-stranded DNA and is therefore a suspected mutagen. However, it is not considered hazardous waste at low concentrations. Guidelines for disposal vary. Those relevant to your institution or place of employment should be followed.
6. The timing of the run and power used will vary depending on the size of the gel, the percentage of agarose used to prepare the gel, and the distance required for the amplicons to be resolved by migration through the gel.
7. Protect your eyes and skin from UV exposure by wearing an appropriate UV protective face shield, long-sleeved lab coat, and gloves.
8. We usually include 3–4 CG sites in primer sequences. CG sites in primers work best to increase specificity of primer binding to the appropriate template when they are located as close as possible to the 3′ end for both M (CG) and U (TG) primers.
9. We recommend inclusion of as many non-CG cytosines as possible within primer binding sequences to increase specificity for the completely modified DNA.

Acknowledgments

We gratefully acknowledge Zack Davenport for his contributions to the artwork. We thank Allison Barratt and Carole Grenier for critical reading of the manuscript. This work was supported by Department of Defense grant W81XWH-11-1-0469, NIH grants R01DK085173 and R01CA142983, and the Gail Parkins Ovarian Cancer Awareness Fund.

References

1. Herman JG et al (1996) Methylation-specific PCR: a novel PCR assay for methylation status of CpG islands. Proc Natl Acad Sci USA 93: 9821–9826
2. Murphy SK et al (2003) Epigenetic detection of human chromosome 14 uniparental disomy. Hum Mutat 22:92–97
3. Li LC, Dahiya R (2002) MethPrimer: designing primers for methylation PCRs. Bioinformatics 18:1427–1431

Chapter 8

Bisulfite Sequencing of Cloned Alleles

Zhiqing Huang, Christopher F. Bassil, and Susan K. Murphy

Abstract

Bisulfite sequencing of cloned alleles is a widely used method for capturing the methylation profiles of single alleles. This method combines PCR amplification of the bisulfite-modified DNA with the subcloning of the amplicons into plasmids followed by transformation into bacteria and plating on selective media. The resulting colony forming units are each comprised of bacterial clones containing the same plasmid reflecting a single allele in the original PCR reaction. Following whole cell PCR and sequencing, the results provide highly detailed information about the status of each CG site within an allele. Sequencing of a large number of individual clones can provide quantitative information, assuming unbiased PCR, subcloning and clone selection. The proportion of methylated cytosine at a particular position within the sequenced alleles can be determined by counting the number of alleles showing methylation at the position of interest and dividing this by the total number of clones sequenced.

Key words DNA methylation, Sodium bisulfite, Cloning, Capillary sequencing

1 Introduction

The cloning and sequencing of bisulfite converted DNA is one of the gold standards of DNA methylation analysis, as the sequencing of subcloned individual DNA molecules provides detailed information on the methylation status of every CG site within a given allele for relatively long stretches of DNA sequence [1–3]. The genomic DNA is first modified by sodium bisulfite. The DNA sequence under investigation is amplified by PCR with primers specific for one strand of the bisulfite converted DNA. The amplified PCR product comprises a pool of DNA molecules representing the individual alleles present within the DNA specimen used for PCR. A portion of the PCR product is subcloned into plasmids and randomly selected clones are sequenced to provide the methylation status of the CG sites within each of the individual DNA molecules. Methylation percentages for each of the CG sites are often calculated according to the number of methylated and unmethylated CG cytosines at a given position across the different clones

Anastasia Malek and Oleg Tchernitsa (eds.), *Ovarian Cancer: Methods and Protocols*, Methods in Molecular Biology, vol. 1049, DOI 10.1007/978-1-62703-547-7_8, © Springer Science+Business Media New York 2013

that are sequenced. Accuracy increases with the number of clones sequenced.

Relative to direct sequencing of a PCR amplicon pool generated from a bisulfite-modified genomic DNA template, sequencing of clones provides a higher resolution result due to the ability to score methylation for single alleles. The sequence data is semi-quantitative and can reveal variable patterns of methylation within a specimen. However, the procedure can be labor intensive. In addition, PCR bias and/or cloning bias may contribute to skewing of results when attempting to quantify methylation [4].

We begin with important considerations for primer design. Subheading 3 is divided into subsections that describe PCR amplification and purification, ligation, transformation and screening, sequencing of the cloned alleles and basic interpretation of results.

To avoid preferential amplification of methylated versus umethylated DNA, the primers for bisulfite sequencing must be designed to anneal to regions devoid of CG dinucleotides. In addition, when selecting primers, a database with information about the presence of polymorphisms (GeneCards, dbSNP, SNP500, SNPbrowser) should be consulted to avoid designing primers that anneal to potential polymorphic sites. Primers for bisulfite sequencing have only three bases and are T-rich due to conversion of non-CG cytosines. This often requires that the primers be greater than 30 bases in length to obtain primer melting temperatures of ~60 °C.

Primer annealing sites can be difficult to identify due to limited availability of regions of sufficient length within an otherwise CG-rich stretch of sequence without inclusion of one or more potentially methylated CG dinucleotide(s). If there are no suitable regions for primer design, the antisense strand derived from the reverse complement of the original input genomic DNA sequence may offer a suitable alternative. The complementary nature of the sense and antisense strands is eliminated following bisulfite modification. However, the same number of CGs and their methylation state (due to the palindromic nature of the methylation status of CG sequence motifs) will be present in both the sense and antisense strands and thus either strand can be used to define the methylation profile of a particular region.

Controls (e.g., no template and unmodified genomic DNA) should be included when running the PCR reactions to insure that there is no contamination and that the amplification is specific to the bisulfite converted DNA.

Bisulfite sequencing is still widely used in research labs, largely because it is straightforward, the primer design is relatively simple, and it provides highly detailed methylation information for the region of interest without the need for specialized instrumentation. This technique is especially useful for studies in which the particular pattern of methylation is of interest, such as studies of site-specific methylation, or for study of allele-specific methylation as is characteristic of the methylation patterns at the regulatory regions associated with genomically imprinted genes, or genes subject to X chromosome inactivation. Limitations of this technique include that it can be time-consuming and expensive depending on the desired number of clones to be sequenced and the number of specimens to analyze. In addition, the accuracy of results obtained can be adversely affected by bias in PCR amplification efficiency and bias in subcloning for alleles of a particular methylation status. Long stretches of thymine nucleotides that are common in bisulfite-modified DNA can also cause problems with the accuracy of the sequencing [5]. Nevertheless, this is the only available technique aside from high throughput bisulfite sequencing approaches that provides allele-specific methylation status at single nucleotide resolution, and thus promises to be a mainstay for analysis of DNA methylation.

2 Materials

2.1 Kits

1. HotStarTaq Polymerase kit (Qiagen, Valencia, USA) or Platinum Taq PCR kit (Invitrogen, Grand Island, USA), containing 10× PCR buffer, 25 mM $MgCl_2$ stock, DNA polymerase and nuclease-free water.
2. Qiagen MinElute PCR Purification kit (Qiagen, Valencia, USA).
3. BigDye® Terminator v3.1 Cycle Sequencing Kit (Applied Biosystems, Foster City, USA).
4. pGEM®-T Easy Vector System II (containing JM109 competent cells) (Promega, Madison, USA).
5. Epitect Unmethylated and Methylated Bisulfite Converted Controls (Qiagen, Valencia, USA).

2.2 Reagent and Supplies

1. Bisulfite converted DNA (20 ng/μl). The bisulfite converted DNA is stable for up to 6 months at −80 °C, up to 3 months at −20 °C and for 1–2 weeks at 4 °C. Avoid freeze-thaws.
2. Forward and revers primers for PCR amplification of target sequence (*see* **Note 1**).
3. T7 and SP6 primers for whole cell PCR amplification.
4. 100 mM dNTP set, PCR grade (Invitrogen, Carlsbad, USA). dNTPs should be stored at −20 °C in 10–20 μl aliquots. Dilute to 10 mM with Nuclease-free water before use.
5. GenePure LE Quick Dissolve Agarose (ISC BioExpress, Kaysville, USA).
6. Parafilm® M Barrier Film (SPI Supplies, West Chester, USA).
7. Ethidium bromide in dropper bottle (0.625 mg/mL) (Genesee Scientific, Research Triangle Park, USA).

8. Sigma GenElute spin columns (Sigma-Aldrich Corp. St. Louis, USA).
9. Phenol:Chloroform:Isoamyl Alcohol solution 25:24:1, Store at 4 °C.
10. 3 M sodium acetate (pH 5.5) (Ambion by Life Technologies, Grand Island, USA).
11. Tris-Borate-EDTA buffer (TBE): 0.089 M Tris-base, 0.089 M Boric acid, 0.002 M EDTA, pH 8.3.
12. 10× OrangeG Gel Loading Buffer. Dissolve 15 mL of glycerol and 100 mg of Orange G powder in water up to final volume 50 mL, vortex to mix. Store at 4 °C.
13. 50 bp DNA Ladder, 1,000 μg/mL (New England Biolabs, Ipswich, USA). Prior to use, add 20 μL ladder to 160 μL nuclease-free water. Add 20 μL OrangeG Gel Loading Buffer. Store at 4 °C.
14. LB agar with 100 μg/mL ampicillin and 60 μg/mL X-gal (Teknova Science Matters, Hollister, USA). Store at 4 °C and protect from light.
15. SOC medium (Sigma-Aldrich Corp. St. Louis, USA). Store at 4°C.

2.3 Equipment

1. Thermocycler.
2. Gel casting tray and gel running boxes for 8 × 10 cm gels.
3. Power supply.
4. UV transilluminator.
5. High throughput capillary sequencer (e.g., Applied Biosytems 3730 xl) and associated software.

3 Methods

3.1 PCR and PCR Products Purification

This protocol is based on using the pGEM®-T Easy Vector System II, HotStarTaq PCR kit and the Qiagen MinElute PCR Purification kit. Use of any other reagents will require optimization.

3.1.1 PCR

Amplify bisulfite-modified genomic DNA (20–50 ng) using the HotStarTaq PCR kit and primers specific to the bisulfite-modified DNA according to the manufacturer's protocol.

1. Prepare the PCR Master Mix. An example for a 25 μL PCR reaction using the Qiagen HotStar Taq PCR kit is shown in Table 1 (*see* **Note 2**):
2. Thoroughly mix the PCR Master Mix by vortexing for several seconds. Spin down briefly to insure liquid is collected at the bottom of the tube.

Table 1
PCR master mix

Stock	Reaction mix volumes (μL)	Final concentration
10× PCR Buffer	2.5	1×
25 mM $MgCl_2$	1.5	1.5 mM
dNTPs (10 mM each)	0.5	0.2 mM each
Forward primer	1	100–500 nM
Reverse primer	1	100–500 nM
HotStarTaq DNA polymerase	0.2	2.0–2.5 U
DNA (to be added last)	1	10–50 ng
Nuclease-free water	17.3	
Total volume	25	

3. Transfer the appropriate amount of PCR Master Mix (25 μl minus the volume of DNA to be added) to reaction wells (*see* **Note 3**).
4. Add template DNA to Master Mix in reaction wells (*see* **Note 4**).
5. Seal the reaction wells. Mix the PCR mixture by vortexing for several seconds. Spin down briefly.
6. Transfer reaction wells containing PCR mixture to a thermocycler. Perform PCR as follows: Initialization step 95°C/15′, then cycling by denaturation step 94°C/30″, annealing step *X*°C/30″ (*see* **Note 5**), extension step 72°C/30″, for 25–35 cycles followed by extension at 72°C for 10′. The samples can be analyzed immediately or can be stored at −20°C prior to use.

3.1.2 Gel Electrophoresis

1. For an 8 × 10 cm, 2% agarose gel, add 50 mL of 1× TBE Buffer to 1.0 g of agarose in a glass beaker (*see* **Note 6**). Swirl gently to mix.
2. Microwave the buffer/gel mixture until the agarose is fully dissolved (usually 1–2 min). Watch closely, as it may be necessary to pause the microwave occasionally for a few seconds to avoid having the mixture boil over.
3. In a fume hood, add one drop of ethidium bromide solution (*see* **Note 7**) to the molten agarose mixture (final concentration 0.5 μg/mL) and swirl gently until fully mixed.
4. Still in the fume hood, carefully pour molten agarose into a gel casting tray with barrier ends and comb(s) in place. Let solidify for 15–20 min.

5. Remove the end barriers from the gel. Fill the gel box with 1× TBE buffer so that the surface of the gel is just submerged in the buffer solution. Carefully remove the comb(s) using a very gentle rocking motion while constantly applying slight upward pressure.
6. Add 10 μL of prepared 50 bp DNA ladder to the desired marker lane(s) for each row of samples to be run.
7. For each of the samples that will be run on the gel, pipet 1 μL of Orange G Gel Loading Buffer onto a short strip of Parafilm® M Barrier Film. The liquid will bead up on the film, making it easy to pipet. Carefully pipet 10 μL of the PCR product onto one of the Orange G drops, pipet up and down to mix, then slowly load the sample into the corresponding well of the gel, making sure to keep the pipet tip within the well while slowly dispensing the sample so that any run over of sample into adjacent wells is prevented. Repeat for the remaining samples.
8. Run gel at an appropriate voltage for the desired time (*see* **Note 8**).

3.1.3 Purification of PCR Products

1. Resolve PCR amplicons on a 2% agarose gel stained with ethidium bromide, as described above (*see* **Note 9**).
2. Excise the band containing the amplicon of interest from the gel (*see* **Note 10**), place the excised gel fragment into a GenElute spin column placed in one of the provided microcentrifuge tubes.
3. Spin in a balanced microcentrifuge at full speed for 15 min. Agarose will be retained on the filter in the spin column while the DNA will pass through the filter with the gel buffer and collect in the microcentrifuge tube. Discard the spin column.
4. Purify the eluted DNA using a standard phenol:chloroform: isoamyl alcohol extraction protocol followed by ethanol precipitation. Briefly, add an equal volume of phenol: chloroform:isoamyl alcohol solution to the DNA from **step 3** under Subheading 3.1.3, Vortex for 10 s followed by centrifugation for 15 min at full speed. Transfer the top (aqueous) layer into a clean tube. Add 1/10 volume 3 M sodium acetate (pH 5.5) and 2.5 volumes of absolute ethanol. Mix by briefly vortexing. Centrifuge for 30 min at full speed at 4°C. Carefully aspirate the ethanol and allow the DNA pellet to air dry. Resuspend the DNA in 10 μl of nuclease-free water.

3.2 Ligation, Transformation and Screening

The presented ligation and cloning protocols are adopted for the pGEM®-T Easy Vector System II, while whole-cell PCR is performed using the Platinum Taq PCR kit. Use of any other reagents will require optimization.

1. Ligate the purified PCR amplicons (1–3 μl) into pGEM®-T Easy plasmids, following the protocol from the manufacturer.
2. Allow the ligation to proceed for 8 h at 16-18°C, or overnight at 4°C.
3. Place 5–10 μl of each ligation reaction into a sterile 1.5 mL microcentrifuge tube on ice.
4. Remove the frozen JM109 High Efficiency Competent Cells from −80°C storage and place in an ice bath until just thawed (about 5 min). Mix the cells by gently flicking the tube.
5. Carefully transfer 50 μl of cells into each tube containing the ligation reaction. Gently flick the tubes to mix and place them on ice for 30 min.
6. Heat-shock the cells for 45–50 s (up to 2 min) in a water bath or heating block at exactly 42°C (do not shake).
7. Immediately return the tubes to ice for 2 min.
8. Add 1,000 μl room temperature SOC medium to the tubes containing the cells transformed with the ligation reactions (*see* **Note 11**)
9. Incubate for 1 h at 37°C with shaking (~150 rpm).
10. Using sterile technique, spread 100–500 μl of each transformation mixture onto LB/ampicillin/X-Gal plates (*see* **Note 12**).
11. Incubate the plates overnight (16–24 h) at 37°C. White colonies generally contain inserts.
12. Prepare reaction mix for appropriate number of PCRs using the Platinum Taq PCR kit according to the manufacturer's instructions.
13. Use whole-cell PCR to amplify the inserted DNA sequence within the plasmids from individual colonies with SP6 and T7 primers (binding sites for these primers are present within the plasmid, flanking the insertion site). The colonies can be picked from the plate using a sterile P-10 pipet tip and immediately transferred into the PCR reaction mix (*see* **Note 13**). Rotate the pipet tip within and against the sides of the reaction well while the tip is submerged in the liquid to transfer as many of the bacterial cells as possible into the PCR reaction mix. Pipet up and down to mix.
14. Perform PCR as follows: Initialization at 94°C for 5′, then 35 cycles of denaturation (94°C/30″), annealing (55°C/30″) and extension (72°C/30-45″), followed by a final extension at 72°C for 5′. Please see comments regarding PCR conditions in **Notes 14** and **15**.
15. Resolve amplicons on 2% agarose gels.
16. Calculate the expected size of the amplicons, including the relevant portions of the plasmid backbone (i.e., all of the T7

Table 2
Sequencing reaction mix (BigDye® Terminator v3.1 Cycle Sequencing Kit)

Stock	Reaction volumes, each
5× BigDye sequencing buffer	2 μL
Primer (10 μM)	1 μL
BigDye Terminator v3.1	1 μL
Eluted PCR amplicons	1–2 μL
Nuclease free water	x
Total volume	10 μL

primer binding site to the insertion site, the insert itself, and other side of the insertion site through the SP6 primer binding site).

17. Purify individual amplicons of the anticipated size using Sigma GenElute spin columns as described above, **Steps 2** and **3** of Subsection 3.1.3.

3.3 Sequencing of Cloned Alleles

The eluted amplicons are directly sequenced using the BigDye® Terminator v3.1 Cycle Sequencing Kit from Applied Biosystems that utilizes the process of "dye terminator sequencing". The forward or reverse PCR primer used to amplify the region of interest (from Section 3.1.1 above) can generally be used for the sequencing reaction. The reactions are run using a capillary sequencing instrument, such as an ABI-3730xl-DNA-Analyzer. Results can be visualized with 4Peaks software (freeware from mekentosj.com) or Finch TV (free for download from PerkinElmer).

1. Prepare sequencing reaction mix according to the supplier's protocol. An example of preparing the reaction mix using the BigDye® Terminator v3.1 Cycle Sequencing Kit is shown in Table 2.
2. Amplify according to the manufacturer's recommendations: Initialization step 96°C/2′, then cycling by denaturation step 96°C/30″, annealing step 50°C/15″, extension step 62°C/240″, for 25–35 cycles.
3. Sequencing is performed in accordance with protocols provided by the equipment supplier.

3.4 Interpreting Results

The sequence obtained for each cloned allele should be inspected to insure that the sequence is clean and specific to the region of interest (*see* **Note 16**). Each clone showing good quality sequence can then be scored for methylation status at each individual CG dinucleotide. Using this technique, methylation status within a clone at a given CG position is a binary variable. Each CG cytosine is either methylated or unmethylated within the given allele.

The combined methylation status for each clone by CG site can be assembled and represented as shown in Fig. 1, where each row corresponds to one of the individual cloned alleles, and each column represents an individual CG site. Typically in such a

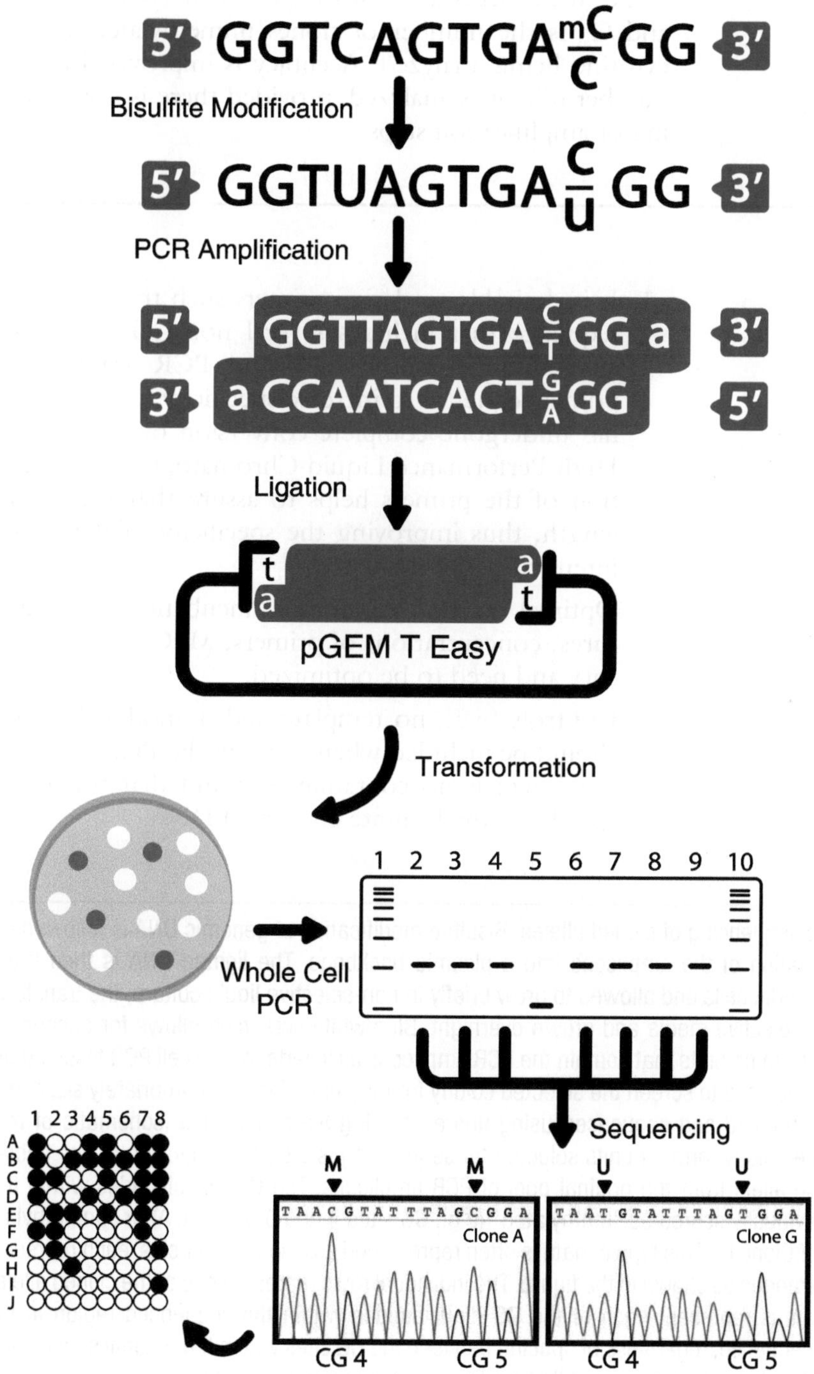

Fig. 1 (continued)

lollipop-style map, filled symbols are indicative of a methylated cytosine while unfilled symbols represent unmethylated cytosines. The methylation status of CG cytosines at a given position within the sequence, given as percent methylation, can be calculated as follows: $\%M = [C^M/(C^M + C^U)] \times 100$, where C^M is the number of clones with methylation at the particular cytosine being analyzed, and C^U is the number of clones unmethylated at the particular cytosine being analyzed. Accuracy is improved by increasing the number of clones analyzed, provided there is not bias in the cloning or amplification steps.

4 Notes

1. It is desirable to design primers such that they will anneal to sequence that includes several non-CG cytosines (thymines after bisulfite modification and PCR amplification) in the primer sequence to increase specificity for genomic DNA that has undergone complete conversion by the sodium bisulfite. High Performance Liquid Chromatography (HPLC) purification of the primers helps to assure that the primers are full length, thus improving the specificity of the primers for the intended target sequence.
2. Optimal reaction conditions (incubation times and temperatures, concentrations of primers, $MgCl_2$, and template DNA) vary and need to be optimized.
3. Controls (e.g., no template and unmodified genomic DNA) should be included when running the PCR reactions to insure that there is no contamination and that the amplification is specific to the bisulfite converted DNA.

Fig. 1 Bisulfite sequencing of cloned alleles. Bisulfite modification of genomic DNA is followed by PCR amplification and ligation of the amplicons into a plasmid backbone. The ligated DNA is then transformed into competent bacterial cells and allowed to grow briefly in non-selective liquid culture; the transformed cells are then plated to selective media and grown overnight. Blue/white screening allows for enhanced selection of (white) colony forming units that contain the PCR amplicons as inserts. Whole cell PCR followed by agarose gel electrophoresis is used to screen the selected colony forming units for the appropriately sized inserts. Positive amplicons are purified and sequenced using fluorescent BigDye sequencing (schematic of results shown). Each one of the colony forming units selected for sequencing is a clonal expansion of one bacterial cell containing a single allele from the original pool of PCR amplicons. The CG dinculeotides within the sequenced region are individually scored as "methylated" (e.g., CG sites 4 and 5 of Clone A) or "unmethylated" (e.g., CG sites 4 and 5 of Clone G). This type of data is often represented as a series of circles, each representing a single CG site, and arranged as shown in the figure. The individual rows represent one of the cloned alleles sequenced while the columns represent each of the CG dinucleotides within the sequenced region in the order they appear in the sequence, regardless of spacing between the CG sites within the original sequence. Filled circles represent methylated CG sites and unfilled circles represent unmethylated CG sites

4. The template DNA required varies and should be optimized. We typically elute 800 ng of bisulfite converted DNA with 40 μL of elution buffer (with the concentration of bisulfite converted DNA at about 20 ng/μL, assuming that all DNA was recovered after the bisulfite modification process) and use 1–3 μL (20–60 ng of input DNA) in each 25 μL PCR reaction.
5. The primer annealing temperatures are a good point at which to start when optimizing the PCR reactions, using the lowest annealing temperature for the primers used. Every effort should be made to try and choose primers with similar annealing temperatures to avoid bias in performance during the PCR reactions.
6. The concentration of TBE used to prepare the gel must match that used as running buffer. If the gel is prepared with 1X TBE, it must be run in 1X TBE running buffer.
7. Ethidium bromide intercalates double stranded DNA and is therefore a suspected mutagen. However, it is not considered hazardous waste at low concentrations. Guidelines for disposal vary. Those relevant to your institution or place of employment should be followed.
8. The timing of the run and power used will vary depending on the size of the gel, the percentage of agarose used to prepare the gel and the distance required for the amplicons to be resolved by migration through the gel.
9. Strong and specific PCR amplicons should be obtained from the bisulfite-modified genomic DNA in order to ensure cloning and sequencing success.
10. Protect your eyes and skin from UV exposure by wearing an appropriate UV protective face shield, long sleeved lab coat and gloves.
11. LB broth may be substituted, but colony number may be lower.
12. High colony density may make selecting individual CFUs difficult; it is better to have fewer CFUs such that each colony represents a clonal expansion of a single bacterial cell.
13. Usually a minimum of 10–20 white colony forming units (CFUs) are selected for analysis.
14. Denaturation at 96°C for 5 min before PCR thermocycling is necessary when performing whole cell PCR to facilitate release of plasmid DNA from the bacterial cells.
15. The extension time for the PCR reaction is size dependent. We typically use 30 s for an amplicon size less than 500 bp and 45 s for amplicons longer than 500 bp.

16. High quality sequence data from BigDye® sequencing typically begins approximately 50–60 bases from the 3′-end of the sequencing primer. The positioning of the sequencing primer should therefore be taken into account with regard to the sequence information desired.

Acknowledgments

We gratefully acknowledge Zack Davenport for his contributions to the artwork. We thank Allison Barratt and Carole Grenier for critical reading of the manuscript. This work was supported by Department of Defense grant W81XWH-11-1-0469, NIH grants R01DK085173 and R01CA142983 and the Gail Parkins Ovarian Cancer Awareness Fund.

References

1. Frommer M, McDonald LE, Millar DS, Collis CM, Watt F et al (1992) A genomic sequencing protocol that yields a positive display of 5-methylcytosine residues in individual DNA strands. Proc Natl Acad Sci USA 89:1827–1831
2. Clark SJ, Harrison J, Paul CL, Frommer M (1994) High sensitivity mapping of methylated cytosines. Nucleic Acids Res 22:2990–2997
3. Feil R, Charlton J, Bird AP, Walter J, Reik W (1994) Methylation analysis on individual chromosomes: improved protocol for bisulphite genomic sequencing. Nucleic Acids Res 22: 695–696
4. Warnecke PM, Stirzaker C, Song J, Grunau C, Melki JR et al (2002) Identification and resolution of artifacts in bisulfite sequencing. Methods 27:101–107
5. Kristensen LS, Hansen LL (2009) PCR-based methods for detecting single-locus DNA methylation biomarkers in cancer diagnostics, prognostics, and response to treatment. Clin Chem 55:1471–1483

Chapter 9

Bisulfite Pyrosequencing

Christopher F. Bassil, Zhiqing Huang, and Susan K. Murphy

Abstract

Bisulfite pyrosequencing is a sequencing-by-synthesis method used to quantitatively determine the methylation of individual CG cytosines from PCR amplicons of a region up to 115 bases in length. The procedure relies on prior bisulfite conversion of all potentially methylated CG cytosines to either cytosine (methylated) or thymine (unmethylated) and involves the stepwise incorporation of deoxynucleotide triphosphates into the growing strand of nascent DNA. The incorporation of these dNTPs results in the proportional release of pyrophosphate, which is converted into ATP to aid in a subsequent conversion of luciferin to oxyluciferin. The amount of light released in the process is proportional to the number of nucleotides incorporated, and the procedure provides a quantitative portrait of the methylation profile for the amplicon in question.

Key words PCR, Pyrosequencing, Sequencing-by-synthesis, Methylation, Epigenetics

1 Introduction

Pyrosequencing is a sequencing-by-synthesis method used to quantitatively determine the methylation of individual CG cytosines from PCR amplicons produced using a bisulfite-modified DNA template. The pyrosequencing approach involves isolating the template strand from its complementary strand following PCR amplification, accomplished as a result of incorporation of biotin at the 5′ end of the primer used to initiate amplification of the particular strand destined to undergo pyrosequencing. Following PCR amplification, the biotin-labeled double-stranded PCR amplicon is bound to streptavidin beads that are then immobilized on vacuum filtration tips that allow for removal of the complementary (non-biotin containing) strand through denaturation and purification. The single-stranded DNA is then annealed to a sequencing primer and undergoes pyrosequencing, allowing for the incorporation of deoxynucleotide triphosphates (dNTPs), one at a time, in a template-dependent, stepwise fashion.

Anastasia Malek and Oleg Tchernitsa (eds.), *Ovarian Cancer: Methods and Protocols*, Methods in Molecular Biology, vol. 1049, DOI 10.1007/978-1-62703-547-7_9, © Springer Science+Business Media New York 2013

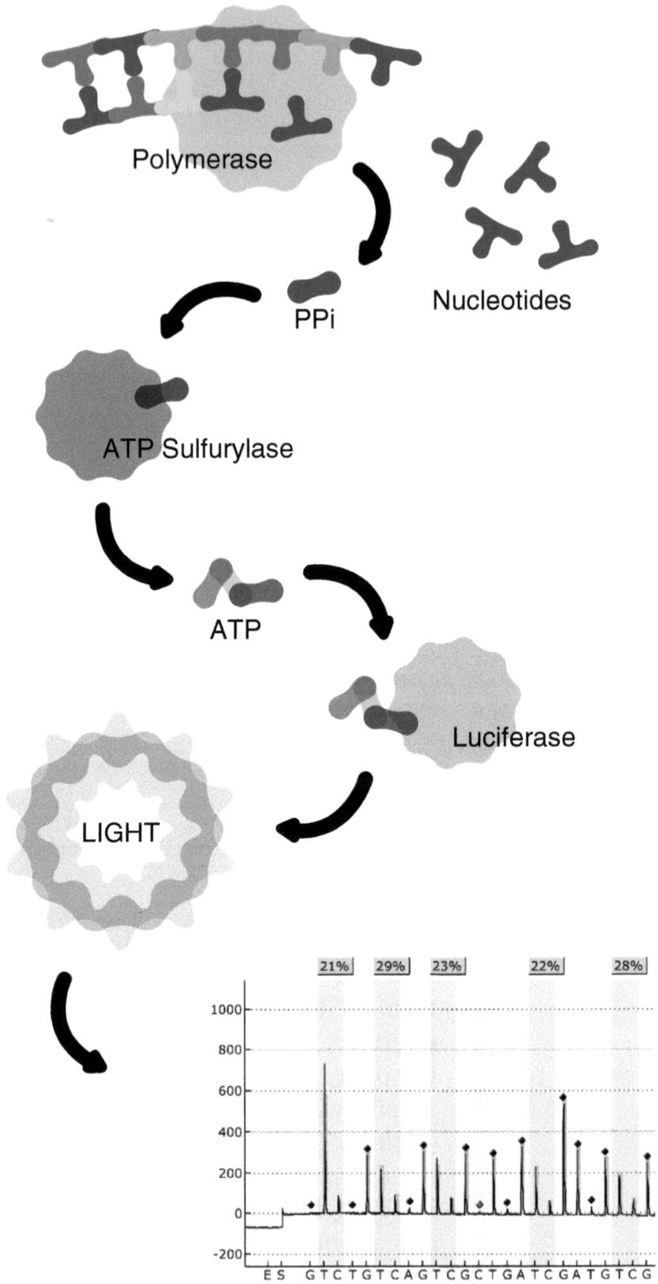

Fig. 1 Bisulfite pyrosequencing. The pyrosequencing reaction uses a single-stranded, biotin-labeled template and involves the addition of a single nucleotide at a time into the reaction mix. Following incorporation of the nucleotide into the nascent complementary strand by DNA polymerase, pyrophosphate is released in a stoichiometric manner and is used to form ATP by ATP sulfurylase. The ATP then fuels production of oxyluciferin from luciferin by luciferase, whereby light is emitted that is proportional to the amount of ATP produced and thus to the number of nucleotides incorporated. The pyrosequencing instrument measures the light produced and plots this on a graph called a pyrogram. Any unincorporated

As each nucleotide is incorporated by the polymerase into the growing strand, pyrophosphate is released. The pyrophosphate is then converted to ATP by ATP sulfurylase and serves as fuel for the luciferase-mediated conversion of luciferin to oxyluciferin, which releases visible light that is proportional to the amount of pyrophosphate initially released and thus to the number of nucleotides incorporated (Fig. 1). Any residual unincorporated nucleotides that remain in the reaction mixture are degraded after each step by apyrase. The intensity of the light emitted for each reaction well is used to both provide information regarding the quantity of template present and also to confirm that the sequence produced matches the sequence of the template. Cytosines that are potentially methylated are treated as variable positions in the sequence, whereby sequential addition of bases corresponding to methylated (C) and unmethylated (T) cytosines provides the means to quantify methylation by measuring peak heights reflecting the incorporation of cytosine relative to the total incorporation for cytosine plus thymine at that particular position. These percentages are automatically calculated by the PyroMark® CpG Software for each of the CG cytosines within the sequence analyzed.

Over 84,000 predesigned pyrosequencing assays are available for purchase through Qiagen (PyroMark® CpG Assays; www.qiagen.com). Alternatively, pyrosequencing assays can be designed using PyroMark® Assay Design Software (Qiagen; Valencia, USA). A thorough description of assay design is beyond the scope of this chapter, but in our experience there are several critical factors to achieve success. The pyrosequencing reaction is carried out at a relatively low temperature and as such is vulnerable to mispriming events from promiscuous priming of the sequencing primer but also potentially from carry forward of any unincorporated biotin-tagged primer or even from template looping. The PyroMark® Assay Design Software detects and evaluates these potential mispriming events. This information is used as part of the criteria for determining the suitability of the assay design. Pyrosequencing

Fig. 1 (continued) nucleotides are degraded by apyrase (not shown) prior to injection of the next nucleotide in to the reaction mix. The *y* axis of the pyrogram represents the light produced and the *x* axis provides a readout of the sequence to analyze. Note that multiple sequential same nucleotides in the template will result in incorporation of a proportional amount of the complementary nucleotide at one pyrogram peak position, such that two of the same nucleotides in a row will produce a peak height that is twice as big as that for a single nucleotide incorporation, and so on. The % methylation measured for each CG cytosine is shown above the pyrogram and is calculated by the software. The single nucleotide width vertical shading at nucleotide position 13 indicates a bisulfite control representing a non-CG cytosine in the original sequence. "E" represents injection of enzyme at the beginning of the run, "S" indicates the injection of substrate, both of which should not produce measurable light using current technology is limited to no more than ~115 bp in length. PCR amplicons for pyrosequencing should be between 150 and 250 bp in length to avoid potential amplification bias and to minimize potential for mispriming [1].

We use Qiagen's Epitect Control DNAs for pyrosequencing assay validation prior to use in evaluating methylation in research specimens by preparing and running replicates of defined mixtures of the fully methylated and unmethylated DNAs as follows: 100%U, 25%M:75%U, 50%M:50%U, 75%M:25%U, and 100%M. This allows us to determine the degree of technical variability, to detect the potential bias in amplification of the methylated versus unmethylated sequence, and to ensure that the assay is able to detect a linear increase in methylation across the dynamic range of the assay.

There are multiple procedural steps required for pyrosequencing, and as such Subheading 3 is broken into subsections that describe the PCR reaction, setting up the pyrosequencing run, procedures for preparing the reagent and capillary tips, preparing the master mix and primer, preparing the nucleotides, preparing the PCR product and adding nucleotides to the tips, performing the dispensation test and preparing the workstation, loading the plate and beginning the run, workstation cleanup, and data analysis and interpretation.

Bisulfite pyrosequencing is particularly useful for not only detailed and accurate quantitative analysis of methylation at specific loci but also analysis of repeat elements, often used as a proxy to assess how methylation is altered throughout the genome. Once assay conditions are optimized, pyrosequencing is amenable to high-throughput analysis of many specimens since the assays are carried out in 48-well or 96-well plate format. We have shown that pyrosequencing can distinguish 5 % differences in methylation using defined mixtures of methylated and unmethylated template DNAs [2]. Pyrosequencing has been used to evaluate DNA methylation profiles in multiple studies of cancer, including gynecologic malignancies [3–6].

2 Materials

2.1 Reagents and Supplies

1. PyroMark® PCR Kit containing 2× PyroMark® PCR Master Mix, 10× CoralLoad™ Concentrate, 25 mM $MgCl_2$ stock, and Nuclease-free water.
2. PCR Primers (one with 5′ biotin label, HPLC purified; *see* Subsection 3.1, PCR, below).
3. 96-well plate.
4. Nuclease-free H_2O.
5. PyroMark® Binding Buffer.
6. PyroMark® Annealing Buffer.

7. GE Healthcare Streptavidin Sepharose™ High-Performance Beads.
8. Pyrosequencing Primer.
9. PyroMark® Gold Q96 CDT Reagents including PyroMark® Enzyme Mixture, PyroMark® Substrate Mixture, and PyroMark® dNTPs (dATPαs, dCTP, dGTP, and dTTP).
10. Plate Sealing Film for Raised Edge Plates (Denville Scientific, Inc.).
11. PyroMark® Wash Buffer, 10×.
12. PyroMark® Denaturation Solution.
13. PyroMark® Q96 HS Plate.
14. PyroMark® Q96 HS Capillary Tips (CDTs).
15. PyroMark® Q96 HS Reagent Tips (RDTs).
16. Aluminum Plate Seals (Greiner Bio-One SILVERseal).

2.2 Equipment

1. PyroMark® Q96 MD Pyrosequencing Instrument.
2. PyroMark® Q96 Vacuum Workstation.
3. 96-well Capacity Thermocycler.
4. Eppendorf MixMate plate mixer (*see* **Note 1**).
5. Heat block, prewarmed to 85 °C.

3 Methods

3.1 PCR

PCR for pyrosequencing requires use of a forward and reverse primer, one of which is modified by the addition of a biotin molecule at the 5′ end. The primer containing the biotin molecule should be the one used to synthesize the strand that will be used as template for pyrosequencing. Without the biotin, the amplified DNA will not be retained on the streptavidin beads for analysis in later steps and will instead pass through the filter probes of the pyrosequencing workstation. Optimization of PCR conditions for the primers is required prior to their use in pyrosequencing. The goal of the optimization is to produce a single, robust band of the correct size as detected by ethidium bromide staining following agarose gene electrophoresis. Due to the added expense of the biotin modification of the primer, we typically order standard primers for use during the PCR optimization process. Once the optimal PCR conditions are defined, we order the appropriate primer with the 5′ biotin modification and with HPLC purification.

1. Prepare the PCR Master Mix in a nuclease-free tube to bring the volume per reaction to 25 μL after the addition of bisulfite modified DNA in **step 2** (*see* Table 1 and **Note 2**).

Table 1
PCR Master Mix

Stock	Reaction mix volumes (μL)	Final concentration
Reverse primer	0.3 μL	120 nM
Forward primer	0.3 μL	120 nM
25 mM $MgCl_2$	1.5 μL	1.5 μM
10× Coral Load™ Concentrate	2.5 μL	1×
2× PyroMark® PCR Master Mix	12.5 μL	1×
DNA (to be add later)	*X*	20–50 ng/reaction
Nuclease-free water	*X*	
Total volume	25 μL	

2. Add bisulfite modified DNA (20–50 ng) to the PCR master mixture in each reaction well. After sealing the tube, vortex, and quick spin to collect contents at the bottom of tubes.
3. Transfer the reaction wells to a thermocycler and perform PCR using the conditions most appropriate for an analysis of the gene in question.
4. After the PCR has finished, the sample may either be removed from the thermocycler for immediate analysis or stored at -20 °C.

3.2 Pyrosequencing: Setting Up the Run

1. Open PyroMark® CpG Software 1.0.11.
2. For a new assay, open a new file in Pyro Q-CpG design folder, right click and choose "New Assay." Copy/paste the sequence into the "sequence to analyze" window and click on "generate dispensation order." Add bisulfite control sites at the orange "T" sites as designated by the software, which are preselected as bisulfite controls and represent non-CG cytosines in the original sequence. The CG sites are highlighted in gray and the BS control sites are in orange.
3. Select "File → New Run" to access the run setup menu. The run setup menu can also be accessed by clicking on the "New Run" icon located beneath the toolbar.
4. There will be three smaller run setup windows that appear on the right of the screen. The upper left screen shows the run name, instrument parameters, plate ID, reagent ID and also has a small window available for entering notes.
5. Enter run name and plate ID in the run setup menu.
6. Select "Instrument Parameters" according to the CDT version used. The parameter information for specific CDT versions

can be found at www.qiagen.com and is based on the lot number of the CDTs purchased.

7. The lower panel on the right-hand side of the screen shows the plate wells. There are three text boxes for each well. The uppermost text box is used to designate which assay you want to run, selected from the pre-entered assay designs. Select the appropriate assay in the Pyro Q-CpG design folder and drag and drop this on the "Assay Name" in the top text box of the first well. Click the box and drag the cursor across all other wells to assign that same assay information via auto-fill, as appropriate.
8. Enter the sample ID into the middle textbox of each well in the "Plate Wells" panel. The lower text box can be used for adding any desired notes.
9. After all of the above information has been entered, the right upper panel will show the well information with the assay design, sample ID, and notes. Double check to ensure that all information is correct.
10. For reagent and capillary tip volume information, select "Tools → Volume Information." Enzyme and substrate volumes are listed under "E-mix" and "S-mix", respectively. Nucleotide volumes for capillary tips are listed according to each base. Note these volumes for a later step in the protocol.

3.3 Cleaning Reagent and Capillary Tips

Cleaning of the reagent and capillary tips should be performed both prior to and after a run (*see* **Note 3**).

1. To wash a reagent (RDT) or capillary (CDT) tip, first rinse the interior of the tip with nuclease-free water five times by filling to the brim with nuclease-free water and inverting to empty.
2. After the tip has been rinsed, finish cleaning by "milking" five times. To milk the tip, first fill to the brim with nuclease-free water and then create a seal at the top by completely covering the opening with your thumb. Then, lightly apply pressure to the top and sides of the tip using the thumb and forefingers of the opposite hand, respectively, until a straight stream of water can be steadily produced.
3. Once tips have been rinsed and milked prior to use in the pyrosequencing run, place each tip upside down on a Kim wipe until use.

3.4 Preparing the PCR Components

1. To prepare the master mix, in a 15-mL conical tube combine 2 μL of Sepharose streptavidin-coated beads, 40 μL of PyroMark® Binding Buffer, and nuclease-free water to bring the volume to 80 μL for each of the reactions after accounting for addition of the PCR product (plus some additional to allow for pipetting error) (*see* **Note 4**).
2. Invert gently several times to mix (do not vortex).

3. Immediately (before the beads settle) pipet the appropriate amount of master mix into each well of a PCR plate for each sample to be analyzed (80 μL minus the amount of PCR product to be added). Place on ice.
4. To dilute the primer for an entire 96-well plate, add 4 μL of appropriate sequencing primer (100 μM) to 1,196 μL of PyroMark® Annealing Buffer and vortex thoroughly. Place on ice.
5. In four separate tubes, prepare each of the four PyroMark® dNTPs by mixing each dNTP with an equal volume of TE Buffer to make a final volume given by "Tools → Volume Information" (*see* **step 10** from Subheading 3.2).
6. Add PCR product (8–10 μL) to the master mix in each well (from **step 3**, Subheading 3.4).
7. Seal the plate thoroughly using an aluminum plate seal.
8. Place the plate on the plate mixer at 1,400 rpm for 7–10 min at room temperature.
9. Load each dNTP mixture into the corresponding CDT in alphabetical order (A, C, G, T). Load the required volumes of enzyme and substrate into the RDT tips. Place each CDT and RDT tip into its corresponding slot in the cartridge (*see* **Note 4**).

3.5 Dispensation Test and Preparing the Pyrosequencing Reactions

1. To insure proper functioning of the tips, a dispensation test, controlled by the software, is performed prior to the actual run whereby reagents and nucleotides are dispensed by the pyrosequencer onto a clear plastic plate cover and should form droplets that are easily visible and of uniform size. Open the outer lid of the PyroMark® Q96 MD. Load the reagent cartridge into the instrument and select "Open Process Chamber" from the software menu. Once the process chamber is open, load a dispensation test plate with a clear plastic cover on top and click on "Close Process Chamber." Then, click on "Test Dispensing Tips" to begin the dispensation test.
2. To prepare the workstation, load troughs 1–4 with 110 mL 70 % EtOH, 90 mL PyroMark® Denaturation Solution, 110 mL nuclease-free water, and 110 mL PyroMark® Wash Buffer, respectively. Load the "Parking" trough with 180 mL nuclease-free water and submerge the filter tips of the vacuum prep tool in the nuclease-free water.
3. Return to the computer, close the "Test Dispensing Tips Finished" message, and open the process chamber lid. The dispensations should appear as six rounded droplets. If any of the droplets are not present or appear aberrant, repeat the dispensation test. If the problem persists after multiple dispensation tests, rinse tips and test for flow-through of liquid using the manual cleaning procedure described above in "Cleaning Reagent and Capillary Tips."

4. Vortex the diluted primer and add 12 μL to each well in a PyroMark® Q96 plate. Once the primer has been plated, slide the PyroMark® Q96 plate into the PyroMark® plate platform in the vacuum workstation.
5. Remove the plate with the PCR product from the vortexer and peel off the aluminum seal. DO NOT quick spin the PCR product plate at this point. Then, check to make sure that the vacuum seal on the liquid waste container at the workstation is tightly sealed.
6. Remove the prep tool from the parking trough and start the pump. Apply a vacuum to the prep tool by turning the workstation to ON. Keep the vacuum ON THROUGH **step 9** so that the beads remain attached to the filter probes. Matching position A1 of the prep tool to position A1 of the PCR product-beads plate, slowly lower the filter probes into the plate wells until the entire PCR product mixture has been aspirated through the filter tips and the streptavidin beads have been immobilized on the probes. Then, gently remove the prep tool from the plate, taking care not to dislodge the streptavidin beads from the filter probes. Aspiration of the liquid and immobilization of the beads on the filter probes should take roughly 15 s.
7. While maintaining the vacuum, place the prep tool filter probes directly into the 110 ml of 70 % EtOH in trough 1. Once fluid is visible in the tubing, continue aspiration for 5 s, then remove the prep tool from the 70 % EtOH while maintaining its orientation and allow the remaining 70 % EtOH to be fully aspirated from the prep tool by the vacuum.
8. Place the prep tool into the 90 mL of PyroMark® Denaturation Solution in trough 2. Once fluid is visible in the tubing, continue aspiration for 5 s, remove the prep tool and allow the Denaturation Solution to be fully aspirated from the prep tool by the vacuum.
9. Place the prep tool into the 110 mL of PyroMark® Wash Buffer in trough 3 and aspirate the Wash Buffer completely. Lift the prep tool out of the Wash Buffer and, while maintaining its orientation, turn the workstation to OFF, stop the pump, and release the vacuum on the liquid waste container by loosening the lid.
10. Lower the prep tool into the primer-loaded PyroMark® Q96 plate in the plate platform of the workstation, so that the filter probes rest in their corresponding wells (A1 to A1). Gently rock the prep tool from side to side to release the beads into the wells.
11. Place the PyroMark® Q96 plate on a prewarmed PyroMark® Q96 Sample Prep Thermoplate. There are two parts to the Thermoplate; the PyroMark® Q96 plate should be sandwiched

between the upper and lower blocks and should be fully covered by the top block. Place the PyroMark® Q96 plate-Thermoplate onto the surface of the heating block at 85 °C for 2 min.

12. After 2 min, switch the heating block off but do not remove the PyroMark® Q96 plate-Thermoplate from the heating block. Allow the PyroMark® Q96 plate-Thermoplate to sit atop the (now cooling) heating block for another 2 min. Then, remove the PyroMark® Q96 plate from between the two blocks of the Thermoplate and let cool to room temperature (~5 min). Once the PyroMark® Q96 plate has reached room temperature, move on to the next part of the protocol.

3.6 Loading the Plate and Beginning the Run

1. Click on "Open Process Chamber" and insert the PyroMark® Q96 plate into the PyroMark® Q96 MD instrument, and select "Close Process Chamber."
2. Begin the run by clicking the "Start Run" arrow button located next to the run parameters.

3.7 Workstation Cleanup

1. Place the filter probes of the prep tool into the 110 mL of nuclease-free water in trough 4 and gently agitate for 10 s.
2. Tighten the vacuum lid on the waste container, start the pump, and turn the workstation to ON to flush the filter probes for ~5 s.
3. Lift the prep tool from the water, and aspirate the water through the prep tool.
4. Stop the pump, turn the workstation to OFF, release the vacuum and return the prep tool into a clean storage box until next use (*see* **Note 5**).

3.8 Data Analysis and Interpretation

1. When the run is complete, the data for each sample will be analyzed by the software and scored as "passed," "check quality," or "fail."
2. Run data for each specimen should be inspected to insure that adequate peak heights were achieved (~150–300 light units for a single-nucleotide incorporation). Low peak heights are more likely to reflect stochastic results from having too little template or loss of beads during the wash steps on the workstation, even if the run was scored as "passed."
3. The pyrogram software output produced for each sample provides a linear representation of the sequence read based on the intensity of light produced after each incorporation. Peak heights will proportionately increase with the number of same sequential nucleotides in the template being sequenced. For example, the template sequence 3′-A-G-G-T-T-T-A-T-5′ will show results in which the first incorporation will be a single

peak height T, the second will be a double peak height C, the third will be a triple peak height A, the fourth will be a single peak height T, and the fifth will be a single peak height A. Deviations in the expected peak heights, based on those anticipated from the input sequence, will trigger the software to score the run as a "check quality" run or a "fail."

4. The pyrosequencing software treats cytosines within "CG" dinucleotide positions within the sequence much like a polymorphic site, since either a C or T is possible at the cytosine position depending on if this particular cytosine was methylated or unmethylated, respectively, in the original sequence. Thus, the sequence to analyze will contain a "T" adjacent to a "C". The light produced from each of these peaks is used to determine the proportion of cytosine that is methylated in the sample at that position by calculating the light intensity produced from incorporation of the C relative to the total produced from combined C + T incorporation. The percent methylation calculated is provided as a visual readout above each CG position within the sequence in the pyrogram.
5. Bisulfite controls are also a necessary component of pyrosequencing and are automatically chosen and inserted into the sequence to analyze by the PyroMark® CpG Software. These controls represent cytosines in the original sequence that are not in CG context and therefore should be fully converted by the bisulfite treatment to uracils (thymine following PCR). A "T" adjacent to a "C" is also used for these positions, just as for CG cytosines (described above), except in this case the results should show near complete incorporation for the "T". The proportion of "C" incorporation at these positions is indicative of the degree to which conversion was incomplete, at least at that position. This is calculated by the software, which has a default threshold setting of 96.5 % conversion (4.5 % incomplete conversion of cytosines) before a sample will fail the run. This threshold setting can be adjusted using the software settings as desired. It is important to note that incomplete conversion will falsely elevate the signals coming from CG positions. In our hands, conversion efficiencies are typically >98 % for high quality, high purity bisulfite modified genomic DNA.

4 Notes

1. It is important to use a mixer that can thoroughly mix the reagents in a 96-well plate while not causing the reagents to spill or splash up onto the sides of the tubes or the plate seal. We have tried several brands and the Eppendorf MixMate works well in our hands.

2. It is strongly recommended to include controls on each plate for both the PCR reactions (e.g., positive control, no template control, etc.) and pyrosequencing reactions (annealing buffer plus template but without primer, primer plus annealing buffer but without template) along with positive and negative controls for methylation status. We use the EpiTect Control DNAs from Qiagen that are provided in bisulfite modified form. These are produced using whole genome amplification followed by treatment with or without the bacterial *Sss*I methyltransferase. *Sss*I methyltransferase enzymatically methylates all CG cytosines throughout the genome to generate the fully methylated DNA while the methylation pattern in the original template is effectively "erased" by the whole genome amplification to produce the unmethylated DNA. These controls are especially useful for assessing assay performance for regions of the genome that normally exhibit endogenous methylation, such as imprinted loci, since it is extremely difficult to obtain naturally occurring DNA specimens that exhibit a complete lack of methylation at these loci for use as unmethylated controls.
3. It is critical to clean the tips well, as unexpected peaks might otherwise be generated in the subsequent sequencing run. These unexpected peaks can be caused by pyrophosphate generated as a result of reagent(s) remaining in unclean tips. We have found that with appropriate handling, CDTs can be cleaned and reused for up to 15 runs and RDTs for up to 8 runs.
4. Due to light sensitivity, minimize exposure of the reagents to light.
5. An empty pipet-tip box can be used as a storage box such that the filter probes are gently inserted into the empty holes and thus kept clean and protected from damage.

Acknowledgments

We gratefully acknowledge Zack Davenport for his contributions to the artwork. We thank Allison Barratt and Carole Grenier for critical reading of the manuscript. This work was supported by Department of Defense grant W81XWH-11-1-0469, NIH grants R01DK085173 and R01CA142983, and the Gail Parkins Ovarian Cancer Awareness Fund.

References

1. Shen L, Guo Y, Chen X, Ahmed S, Issa JP (2007) Optimizing annealing temperature overcomes bias in bisulfite PCR methylation analysis. Biotechniques 42:48–58
2. Murphy SK, Huang Z, Hoyo C (2012) Differentially methylated regions of imprinted genes in prenatal, perinatal and postnatal human tissues. PLoS One 7:e40924
3. Coley HM, Safuwan NA, Chivers P, Papacharalbous E, Giannopoulos T et al (2012) The cyclin-dependent kinase inhibitor p57(Kip2) is epigenetically regulated in carboplatin resistance and results in collateral sensitivity to the CDK inhibitor seliciclib in ovarian cancer. Br J Cancer 106:482–489
4. Feng W, Marquez RT, Lu Z, Liu J, Lu KH et al (2008) Imprinted tumor suppressor genes *ARHI* and *PEG3* are the most frequently down-regulated in human ovarian cancers by loss of heterozygosity and promoter methylation. Cancer 112:1489–1502
5. Mirabello L, Sun C, Ghosh A, Rodriguez AC, Schiffman M et al (2012) Methylation of human papillomavirus type 16 genome and risk of cervical precancer in a Costa Rican population. J Natl Cancer Inst 104: 556–565
6. Lof-Ohlin ZM, Levanat S, Sabol M, Sorbe B, Nilsson TK (2011) Promoter methylation in the PTCH gene in cervical epithelial cancer and ovarian cancer tissue as studied by eight novel Pyrosequencing® assays. Int J Oncol 38: 685–692

Part III

Gene/Genome Expression Assessing

Chapter 10

RNA Networks in Ovarian Cancer

Anastasia Malek

Abstract

Development of ovarian cancer is known to be associated with alterations in the expression of cellular RNAs. Most of the clinical and biological characteristics of ovarian cancer have been correlated with significant changes in the expression of a subset of genes. Over the last few years, considerable resources have been focused on understanding the complex structure and function of noncoding RNAs, and this paradigm is also applicable to ovarian cancer research. The chapter provides a brief review of methodological approaches used to study alterations in protein coding and noncoding RNAs in the context of ovarian cancer.

Key words Ovarian cancer, Transcriptional profiling, Alternative splicing, Noncoding RNA, Computational analysis

1 New Insights into Transcriptome Research

For many years, the central dogma of molecular biology has been that RNA functions mainly as an informational intermediate between a DNA sequence and its encoded protein. One of the great surprises of modern biology was the discovery that protein-coding genes represent only about 2 % of the total genome sequence and that at least 90 % of the human genome is actively transcribed. The human transcriptome is much more complex than a collection of protein-coding genes [1]. Technological advances in last decade have increased our knowledge of posttranscriptional genome functionality and revealed new classes of RNA molecules with unique regulatory activities. Alterations to these molecules may be directly related to the process of malignant transformation.

Ovarian cancerogenesis has several specific biological characteristics. Exfoliation of ovarian cancer cells into the peritoneal cavity and the ability of non-adherent cells to survive define yearly upset of dissemination and its specific patterns. Progression of ovarian cancer is accompanied by a distinct disbalance of epithelial and mesenchymal features. The sensitivity of ovarian cancer to

Anastasia Malek and Oleg Tchernitsa (eds.), *Ovarian Cancer: Methods and Protocols*, Methods in Molecular Biology, vol. 1049, DOI 10.1007/978-1-62703-547-7_10, © Springer Science+Business Media New York 2013

first-line chemotherapy is usually followed by development of chemoresistance and disease recurrence. Despite advances in treatment, ovarian cancer remains the leading cause of death among the gynecologic tumors. The clinical and biological features of ovarian cancer could be due to specific alterations in posttranscriptional genome activity. Understanding the role of RNA networks in ovarian cancer may improve our conceptual understanding and clinical management of this disease. The important laboratory techniques for investigating gene/genome transcriptional products were recently updated and published [2]. This part of the book presents specific applications of known methods with a focus on particular types of RNA molecules and explores the characteristics of these molecules in the context of ovarian cancer research.

2 Array-Based Genome Expression Profiling

The genome-wide transcriptional profiling technique has been well established and is broadly accepted. This approach is used to examine differential gene expression patterns between tumor and normal cells, identify gene expression signatures that correlate with various clinical outcomes, and generate biomarkers that can predict patient responses to surgery and chemotherapy [3]. The basic idea of microarray analysis is simple: membranes or slides are "arrayed" with oligonucleotides or DNA fragments that complement specific gene expression products. RNA is purified from the sample of interest, retro-transcribed into cDNA, labelled, and hybridized to the membrane or slide. The amount of hybridized RNA (or cDNA) indicates the level of RNA expression in the tissue sample or cell line. This technique can measure thousands of genes in a single sample. Assessing a set of samples with the same array platform allows the samples to be grouped based on clinical, histological, or experimental factors and enables expression profiling of one group of samples versus another. The method provides a unique opportunity to explore the influence of various factors on the whole genome expression profile. However, there are several disadvantages to this technique. Most of the commercially available arrays evaluate the expression of 25–35 thousands of genes and it can be difficult to extract meaningful results from large amounts of outcome data. A number of computational algorithms and statistical approaches for gene expression analysis have been developed, and there are a number of internet resources and databases that contain supplementary material to improve the quality of analysis. The effect of luteinizing hormone on the transcriptome profile in ovarian cancer cells is evaluated in Chapter 11 to provide a framework of this analytic approach. Although several aspects should be taken in consideration in order to plan correctly array-based study. First one is the general and comparative nature of the array-based analysis. Arrays-based results may provide an interesting and scientifically reasonable overview of transcriptome alterations; conclusions regarding certain genes require confirmation using other methods. Second, arrays-based approach can evaluate the expression of a finite number of genes, defining the gene may be problematic because small genes can be difficult to detect, one gene can code for several protein products, some genes only code for RNA and two genes can overlap. Third, because array-based analysis has a defined threshold of sensitivity, changes in genes with generally low expression levels may be undetectable.

Other methods, such as subtractive suppression hybridization (SSH) or next-generation sequencing (NGS), may be considered as alternative approaches. SSH allows detection of mRNAs expressed differently between two samples (for instance, cancer and norm) including low-abundance transcripts. The method was introduced quite long ago [4] and has been successfully applied for ovarian cancer research [5]. The main disadvantages are laboriousness and low reproducibility. The emergence of next-generation sequencing technologies has led to dramatic advances in transcriptome studies as well as many other genetic, genomic, and epigenomic approaches [6] The increased efficiency and resolution of next-generation sequencing greatly facilitate the detection of transcriptome alteration. In Chapter 12, readers will find short discussion of main existing NGS platforms as well as the protocol of transcriptome analysis using the Illumina's platform. This approach was applied for study transcriptional events underlying chemoresistance of ovarian cancer [7].

3 Alternative Splicing and Assessment

Alternative RNA splicing is a phenomenon that provides an important dimension to the complexity of genome expression. Pre-mRNA splicing is an essential and tightly regulated process that occurs after transcription in approximately 60 % of all human genes. Because splicing can add or delete functional domains from the protein-coding sequence, physiological activity alternative variants can vary significantly. Splicing is performed by multicomponent complexes (spliceosomes) containing five small nuclear ribonucleoproteins (snRNPs) and over 100 other proteins. The spliceosome recognizes the boundary between exonic and intronic sequences in pre-mRNA and catalyzes the cut-and-paste reaction that removes introns and joins exons. Exon recognition is not trivial because exons are relatively small compared to introns, splice sites are poorly conserved, and introns contain a large number of sequences that resemble splice sites. In addition to sequence-defined events, splicing is regulated by RNA regulatory elements, protein components of spliceosomes, and epigenetic components, such as chromatin structure and histone modifications [8]. Malignant transformation is associated with alterations in the post-transcriptional mRNA splicing process, and these alterations may play a causative role in inducing cancer progression or acting as surrogate markers. Altered expression and functional activity of splicing factors, such as the polypyrimidine tract-binding protein, are associated with ovarian cancer cell proliferation and invasiveness [9]. A high-throughput approach based on reverse transcription PCR has been applied to reveal global alterations in the mRNA splicing process associated with ovarian cancer progression and demonstrated changes in approximately half of all active alternative splicing events [10, 11]. The methodological details of this technique are described in another study [12]. Similar to array-based expression profiling, this approach reveals general shifts in the mRNA splicing activity of cancer cells, although a more detailed analysis is required to explore the splicing alterations of specific genes. Chapter 13 of the book presents an example of a detailed assay. Posttranscriptional processing of survivin mRNA produces five alternative splicing forms with various activities, cellular localizations, and involvement in ovarian cancerogenesis. RT-PCR-based quantitative assessments and siRNA-based evaluation of the functional activity of specific splicing variants are described in detail to provide a tentative framework of this type of investigation. In addition to splicing variability, other aspects of posttranscriptional mRNA processing, including polyadenylation (APA) and mRNA degradation, may be altered in ovarian cancer cells [13]. Global changes in these processes have been assayed by array-based techniques with a corresponding statistical algorithm, while the RT-PCR-based approach can be applied to evaluate point alterations.

4 MiroRNA (miRNA) Profiling

MiRNAs are a class of small regulatory RNA molecules that negatively regulate messenger RNA translation of target genes by sequence complementarity. MiRNA genes represent approximately 1 % of the genome in various species, each with hundreds of different conserved or non-conserved targets. Approximately 30 % of the genes are regulated by at least one miRNA [14]. MiRNAs are generally transcribed by RNA polymerase II as long primary transcripts characterized by hairpin structures (pre-microRNAs) and processed into the nucleus by RNase III Drosha into 70- to 100-nt-long pre-microRNAs. These precursor molecules are exported by an exportin 5-mediated mechanism to the cytoplasm where an additional step mediated by RNAse III Dicer generates a dsRNA approximately 22 nucleotides in length. The mature single-stranded miRNA product is then incorporated into a miRNA-containing ribonucleoprotein complex (miRNP) or miRNA-containing

RNA-induced silencing complex (miRISC), while the other strand is likely degraded. In this complex, the mature miRNA is able to regulate gene expression at the posttranscriptional level by binding with partial complementarity to the 3-UTR of target mRNAs, which leads to some degree of mRNA degradation and translation inhibition [15]. miRNAs are functionally involved in the pathogenesis of ovarian cancer [16, 17]. miRNA let-7 has been shown to be involved in progesterone-mediated control of ovarian cancer progression and is associated with resistance against taxanes. All of the traditional methods of RNA evaluation, including RT-PCR, Northern blot, and in situ RNA hybridization, are applicable for studying miRNAs. Profiling known miRNAs is commonly performed using the array-based technique described in Chapter 14. However, there is potential for cross-hybridization of miRNAs that are highly related in sequence due to their small size, which makes it difficult to definitively distinguish between miRNAs that differ by one or two nucleotides. Deep sequencing can overcome the limitations associated with the array-based technique and may assist in discovering new miRNAs involved in ovarian cancerogenesis [18].

In general, the accepted method of experimental posttranscriptional gene silencing by siRNA is based on the natural phenomenon described previously. Molecular mechanisms and laboratory protocols of artificial siRNA-mediated gene silencing with various technical modifications and possible therapeutic applications are described in detail in the literature. Although describing the proper experimental RNA interference procedure is beyond the scope of the book, several excellent reviews are available [19, 20].

5 Noncoding RNA and Roles in Gene Expression Control

Although the ability of small duplex RNAs to direct epigenetic events and transcriptional gene silencing (TGS) in mammalian cells was first described in 2004 [21], a lack of knowledge regarding the underlying biological mechanisms responsible for this phenomenon has limited research in this area. The exact molecular mechanisms of RNA-mediated transcriptional regulation of gene expression are still not clear. Recent experimental data indicate that small duplex RNAs catalyze the formation of multiprotein complexes containing elements of RNA interference machinery, such as Argonaute proteins (AGO proteins), and epigenetic effectors at the promoter region of a targeted gene. In this nuclear complex, AGO proteins with intrinsic RNA-binding capacity appear to play an essential role by mediating the interactions between regulatory RNA and promoter DNA molecules [22]. Additional investigation of RNA-mediated transcriptional gene regulation requires complex, multistep laboratory approaches that allow simultaneous evaluation of structural components and estimation of their possible interactions and functionality. A detailed analysis of the small RNAs associated with the c-Myc promoter implicated in regulation of transcriptional activity is presented in Chapter 15. Directional RT-PCR, RNA interference (RNAi), and nucleic acid immuneprecipitation are combined to define the presence, structure, and orientation of promoter-associated RNA and to estimate interactions with components of the multiprotein promoter-targeting complex and resulting biological effects.

6 Mathematic Approaches in Transcriptome Research

Despite the discovery several new classes of RNAs in the past decade, we are still far from fully understanding the structural composition and functionality of cellular transcriptomes. The RNA network mediates interactions between the genome and the proteome, although this regulatory system is very complex and contains multiple signalling loops, cross talk, and divergence. System models jointly created by biologists and mathematicians present a way to comprehend the nature of RNA networks and to predict natural behaviors. Several advanced kinetic models describing the interplay of various RNA classes and proteins with an assumption of stochastic and spatiotemporal effects are reviewed in the literature [23]. MiRNA and gene regulatory modules have been explored to model transcriptome regulation networks in various cancer types, including ovarian cancer [24, 25]. Chapter 16 introduces an approach to integrate mRNA and miRNA expression profiling datasets with information regarding miRNA-gene and gene-gene interactions. This method allows evaluation of co-modules that are highly relevant to the biological behavior of ovarian cancer.

Transcriptome research is a rapidly advancing field in molecular biology. It is not possible to present all of the various laboratory approaches in one book. The following chapters introduce the most applicable methods and provide readers with a framework understanding of transcriptome research.

References

1. Sana J, Faltejskova P, Svoboda M, Slaby O (2012) Novel classes of non-coding RNAs and cancer. J Transl Med 10:103
2. Rio DC, Manuel Ares J, Nilsen TW (2010) RNA: a laboratory manual. Cold Spring Harbor Laboratory Press, New York, USA
3. Chon HS, Lancaster JM (2011) Microarray-based gene expression studies in ovarian cancer. Cancer Control 18:8–15
4. Diatchenko L, Lau YF, Campbell AP, Chenchik A, Moqadam F et al (1996) Suppression subtractive hybridization: a method for generating differentially regulated or tissue-specific cDNA probes and libraries. Proc Natl Acad Sci USA 93:6025–6030
5. Tchernitsa OI, Sers C, Zuber J, Hinzmann B, Grips M et al (2004) Transcriptional basis of KRAS oncogene-mediated cellular transformation

in ovarian epithelial cells. Oncogene 23: 4536–4555

6. Dong H, Wang S (2012) Exploring the cancer genome in the era of next-generation sequencing. Front Med 6:48–55
7. Cheng L, Lu W, Kulkarni B, Pejovic T, Yan X et al (2010) Analysis of chemotherapy response programs in ovarian cancers by the next-generation sequencing technologies. Gynecol Oncol 117:159–169
8. Luco RF, Allo M, Schor IE, Kornblihtt AR, Misteli T (2011) Epigenetics in alternative pre-mRNA splicing. Cell 144:16–26
9. He X, Pool M, Darcy KM, Lim SB, Auersperg N et al (2007) Knockdown of polypyrimidine tract-binding protein suppresses ovarian tumor cell growth and invasiveness in vitro. Oncogene 26:4961–4968
10. Klinck R, Bramard A, Inkel L, Dufresne-Martin G, Gervais-Bird J et al (2008) Multiple alternative splicing markers for ovarian cancer. Cancer Res 68:657–663
11. Venables JP, Klinck R, Koh C, Gervais-Bird J, Bramard A et al (2009) Cancer-associated regulation of alternative splicing. Nat Struct Mol Biol 16:670–676
12. Brosseau JP, Lucier JF, Lapointe E, Durand M, Gendron D et al (2010) High-throughput quantification of splicing isoforms. RNA 16: 442–449
13. Singh P, Alley TL, Wright SM, Kamdar S, Schott W et al (2009) Global changes in processing of mRNA 3' untranslated regions characterize clinically distinct cancer subtypes. Cancer Res 69:9422–9430
14. Bartel DP (2004) MicroRNAs: genomics, biogenesis, mechanism, and function. Cell 116:281–297
15. Iorio MV, Croce CM (2009) MicroRNAs in cancer: small molecules with a huge impact. J Clin Oncol 27:5848–5856
16. Mezzanzanica D, Bagnoli M, De Cecco L, Valeri B, Canevari S (2010) Role of microRNAs in ovarian cancer pathogenesis and potential clinical implications. Int J Biochem Cell Biol 42:1262–1272
17. Kuhlmann JD, Rasch J, Wimberger P, Kasimir-Bauer S (2012) microRNA and the pathogenesis of ovarian cancer–a new horizon for molecular diagnostics and treatment? Clin Chem Lab Med 50:601–615
18. Wyman SK, Parkin RK, Mitchell PS, Fritz BR, O'Briant K et al (2009) Repertoire of microRNAs in epithelial ovarian cancer as determined by next generation sequencing of small RNA cDNA libraries. PLoS One 4:e5311
19. Aigner A (2007) Applications of RNA interference: current state and prospects for siRNA-based strategies in vivo. Appl Microbiol Biotechnol 76:9–21
20. Bora RS, Gupta D, Mukkur TK, Saini KS (2012) RNA interference therapeutics for cancer: challenges and opportunities (review). Mol Med Report 6:9–15
21. Morris KV, Chan SW, Jacobsen SE, Looney DJ (2004) Small interfering RNA-induced transcriptional gene silencing in human cells. Science 305:1289–1292
22. Pastori C, Magistri M, Napoli S, Carbone GM, Catapano CV (2010) Small RNA-directed transcriptional control: new insights into mechanisms and therapeutic applications. Cell Cycle 9:2353–2362
23. Zhdanov VP (2011) Kinetic models of gene expression including non-coding RNAs. Phys Rep 500:1–42
24. Zhang W, Edwards A, Fan W, Flemington EK, Zhang K (2012) miRNA-mRNA correlation-network modules in human prostate cancer and the differences between primary and metastatic tumor subtypes. PLoS One 7:e40130
25. Zhang S, Li Q, Liu J, Zhou XJ (2011) A novel computational framework for simultaneous integration of multiple types of genomic data to identify microRNA-gene regulatory modules. Bioinformatics 27:i401–i409

Chapter 11

Microarray-Based Transcriptome Profiling of Ovarian Cancer Cells

Juan Cui, Ying Xu, and David Puett

Abstract

Transcriptome profiling is a powerful method for monitoring genes and their expression levels under a variety of conditions. Completion of the human genome and advances in high-throughput gene microarray instrumentation enables one to collect large amounts of data in a relatively short time. The challenge then becomes that of data analysis to identify patterns in expression changes and, from there, to relate the observed changes to functional compartments and pathways in cells, tissues, and organisms. Using cultured human ovarian cancer cells as an experimental model cellular system, we describe approaches that are used in analysis of the transcriptome, focusing on those genes encoding proteins and microRNAs. Coupled with other approaches described herein, one can also use the transcriptome to identify potential serum biomarkers, thus providing direction to what usually is a laborious search for low abundance proteins.

Key words Transcriptomic analysis, Microarray analysis, Pathway identification, MicroRNAs, Serum biomarker prediction, Ovarian cancer

1 Introduction

Emerging as a widely used approach, transcriptome profiling has become readily available to monitor genome-wide alterations in gene expression. Three major methodologies used for this purpose are DNA microarray, RCR array, and deep sequencing. Using any of these, the experimentalist is able to generate relatively large amounts of data quickly; however, computational techniques are required to sort these large datasets into meaningful biological observations. While there are many software packages available to assist in data reduction and statistical analysis, some tend to be more widely accepted due to their ease of use and reliability, as well as their specific design for varied research purposes. It should be noted that the recently introduced methodology referred to as RNAseq shows increased ability to detect transcripts that are expressed at low levels, but the complexity of analyzing huge sets of data hinders the general use. Most of the current transcriptomic

Anastasia Malek and Oleg Tchernitsa (eds.), *Ovarian Cancer: Methods and Protocols*, Methods in Molecular Biology, vol. 1049, DOI 10.1007/978-1-62703-547-7_11, © Springer Science+Business Media New York 2013

studies are still microarray based, its prevalence resting on the flexibility of the array customization and reasonable cost with good experimental outcomes.

The availability of the recently emerging technologies to elucidate gene expression in cells and tissues offers the possibility of garnering new insights into cell function and drug development for various diseases. Currently there are a number of specialized instruments and facilities capable of producing results using high-throughput techniques for transcriptome profiling. At present, however, the statistical analysis and meaningful interpretation of the voluminous data obtained pose major challenges. Complementing the collection of new microarray data, there are also many resources to download results for subsequent analysis (*see* **Note 1**). In view of the massive data obtainable, it behooves the investigator to rigorously select and use appropriate platforms in order to make meaningful biological interpretations. For this it is imperative that rigorous statistical analyses be conducted to identify important genes and pathways operative in normal and disease states.

In order to illustrate the procedures used in transcriptome profiling, we have chosen to focus on ovarian cancer, the most lethal form of gynecological cancer [1]. The experimental system is that of cultured human ovarian cancer cells responding to a gonadotropic hormone, luteinizing hormone (LH). The presence of LH and its cognate G protein-coupled receptor (LHR) has been suggested to be contributory to the initiation and/or progression of the disease, although this is controversial [2–9]. This choice of an experimental system to analyze also demonstrates the, at times, conflicting results that can emerge in transcriptome profiling [10], thus emphasizing the importance of coupling experimental and computational studies whenever possible.

The cells used in our study were a genetically engineered version of a parent SKOV3 cell line stably expressing functional LHRs [11]. Both the parent cell line, devoid of LHR expression (SKOV3/LHR–), and the LHR-expressing cells (SKOV3/LHR+) were studied. The latter cells were also incubated with LH for various time periods, after which RNA was prepared for transcriptome profiling. The resulting cDNA samples were hybridized to the Affymetrix Human Genome U133 Plus2 Array and analyzed by Almac Diagnostics (Durham, NC, USA). From 54,671 transcripts profiled, 2,373 genes exhibited a twofold or greater change in differential expression when compared between any two groups. An analysis of the data showed that LH itself led to differential expression of 1,783 genes [10]. The application of hierarchical clustering of the 2,373 genes led to the identification of 12 highly correlated expression patterns involving myriad cellular functions. With the present interest on cancer, one can focus on genes that function in cell growth, migration, invasion, apoptosis, and many other processes that are associated with this disease.

Taking into account the strong association of noncoding RNA (microRNA) expression and cancer development/progression, which is one of the key factors regulating gene expression, approaches will be discussed on the analysis of microRNAs and target gene expression from microarray data. In order to profile microRNA expression in ovarian cancer, one can either use the human microRNA array from Affymetrix or the Almac Diagnostic Ovarian Cancer DSA™ specially designed chip by Almac Diagnostics. We chose the latter in the analysis of microRNAs [12] since it has the advantage of gathering extensive mRNA data and microRNA information in ovarian cancer on the same chip, which largely avoids the technical noise associated with profiling those expressions on separate chips. The platform so designed includes over 100,000 transcripts covering ovarian-specific genes and many novel genes not included on standard chips (*see* **Note 2**). Of the genes analyzed, 2,210 and 4,297 were found to be upregulated and downregulated, respectively. Further analysis has revealed groups of genes likely regulated by some microRNAs, while significant correlation of possible microRNA–mRNA pairs can elucidate new regulatory mechanisms. The raw data have been deposited in the GEO database with accession number GSE27328, all MIAME (Minimum Information About a Microarray Experiment) compliant.

Ovarian cancer is associated with a relatively high death rate, attributable in part to the difficulty of early diagnosis. Consequently, the availability of reliable serum biomarkers would represent a major contribution in combating this disease. This chapter also treats recent developments on the feasibility of using transcriptomic analysis to make predictions on gene products (proteins) likely to be found in serum. As experience and confidence grow in using this approach, it may be possible to combine transcriptome profiling and prediction of secreted proteins to greatly accelerate biomarker identification.

2 Materials

2.1 Cell Cultures

The cells were grown in DMEM supplemented with 5 % fetal bovine serum, 10 mmol/L HEPES, 1,000 units/mL penicillin, 1 mg/mL streptomycin, and 2.5 μg/mL amphotericin B at 37 °C with a humidified atmosphere containing 10 % CO_2. All experimental treatments should be done in triplicate (minimum of three times for statistical purposes):

1. The parent line of SKOV3 human ovarian cancer cells (SKOV3/LHR–) was obtained from American Type Culture Collection.
2. These cells were stably transfected to express approximately 12,000 LH receptors per cell (SKOV3/LHR+) [11].

As judged by hormone binding, hormone-mediated increases in cAMP and inositol phosphates, and phosphorylation of the HER2 protein, the receptors were functional.

3. The SKOV3/LHR+ cells were incubated with 13 nM human LH for 0, 1, 4, 8, and 20 h.

2.2 RNA Processing and Hybridization Arrays

There are many different platforms available for transcriptome profiling. The discussion we provide, however, will be focused on the Affymetrix human gene array and the Almac DSA array used in our previous studies [10, 12]:

1. Crude RNA was extracted from confluent cell cultures with Trizol using the protocol established by the Molecular Research Corporation. This RNA fraction was incubated for 30 min at 37 °C with RQ1-DNase from Promega and then further purified using Qiagen RNeasy columns. Quantification was via UV spectrometry, and gel electrophoresis was used to assess quality.
2. cDNA was prepared from the purified RNA using the High-Capacity cDNA Archive kit utilizing random primers and reverse transcriptase from Applied Biosystems, Inc.
3. The cDNA fractions were analyzed on the Affymetrix Human Genome U133 Plus2 Array for mRNA profiling and the specifically designed chip by Almac Diagnostics, Almac Diagnostic Ovarian Cancer DSA™, for microRNA profiling.

2.3 Bioinformatics Toolbox

Numerous software packages are available for analyzing the data, and we have found many to be particularly useful (*see* **Note 3**).

2.3.1 Software (Freely Available or Installed)

1. Bioconductor/R (http://www.bioconductor.org; http://cbio.uct.ac.za/CRAN).
2. Affymetrix Power Tools (APT) (http://www.affymetrix.com/partners_programs/programs/developer/tools/powertools.affx).
3. Cluster 3.0 and Java TreeView for hierarchical clustering (http://www.eisenlab.org/eisen/?page_id=42).
4. Expander (http://acgt.cs.tau.ac.il/expander/).
5. KOBAS: KEGG Orthology-Based Annotation System (http://kobas.cbi.pku.edu.cn/).

2.3.2 Databases and Web Resources Used

1. GEO DataSets (http://www.ncbi.nlm.nih.gov/gds).
2. Stanford Microarray Database (http://smd.stanford.edu/).
3. ArrayExpress (http://www.ebi.ac.uk/arrayexpress/).

4. miRecords database (www.mirecords.biolead.org).
5. miRBase (www.mirbase.org/).
6. TargetScan (www.targetscan.org/).
7. MiRanda (www.microrna.org/microrna/home.do).
8. DAVID Functional Annotation Bioinformatics Microarray Analysis (http://david.abcc.ncifcrf.gov/).
9. Ovarian cancer DSA platform by Almac Diagnostics (Durham, NC, USA) (http://www.almacgroup.com/wp-content/uploads/Ovarian_Cancer_DSA_techsheet2.pdf).
10. Gene marker identification system marker (http://bioinfosrv1.bmb.uga.edu/DMarker/).

2.3.3 Computational and Statistical Algorithms Applied

1. Cluster Analysis and Visualization (http://bonsai.hgc.jp/~mdehoon/software/cluster/manual/index.html).
2. A QUalitative BI-Clustering algorithm (QUBIC) for gene expression analysis (http://csbl.bmb.uga.edu/~maqin/bicluster/).
3. A Support Vector Machine (SVM)-based classification strategy for gene markers identification (http://www.csie.ntu.edu.tw/~cjlin/libsvm/).

3 Methods

3.1 Gene Chip Quality Control

Before proceeding to a detailed analysis of the results, it is most important to ensure that the data obtained from gene microarrays are reliable. The quality control (QC) assessment contains two parts, the gene chip QC and sample integrity assessment.

3.1.1 Quality Metric Assessment

The first step is to assess the quality metrics of each hybridized array comprehensively, including examination of the percentage of the perfect match (PM) probe sets called "present" (detected over background) relative to the total number of probe sets on the array. In our case, the signal value was calculated using an Almac proprietary method that was optimized to provide the most similar results as those obtained with MAS5 [13] for this perfect PM-only chip design. Specifically the algorithm computes RMA (Robust Multi-array Average) [14] background depending on the GC content (in six GC classes: 1:7, 8:10, 11:13, 14:16, 17:19, 20:25). This computed GC Background, instead of the mismatch (MM), is used corresponding to the same GC content as the PM probe. Wilcoxon signed-rank test is applied on each probe set, and a probe set is called present if the *p*-value is less than 0.001. The mean, standard deviation, and lower and upper boundary of two standard deviations are also calculated for each metric (PM-only %P, RMA Background, mean raw intensity). The chip QC metric values were compared against the lower and upper boundary to identify significant deviation. The standard deviations should be small for all three metrics.

3.1.2 Control Gene Examination

Next, a few control genes should be examined to evaluate the chip quality from different aspects, including the following:

1. *Hybridization controls* on most GeneChip® arrays consist of four hybridization controls derived from three *E. coli* genes from the biotin synthesis pathway (bioB, bioC, bioD) and the recombinase gene from P1 bacteriophage (cre). The controls are prepared as a mixture of biotin-labeled cRNA transcripts in staggered concentrations (1.5, 5, 25, and 100 pM for bioB, bioC, bioD, and cre, respectively). The controls are spiked into each sample at the end of sample preparation and thus are used to evaluate hybridization efficiency. Following hybridization, then washing and scanning, the controls should show a generally increasing intensity to reflect their increasing concentrations. The bioB control should be called present at least 50 % of the time (as it is spiked in at the minimum threshold of assay sensitivity), while the other controls should be called present 100 % of the time.
2. *Poly A control genes* are derived from the lys, phe, thr, and dap genes from *Bacillus subtilis* that have been modified by the addition of Poly A tails. These control genes are spiked into the RNA samples at staggered concentrations prior to amplification and as such can be evaluated like internal control genes. For NuGEN RNA Amplification V2 processed samples, the Poly A control genes should all be present and demonstrate overall increasing signal intensities to reflect their increasing concentrations.
3. *GAPDH and β-actin housekeeping genes* can be used to assess the RNA sample and assay quality for GeneChip® arrays. The signal values for the 3′ probe sets are compared to the 5′ probe sets for both GAPDH and β-actin. For at least one of these housekeeping genes, the ratio of the 3′ probe set to the 5′ probe set should generally be no more than 3.0 for samples processed using the Affymetrix® One-cycle cDNA synthesis or the NuGEN™ RNA Amplification V2 protocol.

3.1.3 Data Amount Reduction

Subsequently, hierarchical clustering and principal components analyses were employed to assess the quality of the processed expression data before analysis. For example, only the 26,821 transcripts that passed the background filter, i.e., three times the standard deviation of the average background intensity of the 18 samples, were used for the analysis [10]:

1. *Hierarchical clustering.* A dendrogram/tree is created from the reliably detected transcripts with hierarchical clustering showing the relationships among samples based on the gene expression levels. This allows the identification of spurious samples. Similar samples should cluster together, based on the conditions/groups being assessed. The hierarchical tree as shown in Fig.1a has been created using the Average Link and Cosine correlation metric. Probe sets were selected by the criteria of intensity *p*-value of 0.05 or less and coefficient of variation of 0.3 or greater.
2. *Principal components analysis (PCA)* produces a set of expression patterns through decomposition. Linear combinations of these patterns can be assembled to represent the behavior of all of the samples in a given dataset based on their gene expression patterns. Data reduction characterizes the most abundant themes or building blocks that recur in many genes in the experiment. Again, samples from the same experimental condition should form distinct groups. A plot of the PCA results is shown in Fig. 1b. All of the samples fall into the expected groups, indicating a high level of sample integrity and minimal variation within groups.

   The results of clustering and data reduction were assessed comprehensively to ascertain the suitability of the results for further analysis (*see* **Note 4**).

3.2 Statistical Analyses

Statistical analyses were performed to identify the differentially expressed genes between any two groups, especially at the transition points when LHR and LH are introduced. Before starting this, we need to ensure that:

1. All the gene expression data have been normalized, which is particularly important when combining data from different experiments. The APT package can be used for summarizing probe intensity and quintile normalization (*see* **Note 3**). Other useful packages such as R/Bioconductor Expander [15] can be freely downloaded from their websites (*see* **Note 3**).
2. Genes having very low expression in both sample groups should be removed due to the extremely low signal-to-noise ratio; specifically, a gene was removed if its maximum (Expr. group1, Expr.group2) was below a certain threshold, for example, less than 4.0 (log2 transformed, normalized signal intensity) or within the 5 percentile of the expression range in an array (*see* **Note 5**).

Since the ovarian DSA is a high-density platform including only PM probes, the transcript expression was computed using the

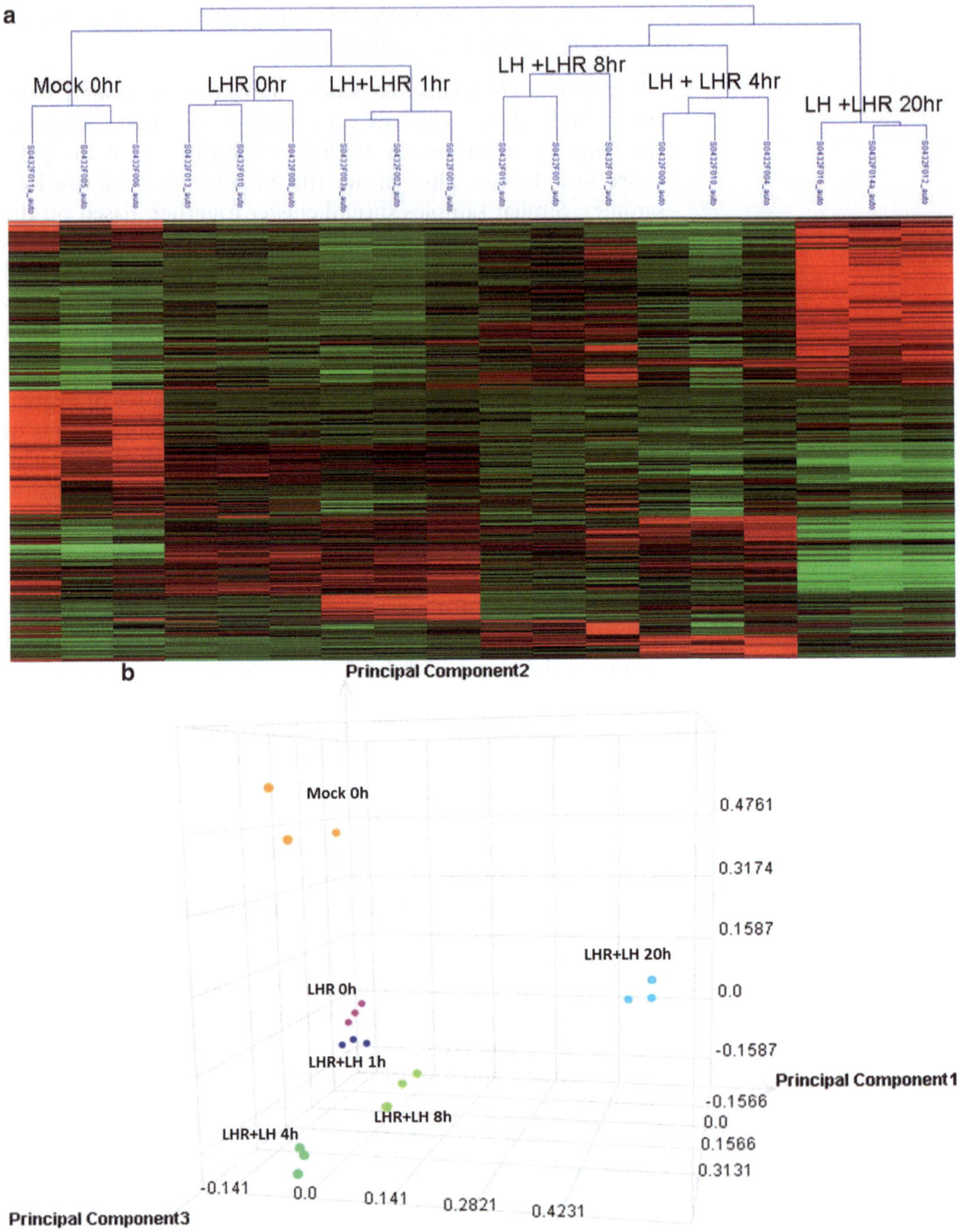

Fig. 1 Microarray data quality control by (**a**) hierarchical clustering and (**b**) PCA. In *Panel A*, the dendrogram/tree is created from the reliably detected transcripts using Average Link and Cosine correlation metric, showing the sample relationship based on the gene expression levels. Similar samples should cluster together. In *Panel B*, the expression patterns were produced through decomposition. Again, samples from the same experimental condition should form distinct groups from others. Overall, the results show all samples are grouped within the expected treatment or time point the results as the study design

PM-only normalization algorithm designed by Almac Diagnostics which is similar to MAS5. Transcripts with the maximum intensity among all 18 samples lower than 10 (without log-transform) were removed, and the geometric mean expression of each transcript was calculated from the triplicates in each group.

The Student's *t*-test and Mann–Whitney test can be used to test the null hypothesis that the means of two normally distributed populations are equal, while the latter one is more suitable for small sample size without requiring a normal distribution. Equal variance is normally considered if there are no evidential clues showing that the two distributions are different. For those with multiple groups (as our study including time points of LHR– control, LHR+, LHR+ treated 1–20 h with LH), ANOVA [16] can be used to examine if the gene expression is altered in any of the transition points when compared against others. Normally, only genes with a differential expression change of more than 1.5-fold (or two-fold), with the p-value < 0.05 adjusted for multiple test by R package, were accepted for further analysis. In our study, we also restrained FDR < 0.1 and more rigorously focused on those expression changes consistently observed at the transition points, which means the expression levels of the triplicate measures of group A are all higher (or lower) than those of group B. Overall, the experimental design, coupled with the statistical significance and fold-change criteria employed, engenders high confidence of selecting reliable differential expressions.

If the data include paired information, for example, the gene expression from a primary tumor and its corresponding normal tissue control, or from cells with treatment and their control, one can take advantage of this information to evaluate if the differential expression is consistent within those samples paired in addition to the general comparison between the tumor and control group. Besides paired *t*-test and Wilcoxon signed-rank test, we have also applied another simple statistical test as follows when dealing with paired samples: Given the hypothesis (H_0) that a particular gene does not show differential expression (more than k-fold change) in treated cells versus its control cells across the majority of the sample pairs (p-value < 0.05), the rejection of this hypothesis means that the gene is differentially expressed in treated cells versus control. Let $N[i]$ and $C[i]$, $i = 1 \ldots m$, be the genes expressions in the i-th pair of control and treated cells and m be the total number of sample pairs. If the hypothesis H_0 is true, then the probability $P(N[i] > C[i]) = P(N[i] < C[i]) = 0.5$, assuming that gene expression is a continuous random variable. Let K be the number of pairs with $N[i]/C[i] > 0.5$, then based on the Central Limit Theorem, the random variable K/m approximately follows a normal distribution with its mean = 0.5 and a standard variation = $0.5/\sqrt{m}$, or $X = 2K/\sqrt{m}$ follows a normal distribution $N(0, 1)$. Thus, the p-value can be estimated as $P(X > 2K_{\exp}/\sqrt{m})$, where $K_{\exp}$ is the experimentally observed number of pairs with $P(N[i] < C[i])$. Again, we consider a gene being differentially expressed if the statistical significance, *p*-value, is less than 0.05 and its fold change is at least 2.0. In some cases, the calculated *p*-value will not be adjusted on the multiple hypotheses testing in order to avoid any loss of genes that may be potentially effective if more rigorous classification analysis is carried out subsequently.

3.3 Co-expression Clustering Analysis

In order to identify expression patterns, it is necessary to perform hierarchical clustering [17]. This procedure also enables one to ascertain important biological functional families and determine cellular pathways. Three of the most popular clustering analyses include the following:

1. *K*-mean clustering: define *k*, the number of clusters in which to partition selected genes or conditions into. The algorithm attempts to minimize intracluster variability and maximize intercluster variability.
2. Hierarchical clustering: produce a gene/condition tree where the most similar expression profiles are joined together.
3. SOM (Self-Organizing Map) clustering: similar to *k*-means but also produces information about similarity between the clusters.

Clustering 3.0, by Michael Eisen, is one of the earliest and most popular programs that implements a hierarchical clustering algorithm and is available (*see* **Note 3**). TreeView is a complementary tool to graphically browse results of clustering (e.g., Fig. 2a), which supports tree-based and image-based browsing of hierarchical trees, as well as multiple output formats for generation of images for publication. A complete online manual is available that provides detailed guidance for data loading, filtering, and adjusting and the setting of the distance/similarity measures in clusters, as well as visualization of hierarchical clustering results with Java TreeView (*see* **Note 6**).

For those who are interested in finding expression patterns within subgroup of the samples, our in-house bi-clustering QUBIC (QUalitative BI-Clustering) program can be used to identify statistically significant bi-clusters in the data [18]. The basic idea of the algorithm is to find all subgroups of genes with similar expression patterns among some (to be identified) subsets of samples, and hence, genes involved in each such pattern can possibly be used as signatures for sample subgrouping such as cancer subtyping or staging. QUBIC can solve the more general form of the bi-clustering problem in a computationally efficient manner (*see* **Note 7**).

In our study on cultured human ovarian cancer cells, SOM [19] was applied, which is a different algorithm from hierarchical clustering but also useful for extracting co-expression patterns associated with LHR expression and LH-mediated activation (Fig. 2b). The commercial package, GeneSpring GX from Agilent and free software Expander [15], integrates different functionalities of doing clustering analysis.

3.4 Functional Enrichment Analysis

Within a given set of genes, possible from the previous clustering analysis, one may apply the gene annotation to examine if certain GO terms (molecular function, biological process, or cellular location) and pathway or functional processes are involved. Different tests such as the hypergeometric test can be carried out with multiple testing corrections to handle multiple GO term testing and correlations between them.

BiNGO is a Java-based tool for GO term enrichment analysis, a plug-in for Cytoscape, which is an open-source bioinformatics software platform for visualizing and integrating molecular

a

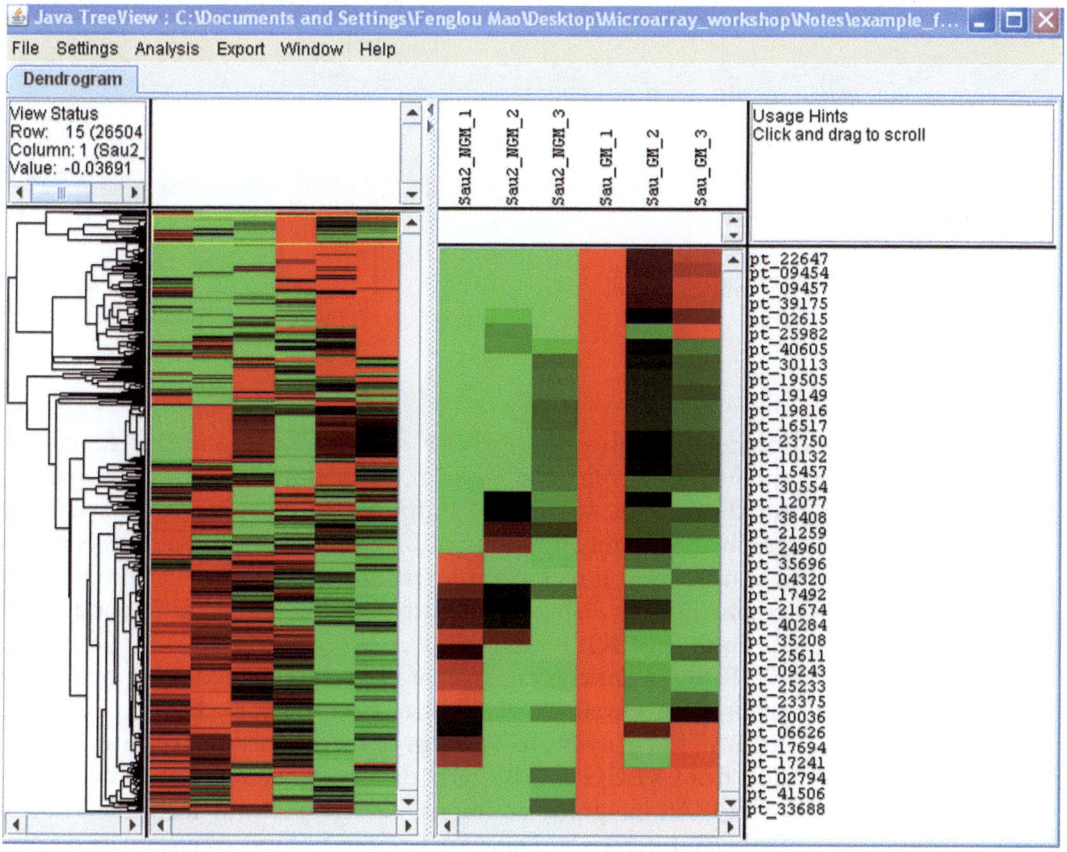

Fig. 2 Output of clustering analyses by (**a**) hierarchical clustering using Cluster 3.0 and visualized in Java TreeView and (**b**) SMO which identified 12 co-expression clusters from the differentially expressed genes. Genes with similar expression pattern cluster together, as shown in each figure

b

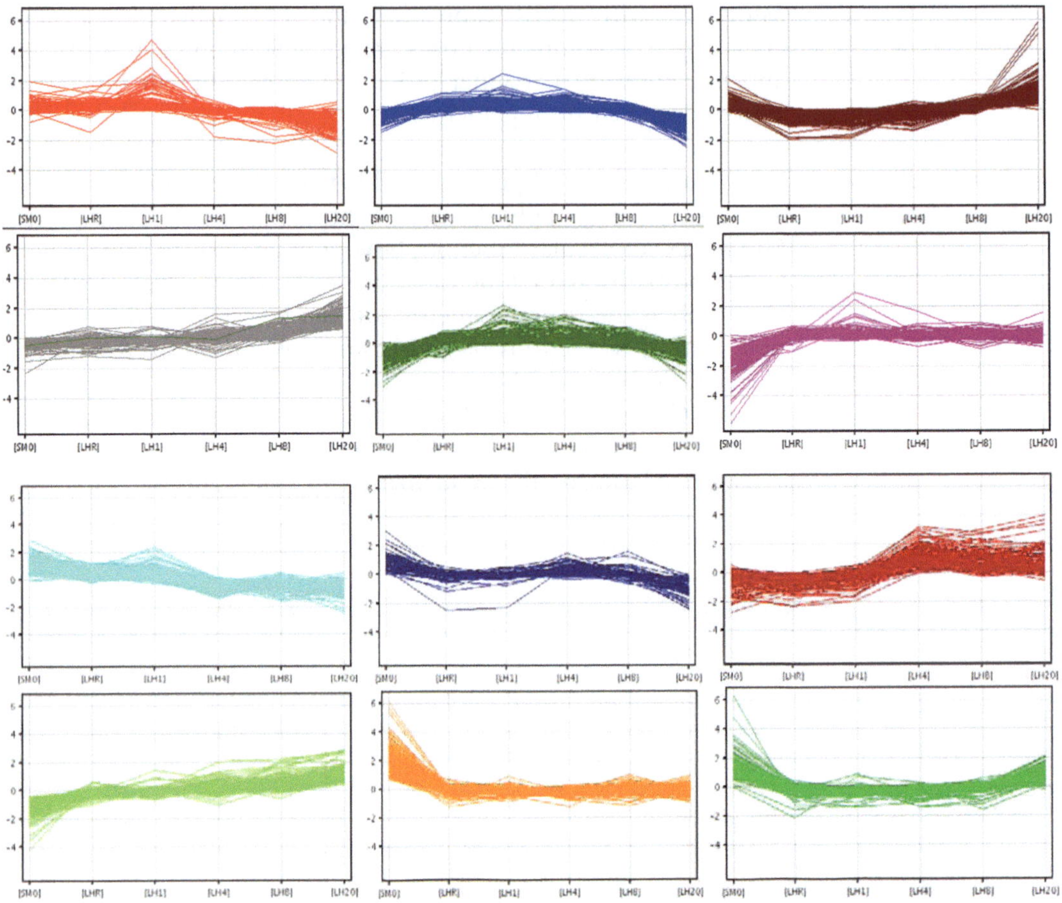

Fig. 2 (continued)

interaction networks. BiNGO maps the predominant functional themes of a given gene set (e.g., derived from microarray analysis) on the GO hierarchy and outputs this mapping as a Cytoscape graph. The main advantage of BiNGO over other GO tools is that it can be used directly and interactively on molecular interactions graphs. Figure 3 shows the output of the GO enrichment analysis through BiNGO.

Pathway enrichment analysis can be conducted using two popular programs available at no charge to the user, DAVID [20] and KOBAS [21] (*see* **Note 3**). Most of these tools use pathway annotation from KEGG and Biocarta databases, while an updated version of KOBAS integrates additional curated pathway from the Human Pathway Interaction Database [22] and others to ensure a comprehensive coverage. If in-house annotation is given, one can calculate the statistical *p*-value for each relevant pathway based on Fisher's exact test on queried genes against the entire human genome.

3.5 Signature Identification from Transcriptome Profiling and Blood-Secreted Prediction

For any two given sample groups, one important research topic is to identify a minimal subset of genes whose expression can discriminate one group from the other, although this was not one of the major questions in our ovarian cancer study. Assuming that one has a set of microarray data from ovarian cancer cases and health groups, or two subtypes of ovarian cancer, here we will demonstrate a Support Vector Machine (SVM)-based strategy to find gene markers (signatures) for ovarian cancer or its subtypes.

The most popular feature (gene) selection tool provided in LIBSVM can be used, which is available (*see* **Note 8**). An *F*-score, defined as follows, is used to measure the discerning power of each feature value to the classification problem:

$$F(i) = \frac{(\overline{x}_i^{+} - \overline{x}_i)^2 + (\overline{x}_i^{-} - \overline{x}_i)^2}{\frac{1}{n_+ - 1}\sum_{k=1}^{n+}\left(x_{k,i}^{+} + -\overline{x}_i^{+}\right)^2 + \frac{1}{n_- - 1}\sum_{k=1}^{n-}\left(x_{k,i}^{-} - \overline{x}_i^{-}\right)}$$

where X_k refers to the training feature values ($k = 1,\ldots, m$); n_+ and n_- are the number of samples in the positive (+) and negative (−) groups of the training dataset, respectively, $\overline{x}_i$, $\overline{x}_i^{+}$ and $\overline{x}_i^{-}$ are the averages of the i-th feature value across the whole training dataset, the positive dataset and the negative dataset, respectively, $x_{k,i}^{+}$ and $x_{k,i}^{-}$ are the i-th feature of the k-th sample in the positive and negative training data, respectively. Generally, the larger an F-score, the more discriminative the corresponding feature is. To find an optimal F-score threshold, one should consider a list of possible

a

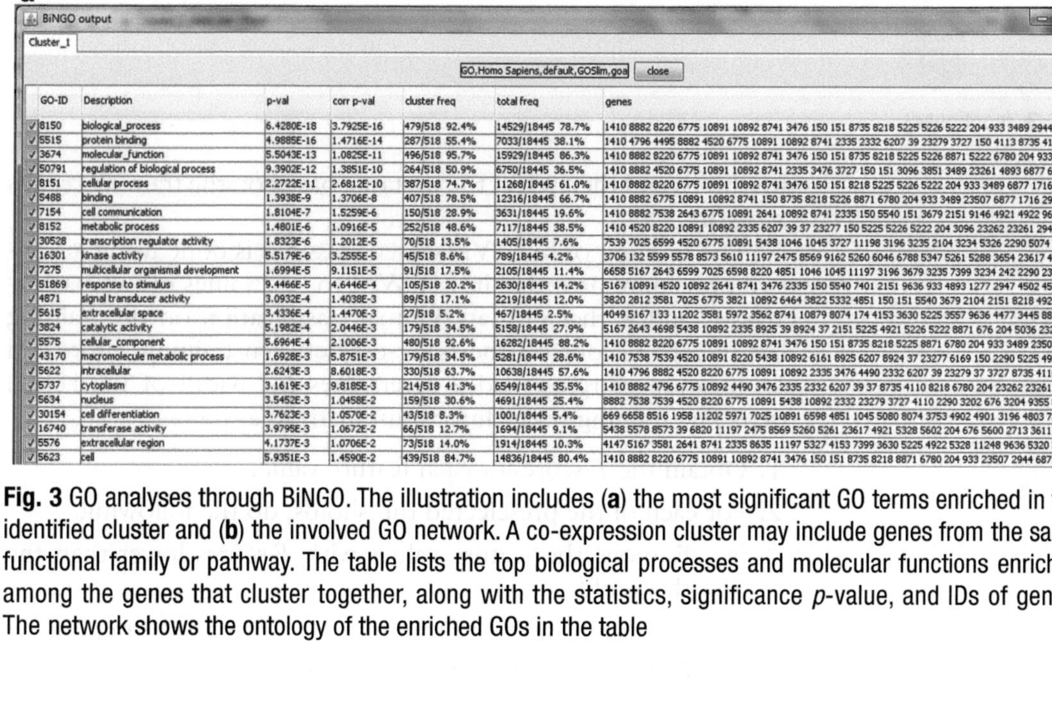

GO-ID	Description	p-val	corr p-val	cluster freq	total freq	genes
8150	biological_process	6.4280E-18	3.7925E-16	479/518 92.4%	14529/18445 78.7%	1410 8882 8220 6775 10891 10892 8741 3476 150 151 8735 8218 5225 5226 5222 204 933 3489 2944 687
5515	protein binding	4.9885E-16	1.4716E-14	287/518 55.4%	7033/18445 38.1%	1410 4796 4495 8882 4520 6775 10891 10892 8741 2335 2332 6207 39 23279 3727 150 4113 8735 4110 8
3674	molecular_function	5.5043E-13	1.0825E-11	496/518 95.7%	15929/18445 86.3%	1410 8882 8220 6775 10891 10892 8741 3476 150 151 8735 8218 5225 5226 8871 5222 6780 204 933 348
50791	regulation of biological process	9.3902E-12	1.3851E-10	264/518 50.9%	6750/18445 36.5%	1410 8882 4520 6775 10891 10892 8741 2335 3476 3727 150 151 3096 3851 3489 23261 4893 6877 6776
8151	cellular process	2.2722E-11	2.6812E-10	387/518 74.7%	11268/18445 61.0%	1410 8882 8220 6775 10891 10892 8741 3476 150 151 8218 5225 5226 5222 204 933 3489 6877 1716 294
5488	binding	1.3938E-9	1.3706E-8	407/518 78.5%	12316/18445 66.7%	1410 8882 6775 10891 10892 8741 150 8735 8218 5226 8871 6780 204 933 3489 23507 6877 1716 2947 6
7154	cell communication	1.8104E-7	1.5259E-6	150/518 28.9%	3631/18445 19.6%	1410 8882 7538 2643 6775 10891 2641 10892 8741 2335 150 5540 151 3679 2151 9146 4921 4922 9636 3
8152	metabolic process	1.4801E-6	1.0916E-5	252/518 48.6%	7117/18445 38.5%	1410 4520 8220 10891 10892 2335 6207 39 37 23277 150 5225 5226 5222 204 3096 23262 23261 2944 68
30528	transcription regulator activity	1.8323E-6	1.2012E-5	70/518 13.5%	1405/18445 7.6%	7539 7025 6599 4520 6775 10891 5438 1046 1045 3727 11198 3196 3235 2104 3234 5326 2290 5074 3202
16301	kinase activity	5.5179E-6	3.2555E-5	45/518 8.6%	789/18445 4.2%	3706 132 5599 5578 8573 5610 11197 2475 8569 9162 5260 6046 6788 5347 5261 5288 3654 23617 4058
7275	multicellular organismal development	1.6994E-5	9.1151E-5	91/518 17.5%	2105/18445 11.4%	6658 5167 2643 6599 7025 6598 8220 4851 1046 1045 11197 3196 3679 3235 7399 3234 242 2290 23617
51869	response to stimulus	9.4466E-5	4.6446E-4	105/518 20.2%	2630/18445 14.2%	5167 10891 4520 10892 2641 8741 3476 2335 150 5540 7401 2151 9636 933 4893 1277 2947 4502 4501 1
4871	signal transducer activity	3.0932E-4	1.4038E-3	89/518 17.1%	2219/18445 12.0%	3820 2812 3581 7025 6775 3821 10892 6464 3822 5332 4851 150 151 5540 3679 2104 2151 8218 4921 41
5615	extracellular space	3.4336E-4	1.4470E-3	27/518 5.2%	467/18445 2.5%	4049 5167 133 11202 3581 5972 3562 8741 10879 8074 174 4153 3630 5225 3557 9636 4477 3445 8822 3
3824	catalytic activity	5.1982E-4	2.0446E-3	179/518 34.5%	5158/18445 27.9%	5167 2643 4698 5438 10892 2335 8925 39 8924 37 2151 5225 4921 5226 5222 8871 676 204 5036 23262 2
5575	cellular_component	5.6964E-4	2.1006E-3	480/518 92.6%	16282/18445 88.2%	1410 8882 8220 6775 10891 10892 8741 3476 150 151 8735 8218 5225 8871 6780 204 933 3489 23507 29
43170	macromolecule metabolic process	1.6928E-3	5.8751E-3	179/518 34.5%	5281/18445 28.6%	1410 7538 7539 4520 10891 8220 5438 10892 6161 8925 6207 8924 37 23277 6169 150 2290 5225 4921 5
5622	intracellular	2.6243E-3	8.6018E-3	330/518 63.7%	10638/18445 57.6%	1410 4796 8882 4520 8220 6775 10891 10892 2335 3476 4490 2332 6207 39 23279 37 3727 8735 4110 82
5737	cytoplasm	3.1619E-3	9.8185E-3	214/518 41.3%	6549/18445 35.5%	1410 8882 4796 6775 10892 4490 3476 2335 2332 6207 39 37 8735 4110 8218 6780 204 23262 23261 489
5634	nucleus	3.5452E-3	1.0458E-2	159/518 30.6%	4691/18445 25.4%	8882 7538 7539 4520 8220 6775 10891 5438 10892 2332 23279 3727 4110 2290 3202 676 3204 9355 8545
30154	cell differentiation	3.7623E-3	1.0570E-2	43/518 8.3%	1001/18445 5.4%	669 6658 8516 1958 11202 5971 7025 10891 6598 4851 1045 5080 8074 3753 4902 4901 3196 4803 7335
16740	transferase activity	3.9795E-3	1.0672E-2	66/518 12.7%	1694/18445 9.1%	5438 5578 8573 39 6820 11197 2475 8569 5260 5261 23617 4921 5328 5602 204 676 5600 2713 3611 425
5576	extracellular region	4.1737E-3	1.0706E-2	73/518 14.0%	1914/18445 10.3%	4147 5167 3581 2641 8741 2335 8635 11197 5327 4153 7399 3630 5225 4922 5328 11248 9636 5320 3489
5623	cell	5.9351E-3	1.4590E-2	439/518 84.7%	14836/18445 80.4%	1410 8882 8220 6775 10891 10892 8741 3476 150 151 8735 8218 8871 6780 204 933 23507 2944 6877 171

Fig. 3 GO analyses through BiNGO. The illustration includes (**a**) the most significant GO terms enriched in the identified cluster and (**b**) the involved GO network. A co-expression cluster may include genes from the same functional family or pathway. The table lists the top biological processes and molecular functions enriched among the genes that cluster together, along with the statistics, significance *p*-value, and IDs of genes. The network shows the ontology of the enriched GOs in the table

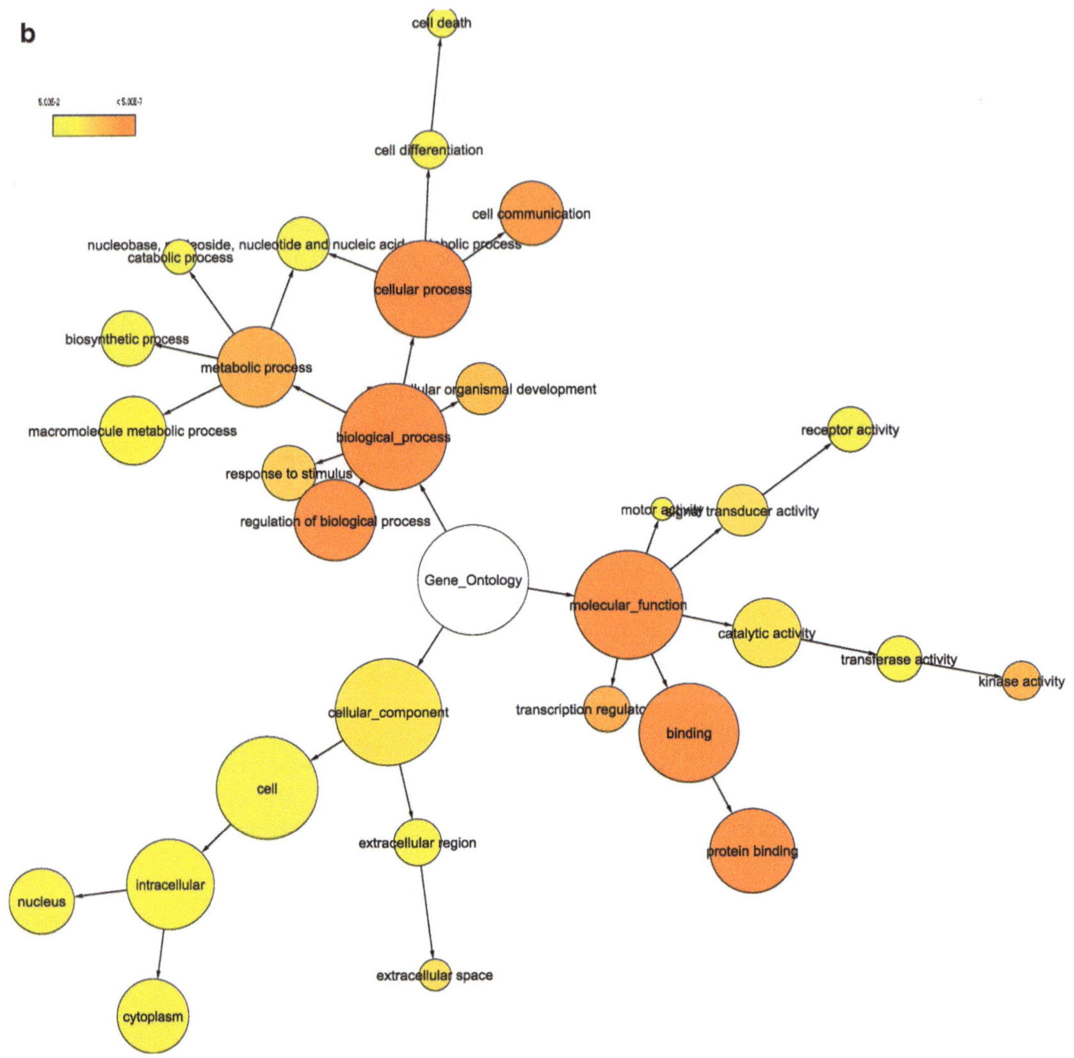

Fig. 3 (continued)

thresholds and then select the best one based on the training results (*see* **Note 9**).

The training of our SVM-based classifier is done using a standard procedure provided in LIBSVM to find values of two parameters, C and γ, that give an optimal classification on the training data, where C controls the trade-off between training errors and classification margins, and γ determines the width of the kernel used. The training procedure is summarized as follows:

1. Obtain the F-score for each feature value.
2. For each of the preselected thresholds, do the following:
   (a) Remove the feature values with F-scores lower than the threshold.
   (b) Randomly split the training data into a sub-training set and a sub-validation set of equal size.

(c) Train an SVM with an RBF kernel on the sub-training set to search for optimal values of C and γ, and then apply it to the sub-validation data and calculate the classification error.

(d) Repeat **steps** (**a–c**) five times and calculate the average validation error.

3. Choose the threshold that gives the lowest average validation error and keep the features with *F*-score above the selected threshold.
4. Retrain an SVM based on the selected features as the final classifier.

An optional SVM recursive feature elimination procedure (RFE-SVM) and an exhaustive search strategy have also been introduced [23, 24]. To further assess the specificity of these marker genes, one can use a biomarker evaluation system to check if the expression pattern of the predicted markers could also be caused by other human diseases (*see* **Note 10**). This database collects the microarray datasets from the GEO [25], Oncomine [26], and SMD [27] for human diseases.

We recently developed a method to predict proteins that are likely to be secreted into the blood, thus enabling the search for serum biomarkers [28, 29]. When coupled with transcriptome profiling, this becomes a powerful approach to add specificity to the search for accurate and reliable disease markers (*see* **Note 11**).

3.6 MicroRNA Target and Functional Analysis

The determination of microRNA function is a challenging prospect in part because a given microRNA can regulate a number of genes. One approach to examine possible microRNA function is to study the biological processes in which its gene targets are involved, which introduces another challenging issue, microRNA target prediction:

1. First, microRNAs and the detailed information of their host gene are available from miRBase [30]. Gene loci thus can be obtained from Ensemble (hg19 version). The microRNA expression profiles can be analyzed to identify differentially expressed microRNAs (Subheading 3.2).
2. Except for the known mRNA targets from the miRecords database [31], there are numerous computational algorithms for predicting microRNA/mRNA interaction on information embodied in the sequence and structure [32], including TargetScan 5.1, miRanda, and miRecord databases. Since most of these programs are questioned by the high false-positive prediction, MiRanda [33] and TargetScan [34] are suggested as the most reliable tools (*see* **Note 12**).
3. To further exclude false predictions, the Spearman's rank Rho coefficient between expression levels of the microRNA and

their targets was calculated based on the following. Given X_i and Y_i with $i = 1 \ldots n$ representing the expression profiles of microRNA and mRNA, where $n = 6$ represents six distinct cellular states in order of LHR−, LHR+, LH1, LH4, LH8, and LH20, the expression level was converted to ranks x_i, and y_i, respectively. The difference, $d_i = x_i - y_i$, between the ranks of each observation was calculated, and the coefficient is given by $\text{rho} = 1 - \frac{6\sum d_i^2}{n(n^2-1)}$, where rho > 0, rho < 0 and rho = 0 represent a positive, negative, or no regulatory effect between microRNA and mRNA. Given the null hypothesis H_0 that x_i and y_i are independent, a two-tailed test was conducted where the *p*-value is given as $p - \text{value} = 2 \cdot \text{P}(\text{Z} \geq |\text{r}|\sqrt{n-1})$. Those correlated pairs with modestly relaxed significance (|rho| > 0.8, *p*-value ≤ 0.05) were the focus for further analysis.

4. Among all possible microRNA–mRNA pairs, significant correlations were detected using (|rho| > 0.8, *p*-value <0.05). It shows that most microRNAs have more positively correlated microRNA–mRNA pairs than negatively correlated pairs. With the cutoffs used above, only 155 genes were retained as high-confident ones, i.e., negatively correlated with microRNA and differentially expressed, for functional analysis. Similarly, the correlation between each microRNA and its host gene was studied (*see* **Note 13**).
5. For each microRNA found to be differentially expressed [12], one can carry out functional enrichment analysis (Subheading 3.4) on its target genes, which can thus provide some indication of the function of the microRNA.

4 Notes

1. Public microarray databases:
   - GEO DataSets, NCBI (National Center for Biotechnology Information):
     http://www.ncbi.nlm.nih.gov/gds
   - SMD, Stanford Microarray Database:
     http://smd.stanford.edu/
   - Oncomine Research Edition, COMPENDIA BIOSCIENCE, INC.:
     https://www.oncomine.org/resource/login.html
   - ArrayExpress, EBI (European Bioinformatics Institute):
     http://www.ebi.ac.uk/arrayexpress/
   - ChipDB, Whitehead Institute for Biomedical Research/MIT Centre for Genome Research:
     http://chipdb.wi.mit.edu/chipdb/public/

- Dragon, Johns Hopkins University: http://pevsnerlab.kennedykrieger.org/dragon.htm

2. The following website provides the detailed information on the ovarian cancer DSA platform used in this study: http://www.almacgroup.com/wp-content/uploads/Ovarian_Cancer_DSA_techsheet2.pdf.
3. Public tools for data analysis:
   - Mev microarray analysis package: http://www.tm4.org/
   - Bioconductor/R: http://www.bioconductor.org and http://cbio.uct.ac.za/CRAN
   - The APT package for summarizing probe intensity and quintile normalization: http://www.affymetrix.com/partners_programs/programs/developer/tools/powertools.affx
   - SIMCA-P: http://www.umetrics.com/default.asp/pagename/software_simcap/c/3
   - Cluster 3.0 and Java TreeView for hierarchical clustering: http://www.eisenlab.org/eisen/?page_id=42
   - Expander: http://acgt.cs.tau.ac.il/expander/
   - DAVID Functional Annotation Bioinformatics Microarray Analysis: http://david.abcc.ncifcrf.gov/
   - KOBAS (KEGG Orthology-Based Annotation System): http://kobas.cbi.pku.edu.cn/
   - Others: http://www.nslij-enetics.org/microarray/soft.html
4. Outlier (either gene or sample) should be removed from further analysis if it fails any control step of the quality control; data normalization across different samples is important and is normally needed after summarizing the probe expression using RMA, either through scaling or quintile normalization depending on the feature of the data.
5. Genes whose expression is significantly missing, for instance, in more than 20 % of the samples, should be removed from clustering analysis. However, it may work for bi-clustering if it is correlated with subtyping.
6. A manual that provides assistance in data loading, filtering, and adjusting; the setting of distance/similarity measures in clusters; and visualization of hierarchical clustering data with Java TreeView is available as follows: http://bonsai.hgc.jp/~mdehoon/software/cluster/cluster3.pdf.
7. A program, QUBIC, which solves the general form of the bi-clustering problem can be accessed at http://csbl.bmb.uga.edu/~maqin/bicluster/.

8. The following site is helpful when seeking an SVM-based strategy to identify gene markers.
9. Within the whole dataset, there should be no bias for dividing the training and testing datasets for signature identification through classification. Random separation for multiple times is normally needed.
10. The website below is useful in determining the specificity of marker genes. http://bioinfosrv1.bmb.uga.edu/DMarker/.
11. This in-house package can be used to identify proteins likely to be secreted into the blood, thus rendering them as potential biomarkers.
12. miRNA database and target prediction tools:
    - miRecords database: www.mirecords.biolead.org
    - miRBase: the microRNA database: www.mirbase.org/
    - TargetScan: www.targetscan.org/
    - MiRanda: www.microrna.org/microrna/home.do
13. One possible explanation for the poor correlations between microRNA and its host gene is that the microRNAs may have their own regulatory elements rather than sharing the same with their host genes. To confirm this possibility, one can search for the transcriptional features in flanking sequences of microRNA precursors such as transcription start sites (TSS), CpG islands, and transcription factor binding sites (TFBS), compared to the same analysis on the host genes. Of course, one cannot exclude the possibility that some microRNAs may regulate their host gene through the mRNA degradation machinery.

Acknowledgements

This research was supported by NIH (DK069711, DK033973, and GM075331) and NSF (DBI-0354771, ITR-IIS-0407204, CCF-0621700, and DBI-0542119).

References

1. American Cancer Society http://www.cancer.org. Cancer Facts and Statistics. Last Revised: 10/13/2010 ed.
2. Kwintkiewicz J, Giudice LC (2009) The interplay of insulin-like growth factors, gonadotropins, and endocrine disruptors in ovarian follicular development and function. Semin Reprod Med 27:43–51
3. Ozols RF, Bookman MA, Connolly DC, Daly MB, Godwin AK et al (2004) Focus on epithelial ovarian cancer. Cancer Cell 5:19–24
4. Mosgaard BJ, Lidegaard O, Kjaer SK, Schou G, Andersen AN (1997) Infertility, fertility drugs, and invasive ovarian cancer: a case-control study. Fertil Steril 67:1005–1012
5. Sanner K, Conner P, Bergfeldt K, Dickman P, Sundfeldt K et al (2009) Ovarian epithelial neoplasia after hormonal infertility treatment: long-term follow-up of a historical cohort in Sweden. Fertil Steril 91:1152–1158
6. Huhtaniemi I (2010) Are gonadotrophins tumorigenic–a critical review of clinical and

experimental data. Mol Cell Endocrinol 329:56–61

7. Leung PC, Choi JH (2007) Endocrine signaling in ovarian surface epithelium and cancer. Hum Reprod Update 13:143–162
8. Ries L, Melbert D, Krapcho M, Stinchcomb D, Howlader N, et al (2008) SEER cancer statistics review http://seer.cancer.gov/csr/1975_2010/. In: Bethesda M (ed), National Cancer Institute.
9. Choi JH, Wong AS, Huang HF, Leung PC (2007) Gonadotropins and ovarian cancer. Endocr Rev 28:440–461
10. Cui J, Miner BM, Eldredge JB, Warrenfeltz SW, Dam P et al (2011) Regulation of gene expression in ovarian cancer cells by luteinizing hormone receptor expression and activation. BMC Cancer 11:280
11. Warrenfeltz SW, Lott SA, Palmer TM, Gray JC, Puett D (2008) Luteinizing hormone-induced up-regulation of ErbB-2 is insufficient stimulant of growth and invasion in ovarian cancer cells. Mol Cancer Res 6:1775–1785
12. Cui J, Eldredge JB, Xu Y, Puett D (2011) MicroRNA expression and regulation in human ovarian carcinoma cells by luteinizing hormone. PLoS One 6:e21730
13. Hubbell E, Liu WM, Mei R (2002) Robust estimators for expression analysis. Bioinformatics 18:1585–1592
14. Irizarry RA, Hobbs B, Collin F, Beazer-Barclay YD, Antonellis KJ et al (2003) Exploration, normalization, and summaries of high density oligonucleotide array probe level data. Biostatistics 4:249–264
15. Shamir R, Maron-Katz A, Tanay A, Linhart C, Steinfeld I et al (2005) EXPANDER–an integrative program suite for microarray data analysis. BMC Bioinformatics 6:232
16. Affymetrix whitepaper: Alternative Transcript Analysis Methods for Exon Arrays (2005) http://media.affymetrix.com/support/technical/whitepapers/exon_alt_transcript_analysis_whitepaper.pdf.
17. Eisen MB, Spellman PT, Brown PO, Botstein D (1998) Cluster analysis and display of genome-wide expression patterns. Proc Natl Acad Sci USA 95:14863–14868
18. Li G, Ma Q, Tang H, Paterson AH, Xu Y (2009) QUBIC: a qualitative biclustering algorithm for analyses of gene expression data. Nucleic Acids Res 37:e101
19. Kohonen T (1982) Self-organized formation of topologically correct feature maps. Biol Cybern 43:59–69
20. Dennis G Jr, Sherman BT, Hosack DA, Yang J, Gao W et al (2003) DAVID: database for annotation, visualization, and integrated discovery. Genome Biol 4:P3
21. Wu J, Mao X, Cai T, Luo J, Wei L (2006) KOBAS server: a web-based platform for automated annotation and pathway identification. Nucleic Acids Res 34:W720–724
22. Schaefer CF, Anthony K, Krupa S, Buchoff J, Day M et al (2009) PID: the pathway interaction database. Nucleic Acids Res 37:D674–679
23. Inza I, Larranaga P, Blanco R, Cerrolaza AJ (2004) Filter versus wrapper gene selection approaches in DNA microarray domains. Artif Intell Med 31:91–103
24. Cui J, Chen Y, Chou WC, Sun L, Chen L et al (2011) An integrated transcriptomic and computational analysis for biomarker identification in gastric cancer. Nucleic Acids Res 39:1197–1207
25. Barrett T, Suzek TO, Troup DB, Wilhite SE, Ngau WC et al (2005) NCBI GEO: mining millions of expression profiles–database and tools. Nucleic Acids Res 33:D562–566
26. Rhodes DR, Yu J, Shanker K, Deshpande N, Varambally R et al (2004) ONCOMINE: a cancer microarray database and integrated data-mining platform. Neoplasia 6:1–6
27. Sherlock G, Hernandez-Boussard T, Kasarskis A, Binkley G, Matese JC et al (2001) The Stanford microarray database. Nucleic Acids Res 29:152–155
28. Liu Q, Cui J, Yang Q, Xu Y (2010) In-silico prediction of blood-secretory human proteins using a ranking algorithm. BMC Bioinformatics 11:250
29. Cui J, Liu Q, Puett D, Xu Y (2008) Computational prediction of human proteins that can be secreted into the bloodstream. Bioinformatics 24:2370–2375
30. Griffiths-Jones S, Grocock RJ, van Dongen S, Bateman A, Enright AJ (2006) miRBase: microRNA sequences, targets and gene nomenclature. Nucleic Acids Res 34:D140–144
31. Xiao F, Zuo Z, Cai G, Kang S, Gao X et al (2009) miRecords: an integrated resource for microRNA-target interactions. Nucleic Acids Res 37:D105–110
32. Dai Y, Zhou X (2010) Computational methods for the identification of microRNA targets. Open Access Bioinformatics 2010:29–39
33. Miranda KC, Huynh T, Tay Y, Ang YS, Tam WL et al (2006) A pattern-based method for the identification of MicroRNA binding sites and their corresponding heteroduplexes. Cell 126:1203–1217
34. Lewis BP, Burge CB, Bartel DP (2005) Conserved seed pairing, often flanked by adenosines, indicates that thousands of human genes are microRNA targets. Cell 120:15–20

Chapter 12

Deep Transcriptome Profiling of Ovarian Cancer Cells Using Next-Generation Sequencing Approach

Lisha Li, Jie Liu, Wei Yu, Xiaoyan Lou, Bingding Huang, and Biaoyang Lin

Abstract

The next-generation sequencing technology allows identification and cataloging of almost all mRNAs, even those with only one or a few transcripts per cell. To understand the chemotherapy response program in ovarian cancer cells at deep transcript sequencing levels, we applied two next-generation sequencing technologies to study two ovarian chemotherapy response models: the in vitro acquired cisplatin-resistant cell line model (IGROV-1-CP and IGROV1) and the in vivo ovarian cancer tissue resistant model. We identified 3,422 signatures (2,957 genes) that are significantly differentially expressed between IGROV1 and IGROV-1-CP cells ($P < 0.001$). Our database offers the first comprehensive view of the digital transcriptomes of ovarian cancer cell lines and tissues with different chemotherapy response phenotypes.

Key words Ovarian cancer, Gene expression, Next-generation sequencing, RNA-seq, Cufflinks, SAMtools

1 Introduction

Gene expression profiling relying on RNA hybridization on high-density arrays has several shortcomings including (1) limited coverage as it relies on sequence-specific probe on the arrays for hybridization and (2) background and cross hybridization which again limited the detection sensitivity to medium- and high-expression transcripts. Digital transcript-counting approaches based on newly developed next-generation sequencing (NGS) overcome many of the inherent limitations of array-based approaches and bypass problems inherent to data analysis from analog measurements in the array-based approaches, including complex normalization procedures and limitations in detecting low-abundance transcripts [1].

There are several platforms of NGS, each with its advantages and disadvantages [2, 3]. The most common platforms are the 454 sequencing (used in the 454 Genome Sequencers, Roche Applied Science, Basel), HiSeq 2000 (Genome Analyzer, Illumina, USA),

Anastasia Malek and Oleg Tchernitsa (eds.), *Ovarian Cancer: Methods and Protocols*, Methods in Molecular Biology, vol. 1049, DOI 10.1007/978-1-62703-547-7_12, © Springer Science+Business Media New York 2013

the SOLiD platform (Applied Biosystems, Foster City, CA, USA), the HeliScope Single Molecule Sequencer technology (Helicos, Cambridge, MA, USA), and the integrated system including DNA nanoballs, nanoarrays, and combinatorial probe-anchor ligation (cPAL™)-based DNA sequencing by Complete Genomics, Inc. (Mountain View, CA, USA). Each of the NGS platforms has their own technical principles and unique characteristics [4]. For example, the Roche 454 platform generates longer read lengths, approaching those of Sanger sequencing (700–1,000 base pairs (bp)), but the sequence capacity is much lower than the that of Illumina (HiSeq) and Life Technologies (SOLiD 5,500), which generate many more sequence reads (800 million to 1 billion reads) but of a much shorter length (<150 bp).

NGS can be used for many applications from whole genome sequencing, targeted genomic sequencing, chromatin immunoprecipitation sequencing (ChIP-seq), RNA-seq, etc. [5]. In this chapter, we will just focus on RNA-seq. RNA-seq, which allows the detection of 0.3 RNA copies per cell [6], is currently the most robust discovery tool for profiling mRNA as well as other species of RNAs (e.g., microRNAs, antisense RNAs, snoRNAs). Furthermore, it has the potential to discover novel transcripts, novel isoforms, new alternatively spliced sites, rare transcripts, and cSNPs (coding region single-nucleotide polymorphisms) in one experiment.

We applied two next-generation sequencing technologies—MPSS (massively parallel signature sequencing) and SBS (sequencing by synthesis)—were used to sequence the transcripts of IGROV1 and IGROV-1-CP cells and to sequence the transcripts of a highly chemotherapy responsive and a highly chemotherapy resistant ovarian cancer tissue [7]. An integrative analysis of the two NGS data sets identified 111 common differentially expressed genes including two bone morphogenetic proteins (BMP4 and BMP7), six solute carrier proteins (SLC10A3, SLC16A3, SLC25A1, SLC35B3, SLC7A5, and SLC7A7), transcription factor POU5F1 (POU class 5 homeobox 1), and KLK10 (kallikrein-related peptidase 10). A further network analysis revealed a subnetwork with three genes BMP7, NR2F2, and AP2B1 that were consistently overexpressed in the chemoresistant tissue or cells compared to the chemosensitive tissue or cells [7]. Our data also provide a comprehensive resource for analyzing novel splicing isoforms and novel transcripts related to chemotherapy response program in ovarian cancers. We are sharing our experience working with RNA-seq including both sample preparation and sequencing as well as data analysis.

Please note that the protocols described in this chapter of RNA-seq were written for Illumina's platform for the reason that we think this platform is best for the RNA-seq analysis as they are more downstream open-source data analysis support. The Life Technologies' SOLiD platform is also very good for RNA-seq but there is less support in terms of downstream data analysis. The SOLiD platform is very good for mutation or variance analysis as they sequenced the DNA in two phases (color space mapping) and therefore provide very high accurate sequencing calls. We did not discuss other platform for RNA-seq analysis in this chapter, because either they are not commonly available yet (e.g., the Pacific Biosciences' platform) or they are not available for RNA-seq (e.g., Complete Genomics' platform).

There are three different flavors for the RNA-seq analysis depending on what the user wants to get out of the data. The first kind of RNA-seq analysis is simply to study the expression of genes as a substitute, and yet more sensitive, approach for gene expression profiling compared with the array technology [1]. We called this type of RNA-seq the expression tag sequencing or end-tag sequencing. In this method, the tags were usually generated by capturing polyadenylated mRNA on a solid support (e.g., oligo-dT-conjugated magnetic beads) and cDNAs were synthesized, then digested with a 4-base pair restriction enzyme cutter (e.g., DpnII). 3′ most (closest to the polyA tail) tags were retained after digestion. A linker, which contains a type III restriction enzyme (e.g., MmeI) that cuts at approximately 25 base pairs from the site, was then ligated to the tags. Digestion with the type III restriction enzyme will generate unique tags for library construction and sequencing. In this method, one can modify the 4-base pair enzyme cutter or the type III restriction enzyme used. The reason for doing so is that some of the mRNAs would not have DpnII site and would be missed from the analysis. An advantage of this method is that it is able to distinguish mRNA isoforms derived from alternative usages polyadenylated sites, which the standard method described below could not.

The second method, which is the most commonly used method, is referred to as the standard RNA-seq. This kind of RNA-seq method aims to get more information than the expression tag sequencing method. It aims to get information about alternative splicing or to identify novel transcripts. In this method, mRNAs were fragmented by chemical or physical means, and the resulting small fragments were used to construct the library for sequencing. Sequence tags could be derived from any regions of mRNAs. Alternatively, total RNAs can also be used after removing ribosomal RNAs using the ribosomal RNA depletion reagents.

Recently, Ruan and Ruan developed a method called RNA-PET (RNA paired-end-tag sequencing), which is a method for full-length mRNA transcripts analysis [8]. Unlike the previously method that sequences randomly sheared shotgun RNA short fragments or only capture the 3′ end, the RNA-PET captures and sequences both the 5′ and 3′ end tags of full-length cDNA fragments, thus RNA-PET sequences can demarcate the boundaries of transcription units, and have the ability to identify fusion transcripts in addition to quantifying gene expressions. As the RNA-PET protocol was described in details by Ruan and Ruan [8], we will not cover it in the chapter. We will focus on the end-tag sequencing and the standard RNA-seq.

2 Materials

2.1 Cells and Tissues

1. The human ovarian carcinoma DDP-resistant cell line IGROV-1-CP (*see* **Note 1**) grown at 37 °C in RPMI 1640 supplemented with 10 % fetal bovine serum, 50 IU/ml penicillin, and 50 μg/ml streptomycin with a humidified atmosphere containing 5 % CO_2. IGROV-1-CP cells are cisplatin-resistant ovarian cancer cells derived experimentally from cisplatin-sensitive parental IGROV-1 cells after prolonged exposure to cisplatin compound and selection of resistant clones [9]. However, they were grown at the same culture media for this experiment to remove any potential media induced changes. In general, IGROV-1-CP is put back to media with cisplatin every 3–5 generations to maintain its cisplatin-resistant properties.
2. Two ovarian cancer tissues were obtained at the Department of Gynecological Oncology, Roswell Park Cancer Institute, with IRB approval and informed consent.

2.2 Sample Preparation

Prepare all solutions using ultrapure water (prepared by purifying deionized water to attain a sensitivity of 18 MΩ cm at 25 °C). Unless otherwise indicated, store reagents at room temperature.

1. *mir*Vana™ miRNA Isolation Kit (Ambion®, Life Technologies, USA).
2. QIAquick PCR Purification Kit (QIAGEN, USA).
3. MinElute PCR Purification Kit (QIAGEN, USA).
4. QIAquick Gel Extraction Kit (QIAGEN, USA).
5. Gene Expression Sample Prep DpnII Kit (Illumina, USA).
6. mRNA-Seq 8 sample prep kit (Illumina, USA).
7. SuperScript II Reverse Transcriptase with 100 mM DTT.
8. Phenol/chloroform/isoamyl alcohol solution (25:24:1).
9. Chloroform/isoamyl alcohol solution (24:1).
10. Solution NaOAc, 3 M, pH 5.2.
11. Ethanol 100 %. Store at −20 °C.
12. Ethanol 70 %.
13. 6 % TBE PAGE gel, 1.0 mm, 10 well.
14. 5× TBE buffer: 0.445 M Tris base, 0.445 M boric acid, 10 mM EDTA (free acid), pH 8.3.

2.3 Sequencing Regents

1. Single-Read Cluster Generation Kit v4 (Illumina, USA).
2. Genomic Sequencing Primer Kit (Illumina, USA).

2.4 Equipment

1. Thermomixer.
2. Room temperature tube rotator.
3. Dark Reader transilluminator.
4. Agilent Technologies 2100 Bioanalyzer or equivalent.
5. PCR thermal cycler.
6. An Illumina-Solexa GAII instrument.

2.5 Bioinformatics Toolbox

1. Goat module (Firecrest v.1.4.0 and Bustard v.1.4.0 programs) of the Illumina pipeline v.1.4.

3 Methods

3.1 Extraction of Total RNA from Tissues and Cell Lines of Interest

This protocol is suitable for 1–2 μg of total RNA. Lower amounts may result in inefficient ligation and low yield. Check total RNA integrity following isolation using an Agilent Technologies 2100 Bioanalyzer. Only RNA with an RNA integrity number (RIN) value greater than 8 should be used. We extracted total RNAs from ovarian cancer tissues and cell lines using mirVana™ miRNA Isolation Kit (Ambion®, Life Technologies, USA). The buffer and solution referred to below are from the kit.

1. Collect 10^5–10^7 cells or 0.5–250 mg tissue; wash cells in cold PBS.
2. Disrupt samples in 1 ml of Lysis/Binding Buffer.
3. Add 1/10 volume of miRNA Homogenate Additive; incubate 10 min on ice.
4. Extract with a volume of acid phenol: chloroform equal to the initial lysate volume.
5. Recover the aqueous phase; transfer the aqueous phase to a fresh tube.
6. Add 1.25 volumes 100 % ethanol, and mix thoroughly.
7. Pass the lysate/ethanol mixture through a filter cartridge.
8. Wash the filter with 700 μl miRNA Wash Solution 1.
9. Wash the filter twice with 500 μl Wash Solution 2 and then 3.
10. Elute RNA with 100 μl 95 °C Elution Solution or Nuclease-free Water.

3.2 Sample Preparation for End-Tag RNA-Seq

This method of RNA-seq should be chosen when the study is only focused on gene expression analysis or is designed to understand alternative polyadenylation of mRNAs. Otherwise, the standard

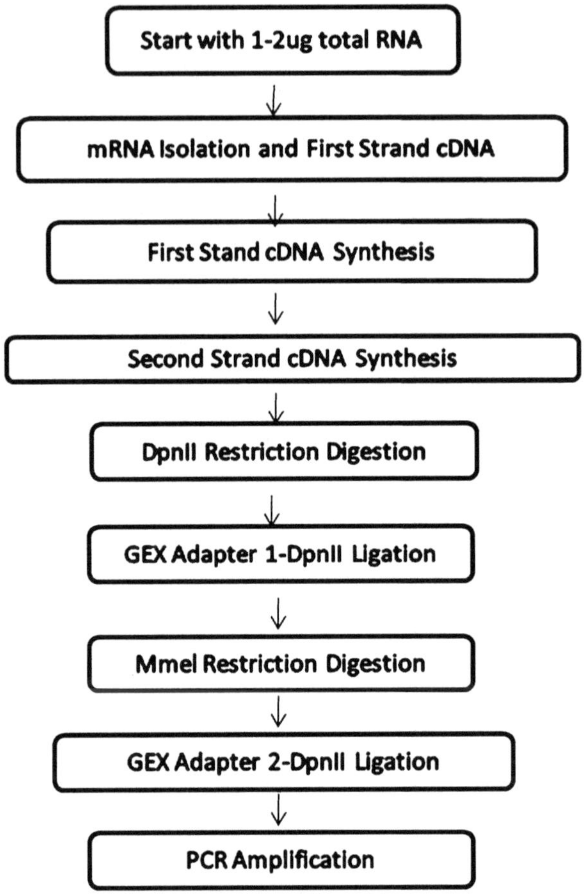

Fig. 1 An outline of the major steps involved in library construction for expression tag sequencing

RNA-seq method should be used as it provided added information about splicing isoforms. The buffer and reagents described in this section are from the Gene Expression Sample Prep DpnII Kit (Illumina, USA) unless alternatives are provided. Overview of consequent manipulations is presented in Fig. 1.

This sample preparation generates a library of 16 base pair (bp) cDNA fragments after the recognition site of DpnII (GATC). After sequencing, a total of 20 base pairs (GATC plus 16 base pairs) can be used to aligning to reference databases. The design of the protocol ensures that the 16 bp fragments are from between the last DpnII site and the polyA tail, and thus the information can be used to infer alternative polyadenylation of mRNAs. The caveat is that not all cDNAs have DpnII sites, and those without a DpnII site would be missed in this analysis. A design with a different 4 bp cutter (e.g., NlaIII, which cuts CATG) can be used as an alternative or complementary approach.

3.2.1 Total RNA Preparation

This step prepares the total RNA for annealing with oligo-dT. Total RNAs are heated to 65 °C to disrupt potential secondary RNA structures that may include polyA tails.

1. Dilute 1–2 μg of total RNA with ultrapure water to 50 μl in a sterile RNase-free 200 μl microtube.
2. Heat the 50 μl of total RNA at 65 °C in a thermal cycler for 5 min to disrupt any secondary structure.
3. Immediately place on ice.

3.2.2 Preparation of the Magnetic Oligo(dT) Beads

Before using the beads to capture mRNAs, it should be washed for several times, as they are stored in storage buffer, which is different from binding buffer.

1. While the RNA is denaturing, thoroughly resuspend the supplied oligo(dT) beads and transfer 50 μl to a 1.5 ml RNase-free, siliconized microtube (*see* **Note 2**).
2. Place the tube on the magnetic stand for 1–2 min. Carefully pipette off the supernatant and discard it (*see* **Note 3**).
3. Wash the beads by resuspending them in 100 μl of GEX binding buffer (Gene Expression Sample Prep DpnII Kit). Add the buffer to the tube while the tube is on the magnetic stand (*see* **Note 4**).
4. Cap the tube, remove it from the magnetic stand, and resuspend the beads. You can resuspend the beads by flicking the tube with your finger or use a vortexer set at 5–6. Centrifuge briefly to collect any beads that may remain in the tube cap.
5. Place the tube back on the magnetic stand for 1–2 min. Carefully pipette off the supernatant and discard it (*see* **Note 3**).
6. Wash with another 100 μl of GEX binding buffer (Gene Expression Sample Prep DpnII Kit) as described in **steps 3–5**.
7. Place the tube back on the magnetic stand for 1–2 min. Carefully pipette off the supernatant and discard it.
8. Resuspend the beads in 50 μl of GEX binding buffer (Gene Expression Sample Prep DpnII Kit).

3.2.3 Isolation of the mRNA

In this step, magnetic beads conjugated with oligo-dT are used to capture mRNAs from total RNA. GEX binding buffer (Gene Expression Sample Prep DpnII Kit) is used for annealing of polyA tails of mRNAs to the oligo-dT on the beads. Beads with attached mRNAs are then washed to remove contaminants that may have bound nonspecifically. Make sure to remove the supernatant completely between each washing step. As an alternative to the protocol described below, Dynal oligo(dT) beads (#610-06, Invitrogen, USA) can be used here with the protocol from the manufacturer.

Illumina did not disclose the components of its buffers used in this protocol. However, Dynabeads oligo-dT uses the binding buffer (Tris–HCl 20 mM, LiCl 1 M, EDTA 2 mM), the washing buffer (Tris–HCl 10 mM, LiCl 0.15 M, EDTA 2 mM), and the elution buffer (Tris–HCl 10 mM).

1. Add 50 μl of diluted total RNA to the tube containing oligo(dT) beads in 50 μl of GEX binding buffer (Gene Expression Sample Prep DpnII Kit).
2. Using the room temperature tube rotator, rotate the tube at room temperature for 5 min.
3. Place the tube on the magnetic stand for 1–2 min. Carefully pipette off the supernatant and discard it.
4. Wash beads by resuspending them in 200 μl of GEX washing buffer (Gene Expression Sample Prep DpnII Kit).
5. Place the tube on the magnetic stand for 1–2 min. Carefully pipette off the supernatant and discard it.
6. Repeat **steps 4** and **5** with another 200 μl of GEX washing buffer (Gene Expression Sample Prep DpnII Kit).
7. Place the tube on the magnetic stand for 1–2 min. Carefully pipette off the supernatant and discard it.
8. Wash the beads by resuspending them in 100 μl of freshly prepared 1× first-strand buffer (Gene Expression Sample Prep DpnII Kit).
9. Repeat **steps** 7 and **8** three additional times for a total of four washes in 100 μl of 1× first-strand buffer (Gene Expression Sample Prep DpnII Kit).
10. Upon completion of the four washes you should have a tube of beads resuspended in 1× first-strand buffer (Gene Expression Sample Prep DpnII Kit).

3.2.4 The First-Strand cDNA Synthesis

The oligo-dT on the magnetic beads is used to both capture the mRNA and also act as a primer for first-strand cDNA synthesis; therefore, no new primers are necessary.

1. Premix the following reagents in the order listed in a separate tube: 29.5 μl of ultrapure water, 10 μl of 5× first-strand buffer (Gene Expression Sample Prep DpnII Kit), 5 μl of 100 mM DTT, 2.5 μl of 10 mM 5mC-dNTP mix, and 1 μl of RNaseOUT (Gene Expression Sample Prep DpnII Kit). The total volume should be 48 μl. Multiply each volume by the number of samples being prepared. Prepare 10 % extra reagent mix if you are preparing multiple samples.
2. Place the tube of beads resuspended in 1× first-strand buffer (Gene Expression Sample Prep DpnII Kit) on the magnetic stand for 1–2 min. Carefully pipette off the supernatant and discard it.

3. Resuspend the beads in 48 μl of the first-strand cDNA synthesis premix outlined in **step 1**. Mix well.
4. Heat the bead/premix tube at 42 °C in a thermal cycler for 2 min.
5. Add 2 μl of SuperScript II Reverse Transcriptase.
6. Incubate at 42 °C in a thermomixer that is constantly mixing at 1,400 rpm for 1 h.
7. Transfer the tube to a 70 °C thermomixer that is programmed to mix at 1,400 rpm for 15 s and then standing for 2 min, for a total of 15 min. Place the tube on ice.

3.2.5 The Second-Strand cDNA Synthesis

In this step, the nick translational replacement of the mRNA to synthesize the second-strand cDNA is used. This approach employs RNase H, which recognizes the mRNA DNA:mRNA hybrid after first-strand cDNA synthesis, and cleaves the RNA at a number of nonspecific sites [10]. After cleavage, the short RNA oligoribonucleotides are still attached to the cDNA and they serve as 3′ OH-primers for the DNA pol I to synthesize the second-strand cDNA. Please note that DNA pol I (not Klenow) is used since the 5′–3′ exonuclease activity is needed to remove RNA in front of the enzyme, allowing the second-strand cDNA to elongate. This strategy was adapted from the publication by D'Alessio, J.M. and G.F. Gerard [11]. Both DNA pol I and RNAse H are added at the same time as D'Alessio and Gerard showed longer stretch of cDNA could be synthesized compared with the method without inclusion of RNAse H [11]. The reaction is carried out at 16 °C for the second-strand cDNA synthesis to prevent spurious synthesis by DNA polymerase I due to its tendency to strand displace (rather than nick translate) at higher temperatures, and then at 37 °C for a short period of time for the RNAse H to remove all remaining RNAs and for DNA pol I to complete the remaining synthesis. After second-strand cDNA synthesis, the double-strand cDNAs are still linked to the magnetic beads via the oligo-dT.

1. Add 31 μl of ultrapure water to the 50 μl of mRNA/cDNA hybrid mix on ice.
2. Add 10 μl GEX second-strand buffer (500 mM Tris–HCl pH 7.8, 50 mM $MgCl_2$, 10 mM DTT) and 3 μl of 10 mM 5mC-dNTP mix.
3. Mix well and incubate on ice for 5 min.
4. Add 5 μl of DNA polymerase I (Gene Expression Sample Prep DpnII Kit or #18010-025, DNA Pol I , 10 U/μL, Invitrogen, CA, USA) and 1 μl of RNase H (Gene Expression Sample Prep DpnII Kit or #18021-014, RNaseH, 2 U/μl, Invitrogen, CA, USA).
5. Mix well and incubate at 16 °C in a thermomixer, programmed to mix at 1,400 rpm for 15 s and stand for 2 min, for a total of 2.5 h.

6. Place the tube on the magnetic stand for 1–2 min. Carefully pipette off the supernatant and discard it.
7. Wash the beads by resuspending them in 750 μl of GEX buffer C (Gene Expression Sample Prep DpnII Kit).
8. Place the tube on the magnetic stand for 1–2 min. Carefully pipette off the supernatant and discard it.
9. Resuspend the beads in 100 μl of fresh working cleaning solution (Gene Expression Sample Prep DpnII Kit).
10. Incubate at 37 °C in a thermomixer, programmed to mix at 1,400 rpm for 15 s, and stand for two minutes, for a total of 15 min.
11. Place the tube on the magnetic stand for 1–2 min. Carefully pipette off the supernatant and discard it.
12. Resuspend the beads in 750 μl of GEX buffer D (Gene Expression Sample Prep DpnII Kit).
13. Repeat **steps 11** and **12** three additional times for a total of four washes in 750 μl of GEX buffer D (Gene Expression Sample Prep DpnII Kit).
14. Upon completion of the four washes you should be left with a tube of beads resuspended in 750 μl of GEX buffer D (Gene Expression Sample Prep DpnII Kit).
15. Place the tube on the magnetic stand for 1–2 min. Carefully pipette off the supernatant and discard it.
16. Resuspend the beads in 100 μl of 1× DpnII buffer (Gene Expression Sample Prep DpnII Kit).
17. Place the tube on the magnetic stand for 1–2 min. Carefully pipette off the supernatant and discard it.
18. Resuspend the beads in 100 μl of 1× DpnII buffer (Gene Expression Sample Prep DpnII Kit).
19. Transfer the bead and 1× DpnII buffer solution (Gene Expression Sample Prep DpnII Kit) to a sterile, RNase-free, siliconized 1.5 ml microtube.

3.2.6 Restriction Digest with DpnII

In this step, DpnII was used to digest the ds cDNA bound to magnetic beads via the oligo-dT. After digestion, the fragment from the last DpnII site of a cDNA to the polyA tail is retained on the beads. They were washed four times with buffer D to remove the beads-free DNA as much as possible.

1. Place the tube of cDNA-attached beads resuspended in 1× DpnII buffer (Gene Expression Sample Prep DpnII Kit) on the magnetic stand for 1–2 min. Carefully pipette off the supernatant and discard it.
2. Resuspend the beads in 99 μl of the DpnII digestion premix (Gene Expression Sample Prep DpnII Kit).

3. Add 1 μl of DpnII enzyme.
4. Incubate at 37 °C in a thermomixer, programmed to mix at 1,400 rpm for 15 s and stand for 2 min, for a total of 1 h.
5. Place the tube on the magnetic stand for 1–2 min. Carefully pipette off the supernatant and discard it.
6. Wash the beads by resuspending them in 750 μl of GEX buffer C (Gene Expression Sample Prep DpnII Kit).
7. Place the tube on the magnetic stand for 1–2 min. Carefully pipette off the supernatant and discard it.
8. Resuspend the beads in 100 μl of fresh working cleaning solution.
9. Incubate at 37 °C in a thermomixer, programmed to mix at 1,400 rpm for 15 s and stand for 2 min, for a total of 15 min.
10. Place the tube on the magnetic stand for 1–2 min. Carefully pipette off the supernatant and discard it.
11. Resuspend the beads in 750 μl of GEX buffer D (Gene Expression Sample Prep DpnII Kit).
12. Repeat **steps 10** and **11** three additional times for a total of four washes in 750 μl of GEX buffer D (Gene Expression Sample Prep DpnII Kit).
13. Upon completion of the four washes you should be left with a tube of beads resuspended in 750 μl of GEX buffer D (Gene Expression Sample Prep DpnII Kit).
14. Store the resuspended beads overnight at 4 °C.

3.2.7 Ligation of GEX DpnII Adapter I

In this step, a defined gene expression adapter (GEX DpnII Adapter I, the sequence is shown below) is ligated to the site of DpnII cleavage. The GEX DpnII Adapter I contains the sequence for the restriction enzyme MmeI, which recognizes TCCRAC (R=A or G) and digests 20 nucleotides after the recognition site. After the Mme I recognition site and at the end of the GEX DpnII Adapter I, it contains a cohesive end of DpnII site. The ligated fragments would still be attached to the beads. The ligation of GEX DpnII Adapter 1 allows the digestion of the ligated fragments in the next step with Mme I to create a library of fragments with 16 bps after the GATC (DpnII enzyme recognition site).

GEX DpnII Adapter I

5′ P-GATCGTCGGACTGTAGAACTCTGAAC-3′

5′-ACAGGTTCAGAGTTCTACAGTCCGAC-3′

The alignment of the sequences used in the DpnII gene expression sample preparation is listed in Fig. 2.

1. Place the tube containing the bead-attached cDNA resuspended in GEX buffer D (Gene Expression Sample Prep DpnII

```
DpnII gene expression

Gex Adapter 1:
5' -------------------A CAGGTTCAGAGTTCTACAGT CCGAC--------------- -------------------- ------ 3'
3' -------------------- ---CAAGTCTCAAGATGTCA GGCTGCTAGp---------- -------------------- ------ 5'
Gex Adapter 2:
5' -------------------- -------------------- -------------------- ----pTCGTATGCCGTCTTC TGCTTG 3'
3' -------------------- -------------------- -------------------- ---NNAGCATACGGCAGAAG ACGAAC 5'
Gex PCR Primer 1:
5' -------------------- -------------------- ----------------------------------------- ------ 3'
3' -------------------- -------------------- -------------------- -----AGCATACGGCAGAAG ACGAAC 5'
Gex PCR Primer 2:
5' AATGATACGGCGACCACCGA CAGGTTCAGAGTTCTACAGT CCGA---------------- -------------------- ------ 3'
3' -------------------- -------------------- -------------------- -------------------- ------ 5'
Result Library:
5' AATGATACGGCGACCACCGA CAGGTTCAGAGTTCTACAGT CCGACGATCNNNNNNNNNNN NNNNNTCGTATGCCGTCTTC TGCTTG 3'
3' TTACTATGCCGCTGGTGGCT GTCCAAGTCTCAAGATGTCA GGCTGCTAGNNNNNNNNNNN NNNNNAGCATACGGCAGAAG ACGAAC 5'
Gex Sequencing Primer:
5' -----------------CGA CAGGTTCAGAGTTCTACAGT CCGACGATC----------- -------------------- ------ 3'
3'-------------------- -------------------- -------------------- -------------------- ------ 5'
```

Fig. 2 Alignments of primers used in the DpnII-based sample preparation for expression end-tag sequencing (Oligonucleotide sequences © 2007–2012 Illumina, Inc. All rights reserved)

Kit) on the magnetic stand for 1–2 min. Carefully pipette off the supernatant and discard it.

2. Resuspend the beads in 100 μl of 1× T4 DNA Ligase Buffer (Gene Expression Sample Prep DpnII Kit).
3. Place the tube on the magnetic stand for 1–2 min. Carefully pipette off the supernatant and discard it.
4. Resuspend the beads in 100 μl of 1× T4 DNA Ligase Buffer (Gene Expression Sample Prep DpnII Kit).
5. Transfer the resuspended beads to a fresh microtube.
6. Place the tube on the magnetic stand for 1–2 min. Carefully pipette off the supernatant and discard it.
7. Add the following in the indicated order to each tube of beads: 36 μl of ultrapure water, 3 μl of GEX DpnII Adapter 1, 10 μl of 5× T4 DNA Ligase Buffer (Gene Expression Sample Prep DpnII Kit), and 1 μl T4 DNA Ligase. The total volume should be 50 μl.
8. Incubate at 20 °C in a thermomixer that is constantly mixing at 1,400 rpm for 2 h.
9. Place the tube on the magnetic stand for 1–2 min. Carefully pipette off the supernatant and discard it.
10. Wash the beads by resuspending them in 750 μl of GEX buffer C (Gene Expression Sample Prep DpnII Kit).
11. Place the tube on the magnetic stand for 1–2 min. Carefully pipette off the supernatant and discard it.
12. Resuspend the beads in 100 μl of fresh working cleaning solution.

13. Incubate at 37 °C in a thermomixer, programmed to mix at 1,400 rpm for 15 s and stand for 2 min, for a total of 15 min.
14. Place the tube on the magnetic stand for 1–2 min. Carefully pipette off the supernatant and discard it.
15. Resuspend the beads in 750 μl of GEX buffer D (Gene Expression Sample Prep DpnII Kit).
16. Repeat **steps 13** and **14** three additional times for a total of four washes in 750 μl of GEX buffer D (Gene Expression Sample Prep DpnII Kit).
17. Upon completion of the four washes you should have a tube of beads resuspended in 750 μl of GEX buffer D (Gene Expression Sample Prep DpnII Kit).
18. Place the tube on the magnetic stand for 1–2 min. Carefully pipette off the supernatant and discard it.
19. Resuspend the beads in 100 μl of 1× restriction buffer (Gene Expression Sample Prep DpnII Kit).
20. Place the tube on the magnetic stand for 1–2 min. Carefully pipette off the supernatant and discard it.
21. Resuspend the beads in 100 μl of 1× restriction buffer (Gene Expression Sample Prep DpnII Kit).
22. Transfer the bead and 1× restriction buffer solution (Gene Expression Sample Prep DpnII Kit) to a fresh, sterile, RNase-free, siliconized 1.5 ml tube.

3.2.8 Restriction Digest with MmeI

In this step, the GEX Adapter I ligated fragments are digested with Mme I to create a library of fragments with 16 bps after the GATC (DpnII enzyme recognition site). They are then dephosphorylated to prevent co-ligation and are prepared for ligation with the GEX Adapter II (sequence listed below) and the aligned sequences in Fig. 2.

GEX Adapter II

5′-CAAGCAGAAGACGGCATACGANN-3′

5′ P-TCGTATGCCGTCTTCTGCTTG-3′

3.2.9 Release the DNA Fragments from Magnetic Beads1

After the digestion, the fragments are now released from the beads. The DNA fragments are 20 bps with 16 bps unique sequences for each fragment after the common GATC (DpnII enzyme recognition site).

1. Place the tube of bead-attached cDNA resuspended in the 1× restriction buffer (Gene Expression Sample Prep DpnII Kit) on the magnetic stand for 1–2 min. Carefully pipette off the supernatant and discard it.
2. Resuspend the beads in 100 μl of the MmeI restriction digest premix (Gene Expression Sample Prep DpnII Kit).

3. Incubate at 37 °C in a thermomixer that is constantly mixing at 1,400 rpm for 1.5 h.
4. Place the tube of MmeI-digested cDNA and beads on the magnetic stand for 1–2 min. Carefully pipette off the supernatant containing cDNA, and transfer it to a sterile, RNase-free, siliconized 1.5 ml microtube (*see* **Note 5**).
5. Discard the tube containing the beads.
6. Add 2 μl of CIAP (Calf Intestinal Alkaline Phosphatase) to the retained supernatant.
7. Dephosphorylate for 1 h at 37 °C.
8. Extract once with 100 μl phenol/chloroform/isoamyl alcohol (25:24:1).
9. Extract once with 100 μl chloroform/isoamyl alcohol (24:1).
10. Add 1 μl of glycogen, 10 μl 3 M NaOAc, and 325 μl of −20 °C 100 % ethanol.
11. Immediately centrifuge to 17,000 × *g* for 20 min.
12. Remove the supernatant and discard it.
13. Wash the pellet with 500 μl of room temperature 70 % ethanol.
14. Remove the supernatant and discard it.
15. Dry the pellet using the speed vac.
16. Resuspend the pellet in 6 μl of ultrapure water.
17. Store overnight at −20 °C.

3.2.10 Ligation of GEX Adapter II

In this step, a second adapter, the GEX Adapter II (Fig. 2), is ligated at the site of *Mme*I cleavage. The GEX Adapter II also contains sequences complementary to the oligos attached to the flow cell surface used for sequencing analysis by the Illumina GAII.

1. To each tube of 6 μl of MmeI-digested and MmeI-resuspended cDNA, add the following in the order listed: 1 μl of GEX Adapter 2 (Gene Expression Sample Prep DpnII Kit), 2 μl of 5× T4 DNA Ligase Buffer (Gene Expression Sample Prep DpnII Kit), and 1 μl of T4 DNA Ligase. The total volume should be 10 μl.
2. Incubate at 20 °C for 2 h in the thermomixer.

3.2.11 Enrichment the Adapter-Ligated cDNA Construct Using PCR

In this step, a PCR reaction was conducted to amplify the adapter-ligated cDNAs using

GEX PCR Primer 1 (5′-CAAGCAGAAGACGGCATACGA-3′) and GEX PCR Primer 2 (5′-AATGATACGGCGACCACCG ACAGGTTCAGAGTTCTACAGTCCGA-3′). The amplification process selectively enriches those cDNA fragments that have adapter molecules on both ends. 15 cycles generally is enough to provide enough enrichment based on empirical experience.

1. Aliquot 47.5 μl of PCR master mix (Gene Expression Sample Prep DpnII Kit) into a sterile, nuclease-free, 200 μl PCR tube.
2. Add 2.5 μl of GEX Adapter 2 ligated cDNA.
3. Amplify the PCR in the thermal cycler using the following protocol: initialization step—98 °C/30″; followed by denaturation step—98 °C/10″, annealing step—60 °C/30″, and extension step—72 °C/15″, for 15 cycles; 72 °C/10″ and hold at 4 °C.

3.2.12 Run the Gel Electrophoresis to Purify the Ligated and PCR Amplified Products (See ***Note 6****)*

In this step, PAGE electrophoresis is used to purify the 86 bps final library constructs (Fig. 2) from other contaminating and undesirable by-products such as adapter self-ligation generated during the sample preparation process. This is important as the sequencing in conducted in parallel in millions of reactions in the flow cells, contaminating products will occupy some of the real estate in the flow cells, reducing the yields of final sequencing outputs.

1. Determine the volume of 1× TBE buffer needed.
2. Dilute the 5× TBE buffer to 1× with Milli-Q water for use in electrophoresis.
3. Assemble the gel electrophoresis apparatus per manufacturer's instructions.
4. Mix 5 μl of 25 bp ladder with 1 μl of 6× DNA loading dye.
5. Mix 50 μl of amplified cDNA construct with 10 μl of 6× DNA loading dye.
6. Load 5 μl of the 25 bp ladder and loading dye mix into one well of the 6 % TBE PAGE gel.
7. Load 25 μl each of the PCR amplified construct and loading dye mix into two wells of the 6 % TBE PAGE gel.
8. Run the gel for 30–35 min at 200 V.
9. Remove the gel from the apparatus.
10. Puncture the bottom of a sterile, nuclease-free, 0.5 ml microtube 4–5 times with a 21-gauge needle.
11. Place the 0.5 ml microtube into a sterile, round-bottom, nuclease-free, 2 ml microtube.
12. Pry apart the cassette and stain the gel with the ethidium bromide in a clean container for 2–3 min.
13. View the gel on a Dark Reader transilluminator to avoid being exposed to UV light. The 25 bp ladder is in 25 bp steps up to 300 bp (*see* **Note 7**).

14. Using a clean scalpel, cut out the 85 bp bands in the sample lanes.
15. Place the gel slice into the 0.5 ml microtube.
16. Centrifuge the stacked tubes at max speed of 17,000 × *g* for 2 min at room temperature to move the gel through the holes into the 2 ml tube.
17. Add 100 μl of 1× gel elution buffer to the gel debris in the 2 ml tube.
18. Elute the DNA by rotating the tube gently at room temperature for 2 h.
19. Transfer the eluate and the gel debris to the top of a Spin-X filter.
20. Centrifuge the filter for 2 min at 17,000 × *g*.
21. Add 1 μl of glycogen, 10 μl of 3 M NaOAc, and 325 μl of −20 °C ethanol.
22. Immediately centrifuge to 17,000 × *g* for 20 min at 4 °C.
23. Remove and discard the supernatant, leaving the pellet intact.
24. Wash the pellet with 500 μl of room temperature 70 % ethanol.
25. Remove and discard the supernatant, leaving the pellet intact.
26. Dry the pellet using the speed vac.
27. Resuspend the pellet in 10 μl resuspension buffer.

3.2.13 The Library Validation

The targeted DNA size should be ~85 bp, and the concentration is determined for the sequencing step (Subheading 3.4).

1. Load 1 μl of the resuspended construct on an Agilent Technologies 2100 Bioanalyzer.
2. Check the size, purity, and concentration of the sample.

3.3 Samples Preparation for Standard Sequencing of mRNA (RNA-Seq)

This is an alternative sample preparation protocol for users who want to get more information than the expression tag sequencing method. Sequencing libraries prepared by this methods cover all regions of mRNAs (in contrast to the 3′ end tag in the previous method described in Subheading 3), and data obtained could be used to identify alternative splicing, to identify novel transcripts, and even to use for identifying SNPs as the whole length of mRNAs are covered and sufficient sequence depth could be achieved for medium to high abundant genes. The buffer and reagents described in this section are all from mRNA-Seq 8 sample prep kit (Illumina, USA), but alternatives are also provided. The outline of the steps is shown in Fig. 3.

The same magnetic beads as described in Subheading 3.2 are used here. This part is similar to described in Subheading 3.2. Alternatively, Dynal oligo(dT) beads (#610-06, Invitrogen, USA) can be used here with the protocol from the manufacturer.

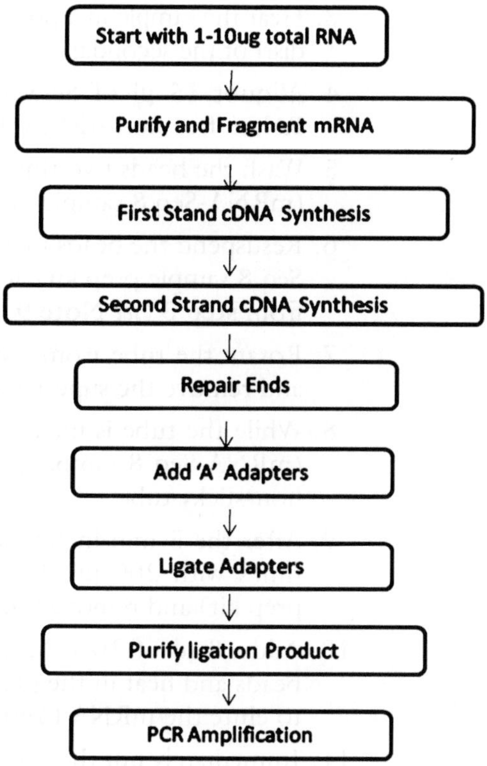

Fig. 3 An outline of the major steps involved in library construction for RNA-seq

3.3.1 Magnetic Beads Washing

1. Place the tube containing the beads on the magnetic stand for at least 1–2 min to separate the beads and the buffer (*see* **Note 2**).
2. Exchange the buffer using a pipette while the tube is on the magnetic stand.
3. Resuspend the beads thoroughly by vortexing with 0.5–1 s pulses (*see* **Note 8**).
4. Centrifuge the samples in a benchtop microcentrifuge for 1–2 s to remove any beads or liquid from the walls of the tube.
5. Repeat **steps 1–4** as required.

3.3.2 The mRNA Purification

This step is similar to Subheading 3.2, except that the mRNAs captured on the beads are eluted in the end, in contrast to the step in Subheading 3.2 that the mRNAs are left to be bound to the beads. The eluted mRNAs are then fragmented in solution in the next step.

1. Preheat one heat block to 65 °C and the other heat block to 80 °C.
2. Dilute the total RNA with nuclease-free water to 50 μl in a 1.5 ml RNase-free non-sticky tube.

3. Heat the sample in a preheated heat block at 65 °C for 5 min to disrupt the secondary structures and then place the tube on ice.
4. Aliquot 15 μl of Sera-Mag oligo(dT) beads into a 1.5 ml RNase-free non-sticky tube.
5. Wash the beads two times with 100 μl of Bead Binding Buffer (mRNA-Seq 8 sample prep kit) and remove the supernatant.
6. Resuspend the beads in 50 μl of Bead Binding Buffer (mRNA-Seq 8 sample prep kit) and add the 50 μl of total RNA sample from **step 3** (*see* **Note 9**).
7. Rotate the tube from **step 6** at room temperature for 5 min and remove the supernatant.
8. While the tube is incubating, aliquot 50 μl of Binding Buffer (mRNA-Seq 8 sample prep kit) to a fresh 1.5 ml RNase-free non-sticky tube.
9. After the 5 min incubation, wash the beads from **step** 7 five times with 200 μl of washing buffer (mRNA-Seq 8 sample prep kit) and remove the supernatant.
10. Add 18 μl of 10 mM Tris–HCl (the elution buffer) to the beads and heat in the preheated heat block at 80 °C for 2 min to elute the mRNA from the beads.
11. Immediately put the tube on the magnet stand and then transfer the supernatant (mRNA) to a fresh 200 μl thin-wall PCR tube. The resulting amount of mRNA should be approximately 18 μl.
12. Optional: The concentration of mRNA can be measured using 1 μl of sample in a QubitH Fluorometer (Invitrogen, CA, USA).

3.3.3 The mRNA Fragmentation

In this step, mRNA is fragment as the Illumina sequencing workflow is optimized with library size below 600 bp. Illumina did not disclose the component of the RNA fragment buffer, but this recipe (200 mM Tris-acetate, pH 8.1, 500 mM KOAc, 150 mM MgOA) works fine. Fragmentation Buffer can also be purchased from Ambion, Invitrogen, USA (#AM8740).

1. Preheat a PCR thermal cycler to 94 °C.
2. Prepare the following reaction mix in a 200 μl thin-wall PCR tube: 2 μl of 10× Fragmentation Buffer (mRNA-Seq 8 sample prep kit or AM8740, Ambion, Invitrogen, USA) plus 18 μl of mRNA. The total volume should be 20 μl.
3. Incubate the tube in a preheated PCR thermal cycler at 94 °C for exactly 5 min.
4. Add 2 μl of Fragmentation Stop Solution (mRNA-Seq 8 sample prep kit or AM8740, Ambion, Invitrogen, USA).
5. Place the tube on ice.

6. Transfer the solution to a 1.5 ml RNase-free non-sticky tube.
7. Add the following to the tube and incubate at −80 °C for 30 min or overnight as desired: 2 μl of 3 M NaOAC, pH 5.2; 2 μl of glycogen (mRNA-Seq 8 sample prep kit or 5 Ug/μl, #AM9510, Ambion, Invitrogen, USA), and 60 μl of 100 % EtOH.

   If you are stopping here, store the samples at −15 to −25 °C.
8. Centrifuge the tube at 14,000 × *g* (20,200 relative centrifugal force) for 25 min at 4 °C in a microcentrifuge.
9. Carefully pipette off the EtOH without dislodging the RNA pellet. The RNA pellet will be small and almost colorless. To avoid dislodging it, remove the EtOH in several steps, removing 90 % at each step and switching to smaller pipette tips for the next step.
10. Without disturbing the pellet, wash the pellet with 300 μl of 70 % EtOH.
11. Centrifuge the pellet and carefully pipette out the 70 % EtOH.
12. Air dry the pellet for 10 min at room temperature.
13. Resuspend the RNA in 11.1 μl of RNase-free water.

3.3.4 The First-Strand cDNA Synthesis

In this step, the fragmented mRNAs are reverse-transcribed into first-strand cDNA using random Hexamer Primers in contrast with the protocol in Subheading 3 in which the oligo-dT on the magnetic beads is used as primer for the first-strand cDNA synthesis.

1. Assemble the following reaction in a 200 μl thin-wall PCR tube: 1 μl of Random Primers (mRNA-Seq 8 sample prep kit or Random Hexamer Primers, 3 Ug/μL, #48190-011, Invitrogen, CA, USA) and 11.1 μl of mRNA. The total volume should be 12.1 μl.
2. Incubate the sample in a PCR thermal cycler at 65 °C for 5 min, and then place the tube on ice.
3. Set the PCR thermal cycler to 25 °C.
4. Mix the following reagents in the order listed in a separate tube: 4 μl of 5× First-Strand Buffer (mRNA-Seq 8 sample prep kit or #18064-014, Invitrogen, CA, USA), 2 μl of 100 mM DTT, 1 μl of 10 mM dNTP Mix, and 0.5 μl of RNase Inhibitor (mRNA-Seq 8 sample prep kit or RNaseOUT (40 U/μL), #10777-019, Invitrogen, CA, USA). Multiply each volume by the number of samples being prepared. Prepare 10 % extra reagent mix if you are preparing multiple samples. The total volume should be 7.5 μl.
5. Add 7.5 μl of mixture to the PCR tube and mix well.

6. Heat the sample in the preheated PCR thermal cycler at 25 °C for 2 min.
7. Add 1 μl SuperScriptII (mRNA-Seq 8 sample prep kit or #18064-014, 200 U/μL, Invitrogen, CA, USA) to the sample and incubate the sample in a thermal cycler with following program: 25 °C/10 min, 42 °C/50 min, 70 °C/15 min, hold at 4 °C.
8. Place the tube on ice.

3.3.5 The Second-Strand cDNA Synthesis

This process removes the RNA template and synthesizes a replacement strand generating double-stranded cDNA.

1. Preheat a PCR thermal cycler to 16 °C.
2. Add 60.4 μl of ultrapure water to the first-strand cDNA synthesis mix.
3. Add the following reagents to the mix: 10 μl of GEX Second-Strand Buffer (500 mM Tris–HCl pH 7.8, 50 mM $MgCl_2$, 10 mM DTT) and 3 μl of 10 mM dNTP Mix.
4. Mix well and incubate on ice for 5 min or until well chilled.
5. Add the following reagents: 1 μl of RNaseH (mRNA-Seq 8 sample prep kit or #18021-014, RNaseH, 2 U/μL, Invitrogen, CA, USA) and 5 μl of DNA Pol I (mRNA-Seq 8 sample prep kit or #18010-025, DNA Pol I, 10 U/μL, Invitrogen, CA, USA).
6. Mix well and incubate at 16 °C in a thermal cycler for 2.5 h.
7. Follow the instructions in the QIAquick PCR Purification Kit to purify the sample and elute in 75 μl of QIAGEN EB buffer (QIAquick PCR Purification Kit).
8. At this point, the sample is in the form of double-stranded DNA.

The protocol can be safely stopped here. If you are stopping, store the samples at −15 to −25 °C.

3.3.6 End Repair

In this step, the overhangs are converted into blunt ends using T4 DNA polymerase and Klenow DNA polymerase. The 3′ to 5′ exonuclease activity of these enzymes removes 3′ overhangs and the polymerase activity fills in the 5′ overhangs.

1. Preheat one heat block to 20 °C and the other heat block to 37 °C.
2. Prepare the following reaction mix in a 1.5 ml RNase-free non-sticky tube: 75 μl of Eluted DNA, 10 μl of 10× End-Repair Buffer (mRNA-Seq 8 sample prep kit, Illumina, USA), 4 μl of 10 mM dNTP Mix, 5 μl of T4 DNA polymerase, 1 μl of Klenow DNA polymerase, 5 μl of T4 PNK. The total volume should be 100 μl.
3. Incubate the sample in a heat block at 20 °C for 30 min.

4. Follow the instructions in the QIAquick PCR Purification Kit to purify the sample and elute in 32 μl of QIAGEN EB buffer (QIAquick PCR Purification Kit).

   The protocol can be safely stopped here. If you are stopping, store the samples at −15 to −25 °C.

3.3.7 Adenylation of the 3′ Ends

In this step, an "A" base was added to the 3′ end of the blunt phosphorylated DNA fragments, using the polymerase activity of Klenow fragment (3′–5′ Exo Minus). It prepares the DNA fragments for ligation to the adapters, which have a single "T" base overhang at their 3′ end.

1. Prepare the following reaction mix in a 1.5 ml RNase-free non-sticky tube: 32 μl of Eluted DNA, 5 μl of A-Tailing Buffer, 10 μl of 1 mM dATP, and 3 μl of Klenow Exo (3′–5′ Exo Minus). The total volume should be 50 μl.
2. Incubate the sample in a heat block at 37 °C for 30 min.
3. Follow the instructions in the MinElute PCR Purification Kit to purify the sample and elute in 43 μl of QIAGEN EB buffer (MinElute PCR Purification Kit).

The protocol can be safely stopped here. If you are stopping, store the samples at −15 to −25 °C.

3.3.8 The Adapters Ligation

In this step, adapters with a T-base overhang are ligated to the ends of the DNA fragments, which containing an overhanging A base. The Adapter sequences are shown in Fig. 4.

1. Prepare the following reaction mix in a 1.5 ml RNase-free non-sticky tube: 43 μl of Eluted DNA, 5 μl of 10× Rapid T4 DNA Ligase Buffer, 1 μl of PE Adapter Oligo Mix, and 1 μl of T4 DNA Ligase. The total volume should be 50 μl.
2. Incubate the sample at room temperature for 15 min. Then incubate at 4 °C overnight.
3. Follow the instructions in the MinElute PCR Purification Kit to purify the sample and elute in 10 μl of QIAGEN EB buffer (MinElute PCR Purification Kit) (*see* **Note 10**).

   The protocol can be safely stopped here. If you are stopping, store the samples at −15 to −25 °C.

3.3.9 The cDNA Templates Purification

In this step, cDNA fragments in the size range of 200 bp (±25 bp) are isolated from gel. The size range is selected for based on Illumina's platform to allow counting depth as well as to allow sequencing of up to 175 bp for each fragment.

1. Prepare a 50 ml, 2 % agarose gel with distilled water and TAE (1×, 40 mM Tris-acetate, 1 mM EDTA, pH 8.2–8.4). Final concentration of TAE should be 1× at 50 ml.
2. Load the samples as follows (*see* **Note 11**):

```
Adapter:
5' -------------------- -----ACACTCTTTCCCTAC ACGACGCTCTTCCGATCT (-) -------------------- -------------- 3'
3' -------------------- -----TGTGAGAAAGGGATG TGCTGCGAGAAGGCTAGp (-) -------------------- -------------- 5'
Adapter:
5' -------------------- -------------------- ------------------ (-) pGATCGGAAGAGCTCGTATG CCGTCTTCTGCTTG 3'
3' -------------------- -------------------- ------------------ (-) TCTAGCCTTCTCGAGCATAC GGCAGAAGACGAAC 5'
PCR Primer:
5' AATGATACGGCGACCACCGA GATCTACACTCTTTCCCTAC ACGACGCTCTTCCGATCT (-) -------------------- -------------- 3'
3' -------------------- -------------------- ------------------ (-) -------------------- -------------- 5'
PCR Primer:
5' -------------------- -------------------- ------------------ (-) -------------------- -------------- 3'
3' -------------------- -------------------- ------------------ (-) TCTAGCCTTCTCGAGCATAC GGCAGAAGACGAAC 5'
Result Library:
5' AATGATACGGCGACCACCGA GATCTACACTCTTTCCCTAC ACGACGCTCTTCCGATCT (N) AGATCGGAAGAGCTCGTATG CCGTCTTCTGCTTG 3'
3' TTACTATGCCGCTGGTGGCT CTAGATGTGAGAAAGGGATG TGCTGCGAGAAGGCTAGA (N) TCTAGCCTTCTCGAGCATAC GGCAGAAGACGAAC 5'
Genomic DNA Sequencing Primer:
5' -------------------- -----ACACTCTTTCCCTAC ACGACGCTCTTCCGATCT (-) -------------------- -------------- 3'
3' -------------------- -------------------- ------------------ (-) -------------------- -------------- 5'
```

Fig. 4 Alignments of primers used in the mRNA-seq sample preparation and sequencing (Oligonucleotide sequences © 2007–2012 Illumina, Inc. All rights reserved)

(a) 2 μl 100 bp DNA ladder (15628-019, Invitrogen, CA, USA) in the first well.

(b) 10 μl DNA elute from the ligation step mixed with 2 μl of 6× DNA loading dye (R0611, Thermo Scientific, USA) in the second well.

(c) 2 μl 100 bp DNA ladder (15628-019, Invitrogen, CA, USA) in the third well using ladders on both sides of a sample help locate the gel area to be excised as the band is not visible.

3. Run the gel at 120 V for 60 min.
4. Excise a region of gel with a clean gel excision tip and remove the gel slice by centrifuging it into a microcentrifuge tube.
5. Follow instructions in the QIAquick Gel Extraction Kit to purify the sample and elute in 29 μl of QIAGEN EB buffer (QIAquick PCR Purification Kit). (Be sure to add isopropanol per manufacturer's instructions.)

   The protocol can be safely stopped here. If you are stopping, store the samples at −15 to −25 °C.

3.3.10 Enrichment the Purified cDNA Templates

In this step, the cDNA fragments are enriched by PCR. The primer sequences are listed below and their alignments are shown in Fig. 4.

PCR primers: 5′-AATGATACGGCGACCACCGAGATCTAC ACTCTTTCCCTACACGACGCTCTTCCGATCT-3′ 5′-CAAGCAGAAGACGGCATACGAGCTCTTCCGATCT-3′.

1. Prepare the following PCR reaction mix in a 200 μl thin-wall PCR tube (make 10 % extra reagent for multiple samples): 10 μl of 5× Phusion Buffer (#F-530, NEB, USA), 1 μl of PCR Primer PE 1.0 (mRNA-Seq 8 sample prep kit, Illumina, USA), 1 μl of PCR Primer PE 2.0 (mRNA-Seq 8 sample prep kit, Illumina, USA), 1.25 μl of 10 mM dNTP Mix (mRNA-Seq 8

sample prep kit, Illumina, USA), 0.5 μl of Phusion DNA polymerase (#F-530, NEB, USA), and 7 μl water. The total volume should be 20.75 μl.

2. Add 29 μl of purified ligation mix (from **step 5** of the previous section) to the 200 μl PCR tube.
3. Amplify using the following PCR process: (a) 30 s at 98 °C; (b) 15 cycles of 10 s at 98 °C, 30 s at 65 °C, and 30 s at 72 °C; (c) 5 min at 72 °C; and (d) hold at 4 °C.
4. Follow the instructions in the QIAquick PCR Purification Kit to purify the sample and elute in 30 μl of QIAGEN EB buffer (QIAquick PCR Purification Kit).

   The protocol can be safely stopped here. If you are stopping, store the samples at −15 to −25 °C.

3.4 Sequencing on Solexa GAII

DNA samples prepared by either method from Subheadings 3.2 or 3.3 can be further processed equally starting from here for sequencing. But the sequencing primer for DNAs from Subheading 3.2 is the GEX sequencing primer and it is the genomic sequencing primer for DNAs prepared in Subheading 3.3.

GEX Sequencing Primer:

5′-CGACAGGTTCAGAGTTCTACAGTCCGACGATC-3′

Genomic sequencing primer:

5′-ACACTCTTTCCCTACACGACGCTCTTCCGATCT-3′

Generating clusters involves four main steps: amplification, linearization, blocking, and primer hybridization. 8 pM final DNA concentration was applied according to manufacturer's recommendation (Illumina Inc.). After cluster generation and primer hybridization, 36 cycles was carried out on the Genome Analyzer following manufacturer's instructions. Images deconvolution and quality values calculation were performed using the Goat module (Firecrest v.1.4.0 and Bustard v.1.4.0 programs) from Illumina pipeline v.1.4.

3.5 RNA-Seq Data Analysis

In this section we will introduce some basic computational tools for RNA-seq data analysis. The RNA-seq data analysis pipeline usually consists of two steps: (1) alignment of the sequence tags to a reference sequence database or reference genome and (2) assignment of tags to genes and quantification of expression based on counts of sequence tags.

3.5.1 Alignment of Sequence Tags

There are several steps in the data analysis to process raw reads produced by Solexa GA II to quantify gene expression (Fig. 5). Sequence tags can be mapped to transcriptome using alignment programs such as SOAP2 [12], Novocraft (Novocraft, 2010), MAQ [13], and Bowtie [14]. Among these mapping tools, SOAP2

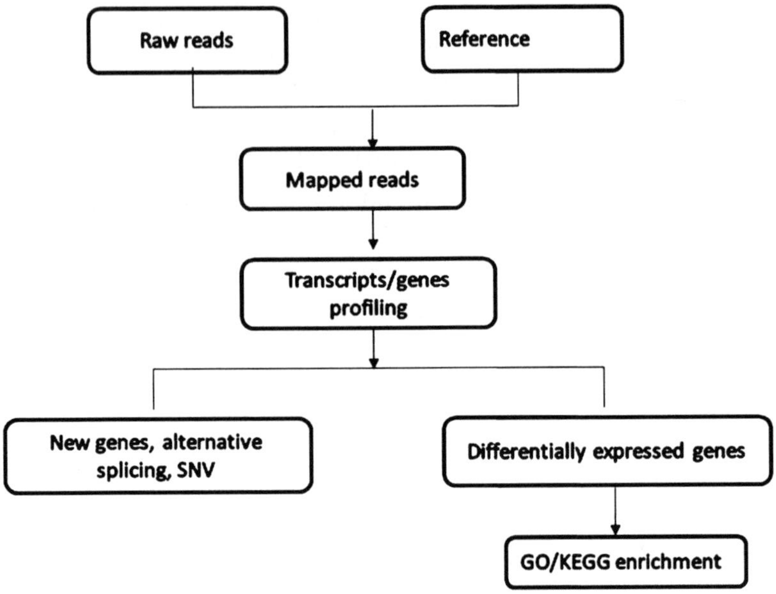

Fig. 5 An outline of the major steps for the RNA-seq data analysis

and Bowtie are used more often than the others. SOAP2 is faster but requires large memory than Bowtie. Bowtie has more output options and more processed files so that the users could choose according to their needs. For example, Bowtie takes an indexed reference genome and a set of reads as inputs and then outputs a list of alignments in SAM format. Bowtie works very efficient when aligning short reads to large genomes [14].

There are two basic steps for Bowtie alignment: (1) build an indexed reference database and (2) alignment of the short sequence tags to the indexed reference databases. The commands are described below and more information can be found at http://bowtie-bio.sourceforge.net/manual.shtml.

1. **bowtie-build [options]* <reference_in><ebwt_base>**
   Bowtie builds the index file from a set of DNA sequences using command bowtie-build.
   The "reference_in" is the reference sequence file. File "ebwt_base" is the base name that you can specify for your output index file, for example, if ebwt_base be the text string "NAME." The index files would be NAME.1.ebwt, NAME.2.ebwt, NAME.3.ebwt, NAME.4.ebwt, NAME.rev.1.ebwt, and NAME.rev.2.ebwt.
2. **bowtie [options]* <ebwt> {-1 <m1> -2 <m2> | --12 <r> | <s> [<hit>]**
   It is used to align reads to indexed reference database. ebwt is the name of the indexed database to be searched. Bowtie

offers the ability to do paired-end alignment. The file m1 and m2 is the paired-end file name, **<r>** is comma-separated list of files containing a mix of unpaired and paired-end reads in tab-delimited format, **<s>** is a comma-separated list of files containing unpaired reads to be aligned, and <hit> is file to write alignments to.

Options for input files include –q for FASTQ files as input query file and -f for FASTA type query file. Options for alignment parameters include -v <int> for reporting alignments with at most <int> mismatches. -n option used for specifying the maximum number of mismatches permitted in the "seed." The "seed" is the first L base pairs of the read (where L is set with -l/--seedlen).

You can use the option for the outputs --al <filename> to write all reads for which at least one alignment was reported to a file with name <filename> and --un<file name> to write all reads that could not be aligned to a file with name <filename>.

Usually, we can use option -s to take SAM format as alignment output. The SAM format alignment could be input file of other NGS analysis software such as Cufflink and SAMtools, which we will describe below.

3.5.2 To Use SAMtools for Manipulating Sequence Alignment Files

It is worth mentioning a tool useful for manipulating sequence alignment files named SAMtools (http://samtools.sourceforge.net/samtools.shtml). It can be used to import from and export to the SAM/BAM (Sequence Alignment/Map) format and provides various utilities to perform sorting, merging and indexing, and generating alignments in a per-position format.

3.5.3 Assignment of Tags to Transcripts and Quantification of Sequence Tags

After mapping reads to reference genomes, the mapped reads are assigned to transcripts for expression quantification. Typically, only unique mapped reads are used here. The reads that mapped to multiple locations of the genome or multiple transcripts can be discarded or be reassigned according to certain criteria. Statistics algorithms used to detect significant differential expression include baySeq (www.bioconductor.org/packages/release/bioc/html/baySeq.html) [22], DEGseq (http://www.bioconductor.org/packages/release/bioc/html/DEGseq.html) [15], Cufflinks (http://cufflinks.cbcb.umd.edu) [16], ERANGE (http://woldlab.caltech.edu/rnaseq) [17], and edgeR (http://www.bioconductor.org/packages/release/bioc/html/edgeR.html) [18]. A recent survey compared baySeq, DEGseq, and edgeR [19]. According to their comparison, DEGseq is the easiest to use. BaySeq in general takes much longer to run with the recommended number of iterations for the bootstrap. edgeR is the most flexible package and can handle both Poisson data and over-dispersed data without the need to prespecify the model. BaySeq also includes these two models but one needs to prespecify which to use. DEGseq does not handle over-dispersed data. Over-dispersion is extremely common among biological samples. edgeR provides estimates of the over-dispersion parameter, which can be helpful in determining if a Poisson model is appropriate when applying the other two packages. edgeR normalizes the data by scaling the number of reads to a common value across all samples. The users can choose any of these software tools and apply to their own data.

For users that do not have much Unix or programming experience, DEB, a web interface for RNA-seq digital gene expression analysis, developed at the University of Florida, can be used (http://www.ijbcb.org/DEB/php/onlinetool.php). It provides three algorithms (baySeq, DEGseq, and edgeR) and different FDR thresholds for the users to choose from [20]. Another useful tool is the Galaxy portal (https://main.g2.bx.psu.edu/), hosted at Penn State Univ., which allows mapping and manipulation of sequencing reads online, and to do RNA-seq analysis using Cufflinks tools, which we will describe their command line usage below.

1. Use Cufflinks for transcripts assembly for RNA-Seq data
   Cufflinks is a computational tool for transcripts assembly and quantification from RNA-Seq reads. It also estimates their abundances and tests for differential expression and regulation in RNA-Seq samples. It takes aligned RNA-Seq reads as input and assembles the alignments into a parsimonious set of transcripts. Cufflinks then estimates the relative abundances of these transcripts based on how many reads support each one, taking into account biases in library preparation protocols. The advantage of Cufflinks is that it is not restricted by prior gene annotations and it accounts for alternative transcription and splicing.

   The command line for usage:

   cufflinks [options]* <aligned_reads.(sam/bam)>

   The argument <aligned_reads.(sam/bam)> is the alignment file with standard SAM format, which could be the output of Bowtie. Options in Cufflinks include –o followed by the name of directory in which cufflinks writes all output.

   When one wants to use a known reference annotation (a GFF file) to estimate isoform expressions, one can use the option -G/--GTF <reference_annotation.(gtf/gff)>. However, with this option, it will not assemble novel transcripts and it will ignore alignments not structurally compatible with any reference transcripts.

   When one wants to identify novel transcripts and novel isoforms accounting for the RNA-seq data from a reference genome, one can use the option -g <referenceannotation.(gtf/gff)>, which Cufflinks will use the supplied reference annotation (GFF) to guide reference annotation based transcript (RABT) assembly.

Cufflinks produces three output files:

Transcripts.gtf: It is a gtf format file contains Cufflinks' assembled isoforms. The first 7 columns are standard GTF, and additional attributes (e.g., "gene_id," and "transcript_id") can be added to column 8.

isoforms.fpkm_tracking: This file contains the estimated isoform-level expression values in the generic FPKM (fragments per kilobase of exon per million fragments mapped) tracking format.

genes.fpkm_tracking: This file contains the estimated gene-level expression values in the generic FPKM tracking format.

2. Use Cuffdiff for quantification of RNA-Seq data
The "Cuffdiff" program in Cufflinks can be used to quantify RNA-seq data to find significant changes in transcript expression, in splicing, and in promoter usages.
From the command line, run Cuffdiff as follows:

cuffdiff [options]* <transcripts.gtf>

sample1_replicate1.sam[,...,sample1_replicateM]> <sample2_replicate1.sam[,...,

sample2_replicateM.sam]>... [sampleN.sam_replicate1.sam

[,...,sample2_replicateM.sam]]

Cuffdiff takes a transcript GTF files (e.g., a GTF produced by cufflinks), along with two or more SAM files for two or more samples to be compared. Replicate RNA-seq data from a sample could be supplied by the replicate SAM files for the sample as a single comma-separated list.

Cuffdiff will output five result files including FPKM tracking files and then the quantification results based on spliced transcripts, primary transcripts, genes, and coding sequences (four files are created:isoform_exp.diff, gene_exp.diff, tss_group_exp.diff, cds_exp.diff). Additionally, Cuffdiff also produce three additional files: (1) splicing.diff, for quantification of differential splicing between isoforms processed from a single primary transcript; (2) cds.diff, for quantification of differential CDS output between samples; and (3) promoters.diff, for quantification of differential promoter usages between samples.

3.5.4 Two Commonly Used Pipelines for RNA-Seq Data Analysis

1. The Bowtie -> Tophat -> Cufflinks pipeline
The most common pipeline used in the RNA-seq analysis use Bowtie, Tophat, and Cufflinks to align RNA-seq reads to the genome, to determine and align reads to splice junctions, and to calculate FPKM/RPKM (fragments/reads per kilobase of exon per million fragments/reads mapped), respectively. This is also the pipeline that we would recommend.

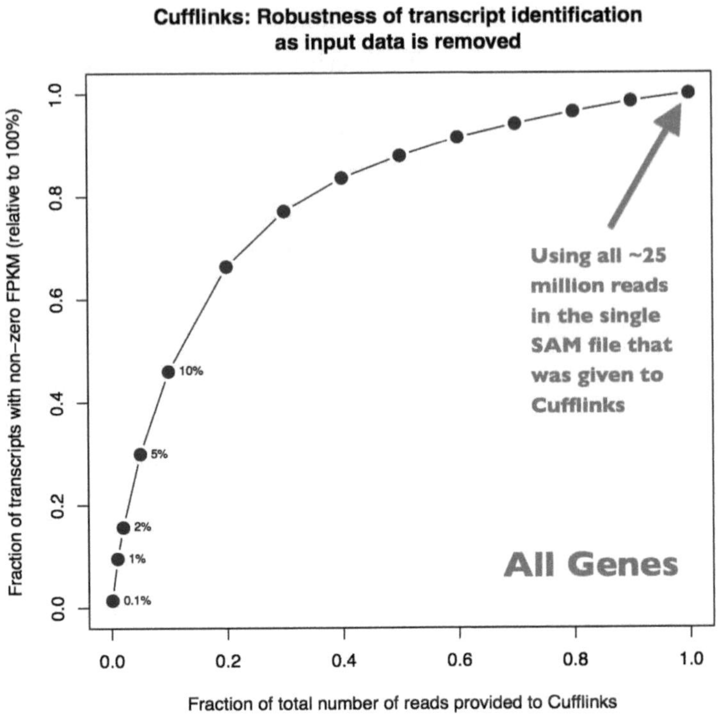

Fig. 6 Shows a simulation of percentage of genes identified with different numbers of input reads of a RNA-seq experiment of mouse heart tissues. At least 25 million reads are needed to identify close to 100 % of expressed transcripts (Taken from http://dingo.ucsf.edu/twiki/bin/view/Cores/BioinformaticsCore/EvaluationsForB2B)

A key question in RNA-seq analysis is how much reads do we need. Figure 6 showed a simulation of percentage of genes identified for the number of input reads of a RNA-seq experiment of mouse heart tissues. At least 25 million reads are needed to identify close to 100 % of expressed transcripts.

2. The Bowtie -> HTseq-count -> (baySeq, DEGseq, and edgeR) pipeline

   A good alternative pipeline for those who are interested only using RNA-seq for gene expression profiling (not interested in splicing junction analysis) is to use Bowtie align RNA-seq reads to the genome, next to use the HTSeq-count (http://www-huber.embl.de/users/anders/HTSeq/doc/overview.html) to obtain a list of counts of number of reads inside each genomic feature, then to use one of the three algorithms (baySeq, DEGseq, and edgeR) to do the counting (to assess differential expression).

   Kvam et al. recently compared several statistical methods for detecting differentially expressed genes from RNA-seq data [21]. They used simulation studies to compare the four

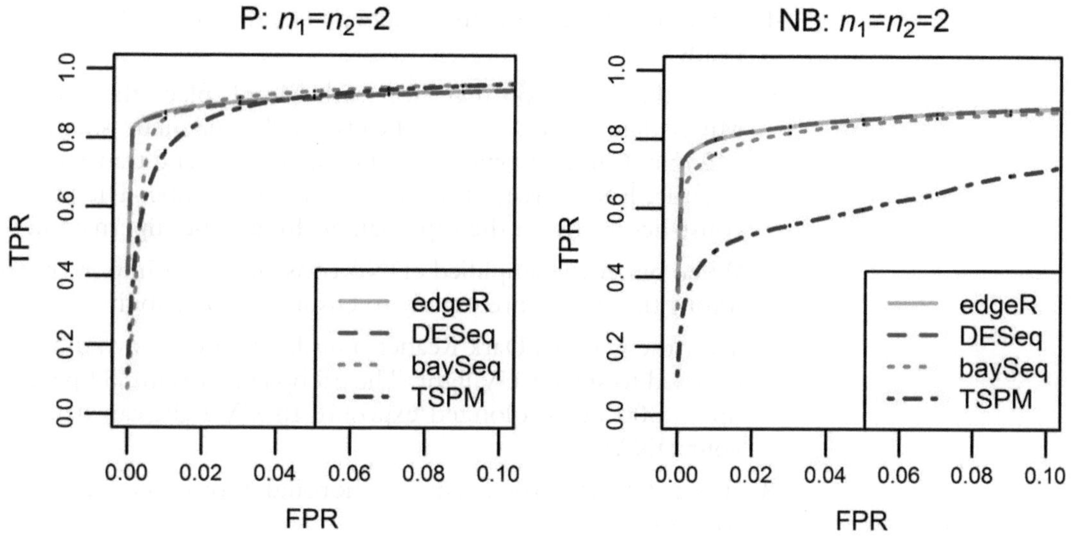

Fig. 7 Mean receiver operating characteristic (ROC) curves, based on 100 simulations to compare the performance of edgeR, DESeq, baySeq, and TSPM in detecting differential expression. Simulation based on Poisson (*left panel*) or NB (*right panel*) distribution. Parameters for Poisson or NB distributions were empirically estimated. Vertical bars at odd levels of false positive rate (FPR) are ±2 times the standard error to the value of the estimated corresponding true positive rate (TPR) (Adapted from Fig. 3 of Kvam et al. [21])

statistical methods TSPM (http://www.stat.purdue.edu/~doerge/software/TSPM.R), edgeR [18], DESeq [15], and baySeq [22] for RNA-seq analysis. Simulation study is very good way to examine properties of certain statistical methods true positives are known beforehand based on the simulation rules. They showed that baySeq performs best in terms of ranking genes according to their significance of differential expression, especially for smaller values of FPR (false positive rate) (Fig. 7) [21]. They also found that both edgeR and DESeq perform similarly and close to baySeq [21]. However, TSPM performs poorly especially when the number of replicates is small.

4 Notes

1. IGROV-1-CP was kindly provided by Dr. Stephen Howell's Lab at Moores UCSD Cancer Center, San Diego.
2. Use 1.5 ml sterile, RNase-free, siliconized microtubes for all steps through the MmeI digestion to prevent the magnetic beads from sticking to the tubes.
3. Do not allow the beads to dry during the entire process. During all wash steps, add buffers to the tube containing the beads while the tube is on the magnetic stand.

4. While the tube is on the magnetic stand, do not disturb the beads.
5. After the restriction digestion with MmeI, place the tube of MmeI-digested cDNA and beads on the magnetic stand for 1–2 min. Carefully pipette off the supernatant and transfer it to a sterile, RNase-free, siliconized 1.5 ml microtube. The library construct is now in the supernatant. Retain the supernatant.
6. When purify the amplified cDNA constructs, it is important to follow this procedure exactly to ensure reproducibility.
7. View the gel on a Dark Reader transilluminator to avoid being exposed to strong UV light. The 25 bp ladder is in 25 bp steps up to 300 bp. Prolonged exposure to UV light can damage your DNAs.
8. It is critical that the beads are thoroughly resuspended in the solution.
9. We recommend that you dilute 1–10 μg of total RNA.
10. This protocol requires a MinElute column rather than a normal QIAquick column.
11. For handling multiple samples, leave one empty lane between samples and ladders to prevent cross contamination. Do not run more than two samples on the same gel to avoid contamination.

References

1. Lin B et al (2005) Evidence for the presence of disease-perturbed networks in prostate cancer cells by genomic and proteomic analyses: a systems approach to disease. Cancer Res 65(8):3081–3091
2. Lin B, Wang J, Cheng Y (2008) Recent patents and advances in the next-generation sequencing technologies. Recent Pat Biomed Eng 1:60–67
3. Niedringhaus TP et al (2011) Landscape of next-generation sequencing technologies. Anal Chem 83(12):4327–4341
4. Mardis ER (2008) Next-generation DNA sequencing methods. Annu Rev Genomics Hum Genet 9:387–402
5. Cheng L, Xu H, Lin B (2012) The application of the next-generation sequencing technologies in cancer research. In: Juan H-F, Huang H-C (eds) Systems biology-applications in cancer-related research. World Scientific, Singapore
6. Kim JB et al (2007) Polony multiplex analysis of gene expression (PMAGE) in mouse hypertrophic cardiomyopathy. Science 316(5830): 1481–1484
7. Cheng L et al (2010) Analysis of chemotherapy response programs in ovarian cancers by the next-generation sequencing technologies. Gynecol Oncol 117(2):159–169
8. Ruan X, Ruan Y (2011) Genome wide full-length transcript analysis using 5′ and 3′ paired-end-tag next generation sequencing (RNA-PET). Methods Mol Biol 809:535–562
9. Benard J et al (1985) Characterization of a human ovarian adenocarcinoma line, IGROV1, in tissue culture and in nude mice. Cancer Res 45(10):4970–4979
10. Okayama H, Berg P (1982) High-efficiency cloning of full-length cDNA. Mol Cell Biol 2(2):161–170
11. D'Alessio JM, Gerard GF (1988) Second-strand cDNA synthesis with E. coli DNA polymerase I and RNase H: the fate of information at the mRNA 5′ terminus and the effect of E. coli DNA ligase. Nucleic Acids Res 16(5):1999–2014
12. Li R et al (2008) SOAP: short oligonucleotide alignment program. Bioinformatics 24(5): 713–714
13. Li H, Ruan J, Durbin R (2008) Mapping short DNA sequencing reads and calling variants

using mapping quality scores. Genome Res 18(11):1851–1858
14. Langmead B et al (2009) Ultrafast and memory-efficient alignment of short DNA sequences to the human genome. Genome Biol 10(3):R25
15. Wang L et al (2010) DEGseq: an R package for identifying differentially expressed genes from RNA-seq data. Bioinformatics 26(1): 136–138
16. Trapnell C et al (2010) Transcript assembly and quantification by RNA-Seq reveals unannotated transcripts and isoform switching during cell differentiation. Nat Biotechnol 28(5): 511–515
17. Mortazavi A et al (2008) Mapping and quantifying mammalian transcriptomes by RNA-Seq. Nat Methods 5(7):621–628
18. Robinson MD, McCarthy DJ, Smyth GK (2010) edgeR: a Bioconductor package for differential expression analysis of digital gene expression data. Bioinformatics 26(1):139–140
19. Gao D et al (2010) A survey of statistical software for analysing RNA-seq data. Hum Genomics 5(1):56–60
20. Yao JQ, Yu F (2011) DEB: A web interface for RNA-seq digital gene expression analysis. Bioinformation 7(1):44–45
21. Kvam VM, Liu P, Si Y (2012) A comparison of statistical methods for detecting differentially expressed genes from RNA-seq data. Am J Bot 99(2):248–256
22. Hardcastle TJ, Kelly KA (2010) baySeq: empirical Bayesian methods for identifying differential expression in sequence count data. BMC Bioinformatics 11:422

Chapter 13

Assessment of mRNA Splice Variants by qRT-PCR

Ileabett M. Echevarria Vargas and Pablo E. Vivas-Mejía

Abstract

Alternative splicing is an essential process for the generation of protein diversity. The physiological role, cellular localization, and abundance of splice variant products compared to the wild-type protein may be completely different. This is illustrated by the five splice variants of the antiapoptotic protein survivin that are more abundant in cancerous cells compared with normal tissues. Interestingly, some survivin splice variants have been associated with drug resistance. Herein, we describe a SYBR green I-based real-time PCR method to assess the messenger RNA levels of the human survivin splice variants in taxane-sensitive versus taxane-resistant ovarian cancer cells and in human ovarian cancer samples. Furthermore, in this chapter, we describe the quantification of survivin splice variants by real-time quantitative PCR (qPCR) after in vitro and in vivo small interference RNA (siRNA)-mediated silencing of survivin splice variants.

Key words SYBR green I-based PCR, Small interference RNA, Real-time PCR, Splice variants, Drug resistance, Ovarian cancer, Survivin

1 Introduction

Survivin, a protein highly expressed in human cancers, is associated with chemotherapy resistance [1–5]. Survivin plays a dual intracellular role as an antiapoptotic protein and as a regulator of mitosis [1, 6]. Alternative splicing of the human survivin gene (*BIRC5*) generates five splice variants, including wild-type (WT) survivin (142 aa), survivin 2α (74 aa), survivin 2B (165 aa), survivin ΔEx3 (137 aa), and survivin 3B (120 aa) (*see* Fig. 1) [7–10]. The expression levels and the subcellular localization patterns of each survivin isoform have been shown to be associated with their functional properties [1, 7, 11, 12]. For example, it has been reported that, compared with their taxane-sensitive counterparts, taxane-resistant ovarian cancer cells express higher survivin 2B messenger RNA (mRNA) levels [13]. In vitro and in vivo small interference RNA (siRNA)-mediated silencing of survivin 2B induced similar effects as siRNA-mediated targeting of all of survivin splice variants [13]. The antitumor effect of the survivin-directed siRNAs was further

Anastasia Malek and Oleg Tchernitsa (eds.), *Ovarian Cancer: Methods and Protocols*, Methods in Molecular Biology, vol. 1049, DOI 10.1007/978-1-62703-547-7_13, © Springer Science+Business Media New York 2013

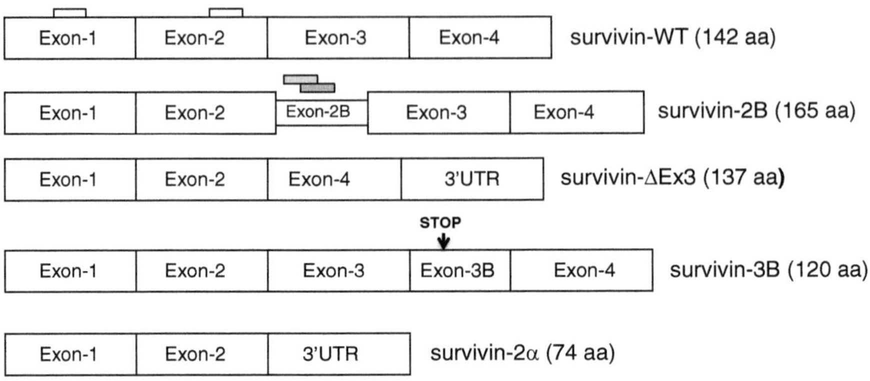

Fig. 1 Splicing of the human survivin pre-mRNA produces five different splice variants. The *empty boxes* on the survivin WT cartoon indicate the approximate location of the siRNAs to inhibit all survivin splice variants (Total siRNA). The *black box* on survivin 2B cartoon indicates the location of the survivin 2B-targeted siRNAs. Reproduced from Vivas-Mejía et al. [13]

enhanced in combination with chemotherapy [13]. A significant association was observed between survivin 2B expression and progression-free survival in epithelial ovarian cancers [13]. Currently, several therapies targeting survivin are being investigated, some of them in clinical trials [14]. However, studies proposing survivin as a prognostic or diagnostic marker or a therapeutic target should consider the differential expression levels of individual survivin splice variants, not only in ovarian cancer but also in many other cancers.

Real-time polymerase chain reaction (PCR) has the capacity to detect the amount of PCR product at every cycle by fluorescence [15]. Previously, we used real-time PCR to identify survivin splice variants after siRNA-based silencing experiments [13]. Here, we describe a real-time PCR-based method to assess the in vitro and in vivo levels of survivin splice variants in ovarian cancer cells and human ovarian cancer tissues.

Two common methods used to perform real-time PCR experiments are Taqman assays and SYBR-I-based PCR [15]. While the Taqman probes use a dual specific labeled probe, in addition to the pair of primers per gene, the SYBR-I-based PCR rely on the intercalation of the SYBR-I dye into the double-strand DNA produced during the PCR reaction [15]. Although Taqman probes are more specific than SYBR PCR, the ability to view melt curves with the SYBR method is an added advantage to determine the specificity of amplification [15]. In this study, we used SYBR-based PCR to assess the alternative splicing variability of gene transcripts because it is also relatively simple and less expensive compared to labeled Taqman probes [15].

2 Materials

Prepare all solutions using ultrapure water (prepared by purifying deionized water to attain a sensitivity of 18 MΩ cm at 25 °C) and analytical grade reagents. When RNase-free conditions are necessary, all buffers must be prepared with RNase-free reagents and DEPC treated water.

2.1 Cell Culture

The specific taxane-sensitive and taxane-resistant ovarian cancer cell lines (SKOV3ip1, SKOV3.TR, HEYA8, and HEYA8.MDR) have been described previously [16, 17] and are not commercially available. However, other ovarian cancer cells available in the American Type Culture Collection (ATCC) or in the European Collection of Cell Cultures (ECACC) can be used, including A2780, A2780CIS, SKOV3, OV-90, and NIH:OVCAR-3. Researchers can also make their own drug-resistant ovarian cancer cells.

1. Roswell Park Memorial Institute-1640 (RPMI) supplemented with 10 % Fetal Bovine Serum (FBS). Store at 4 °C.
2. Phosphate-Buffered Saline buffer (PBS).
3. Trypsin solution (0.25 %) and ethylenediaminetetraacetic acid (EDTA, 1 mM).
4. Cell culture materials (15 and 50 ml conical tubes, 1, 5, 10, and 25 ml pipettes, culture flasks, or plates).

2.2 RNA Extraction

1. RNaseZAP.
2. TRIzol reagent.
3. Dounce homogenizer.
4. Isopropanol.
5. Chloroform.
6. Ethanol 75 %.
7. 1.5 ml nuclease-free tubes.
8. RNase-free water.
9. Filter tips (0.5–10, 10–100, and 100–1,000 μl).

2.3 Complementary (c)DNA Synthesis (see Note 1)

1. 500 μg/ml oligo $(dT)_{12\text{-}18}$.
2. dNTP mix: 10 mM each dNTP at pH 7.
3. 5× First-strand buffer: 250 mM Tris–HCl, 375 mM KCl, 15 mM $MgCl_2$, pH 8.3.
4. 0.1 M Dithiothreitol (DTT).
5. SuperScript II.

6. Nuclease-free water.
7. Nuclease-free microcentrifuge tubes.

2.4 Real-Time PCR Amplification

1. 2× SYBR green PCR master mix (Applied Biosystems, Carlsbad, CA).
2. 10 μM forward primers and 10 μM reverse primers.
3. 96-well real-time PCR plate.
4. 96-well plate adhesive plastic lid.

2.5 In Vitro siRNA-Based Silencing of Specific Survivin Splice Variants

1. Optimem + GlutaMax 1×.
2. Negative control siRNA, total survivin, and survivin 2B siRNAs (*see* **Note 2**).
3. HiPerFect transfection reagent (Qiagen, Valencia, CA) (*see* **Note 3**).
4. Six-well plates.

2.6 In Vivo Silencing of Survivin Splice Variants with Liposomal-Incorporated siRNAs

1. Female athymic nude mice (NCr-nu, 8–12 weeks old; Taconic, Germantown, NY).
2. Syringes 30G.
3. PBS.
4. Hank's Balanced Salt Solution (HBSS) serum free (with Ca^{2+} and Mg^{2+}).
5. 1,2-Dioleoyl-*sn*-glycerol-3-phosphocholine (DOPC)
6. *t*-Butyl alcohol.
7. Tween 20.

2.7 Equipment and Software

1. Laminar flow bench and cell culture incubator.
2. Mini plate spinner MPS 1000 (Labnet, Woodbridge, NJ) or A-2-MTP rotor 5430/5430R centrifuge (Eppendorf, Hauppauge, NY).
3. Centrifuge 5430 R (Eppendorf) or any equivalent centrifuge with capability to reach 12,000 × *g* at 4 °C.
4. NanoDrop 2000 spectrophotometer (Thermo Scientific, Wilmington, Delaware) or an equivalent spectrophotometer with high accuracy and reproducibility.
5. Heating blocks.
6. StepOne plus real-time PCR thermal cycle system (Applied Biosystems) or any equivalent real-time PCR instrument (please read carefully the instrument parameters and settings before starting).
7. StepOne software v2.1 (each PCR instrument includes its own software).
8. Acetone/dry ice bath.

3 Methods

3.1 Cell Culture Conditions

Maintain ovarian cancer cell lines by culturing in RPMI-1640 medium supplemented with 10 % FBS in 5 % CO_2/95 % air at 37 °C. Perform all in vitro assays at 70–80 % cell density. Procedure for cell culture and passaging:

1. Wash the cell monolayers with PBS without Ca^{2+} or Mg^{2+}.
2. Pipette trypsin solution onto the washed cell monolayer using 1 ml per 25 cm^2 of surface area. Place flask in the incubator (37 °C) for 5–10 min.
3. Examine the cells using an inverted microscope to ensure that all the cells are detached and floating. The side of the flasks may be gently tapped to release any remaining attached cells.
4. Resuspend the cells in equal volume of serum-containing RPMI to inactivate the trypsin, and centrifuge at 1,000 rpm for 5 min.
5. Discard the supernatant and resuspend cells in the appropriate media for cell passage or for siRNA transfection.

3.2 RNA Extraction

Before starting, clean the working area and all the reagents and materials with RNaseZAP. Always wear gloves, avoid speech over open tubes, and use aerosol-barrier tips and fresh solutions (maintain all of these precautions for cDNA synthesis and real-time PCR procedures). Please read the protocol enclosed with the TRIzol reagent for full details.

1. For RNA extraction from tissue, remove the tissue samples from −80 °C freezer and thaw slowly on ice. Take approximately 35 mg of tumor tissue (mouse or human tumor samples). For RNA extraction from cell growth cultures, wash cells (approximately 1×10^7 cells) with chilled PBS twice.
2. Add 1 ml of TRIzol and homogenize. For homogenizing tumor tissue, use a dounce homogenizer (20 strokes).
3. Place the sample in a 1.5 ml microcentrifuge tube and incubate for 5 min at room temperature.
4. Add 200 μl of chloroform and shake for 15 s. Incubate for 3 min at room temperature.
5. Centrifuge the sample at 12,000 × *g* for 15 min at 4 °C.
6. Transfer the upper aqueous phase (containing the RNA) into a new 1.5 ml microcentrifuge tube.
7. Add 500 μl of isopropanol and incubate for 10 min at room temperature. This step allows precipitation of the RNA.
8. Centrifuge the samples at 12,000 × *g* for 15 min at 4 °C. Carefully, observe a gel-like pellet in the bottom of the tube.

9. Remove the supernatant, wash the pellet with 1 ml of 75 % ethanol, and mix the sample by vortex.
10. Centrifuge the sample at 7,500 × *g* for 5 min at 4 °C.
11. Remove the supernatant and air-dry the RNA pellet for 10 min.
12. Dissolve the RNA pellet using RNase-free water; incubate for 10 min at 60 °C.
13. Determine the quality and concentration of the RNA with the NanoDrop. A 260/280 ratio of 1.8:2.1 is necessary for cDNA synthesis (*see* **Note 4**).

3.3 cDNA Synthesis

Before starting, read carefully the protocol enclosed with the SuperScript II reverse transcriptase. The main points are listed here (*see* **Note 1**):

1. In a nuclease-free microcentrifuge tube, combine 1 μl of oligo $(dT)_{12-18}$, 1.0 μg of total RNA, 1 μl of 10 mM dNTPs, and nuclease-free water up to 13 μl of total volume.
2. Heat the reaction to 65 °C for 5 min; briefly centrifuge the tube, and quickly place the tube on ice.
3. Add 4 μl of 5× First-strand buffer and 2 μl of 0.1M DTT, mix, and incubate for 2 min.
4. Add 1 μl (200 units) of SuperScript II RT and mix gently by pipetting. The final total volume in the tube will be 20 μl.
5. Incubate to 40 °C for 2 h.
6. Stop the reaction by heating the sample to 70 °C for 15 min (*see* **Note 5**).

3.4 Real-Time PCR Primer Design

Primer design is the most important part of qPCR analysis [15]. As SYBR green I dye assay will detect all double-stranded DNA, including nonspecific reaction products, a well-designed primer is essential for accurate quantitative results. An ideal pair of primers for SYBR-I-based qPCR should meet some important criteria including the amplicon length (60–200 bp), primer length (19–23 bp), GC content (35–65 %), melting temperature (50–68 °C), complementarities (avoiding primer self- or cross-annealing stretches greater than 4 bp), specificity (BLAST primer sequence against entire mRNA database), single-nucleotide polymorphisms (SNP) (primer sequences should not include known SNPs), and 3′-end stability (runs of three or more of C's or G's at the 3′ end of the primer should be avoided). Herein, to amplify all survivin splice variants at the same time, we designed primers in the region containing exons 1 and 2 that are commons to all survivin isoforms (*see* Fig. 1). To amplify survivin WT, survivin 3B, and survivin ΔEX3, we used a common forward primer described by Knauer et al. [10]. The reverse primer for survivin WT was designed in the exon 3 and 4 junction, and for survivin ΔEX3, in the 3′-UTR region (*see* Fig. 1). The reverse primer for survivin 2B and the primers for survivin 3B were described by Knauer et al. [10]. The primers to amplify survivin 2α were from Caldas et al. [8]. Primers were designed with the Internet-free Primer3 v.0.4.0 software at http://fokker.wi.mit.edu/primer3/ [18] with the following parameters (*see* **Note 6**):

- Product size range 100–200
- Primer size minimum 19, optimum 20, maximum 21
- Primer Tm minimum 59, optimum 60, maximum 61
- Other parameters as default values

Table 1 includes the accession number (which identifies each gene in The National Center for Biotechnology Information, NCBI) and the oligonucleotide sequences to specifically amplify each survivin splice variant. In addition, a pair of primers for an internal standard or control gene should be used [15]. Here, β-actin is used as the internal standard (*see* Table 1 and **Note 7**). For all primers a BLAST with the primer designing tool-NCBI (http://www.ncbi.nlm.nih.gov/tools/primer-blast/) was performed to ensure that each pair of primers amplifies only one survivin splice variant.

3.5 Real-Time PCR Amplification

We describe here the use of SYBR-I PCR master mix. As we mentioned above, SYBR-I is a dye which binds nonspecifically to double-stranded DNA [15]. Any unspecific DNA product in the PCR reaction (including primer-dimers) contributes to increases in fluorescence, which is detected by the real-time PCR instruments. Thus, before setting up the real-time PCR reaction, it is necessary to optimize the annealing temperature and concentration for each pair of primers (*see* **Note 8**). Therefore, perform a real-time PCR reaction (in triplicate) followed by a melt-curve analysis (*see* **Note 9**) following **steps 4–9**.

1. Set up the PCR machine program with the following thermal settings: 1 cycle of 15′/95 °C; 40 cycles of 15″/94 °C, 30″/X°C (X = 60 °C for total survivin, X = 58 °C for wild-type survivin, survivin 2B, and ΔEx3; 50 °C for survivin 2α, 54 °C for survivin 3B; and 60 °C for β-actin), for 30″/72 °C. For melt-curve analysis, perform 1 cycle at 55–95 °C (in 0.5 °C increments) for 30″.
2. Prepare a master mix by adding (per reaction) 12.5 μl of 2× SYBR green, 1 μl of forward primer, 1 μl of reverse primer, and 3.5 μl of water. Adjust volumes according to the number of replicates and samples (including negative controls) (*see* **Note 10**).
3. In a 96-well real-time PCR plate, mix 18 μl of master mix (**step 2**) and 2 μl of cDNA (from Subheading 3.2, **step 6**) to obtain 20 μl total volume. Once all reactions are completed, cover the plate with an adhesive plastic lid.

Table 1
Oligonucleotides (primers) used for SYBR-I-based real-time PCR experiments

Gene	Reference sequence	Forward primer	Reverse primer
Survivin WT	NM_001168	GACCACCGCATCTCTACATTC	TGCTTTTTATGTTCCTCTATGGG
Survivin 2B	NM_001012271	GACCACCGCATCTCTACATTC	AAGTGCTGGTATTACAGGCGT
Survivin ΔEx3	NM_001012270	GACCACCGCATCTCTACATTC	ATTGTTGGTTTCCTTTGCATG
Survivin 3B	AB154416.1	GAGGCTGGCTTCATCCACTG	GCTCTCTCAATTTTGTTCTTG
Survivin 2α	AY927772	GCTTTGTTTTGAACTGAGTTGTCAA	GCAATGAGGGTGGAAAGCA
Total survivin	NM_001168	AGCCCTTTCTCAAGGACCAC	CAGCTCCTTGAAGCAGAAGAA
β-actin	NM_001101.3	ATAGCACAGCCTGGATAGCAACGTAC	CACCTTCTACAATGAGCTGCGTGTG

Table 2
Example of a SYBR real-time PCR experiment

	1	2	3	4	5
Cell line	**Ct (β-actin)**	**Ct (T survivin)**	**ΔCt**	**ΔΔCt**	**RQ**
SKOV3ip1	23.04	25.19	2.15	0	1
SKOV3.TR	22.95	24.78	1.83	-0.32	1.25
HEYA8	22.89	25.77	2.88	0.7	0.62
HEYA8.TR	21.79	23.99	2.2	0.05	0.97
A2780PAR	22.6	24.69	2.09	-0.06	1.04
A2780CP20	21.52	23.56	2.4	0.25	0.84

4. Centrifuge the plate in a mini plate spinner.
5. Place the plate in the PCR machine and start the program. The software must be in active mode to collect the amplification and melt-curve.
6. With the Step One Software version 2.1, determine the best concentration and annealing temperature for each pair of primers, based in the threshold cycle (Ct) values (*see* **Note 11**) and melt-curve graphs. The melt-curve should display single sharp peaks (*see* **Note 12**).
7. Repeat **steps 4–9** with the real samples.
8. Using the Step One Software version 2.1, or equivalent software, determine the threshold cycle corresponding to each sample and analyze the relative expression using the ΔΔCt method (*see* **Note 13**).
9. The relative expression of each survivin splice variant can be calculated mathematically or in the excel program with the Ct values. The following steps describe the use of the ΔΔCt method to calculate the relative abundance of total survivin in a panel of six ovarian cancer cell lines. Table 2 shows the results of one SYBR real-time PCR experiment to assess the survivin mRNA expression levels in a panel of six ovarian cancer cell lines.
10. Normalize the average Ct of the gene of interest (total survivin) to the internal control (β-actin) for each sample (*column 2 minus column 1, see* Table 2 and **Note 14**):

$$\Delta Ct = Ct(\text{Total survivin}) - Ct(\beta\text{actin})$$

11. Calculate the differences between the ΔCt of each sample and the ΔCt of the control sample (*column 3,* Table 2). This is ΔΔCt (*column 4,* Table 2):

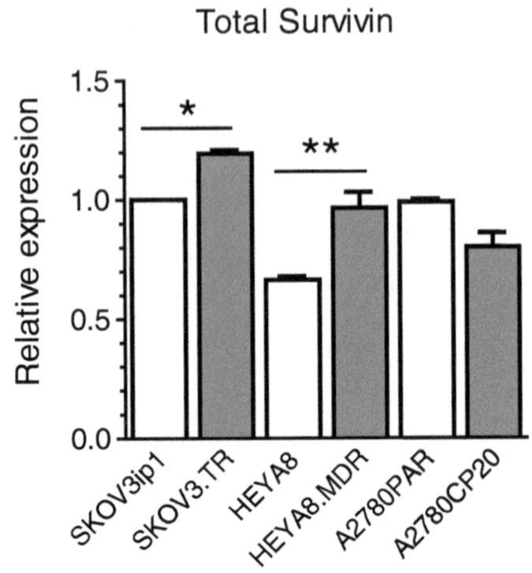

Fig. 2 Relative survivin mRNA levels in a panel of ovarian cancer cells. RNA isolation, cDNA synthesis, and SYBR green I-based PCR were performed as described in Subheadings 3.2, 3.3, and 3.4, respectively. β-actin was used as the internal standard. Survivin expression levels were calculated with the ΔΔCt method. Total survivin mRNA values were expressed relative to the SKOV3ip1 cells. Columns represent the means of triplicates ±S.D. $^{*}p<0.05$, $^{**}p<0.01$. Reproduced from Vivas-Mejía et al. [13]

$$\Delta\Delta Ct = \Delta Ct(\text{cell line}) - \Delta Ct(\text{SKOV3ip1})$$

12. Calculate the relative quantification (RQ) or fold change (*column 5*, Table 2) (*see* Fig. 2).

$$RQ = 2^{-\Delta\Delta Ct}$$

3.6 In Vitro siRNA-Based Silencing of Survivin Splice Variants

Here we used siRNAs to silence total survivin and survivin 2B. Specific siRNAs should be designed to silence other survivin splice variants (*see* **Note 15**):

1. Resuspend ovarian cancer cells in RPMI-1640 supplemented with 10 % FBS at 3×10^4 cells/ml.
2. Plate 2 ml of cells in six-well plates. Incubate plates to 37 °C for 24 h.
3. The siRNA/HiPerFect ratio should be optimized for each cell line. For HEYA8.MDR cells a 1:3 siRNA/HiPerFect ratio was used (*see* **Note 16**). Carefully read the protocol enclosed with the HiPerFect transfection reagent with the following indications:
4. Resuspend siRNAs, negative control, and each survivin splice variant siRNAs, at a stock concentration of 1 μg/μl with DNA-free water.

5. In a 1.5 ml tube, mix 3 μl each siRNA, 9 μl of HiPerFect, and 88 μl Optimem. Mix using vortex (30 s) and let stand 10–20 min at room temperature.
6. Take the six-well plate containing the cells (**step 2**), remove the RPMI medium, and add 1,900 μl of Optimem medium.
7. Add 100 μl of siRNA transfection mix (**step 5**) to the cells drop by drop. Mix by gentle rotation of the plate. Incubate the plate for 48 h in 5 % CO_2/95 % air at 37 °C.
8. Collect the cells and isolate total RNA as described in Subheading 3.2. Perform the cDNA synthesis and real-time PCR as described in Subheadings 3.3 and 3.4.
9. Calculate the changes in expression of each survivin splice variant using the relative value of control siRNA as 100 % of expression.

3.7 In Vivo Silencing of Survivin Splice Variants with siRNA-Loaded Liposomes

1. Use female immunocompromised athymic nude mice (NCr-nu, 8–12 weeks old) to establish ovarian cancer xenografts. Nude mice should be kept in barrier animal facilities maintained at a 12 h light/dark cycle. House the mice at 5 per cage with free access to food and water.
2. Trypsinize ovarian cancer cells (60–80 % confluence) and centrifuge at 1,000 rpm for 5 min at 4 °C.
3. Wash two times with PBS.
4. Dilute cells at a concentration of 5×10^5–1×10^6 cells/ml in HBSS (*see* **Note 17**). HEYA8.MDR cells were used at 1×10^6 cells/ml.
5. Inject 200 μl of cells per mouse into the peritoneal cavity.
6. After 3–4 weeks of the tumor implantation, proceed with the liposomal-siRNA injections. At these stage cells have formed tumors, which can be assessed by palpation of the peritoneal area (*see* **Note 18**).
7. Mix siRNA and 1,2-dioleoyl-sn-glycerol-3-phosphocholine (DOPC) in the presence of excess *t*-butyl alcohol at a ratio 1:10 (w/w) siRNA/DOPC.
8. Add Tween 20 to the mixture at a ratio of 1:10 (v/v) (Tween 20:siRNA/DOPC).
9. Vortex the mixture and freeze in acetone/dry ice bath. Lyophilize the mixture.
10. Resuspend the siRNA-lipid mixture to a final siRNA concentration of 25 μg/ml in PBS without Ca^{2+} and Mg^{2+}.
11. Inject 200 μl (5 μg siRNA) of liposomal siRNA into the peritoneal cavity of nude mice bearing tumors.

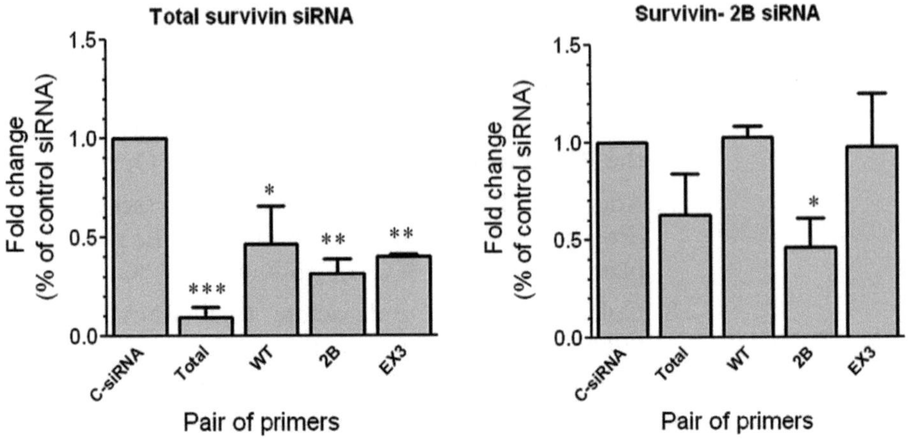

Fig. 3 Real-time PCR with total RNA isolated from tumor tissues. Mice were treated as described in Subheading 3.6. RNA isolation, cDNA synthesis, and SYBR green I-based PCR were performed as described in Subheadings 3.2, 3.3, and 3.4, respectively. Survivin expression levels were calculated with the ΔΔCt method and expressed relative to the control siRNA-treated mice. Columns represent the means of triplicates ±S.D. $^{*}p<0.05$, $^{**}p<0.01$, $^{***}p<0.001$. Reproduced from Vivas-Mejía et al. [13]

12. Two to three days after injection, sacrifice the animal, remove the tumor, and store at −80 °C for total RNA isolation. Perform RNA isolation, cDNA synthesis, and real-time PCR as described in Subheadings 3.2, 3.3 and 3.4.
13. Calculate changes in the expression of each survivin splice variant using the control group of mice (mice injected with liposomal-control siRNA) as 100 % relative mRNA expression levels (*see* Fig. 3).

4 Notes

1. To synthesize cDNA, we used reagents purchased from Life Technologies (former Invitrogen, Grand Island, NY). However, any other well-optimized cDNA synthesis kit can be used. All reagents must be stored at −20 °C.
2. To simultaneously silence all survivin splice variants, the siRNA should bind to any region encompassing the exon 1 and exon 2 (accession number, NM_001168). These exons are common to all survivin isoforms (*see* Fig. 1). The siRNA sequence used here was 5′-CAGACTTGGCCCAGTGTTT-3′. To target survivin 2B specifically (accession number, NM_001012271) (*see* Fig. 1), the following sequence was used: 5′-AATACCAGCACTTTGGGAG-3′.
3. All our procedures have been optimized with the use of HiPerFect transfection reagent. We recommended this

reagent, because it has been shown to cause less toxicity in our cell lines.

4. There are other methods to measure the RNA quality: (a) separating an aliquot of the sample on a denaturing polyacrylamide gel, staining with ethidium bromide, and visualizing the RNA in an UV transilluminator; (b) with the use of an Agilent 2100 bioanalyzer.
5. The cDNA can be stored at −20 °C (1–2 weeks).
6. Other Internet tools can be used to design primers including the primer designing tool-NCBI (http://www.idtdna.com/Primerquest/Home/Index), the IDT PrimerQuest (http://www.idtdna.com/Scitools/Applications/Primerquest/a), and the primer3web version 4.0 (http://frodo.wi.mit.edu/) tool that allow to visualize primers positions in the mRNA sequence and select primers for certain splice variants.
7. The internal standard for PCR reactions should be amplified simultaneously with the gene of interest. In addition, the expression of the internal standard should not be altered by the experiment and should be amplified at the same level or more than the gene of interest. Finally, the amplification product of the internal standard and the gene of interest should be very similar in size.
8. The optimal primer concentration is determined by independently varying forward and reverse primer concentrations. Generally, three different concentrations of each primer are tested, which generate a matrix of nine different PCR reactions of primer forward and primer reverse ratios (all in nM concentrations) as follows: 50/50, 50/200, 50/600, 200/50, 200/200, 200/600, 600/50, 600/200, and 600/600. For the first three PCR reactions, decrease 2 °C, and for the last three reactions, increase 2 °C in the annealing temperature. This strategy will identify the concentration and annealing temperature for each pair of primers.
9. The melting temperature (T_m) of each product is defined as the temperature at which the corresponding maximum peak occurs. The melt-curve should display a single sharp peak in each reaction. The StepOne plus and other real-time PCR instruments include default protocols, which contain the melt-curve analysis at the end of the PCR cycles. Primer concentrations should also be optimized for real-time PCR experiments. The optimal primer concentration for each survivin splice variant is 200 nM (final concentration).
10. Negative controls should include PCR reactions without cDNA (for detecting contamination or nonspecific amplification) and without enzyme (to determine that any amplification that

occurs in the sample is derived from the synthesized cDNA and not genomic DNA).

11. The Ct values are defined as the number of cycles required for the fluorescent signal to exceed the background level. Therefore, the more cDNA is present in a sample, the lower the Ct values, as the threshold is reached earlier.
12. The primer concentrations selected should provide the lowest Ct and highest fluorescence intensity values. Strong amplification of negative control reactions (generally, Ct higher than 35, i.e., 32) indicates that significant nonspecific amplification is occurring. Equally, more than one pick in the melt-curve analysis is indicative of PCR artifacts including primer dimmers or unspecific PCR products. In general, these artifacts have lower melting temperatures than the target amplicon.
13. The ΔΔCt method allows calculation of the relative abundance of each transcript [19]. Another method, commonly used to calculate the mRNA expression levels, is a standard plot of serial cDNA dilutions of each transcript versus the Ct values, followed by interpolating in the graph, the Ct values for each unknown sample [19].
14. In real-time PCR, the control sample is known as the calibrator. This is the sample taken as reference, and its relative abundance is expressed as 1 or 100 %. Here, the calibrator was the SKOV3ip1 cell line.
15. Many pharmaceutical companies have their own tools to design siRNAs. Other Internet tools are also available: http://sirna.wi.mit.edu/ or https://www.genscript.com/ssl-bin/app/rnai. However, these tools, in general, use the mRNA sequence of the most frequently occurring transcript. For example, the commercially available siRNAs for survivin (BIRC5) are directed to WT survivin (NCBI accession number NM_001168). For silencing specifically other splice variants, use their own NCBI accession numbers (i.e., for survivin 2B, NM_001012271). Then, by aligning the sequences of all splice variants, corroborate that the siRNA sequence is not complementary to the mRNA of any other splice variant. If the siRNA targets more than one splice variant, design the siRNA manually. Rules for selecting siRNA targets on mRNA sequences are available at http://www.rnaiweb.com/RNAi/siRNA_Design/.
16. Some cell lines are difficult to transfect with HiPerFect or any other transfection reagent. Electroporation is commonly used to transfect those cells.
17. The number of inoculated cells depends on the rate of cell growth and in the tumorigenic capacity of the cells.

18. To monitor tumor growth in mice, several "labeled" tumor models have been developed. These models involve the creation of tumor cell lines that carry a foreign protein such as green fluorescence protein (GFP), red fluorescence protein (RFP), or firefly luciferase, which allows noninvasive monitoring of tumor growth.

Acknowledgments

We would like to thank Surangani Dharmawardhane Flanagan, Ph.D., for critical reading of the manuscript. This work was funded, in part, by the University of Puerto Rico Comprehensive Cancer Center seed funds to P.E.V.M. and a scholarship to I.M.E.V. from the NIH, Minority Biomedical Research Support-Research Initiative for Scientific Enhancement (MBRS-RISE) Program (R25-GM061838).

References

1. Cheung CH et al (2011) Investigation of survivin: the past, present and future. Front Biosci 16:952–961
2. Liguang Z et al (2007) Survivin expression in ovarian cancer. Exp Oncol 29:121–125
3. Ferrandina G et al (2005) Survivin expression in ovarian cancer and its correlation with clinico-pathological, surgical and apoptosis-related parameters. Br J Cancer 92:271–277
4. Carrasco R et al (2011) Antisense inhibition of survivin expression as a cancer therapeutic. Mol Cancer Ther 20:221–232
5. Pennati M, Folini M, Zaffaroni N (2007) Targeting survivin in a cancer therapy: fulfilled promises and open questions. Carcinogenesis 28:1133–1139
6. Vader G et al (2006) Survivin mediates targeting of the chromosomal passenger complex to the centromere and midbody. EMBO Rep 7:85–92
7. Sampath J, Pelus LM (2007) Alternative splice variants of survivin as potential targets in cancer. Curr Drug Discov Technol 4:174–191
8. Caldas H, Honsey LE, Altura RA (2005) Survivin 2α: a novel survivin splice variant expressed in human malignancies. Mol Cancer 4:11–19
9. Mahotka C et al (1999) Survivin-ΔEx3 and Survivin-2B: two novel splice variants of the apoptosis inhibitor survivin with different antiapoptotic properties. Cancer Res 59: 6097–6102
10. Knauer SK et al (2007) The survivin isoform survivin-3B is cytoprotective and can function as a chromosomal passenger complex protein. Cell Cycle 6:1502–1509
11. Mahotka C et al (2002) Differential subcellular localization of functionally divergent survivin splice variants. Cell Death Differ 9:1334–1342
12. Stauber RH, Mann W, Knauer SK (2007) Nuclear and cytoplasmic survivin: molecular mechanism, prognostic, and therapeutic potential. Cancer Res 67:5999–6002
13. Vivas-Mejía PE et al (2011) Silencing survivin splice variant 2B leads to antitumor activity in taxane-resistant ovarian cancer. Clin Cancer Res 17:3716–3726
14. Doolittle H, Morel A, Talbot D (2010) Survivin-directed anticancer therapies-a review of pre-clinical data and early-phase clinical trials. Eur Oncol 6:10–14
15. Ponchel F et al (2003) Real-time PCR based on SYBR-Green I fluorescence: an alternative to the TaqMan assay for a relative quantification of gene rearrangements, gene amplifications and micro gene deletions. BMC Biotechnol 3:18
16. Lamendola DE et al (2003) Molecular description of evolving paclitaxel resistance in the SKOV-3 human ovarian carcinoma cell line. Cancer Res 63:2200–2205
17. Thaker PH et al (2005) Antivascular therapy for orthotopic human ovarian carcinoma through blockade of the vascular

endothelial growth factor and epidermal growth factor receptors. Clin Cancer Res 11:4923–4933
18. Rozen S, Skaletsky HJ (2000) Primer3 on the WWW for general users and for biologist programmers. In: Krawetz S, Misener S (eds) Bioinformatics methods and protocols: methods in molecular biology. Humana Press, Totowa, NJ, pp 365–386
19. Schmittgen TD, Livak KJ (2008) Analyzing real-time PCR data by the comparative Ct method. Nat Protoc 3:1101–1108

Chapter 14

MicroRNA Profiling in Ovarian Cancer

Marilena V. Iorio and Carlo M. Croce

Abstract

The evaluation of microRNA profiles has represented one of the first approaches to investigate the aberrant microRNA expression in different human cancers, providing the first experimental evidence of the involvement of these small noncoding RNAs in the tumorigenic process. Currently, these and other methods have been applied to the search of new molecular biomarkers of diagnosis, prognosis, and response to therapy prediction.

Here, we described the approach we used for the determination of a miRNA signature unique for human ovarian cancer, first performing a large-scale screening using a custom-made microarray platform, and then validating the obtained data by Northern blot or real-time PCR.

Key words MicroRNAs, Ovarian cancer, Expression profiling, Signature, Biomarker, Diagnosis

1 Introduction

1.1 MicroRNA Profiles in Human Cancer: Rational and Methodological Approaches to Use Them as Diagnostic, Prognostic, and Predictive Biomarkers

At present, we can certainly state that alterations in microRNA expression are not isolated events but the rule in human cancer, indeed microRNA genes are often located in fragile regions of the genome, involved in chromosomal alterations, such as deletion or amplification, in many different human tumors [1]. The first evidence of the involvement of microRNAs in human cancer derived from studies on chronic lymphocytic leukemia (CLL), where the deletion of chr. 13q14 causes loss of two oncosuppressor microRNA genes, miR-15a and miR-16-1 [2]. After these early studies, platforms to assess the global expression of microRNA genes in normal and diseased tissues have been developed, as an attempt to establish whether microRNA profiling could be used for tumor classification, diagnosis, and prognosis [3]: after an extensive use of custom-made [4] and then commercial miRNA microarrays, and bead-based flow cytometric miRNA analysis methods [5], the last generation of large-scale profiling method is represented by the high-throughput deep sequencing [6, 7].

Anastasia Malek and Oleg Tchernitsa (eds.), *Ovarian Cancer: Methods and Protocols*, Methods in Molecular Biology, vol. 1049, DOI 10.1007/978-1-62703-547-7_14, © Springer Science+Business Media New York 2013

Genome-wide profiling showed that miRNA expression signatures allowed different types of cancer to be discriminated with high accuracy (even higher than mRNA profiles). Beside the expression profile studies based on microarray platforms, many other methods for detecting microRNAs have been developed, as quantitative real-time PCR (QRT-PCR) [8, 9], in situ hybridization [10–13], and high-throughput sequencing [14]. The most important disadvantage of microarray technologies resides in the nonquantitative nature of this method, which therefore requires further experimental validation. Real-Time PCR is extremely sensitive and accurate, however it is a more expensive and low-throughput method. In situ hybridization, based on the detection of specific miRNAs by hybridizing a complementary strand (probe) to the sequence of interest in morphologically preserved tissue sections or cell preparations, is certainly highly sensitive and allows the analysis at a single cell or subcellular level. However, it represents a technically challenging, semiquantitative, and low-throughput method. Finally, whereas all these techniques are restricted to detection and profiling of previously identified miRNA sequences, sequence-based methods allow the identification of unknown microRNAs. Indeed, initially used to detect microRNAs expressed at a low level, and extremely expensive and time consuming, since 2007 deep sequencing methods, which rely on next generation sequencing machines, fast and accurate, have led to the discovery of new microRNAs. Recently, these methods have been used to reveal the differential expression of miRNAs in ovarian cancer [14].

Most used methods to detect microRNAs are summarized in Table 1.

In summary, to be successful at narrowing down the biology of a specific tumor to enable more accurate diagnoses, which would be of immense benefit to both doctors and patients, the accuracy of the method is of vital importance. And, similar to all big innovations, also for the use of microRNA signatures in clinics there are some kinks that need to be addressed. Reported lack of consistency between different studies, for example, certainly gives rise to some concern. Such differences typically arise from sample selection or preparation, experimental design, and/or data analysis [15]. Indeed, the use of different controls for data normalization can explain some of the observed variability across studies [16]. Another possibility that must be considered is the dynamic and immediate regulation in miRNA levels in stress response [17] and in hypoxia [18]; thus, time of collection and processing could impact miRNA levels.

Besides the potential to distinguish between normal and cancerous tissue and identify tissues of origin, miRNA signatures can also discriminate different subtypes of a particular cancer and predict cancer prognosis and/or response to specific therapies [19–21].

Table 1
Methods of miRNA detection

Method	Positive aspects	Negative aspects	Reference
Microarray	High-throughput screening	Nonquantitative Higher amount of material required	Liu et al. [4] Lu et al. [5]
Northern blot	Quantitative Mature and precursor forms visualized on the same membrane	Higher amount of material required Low-throughput screening, mainly used for validation Use of radioactive material	Iorio et al. [22]
Real-time PCR	Quantitative Sensitive Low amount of material required	More expensive Low-throughput screening	Chen et al. [8] Raymond et al. [9]
In situ hybridization	Sensitive Analysis at subcellular level	Semiquantitative Low-throughput screening	Obernosterer et al. [10] Pena et al. [11] Nuovo et al. [12] de Planell-Saguer et al. [13]
Deep sequencing	High-throughput screening Discovery of new miRNAs	Expensive More time consuming (but new platforms are fast and accurate)	Wyman et al. [14]

1.2 MicroRNAs in Human Ovarian Cancer

The first report describing an aberrant expression of microRNAs in human ovarian cancer was published in 2007 by Iorio and collaborators from Dr. Croce's group [22], which was performed using a custom microarray platform [4] (Ohio State Comprehensive Cancer Center, version 2.0) (detailed description of the techniques applied in this study are reported in Subheading 3).

Comparing miRNA profiles between EOC surgical specimens and cell lines versus normal ovary, we found 29 differentially expressed miRNAs, differentiating normal versus tumor with a classification rate of 89 %. Moreover, we identified miRNA expression profiles of distinct histotypes of ovarian carcinomas.

Notably, the four miRNAs up-modulated in EOC versus normal ovary were found to be genetically amplified in a study performed by Zhang et al., whereas 10 of the 25 downmodulated miRNAs were genetically deleted [23]. Moreover, also epigenetic alterations as DNA methylation can affect miRNA expression. In contrast, somatic mutations do not seem to be involved in miRNA gene inactivation, at least in EOC.

A couple of years later Zhang et al. [24] found a global down-regulation of the differentially expressed miRNAs in association with OSE malignant transformation and EOC progression, in agreement with the previous report [22]. 25 % of down-regulated miRNAs were aggregated in clusters on three chromosomes: 14, 19, and X. In particular, a cluster of eight miRNAs localized on chr.14 has been found to be down-regulated in advanced relative to early-stage EOC, and in invasive colon and breast cancer. The same cluster is silenced by epigenetic mechanisms in EOC and bladder cancer. Interestingly, Bagnoli et al. also identified a chrXq27.3 microRNA cluster associated with early relapse in advanced stage ovarian cancer patients and response to front-line therapy [25].

Besides the use of different technologies, different normal counterparts have also been used to detect miRNA aberrantly expressed in EOC cell lines or surgical samples. In particular for cancers of epithelial origin, the choice of an appropriate control for evaluating differential miRNA, as well as gene, expression profiles between "normal" and EOC is crucial. Studies of EOC have relied on a variety of sources of "normal" cells for comparison with tumors, including whole ovary samples, short-term culture of OSE, and immortalized OSE cell lines, with pros and cons: whole ovary has a large stromal component, whereas immortalization results in further changes in expression profile [26, 27].

The best approach is probably represented by the so-called brushing technique, which allows the collection of OSE without stroma and provides a relatively pure sample of OSE that is not exposed to culture conditions. However, this certainly requires a higher number of samples as starting material. These results suggest that the selection of a normal control to compare to EOC samples in profiling studies can strongly influence the miRNAs that are identified as differentially expressed, same concern raised for gene expression analysis.

Notably, many of the microRNAs we found differentially expressed in our study [22] were later validated also by other groups using different normal controls and techniques and, even more importantly, have been demonstrated to be actually involved in the biology of human EOC.

Considering the potential role of microRNAs as prognostic or predictive biomarkers, efforts have been made to identify miRNA signatures in EOC and to determine whether dysregulated miRNAs may be associated with patient outcome [28–30] or response to therapy [31, 32].

2 Material

2.1 miRNA Microarray Hybridization and Quantification [4]

2.1.1 RNA Isolation

1. Tryzol.
2. Chloroform.
3. Isopropanol.
4. Ethanol 75 %.
5. RNAse-free water.

2.1.2 RNA Labelling and Hybridization

1. Labelling Kit, including (3′-(*N*)8-(A)12-biotin-(A)12-biotin-5′) oligonucleotide primer and Reverse Transcription Kit.
2. Custom microRNA microarray (Ohio State Comprehensive cancer Center).
3. Hybridization in 6× SSPE (0.9 M sodium chloride, 60 mM sodium phosphate, 8 mM EDTA)/30 % formamide.

2.1.3 Signal Detection and Computational Data Analysis

1. Streptavidin-Alexa647 conjugate.
2. Axon 4000B scanner.
3. Genepix software (Axon Instruments, Sunnyvale, CA).
4. BrB array-tool [33].

2.2 Northern Blotting

2.2.1 RNA Gel

1. 15 % Polyacrylamide, 7 M Urea Criterion precasted gels (Bio-Rad, Hercules, CA).
2. TBE-Urea sample buffer (Bio-Rad).
3. 1× TBE as running buffer.
4. Vertical electrophoresis system (Bio-Rad).

2.2.2 Blotting, Labelling, and Hybridization

1. Hybond-N+ membranes (Amersham, Piscataway, NJ).
2. [gamma-32P]-ATP.
3. Polynucleotide Kinase (Roche).
4. ULTRAhyb-Oligo hybridization buffer (Ambion, Austin, TX).
5. 2× SSPE, 0.5 % SDS, 0.1 % SDS.

2.3 Real-Time PCR

2.3.1 Reverse Transcription

1. TaqMan microRNA Reverse Transcription Kit (Applied Biosystem, Foster City, CA).
2. GeneAmp PCR 9700 Thermocycler (Applied Biosystem) or other thermocycler.

2.3.2 Real-Time PCR

1. TaqMan microRNA Assay (Applied Biosystems).
2. ABI Prism 7900HT Sequence detection system (Applied Biosystems).

2.3.3 Data Analysis

SDS software.

3 Methods

The choice of miRNA detection method should be mainly driven by the following considerations: aim of the study (first, whether it is a large screening study or a validation analysis), the amount of the starting material available, the need to analyze the microRNA, subcellular location or to discover new microRNAs (*see* also Table 1).

3.1 miRNA Microarray Hybridization and Quantification

3.1.1 RNA Isolation (See Note 1)

1. Add Trizol to cell or tissue and incubate the homogenized sample for 5 min at RT.
2. Add 0.2 mL Chloroform per 1 mL Trizol, cap the tube securely, shake tube vigorously by hand for 15 s, incubate for 2–3 min at RT.
3. Centrifuge the sample at 12,000 × *g* for 15 min at 4 °C (Note: the mixture separates into a lower red phenol–chloroform phase, an interphase, and a colorless upper aqueous phase. RNA remains exclusively in the aqueous phase. The upper aqueous phase is ~50 % of the total volume).
4. Remove the aqueous phase avoiding to draw any of the interphase or organic layer and place it into a new tube.
5. Add the same volume (approximately 0.5 mL per 1 mL Trizol) of 100 % isopropanol to the aqueous phase, incubate at room temperature for 10 min.
6. Centrifuge at 12,000 × *g* for 10 min at 4 °C.
7. Remove the supernatant from the tube.
8. Wash the pellet with 0.5–1 mL of 75 % ethanol, vortex the sample briefly, then centrifuge the tube at 7,500 × *g* for 5 min at 4 °C and discard the wash, vacuum or air dry the RNA pellet for 5–10 min.
9. Resuspend the RNA pellet in RNase-free water, incubate in a water bath or heat block set at 55–60 °C for 10–15 min and store at −80 °C.

3.1.2 RNA Labelling and Hybridization

1. Add 5 μg of total RNA to reaction mix in a final volume of 12 μL, containing 1 μg of [3′-(*N*)8-(A)12-biotin-(A)12-biotin-5′] oligonucleotide primer.
2. Incubate the mixture for 10 min at 70 °C and chilled on ice.
3. With the mixture remaining on ice, add 4 μL of 5× first-strand buffer, 2 μL of 0.1 M DTT, 1 μL of 10 mM dNTP mix, and 1 μL of SuperScript II RNaseH$^-$ reverse transcriptase (200 U/μL) to a final volume of 20 μL, and incubate the mixture for 90 min in a 37 °C water bath.
4. After incubation for first-strand cDNA synthesis, add 3.5 μL of 0.5 M NaOH/50 mM EDTA into 20 μL of first-strand

reaction mix and incubate at 65 °C for 15 min to denature the RNA/DNA hybrids and degrade RNA templates.

5. Add 5 μL of 1 M Tris–HCl (pH 7.6) to neutralize the reaction mix, and store labelled targets in 28.5 μL at 80 °C until chip hybridization.

3.1.3 Microarrays Hybridization

The microarrays are hybridized in 6× SSPE (0.9 M sodium chloride/60 mM sodium phosphate/8 mM EDTA, pH 7.4)/30 % formamide at 25 °C for 18 h, washed in 0.75× TNT (Tris–HCl/sodium chloride and /Tween 20) at 37 °C for 40 min.

3.1.4 Signal Detection and Computational Data Analysis (See ***Notes 2*** *and* ***3****)*

1. Detect hybridization signals with Streptavidin-Alexa647 conjugate and quantify scanned images (Axon 4000B) using the Genepix 6.0 software (Axon Instruments, Sunnyvale, CA).
2. Analyze microarray images by using GENEPIX PRO. Average values of the replicate spots of each miRNA are background subtracted, normalized, and subjected to further analysis (*see* **Note 4**).
3. Differentially expressed miRNAs are identified by using the *t*-test procedure within significance analysis of microarrays (SAM), a method developed at Stanford University Labs based on recent paper of Tusher et al. [34].
4. PAM program might be also applied to identify miRNA signatures. This software performs sample classification from gene expression data, via the "nearest shrunken centroid method" of Tibshirani et al. [35].

Other bioinformatic methods are available for microarray data analysis.

3.2 Northern Blotting

1. Isolate RNA as described in Subheading 3.1.1 and dissolve in RNA samples (10 μg each) were in TBE-Urea Buffer.
2. Incubated at 70 °C for 5 min and run on 15 % Polyacrylamide, 7 M Urea Criterion precasted gels (Bio-Rad, Hercules, CA).
3. Transfer samples onto Hybond-N+ membranes (Amersham, Piscataway, NJ).
4. 200 ng of each probe are end labelled with 100 μCi [gamma-^{32}P]-ATP using the polynucleotide kinase (Roche). The oligonucleotides used as probes should be antisense to the sequence of the mature microRNAs (*see* **Note 5** for examples).
5. Perform the hybridization at 37 °C in ULTRAhyb-Oligo hybridization buffer (Ambion, Austin, TX) for 16 h.
6. Wash membranes at 37 °C, twice with 2× SSPE and 0.5 % SDS and evaluate results in according with standard protocol established in laboratory.
7. Blots were stripped in boiling 0.1 % SDS for 10 min before re-hybridization.

3.3 Real-Time PCR

Real-time PCR is certainly more accurate than Northern blot, it requires a lower amount of material to be performed and it is faster. Moreover, it does not require the use of radioactive material.

1. Isolate RNA as described in Subheading 3.1.1.
2. Use TaqMan MicroRNA Assay to detect and quantify microRNA of interest on Applied Biosystems real-time PCR instruments in accordance with manufacturer's instructions (Applied Biosystems, Foster City, CA). Comparative real-time PCR should be performed in triplicate, including no-template controls.
3. Run RT reactions, including no-template controls and RT minus controls, were run in a GeneAmp PCR 9700 Thermocycler (Applied Biosystems).
4. Normalize results using 18S rRNA as a reference. It is important to underline that currently, the preferred housekeeping for miRNA expression normalization are represented by small RNA as U44 or U48 (*see* **Note 6**).
5. Gene expression levels is quantified using the ABI Prism 7900HT Sequence detection system (Applied Biosystems). Relative expression is calculated using the comparative C_t method.

4 Notes

1. When investigating microRNAs modulated in human specimens, take into consideration the quality and the amount of the starting material, the extraction method and—especially concerning human EOC—the importance of using the appropriate normal control.
2. When using a microarray platform, be extremely accurate in analyzing samples processed with homogenous procedures to avoid unwanted biased results (as clusterization of samples belonging to different batches, or run on the platform not at the same time, or extracted with different protocols, etc.).
3. When using a microarray platform, be extremely accurate in data filtering and normalization.
4. We performed a global median normalization of Ovary microarray data by using BRB ArrayTools developed by Richard Simon and Amy Peng Lam [33]. Absent calls were thresholded to 4.5 before subsequent statistical analysis. This level is the average minimum intensity level detected in the experiments. miRNA nomenclature was according to the Genome Browser (http://genome.ucsc.edu) and the miRNA database at Sanger Center (http://microrna.sanger.ac.uk/); in case of discrepancies the miRNA database was followed.

5. The oligonucleotides used as probes in our study were antisense to the sequence of the mature microRNAs: (miR Registry at http://www.sanger.ac.uk/Software/Rfam/mirna/) miR-200a: 5′-ACA TCG TTA CCA GAC AGT GTT A-3′; miR-141: 5′-CCA TCT TTA CCA GAC AGT GTT A-3′; miR-199a: 5′-GAA CAG GTA GTC TGA ACA CTG GG-3′; miR-125b1: 5′-TCA CAA GTT AGG GTC TCA GGG A-3′; miR-145: 5′-AAG GGA TTC CTG GGA AAA CTG GAC-3′; miR-222: 5′-GAG ACC CAG TAG CCA GAT GTA GCT-3′; miR-21: 5′-TCA ACA TCA GTC TGA TAA GCT A-3′.
6. If choosing QRT-PCR as detection method, be aware of the difficult choice of the housekeeping controls, which can different depending on tissue and tumor type, thus requiring an accurate validation.

References

1. Calin GA, Sevignani C, Dumitru CD, Hyslop T, Noch E, Yendamuri S, Shimizu M, Rattan S, Bullrich F, Negrini M, Croce CM (2004) Human microRNA genes are frequently located at fragile sites and genomic regions involved in cancers. Proc Natl Acad Sci USA 101:2999–3004
2. Calin GA, Dumitru CD, Shimizu M, Bichi R, Zupo S, Noch E, Aldler H, Rattan S, Keating M, Rai K, Rassenti L, Kipps T, Negrini M, Bullrich F, Croce CM (2002) Frequent deletions and down-regulation of micro-RNA genes miR15 and miR16 at 13q14 in chronic lymphocytic leukemia. Proc Natl Acad Sci USA 99:15524–15529
3. Calin GA, Croce CM (2006) MicroRNA signatures in human cancers. Nat Rev Cancer 6:857–866
4. Liu CG, Calin GA, Meloon B, Gamliel N, Sevignani C, Ferracin M, Dumitru CD, Shimizu M, Zupo S, Dono M et al (2004) An oligonucleotide microchip for genome-wide microRNA profiling in human and mouse tissues. Proc Natl Acad Sci USA 101: 9740–9744
5. Lu J, Getz G, Miska EA, varez-Saavedra E, Lamb J, Peck D, Sweet-Cordero A, Ebert BL, Mak RH, Ferrando AA, Downing JR, Jacks T, Horvitz HR, Golub TR (2005) MicroRNA expression profiles classify human cancers. Nature 435:834–838
6. Creighton CJ, Reid JG, Gunaratne PH (2009) Expression profiling of microRNAs by deep sequencing. Brief Bioinform 10:490–497
7. Farazi TA, Horlings HM, Ten Hoeve JJ, Mihailovic A, Halfwerk H, Morozov P, Brown M, Hafner M, Reyal F, van Kouwenhove M, Kreike B, Sie D, Hovestadt V, Wessels LF, van de Vijver MJ, Tuschl T (2011) MicroRNA sequence and expression analysis in breast tumors by deep sequencing. Cancer Res 71: 4443–4453
8. Chen C, Ridzon DA, Broomer AJ, Zhou Z, Lee DH, Nguyen JT, Barbisin M, Xu NL, Mahuvakar VR, Andersen MR, Lao KQ, Livak KJ, Guegler KJ (2005) Real-time quantification of microRNAs by stem-loop RT-PCR. Nucleic Acids Res 33:e179
9. Raymond CK, Roberts BS, Garrett-Engele P, Lim LP, Johnson JM (2005) Simple, quantitative primer-extension PCR assay for direct monitoring of microRNAs and short-interfering RNAs. RNA 11:1737–1744
10. Obernosterer G, Martinez J, Alenius M (2010) Locked nucleic acid-based in situ detection of microRNAs in mouse tissue sections. Nat Protoc 2:1508–1514
11. Pena JT, Sohn-Lee C, Rouhanifard SH, Ludwig J, Hafner M, Mihailovic A, Lim C, Holoch D, Berninger P, Zavolan M, Tuschl T (2009) miRNA in situ hybridization in formaldehyde and EDC-fixed tissues. Nat Methods 6:139–141
12. Nuovo G, Lee EJ, Lawler S, Godlewski J, Schmittgen T (2009) In situ detection of mature microRNAs by labeled extension on ultramer templates. Biotechniques 46: 115–126
13. de Planell-Saguer M, Rodicio MC, Mourelatos Z (2010) Rapid in situ codetection of noncoding RNAs and proteins in cells and formalin-fixed paraffin-embedded tissue sections without protease treatment. Nat Protoc 5: 1061–1073

14. Wyman SK, Parkin RK, Mitchell PS, Fritz BR, O'Briant K, Godwin AK, Urban N, Drescher CW, Knudsen BS, Tewari M (2009) Repertoire of microRNAs in epithelial ovarian cancer as determined by next generation sequencing of small RNA cDNA libraries. PLoS One 4:e5311
15. Xu JZ, Wong CW (2010) Hunting for robust gene signature from cancer profiling data: sources of variability, different interpretations, and recent methodological developments. Cancer Lett 296:9–16
16. Peltier HJ, Latham GJ (2008) Normalization of microRNA expression levels in quantitative RT-PCR assays: identification of suitable reference RNA targets in normal and cancerous human solid tissues. RNA 14:844–852
17. Marsit CJ, Eddy K, Kelsey KT (2006) MicroRNA responses to cellular stress. Cancer Res 66:10843–10848
18. Kulshreshtha R, Ferracin M, Wojcik SE, Garzon R, Alder H, Agosto-Perez FJ, Davuluri R, Liu CG, Croce CM, Negrini M, Calin GA, Ivan M (2007) A microRNA signature of hypoxia. Mol Cell Biol 27:1859–1867
19. Rossi S, Shimizu M, Barbarotto E, Nicoloso MS, Dimitri F, Sampath D, Fabbri M, Lerner S, Barron LL, Rassenti LZ et al (2010) microRNA fingerprinting of CLL patients with chromosome 17p deletion identify a miR-21 score that stratifies early survival. Blood 116:945–952
20. Dillhoff M, Liu J, Frankel W, Croce C, Bloomston M (2008) MicroRNA-21 is overexpressed in pancreatic cancer and a potential predictor of survival. J Gastrointest Surg 12:2171–2176
21. Schetter AJ, Leung SY, Sohn JJ, Zanetti KA, Bowman ED, Yanaihara N, Yuen ST, Chan TL, Kwong DL, Au GK et al (2008) MicroRNA expression profiles associated with prognosis and therapeutic outcome in colon adenocarcinoma. JAMA 299:425–436
22. Iorio MV, Visone R, Di Leva G, Donati V, Petrocca F, Casalini P, Taccioli C, Volinia S, Liu CG, Alder H, Calin GA, Ménard S, Croce CM (2007) MicroRNA signatures in human ovarian cancer. Cancer Res 67:8699–8707
23. Zhang L, Huang J, Yang N, Greshock J, Megraw MS, Giannakakis A, Liang S, Naylor TL, Barchetti A, Ward MR, Yao G, Medina A, O'brien-Jenkins A, Katsaros D, Hatzigeorgiou A, Gimotty PA, Weber BL, Coukos G (2006) microRNAs exhibit high frequency genomic alterations in human cancer. Proc Natl Acad Sci USA 103:9136–9141
24. Zhang L, Volinia S, Bonome T, Calin GA, Greshock J, Yang N, Liu CG, Giannakakis A, Alexiou P, Hasegawa K, Johnstone CN, Megraw MS, Adams S, Lassus H, Huang J, Kaur S, Liang S, Sethupathy P, Leminen A, Simossis VA, Sandaltzopoulos R, Naomoto Y, Katsaros D, Gimotty PA, DeMichele A, Huang Q, Bützow R, Rustgi AK, Weber BL, Birrer MJ, Hatzigeorgiou AG, Croce CM, Coukos G (2008) Genomic and epigenetic alterations deregulate microRNA expression in human epithelial ovarian cancer. Proc Natl Acad Sci USA 105:7004–7009
25. Bagnoli M, De Cecco L, Granata A, Nicoletti R, Marchesi E, Alberti P, Valeri B, Libra M, Barbareschi M, Raspagliesi F, Mezzanzanica D, Canevari S (2011) Identification of a chrXq27.3 microRNA cluster associated with early relapse in advanced stage ovarian cancer patients. Oncotarget 2:1265–1278
26. Zorn KK, Jazaeri AA, Awtrey CS, Gardner GJ, Mok SC, Boyd J, Birrer MJ (2003) Choice of normal ovarian control influences determination of differentially expressed genes in ovarian cancer expression profiling studies. Clin Cancer Res 9:4811–4818
27. Farley J, Ozbun LL, Birrer MJ (2008) Genomic analysis of epithelial ovarian cancer. Cell Res 18:538–548
28. Yang N, Kaur S, Volinia S, Greshock J, Lassus H, Hasegawa K, Liang S, Leminen A, Deng S, Smith L, Johnstone CN, Chen XM, Liu CG, Huang Q, Katsaros D, Calin GA, Weber BL, Bützow R, Croce CM, Coukos G, Zhang L (2008) MicroRNA microarray identifies Let-7i as a novel biomarker and therapeutic target in human epithelial ovarian cancer. Cancer Res 68:10307–10314
29. Peng DX, Luo M, Qiu LW, He YL, Wang XF (2012) Prognostic implications of microRNA-100 and its functional roles in human epithelial ovarian cancer. Oncol Rep 27:1238–1244. doi:10.3892/or.2012.1625
30. Hu X, Macdonald DM, Huettner PC, Feng Z, El Naqa I, Schwarz JK, Mutch DG, Grigsby PW, Powell SN, Wang X (2009) A miR-200 microRNA cluster as prognostic marker in advanced ovarian cancer. Gynecol Oncol 114:457–464
31. Marchini S, Cavalieri D, Fruscio R, Calura E, Garavaglia D, Nerini IF, Mangioni C, Cattoretti G, Clivio L, Beltrame L, Katsaros D, Scarampi L, Menato G, Perego P, Chiorino G, Buda A, Romualdi C, D'Incalci M (2011) Association between miR-200c and the survival of patients with stage I epithelial ovarian cancer: a retrospective study of two independent tumour tissue collections. Lancet Oncol 12:273–285
32. Leskelä S, Leandro-García LJ, Mendiola M, Barriuso J, Inglada-Pérez L, Muñoz I, Martínez-Delgado B, Redondo A, de Santiago J, Robledo M, Hardisson D, Rodríguez-Antona C (2010) The miR-200 family controls

beta-tubulin III expression and is associated with paclitaxel-based treatment response and progression-free survival in ovarian cancer patients. Endocr Relat Cancer 18:85–95
33. Wright GW, Simon RM (2003) A random variance model for detection of differential gene expression in small microarray experiments. Bioinformatics 19:2448–2455
34. Tusher VG, Tibshirani R, Chu G (2001) Significance analysis of microarrays applied to the ionizing radiation response. Proc Natl Acad Sci USA 98:5116–5121
35. Tibshirani R, Hastie T, Narasimhan B, Chu G (2002) Diagnosis of multiple cancer types by shrunken centroids of gene expression. Proc Natl Acad Sci USA 99:6567–6572

Chapter 15

Detailed Analysis of Promoter-Associated RNA

Sara Napoli

Abstract

The detailed analysis of noncoding RNA is an upcoming necessity due to a plethora of recently identified components of this class of molecules. The investigation of their structure, directionality, intracellular localization, interaction with other cellular elements is useful to understand the role they play in transcriptional regulation. In this chapter, we describe some techniques, meant to determine very important features of promoter-associated RNAs, in order to clarify their functionality.

Key words Noncoding RNA, Directional RT-PCR, Chromatin immunoprecipitation, RNA immunoprecipitation

1 Introduction

In the last few years, interesting studies led to the generalized conviction that short and long noncoding RNAs (ncRNAs) are spread out all over the genome, both in intergenic regions and in association with transcribed genes. Even if we cannot still classify all these species of molecules in discrete classes with distinct physical and functional features, there are several examples of possible roles played by ncRNAs. As already known for decades, natural ncRNAs can interact with proteins and likely other RNA molecules to take part in complexes with specific function (as ribosomes), binding proteins to modulate their activity or catalyzing biological reactions [1].

Something new is the identification of endogenous ncRNAs playing a role in the modulation of transcription in a gene-specific manner. Natural ncRNAs transcribed in consequence of precise stimuli, as for instance in the case of cyclin D1 gene upon DNA damage [2], can activate a specific repressor protein, inducing its allosteric conformational change, to regulate the expression of only a given gene, among all the targets of that repressor. Sometimes a weak promoting region, regulating the expression of an ncRNA,

Anastasia Malek and Oleg Tchernitsa (eds.), *Ovarian Cancer: Methods and Protocols*, Methods in Molecular Biology, vol. 1049, DOI 10.1007/978-1-62703-547-7_15,

is juxtaposed to a major promoter responsible for transcription of important genes. The activity of the ncRNA promoter can be dependent, for example, on the status of the cell cycle. The presence or not of the ncRNA can regulate, in turn, the expression of the downstream protein-coding gene. One possible mechanism is the direct interaction of the ncRNA with proteins involved in RNA transcription, as general transcription factors or RNA polymerase. In this case the specificity of action is granted by the position where the ncRNA is produced, which induces interference only at the transcription start site (TSS) of the neighbor gene [3]. ncRNAs represent an additional layer of complexity of the transcriptional regulation of important genes in adaptation to a particular cell context.

Another important function ruled out by endogenous ncRNAs is the recruitment of remodeling chromatin proteins sequence specifically, silencing certain genes in long-lasting manner. It is the case of many tumor suppressor genes that inhibit normal cellular growth and which are frequently silenced epigenetically in cancer. Many oncosuppressor genes have nearby antisense RNAs. For example p15, a cyclin-dependent kinase, presents an antisense partner, p15AS, which induces its stable and irreversible silencing, both in *cis* and in *trans*, through changes in the methylation pattern of H3 [4]. Many natural antisense transcripts (NAT) are reported also for p21 in the EST database. The degradation of one of them induced by siRNA, reverts the suppressive H3K27me3 mark at the p21 promoter resulting in gene reactivation [5].

Endogenous ncRNAs may also be constitutively transcribed with low frequency in correspondence of promoting regions of protein-coding genes. Here, they sustain the job of transcriptional machinery and so their expression is frequently correlated to the level of expression of the main gene.

It is the case of the oncogene c-MYC, a transcription factor often overexpressed in tumors. In the interest of this book, genomic analyses have consistently identified region 8q24, containing the c-Myc locus, as the most recurrently gained genomic region (≥60 %) in HGSOC (high-grade serous ovarian cancer), which is often accompanied by high-level of c-Myc gene. In particular, Myc is able to drive tumorigenesis, along with other relevant genetic alterations, transforming normal human fallopian tubes epithelial cells (FTSECs) into high-grade serous carcinomas [6]. In vitro 3D models of early-stage epithelial ovarian cancer, reflecting genetic and phenotypic heterogeneity of the disease, can be established by the overexpression of c-MYC oncogene in hTERT immortalized normal primary ovarian epithelial cells. Molecular genetic characteristics of these models correlate with molecular and clinical features of primary EOCs, since tumors with "c-MYC-like" signatures are more likely to be high grade [7].

A ncRNA transcribed in correspondence of Myc promoter overlaps the transcription starting site (TSS). It seems to behave as a trail for RNA pol II and general factors, in particular TFIIB, to form the preinitiation complex (PIC) and start Myc transcription correctly [8]. The important function exerted by that promoter-associated ncRNA (paRNA) is clearly demonstrated by the complete loss of transcriptional efficiency of c-MYC promoter when an siRNA is directed against its paRNA. The impairment in transcription is dependent on the binding between the siRNA and the paRNA but not on the degradation of the last one. In fact, the interaction was shown to be Ago2-mediated but not due to its slicer activity, implicating that the main reason of transcription inhibition is not paRNA digestion, but the disruption of the interaction between paRNA and RNA polymerase. The presence of an ncRNA overlapping the TSS of c-MYC is necessary for the correct transcription of the oncogene, since it mediates the RNA pol II and TFIIB recognition of the correct TSS. The interference with paRNA–RNA pol II binding destabilizes the constitution of PIC and in consequence impairs MYC transcription initiation. The ncRNA associated to Myc promoter is a nice example of a most general class of molecules. Natural ncRNAs may be produced in a regulated manner to assist the right transcription of certain protein-coding genes, influencing them both positively and negatively through the interaction with multiple proteins. In order to study the mechanism of action of such a variegate class of molecules, new complex techniques of biochemistry and molecular biology have been developed. The aim of this chapter is to describe in the simplest way and elucidate the trickiest steps of sophisticated experimental methods, necessary to understand the role of rare ncRNAs and their interaction with DNA and proteins in hyper-structured complexes.

The approach we describe here includes following consequent steps:

1. Directional RT-PCR.

   PCR-based amplification allows detecting ncRNA associated to a promoter region, to define its presence and orientation (sense/antisense). In order to perform directional RT-PCR, researcher should design and use primers as for a common PCR, with the exception that they will be added to the reaction in two subsequent steps: the first gene-specific primer is used to perform RNA retrotranscription and the second one is added only during the following amplification step. Results of this experiment are semiquantitative if the PCR conditions have been previously checked to amplify known increasing amount of transcript in proportional manner. Real-time PCR can be also performed following an analogous experimental protocol, even if sometimes can be hard quantifying a very low-expressed transcript. In case you nicked and proved presence, position and direction of ncRNA of interest, you may further investigate if this ncRNA does mediate interaction of some proteins, such as chromatin components or transcription factors, with associated promoter region.

2. siRNA interference of promoter-associated RNA followed by chromatin immunoprecipitation.
   Design of siRNA directed against promoter-associated RNA and siRNA transfection procedure are the same like for routinely performed mRNA silencing. These techniques are beyond the scope of this chapter. After promoter-associated RNA is targeted by an siRNA, binding to this promoter of transcription factors, histones, or chromatin remodeling proteins can be assayed by ChIP with corresponding antibodies. Results will show if promoter-associated RNA mediates the binding of some proteins to DNA, and if an siRNA can interfere with this mechanism. The next question to gain insight into promoter-associated RNA gene regulatory function will be about its physical binding with regulated proteins.
3. RNA immunoprecipitation.
   Immunoprecipitation of a protein is performed in RNA preservative conditions. At the end of the purification RNA can be extracted. The presence into the pull-down fraction of the promoter-associated RNA can be assayed by directional RT-PCR to show its direct interaction with selected proteins. Result of this technique can simply describe the interaction between two molecular species but is not able to quantify such interaction.

2 Materials

Prepare all solutions using ultrapure water, prepared by purifying deionized water to attain a sensitivity of 18 MΩ cm at 25 °C and analytical grade reagents. When RNAse-free conditions are necessary, all buffers must be prepared with RNAse-free reagents and DEPC-treated water. Prepare and store all reagents at 4 °C temperature (unless indicated otherwise).

2.1 Directional RT-PCR

1. TRIzol® (Life technologies, Grand Island, NY, USA) (*see* **Note1**).
2. Chloroform.
3. Isopropanol.
4. Ethanol 75 %.
5. Superscript III One-step RT-PCR kit (Invitrogen, Life technologies, Grand Island, NY, USA): it has very high performance, even if you uncouple the primers for retrotranscription and amplification, as suggested for directional RT-PCR.

6. Primers designed for (a) RT either sense or antisense-orientated ncRNA, (b) following qPCR.
7. Tris-borate-EDTA (TBE) buffer: 89 mM Tris–base, 89 mM boric acid, 2 mM EDTA, pH 8.0.
8. Agarose gel: 2 % in TBE.
9. RNAse-free tips and eppendorfs.

2.2 Chromatin Immunoprecipitation After Transfection of siRNA Directed Against Promoter-Associated RNA

1. Formaldehyde 37 %.
2. 1.25 M Glycine (10×): 1.38 g in 100 ml of nuclease free water.
3. Protease inhibitors cocktail (200×).
4. ChIP lysis buffer: SDS 1 % (w/v), 10 mM EDTA, 50 mM Tris–HCl (pH 8.1).
5. ChIP grade (or IP grade) antibody.
6. ChIP dilution buffer: SDS 0.01 % (w/v), Triton-X 100 1.1 % (v/v), 1.2 mM EDTA, 16.7 mM Tris–HCl, 167 mM NaCl (pH 8.1).
7. Protein G Agarose Beads.
8. Low Salt washing buffer: SDS 0.1 % (w/v), Triton-X 100 1 % (v/v), 2 mM EDTA, 20 mM Tris–HCl, 150 mM NaCl (pH 8.1).
9. High Salt washing buffer: SDS 0.1 % (w/v), Triton-X 100 1 % (v/v), 2 mM EDTA (pH 8.0), 20 mM Tris–HCl (pH 8.1), 500 mM NaCl.
10. LiCl buffer: 0.25 M LiCl, IGEPAL-CA 630 1 % (w/v), deoxycholic acid 1 % (v/v), 1 mM EDTA, 10 mM Tris–HCl (pH 8.1).
11. Tris–EDTA (TE) buffer: 10 mM Tris–HCl, 1 mM EDTA, pH 8.1.
12. Elution buffer: SDS 1 % (w/v), 0.1 M $NaHCO_3$.
13. RNAse.
14. 5 M NaCl.
15. Proteinase K.
16. DNA purification kit.
17. Primer for qPCR amplification of DNA region tested for ncRNA-associated binding with protein of interest.

2.3 RNA Immunoprecipitation (See Ref. 3)

1. RIP lysis buffer: 50 mM HEPES, 1 mM EDTA, Triton-X 1 % (v/v) (pH 8.0).
2. RNAse inhibitor.
3. DNAse I (RNAse free).
4. DNAse I buffer 10×: Triton-X 5 %(v/v), 250 mM $MgCl_2$, 250 mM $CaCl_2$.

5. Protein G Agarose Beads.
6. ChIP grade (or IP grade) antibody.
7. Binding buffer: 50 mM HEPES, Triton-X 0.5 % (v/v), 25 mM $MgCl_2$, 5 mM $CaCl_2$, 20 mM EDTA (pH 8.0) (pH 8.0).
8. FA500 buffer: 50 mM HEPES, Triton-X 1 % (v/v), deoxycholic acid 0.1 % (w/v), 500 mM NaCl, 1 mM EDTA (pH 8.0).
9. LiCl buffer: 0.25 M LiCl, Triton-X 1 % (v/v), deoxycholic acid 0.5 % (w/v), 10 mM Tris–HCl (pH 8.1).
10. TES buffer: 10 mM Tris–HCl, 10 mM NaCl, 1 mM EDTA (pH 8.1).
11. RIP elution buffer: 100 mM Tris–HCl, 10 mM EDTA, SDS 1 % (w/v) (pH 7.8).
12. 5 M NaCl.
13. Proteinase k.
14. TRIzol® (Life technologies, Grand Island, NY, USA), Chloroform, Isopropanol, Ethanol 75 % for RNA extraction.
15. Primers and Superscript III One-step RT-PCR kit for directional RT-PCR.

2.4 Equipment

1. Agarose Electrophoresis Equipment.
2. Dark Reader transilluminator.
3. Sonicator.
4. PCR thermal cycle system.
5. Spectrophotometer with high accuracy and reproducibility.
6. Centrifuge with capability to reach 12,000 × *g* at 4 °C.

3 Methods

3.1 Directional RT-PCR

ncRNAs are rare transcripts transcribed all over the genome, often overlapping other transcripts, either mRNAs or other ncRNAs, transcribed in the opposite direction. Directional RT-PCR is a simple technique that allows you to discriminate the directionality of a transcript. It consists in a two-steps protocol: retrotranscription by a direction-specific primer and then amplification of cDNA adding a second primer to amplify cDNA. The design of the primers must be performed according common rules for PCR primers design, and also optimal annealing temperature and extension time are not different from a common PCR. The researcher who wants to understand if a certain transcript is transcribed in sense or antisense direction must retrotranscribe RNA by either forward primer or reverse primer. At the end of retrotranscription the lacking primer must be added for the amplification phase. If a signal is amplified after retrotranscription with forward primer but not with reverse

Table 1
Master mix for directional RT-PCR

	Starting concentration	Volume (μl)	Final concentration
Mix	2×	10	1×
Primer to retrotranscribe	10 μM	0.4–0.8	0.2–0.4 μM
Superscript III enzyme mix		0.5	
Water		to 18.4	
RNA	40 ng/μl	2.5–5	100–200 ng

primer, antisense transcription occurs in the analyzed region. If a signal is amplified after retrotranscription with reverse primer but not with forward primer, sense transcription occurs in the analyzed region. A signal can be obtained also in both reactions. In this case bidirectional transcription occurs. In order to exclude that the amplified amplicon can be contaminated by amplification of residual genomic DNA, a PCR reaction must be run in parallel, assembling the reaction as previously described but avoiding the starting step of retrotranscription (50 °C for 30′). In this case a positive control of genomic DNA (100 ng) must be included.

1. Lyse cells adding 1 ml of Trizol/10 sq cm of plating area, or every 1 million cells, pipet vigorously and transfer the lysate in 1.5 ml eppendorf.
2. Proceed with chloroform extraction immediately, otherwise keep the lysate at −80 °C (*see* **Note 1**). Check RNA concentration and quality (*see* **Note 2**). Prepare RNA dilutions at the concentration 40 ng/μl in RNAse-free water.
3. Prepare RT-PCR reaction mix using Superscript III One-step RT-PCR kit and in according with kit supplier protocol. Assemble RT-PCR reaction on ice, keeping every reagent cold and in RNAse-free conditions; use only RNAse-free tips and eppendorfs. Prepare the master mix on ice, adapting what is indicated in Table 1, for the necessary number of reactions (*see* **Note 3**). Aliquot the master mix in the 0.2 μl tubes and then add the RNA.
4. Retrotranscribe RNA in primer-specific manner at 50 °C for 30′.
5. Denature cDNA and inactivate retrotranscriptase activity at 94 °C for 8′.
6. Cool the samples to 4 °C. Spin down the tubes quickly and then add 1.6 μl of the left primer (2.5–5 μM) to each tube, one by one. Vortex briefly and spin down the tubes.

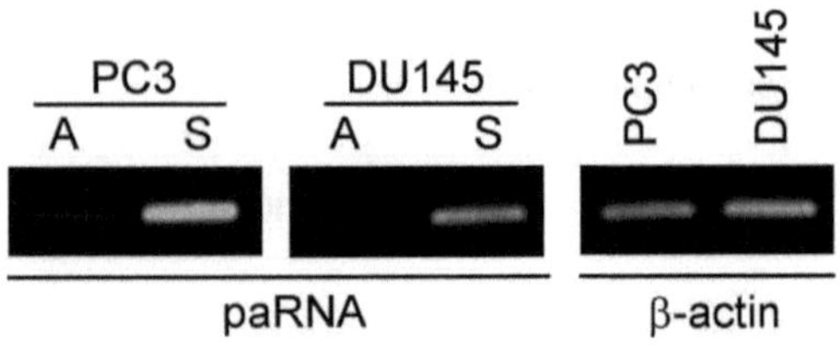

Fig. 1 Gel electrophoresis of directional RT-PCR products. Antisense and sense transcripts were analyzed in the promoter region of gene c-Myc in two prostate cancer cell lines, PC3 and DU145. High level of promoter-associated RNA was found in sense direction (S) both in PC3 and in DU145. Very low level of the antisense transcript (A) was detected in the same region in PC3, while in DU145 the antisense transcript is almost absent. Beta-actin mRNA was amplified as control

7. Perform PCR reaction, according the following program: Hot Start Taq activation 95 °C/2′, Denaturing step 95 °C/15″, Annealing step 55–60 °C/30″, Elongating step 72 °C/15″–60″. Repeat from denaturing to elongating step for 30–35 cycles. Final elongation step 72 °C/10′. Annealing temperature is 5° lower than the primers' melting temperature while elongation time is 60″/kb amplicon length (*see* **Note 4**).
8. Check the presence of the amplicon on a 2 % agarose minigel, running at 90 V for 30′ (Fig. 1) (*see* **Note 5**).

3.2 Chromatin Immunoprecipitation After Transfection of siRNA Directed Against Promoter-Associated RNA

In order to understand if an siRNA is able to disrupt a protein–DNA complex, mediated by ncRNA, cells can be transfected with an siRNA directed against a given promoter-associated RNA. Cells are transfected with either active siRNA or an irrelevant control. The amount of siRNA to transfect must be previously experimentally determined, measuring the transcriptional perturbation of the target gene. Consider that the promoter-directed siRNAs activity on target gene transcription is not necessarily due to the cleavage of paRNA, but even only to its binding, so the measure of paRNA level upon siRNA transfection might not properly reflect the siRNA activity. Cells are cross-linked to stabilize the complexes formed on the chromatin and then lysed. Immunoprecipitation of a given protein is then performed adding the suitable antibody to the lysate. The amount of antibody to add must be previously determined by titration. Consider that along with the experimental samples which you are interested in, a positive and negative controls must be processed. The first is represented by an aliquot of chromatin which will be immunoprecipitated with an antibody recognizing a protein surely bound to the analyzed promoter. The negative control is an aliquot of chromatin incubated with IgG, which eventually measures the unspecific signal. A fixed volume of lysate must be saved before adding the antibody, in order to check if the input, the total amount of chromatin loaded into the

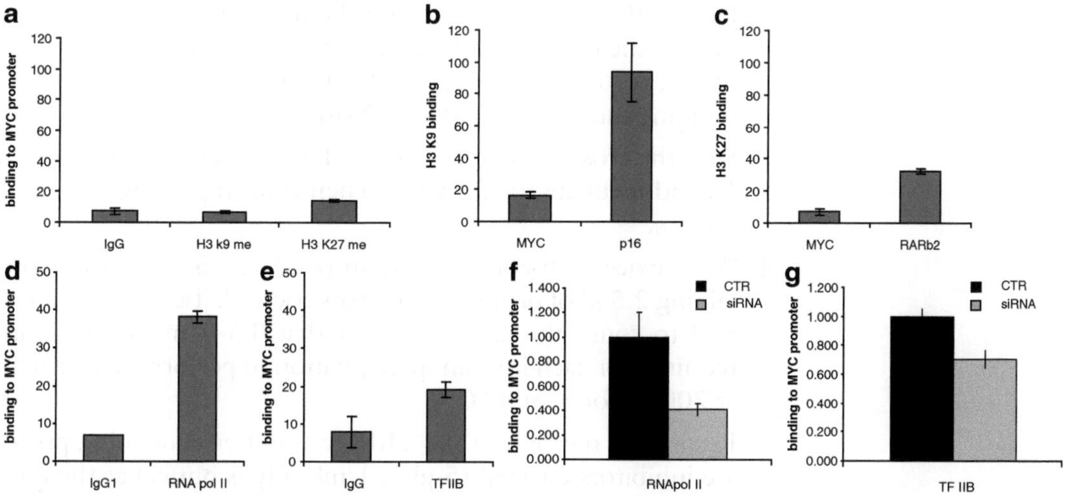

Fig. 2 Chromatin immunoprecipitation of some proteins and histone modifications to assess their association with Myc promoter. (**a**) H3K9 dimethylated and H3K27 trimethylated, two histone marks of silent chromatin, were immunoprecipitated and their binding to MYC promoter was measured by qRT and normalized to the input. No enrichment of H3k9me or H3K27me was detected at MYC promoter since the amount of DNA coprecipitated with the proper antibody is not significant higher than the background coprecipitated with IgG, the negative control. To check if the immunoprecipitation of H3K9me or H3K27me (**c**) worked properly, the same DNA was amplified with primers recognizing a portion of p16 promoter (**b**) or RARb2 promoter (**c**) that were known to be bound, respectively, by H3K9me and H3K27me. (**d**) RNA polymerase II and (**e**) the general transcription factor TFIIB were bound to MYC promoter, since it is a gene highly transcribed, as shown by the enrichment of MYC promoter in the fraction co-immunoprecipitated with RNA pol II or TFIIB compared to the background given by the negative control IgG. The transfection with an siRNA targeting the transcription starting site of MYC impairs the binding of RNA pol II (**f**) and TFIIB (**g**) to MYC promoter, as shown by the reduction in MYC promoter enrichment, obtained with both the antibodies, in the sample transfected with the active siRNA compared to the sample transfected with an irrelevant siRNA

immunoprecipitation, was comparable among all the processed samples. DNA coprecipitated with the protein is finally extracted and analyzed by PCR, to assess if the protein analyzed was bound to a certain DNA sequence. Two additional controls must be considered during the detection step. A region known to be bound by the analyzed protein should be amplified as positive control, and another one surely not bound by the protein must be amplified as negative control. The final amount of DNA coprecipitated with the protein must be normalized for the amount of the amplicon detected in the input, in order to compare the DNA enrichment in different samples (Fig. 2).

1. Seed cells at 80 % confluence in 6-well plate, 2 wells per each group of transfection. 24 h later transfect the cells with 50–100 nM of the siRNA directed against promoter-associated RNA or irrelevant control siRNA. The day after transfection, detach the cells, and reseed them in 100 mm dishes for 48–72 h (*see* **Note 6**).

2. Detach the cells and resuspend them in a 15 ml conical tube. Add to the cells formaldehyde 37 % to the final concentration of 1 %, vortex and incubate at RT for 10′ in order to cross-link proteins and nucleic acids (*see* **Note 7**).
3. Stop the cross-linking, by glycine 10× at final concentration of 1× and incubate for 5′ at RT. Then centrifuge at RT for 5′ at 700 × *g*.
4. Wash twice with cold PBS. Resuspend in 0.5 ml of PBS containing 2.5 μl of protease inhibitors cocktail. Take an aliquot of 5 μl to count the cells. Consider that 0.5–1 million cells are required for each immunoprecipitation to perform. Centrifuge at 700 × *g* for 5′ at 4 °C.
5. Resuspend the cells in the ChIP lysis buffer containing protease inhibitors cocktail (5 μl in 1 ml of lysis buffer) at the concentration of 5–20 million/ml (*see* **Note 8**). At this step the procedure can be stopped and the lysate saved at −80 °C.
6. In order to physically share the chromatin, sonicate the lysate for 8–12 times for 10″ each, at low energy, paused by 30″ of resting between one pulse and the other. Keep the lysate on ice during all the sonication procedure, in order to limit heat production (*see* **Note 9**).
7. Centrifuge the sonicated lysate at 12,000 × *g* for 10′ at 4 °C. The supernatant contains the fragmented chromatin: recover it and subdivide the supernatant in 100 μl—aliquots that can be saved at −80 °C (*see* **Note 10**). The pellet contains only insoluble debris and can be discarded.
8. Prepare the dilution buffer for all the samples which must be processed, adding the protease inhibitor cocktail 200× at the final concentration 1× (*see* **Note 11**).
9. Dilute the chromatin (100 μl from **step** 7) to 1 ml with the dilution buffer. Add 50 μl of protein G to preclear the sample, to discard any lysate component which could aspecifically bind protein G. Incubate for 1 h at 4 °C on a rotating platform, to mix homogenously the samples (*see* **Note 12**).
10. Centrifuge for 1′ at 4,000 × *g* at 4 °C to pellet the protein G agarose and all the material nonspecifically bound to it. Recover the precleared chromatin contained in the supernatant and transfer it in a clean tube. Save 10 μl of the sample as input control. Pay attention not to disturb the pellet of protein G agarose, which can be discarded.
11. Add the antibody to the precleared chromatin and incubate overnight at 4 °C on rotating platform (*see* **Note 13**).
12. Add 50 μl of protein G agarose and incubate for 1 h at 4 °C on rotating platform to recover the antibody and the captured protein. Centrifuge for 1′ at 4,000 × *g* at 4 °C to pellet the

protein G–antibody–protein–DNA complex. Carefully remove all the supernatant containing unbound chromatin (*see* **Note 14**). Pay attention not to disturb the pellet.

13. Wash the pellet with 1 ml of Low Salt washing buffer, on rotation for 5′ at RT. Pellet again by centrifugation at 4,000 × *g* for 1′ (*see* **Note 15**). Repeat twice.
14. Wash once with High Salt washing buffer, as described at **step 13**.
15. Wash twice with TE buffer, as described at **step 13**.
16. In order to elute the protein–DNA complex from the antibody, prepare 100 μl of elution buffer per each sample to elute and each input control. Add 50 μl of elution buffer to the beads and incubate under agitation for 15′ at RT. Centrifuge and collect the supernatant in a clean tube. Repeat with the left 50 μl and pull together.
17. Add 8 μl of 5 M NaCl (to the 100 μl from **step 16**) and incubate at 65 °C for 4–5 h to revert the cross-linking, due to treatment with formaldehyde (**step 2**).
18. In order to digest RNA, add 10 μg of RNAse A and incubate 30′ at 37 °C.
19. In order to digest proteins add 4 μl of 0.5 M EDTA, 8 μl of Tris–HCl pH 6.5, and proteinase K and incubate at 45 °C for 1–2 h.
20. Recover DNA on spin columns for purification of DNA after enzymatic reactions.
21. Perform qRT for the analyzed promoter region to quantify the variation in protein binding to the promoter upon interference with the ncRNA present in that region. The design of primers must consider that after sonication DNA was fractionated in fragment between 1,000 and 200 bp, for this reason the amplicon to analyze should not be usually much longer than 200 bp. To assess if the protein was bound to a certain DNA sequence, the operator must amplify a region surrounding the consensus sequence for the protein binding. The quantification can be performed normalizing each immunoprecipitated sample with the input control.

3.3 RNA Immunoprecipitation

RNA immunoprecipitation is a technique to assess if a certain protein is able to bind a particular RNA molecule, especially an ncRNA. It is not dissimilar by the previously described chromatin immunoprecipitation, except for the RNA preservative conditions maintained all along the procedure, that allow the operator, in the end, to evaluate the binding to a given protein of RNA molecules instead of DNA.

Also in this case the operator must include a negative control, as IgG, an antibody that does not recognize any protein and in

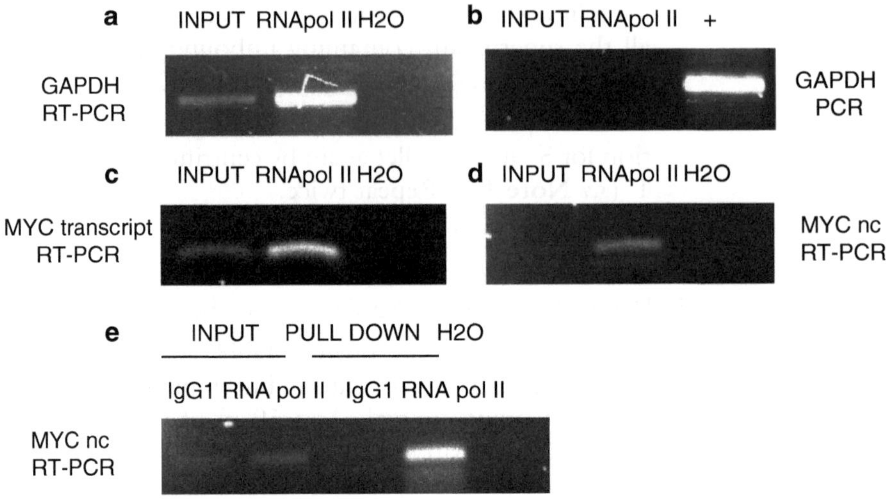

Fig. 3 RIP for ncRNA overlapping MYC transcription starting site and its proper controls. GAPDH and MYC transcripts (**a**, **c**) were used as positive controls since they are bound to RNA polymerase II, as all mRNAs. The RT-PCR was performed on input control and pull-down, a non-template control was also included. In order to exclude contamination by genomic DNA a PCR was performed on input and pull-down RNA samples, without any signal, excluding completely the presence of DNA traces. A positive control of genomic DNA was included in the PCR, to show the efficiency of the reaction (**b**). Also the ncRNA associated to MYC promoter can coprecipitate with RNA pol II (**d**). The ncRNA is so low expressed that it is hard to detect in the input control, while it is evident in the fraction enriched by RNA pol II pull-down. The specificity of ncRNA binding to RNA pol II is clear in *panel* (**e**) where the negative control, IgG, was included in parallel to the RNA pol II pull-down

consequence of that should not coprecipitate RNA. A positive control may also be useful, even if sometimes it is hard to identify a protein surely bound to the RNA molecule under inspection. A proper control is often the RNA polymerase, if it is known, transcribing that particular class of RNA molecules.

During the detection step, the operator must consider to include a control which is not retrotranscribed, to exclude contamination of genomic DNA (Fig. 3).

1. 5 million of cells are cross-linked as already described at **step 2** of Subheading 3.2. Stop cross-linking with glycine at final concentration 3×.
2. Wash cells in PBS, centrifuge and resuspend in 500 μl of RIP lysis buffer containing protease inhibitor cocktail at final concentration 1× and 50 U of RNAse inhibitor.
3. Sonicate in accordance to what already explained at **step 6** of Subheading 3.2.
4. Centrifuge the lysate at 12,000 × *g* for 10′ at 4 °C. Recover the supernatant and transfer it in a clean tube. It is supposed to contain all the RNA molecules, also the ones bound to chromatin, which was shared to make them soluble. The pellet will contain insoluble debris and can be discarded.

5. To digest DNA, add the following reagents to the lysate, adjusting their concentration to the indicated values: 0.5 % Triton-X, 25 mM $MgCl_2$, 5 mM $CaCl_2$, 50 U RNAsin, 1× protease inhibitor cocktail, 30 U DNAse I RNAse free; incubate for 15′ at 37 °C. Stop the digestion, adding EDTA to final concentration of 20 mM.
6. Preclear the sample with 50 μl of protein G, on rotating platform for 2 h at 4 °C.
7. Spin down then transfer the supernatant in a clean tube and save 50 μl as input control.
8. Add the antibody (8–10 μg) to the precleared lysate and incubate at 4 °C on rotating platform for 2 h.
9. Add 50 μl of protein G and incubate at 4 °C on rotating platform for 1 h. Spin down the beads at 5,000 × *g* for 1′, remove carefully the supernatant.
10. Wash the beads twice with binding buffer, twice with FA500 buffer, twice with LiCl buffer and twice with TES buffer. Each wash cycle consist of 5′ on rotation with 1 ml of cold buffer; spin down at 5,000 × *g* for 1′ between one wash and the following one.
11. Add 75 μl of RIP elution buffer to recover the complex protein–RNA which was captured by the antibody (*see* **Note 16**).
12. Adjust NaCl to 200 mM and treat with 20 μg of proteinase k for 1 h at 42 °C and 1 h at 65 °C.
13. Then extract RNA with Trizol/chloroform (*see* **Note 17**). The amount of RNA obtained will be very small, so the operator can even avoid to quantify it.
14. Perform directional RT-PCR to evaluate if the ncRNA of interest interacts to the immunoprecipitated protein directly (*see* **Note 18**). Use primers and PCR conditions indicated in Subheading 3.1. Retrotranscribe the same volume of RNA, regardless the RNA concentration, in order to compare the enrichment of an RNA molecule in the sample where the protein of interest was immunoprecipitated and the controls.

4 Notes

1. TRIzol® reagent is extensively referred to give high-quality, intact RNA from many kinds of biological materials. This reagent is very useful because it allows you to lyse the cells very quickly, directly into the plate, increasing the amount of intact RNA extracted. The most time elapses between cells are detached and RNA is preserved, the highest is the risk of RNA degradation. Lysate obtained by TRIzol® can also be saved at

–80 °C for even 1 year before performing chloroform extraction, without any loss of material.

2. If RNA is contaminated by alcohol, phenols, etc. (Ads 260/230 < 1.6) proceed to reprecipitate your RNA.
3. If the ncRNA to amplify is a sense transcript, retrotranscribe with reverse primer, if it is an antisense transcript with the forward primer. The directionality of ncRNA must be previously determined by two RT-PCR performed in parallel, retrotranscribing with either forward or reverse primer.
4. The amount of RNA, the primers concentration and the number of cycles to perform must be experimentally established, because they depend on the amount of the ncRNA and on the efficiency of primers amplification.
5. If contamination of genomic DNA is evident, go back to the mother RNA, digest with DNAse for 15′ at RT, then reprecipitate RNA and repeat the directional RT-PCR reaction.
6. The best timing for ChIP experiment after siRNA transfection depends on the ncRNA under investigation. Generally, the interference with ncRNA localized onto the chromatin requires longer time then common posttranscriptional gene silencing. However, the best timing must be experimentally validated.
7. Cross-linked cells are especially sticky. The cross-linking of attached cells in the dish can reduce the recovery of cells, for this reason can be preferred cross-linking cells already detached and pulled in a tube.
8. The amount of cells to use for a single chromatin immunoprecipitation depends on the abundance of the protein we want to immunoprecipitate and on the efficiency of the antibody. For this reason it must be empirically determined in the particular cell model used. In general, start from 1 million cells/IP.
9. The first time the experiment is performed in a certain cellular model, the optimal sonication must be experimentally determined. Lysates from different amount of cells must be sonicated with variable number of pulses. After that cross-linking must be reverted, DNA purified resuspended in 100 μl of water and 1/10th must be loaded onto a 2 % agarose gel to see the size of the shared chromatin. A smear between 500 and 200 bp is acceptable.
10. Transfer all the supernatant in a clean tube, pipet to homogenize the shared chromatin and then aliquot.
11. ChIP dilution buffer contain SDS that precipitates at low temperature. Keep the buffer in a water bath at 37 °C, to completely redissolved SDS before use.

12. Protein G is an inhomogeneous solution, so to distribute it properly in each sample, cut off the edge of the tip and pipet slowly.
13. The correct amount of antibody must be empirically evaluated by a previous titration. However, usually 8–10 μg of ChIP grade antibody should work properly.
14. It is recommended to keep the supernatant because it can be reincubated with another antibody, to check the binding of another protein, if it is not supposed to interact with the first one previously immunoprecipitated. This re-incubation can be actually done several times.
15. If all the buffers are kept cold, the centrifugations can be even not refrigerated.
16. Add to the input 25 μl of 3× RIP elution buffer, to adjust the buffer component concentration.
17. RNA amount extracted after immunoprecipitation is very low, so you can couple microscale spin column-based purification kit (f.i. RNAqueous, Ambion) to Trizol extraction.
18. Since the signal of the ncRNA detected bound to an immunoprecipitated protein can be very weak, a step of nested PCR can help to obtain a more robust result.

References

1. Goodrich JA, Kugel JF (2006) Non-coding-RNA regulators of RNA polymerase II transcription. Nat Rev Mol Cell Biol 7(8): 612–616
2. Wang X et al (2008) Induced ncRNAs allosterically modify RNA-binding proteins in cis to inhibit transcription. Nature 454(7200):126–130
3. Martianov I et al (2007) Repression of the human dihydrofolate reductase gene by a non-coding interfering transcript. Nature 445(7128):666–670
4. Yu W et al (2008) Epigenetic silencing of tumour suppressor gene p15 by its antisense RNA. Nature 451(7175):202–206
5. Morris KV et al (2008) Bidirectional transcription directs both transcriptional gene activation and suppression in human cells. PLoS Genet 4(11):e1000258
6. Karst AM, Levanon K, Drapkin R (2011) Modeling high-grade serous ovarian carcinogenesis from the fallopian tube. Proc Natl Acad Sci USA 108(18):7547–7552
7. Lawrenson K et al (2011) Modelling genetic and clinical heterogeneity in epithelial ovarian cancers. Carcinogenesis 32(10):1540–1549
8. Napoli S et al (2009) Promoter-specific transcriptional interference and c-myc gene silencing by siRNAs in human cells. EMBO J 28(12):1708–1719

Chapter 16

Integrating Multiple Types of Data to Identify MicroRNA–Gene Co-modules

Shihua Zhang

Abstract

MicroRNAs (miRNAs) and genes work cooperatively to form the kernel part of gene regulatory system and affect many crucial biological processes. However, the detailed combinatorial roles of most miRNAs and genes in cellular processes and diseases are still unclear. The huge amount of diverse functional genomic data provides unprecedented opportunities to study the miRNA–gene co-regulations. How to integrate diverse genomic data to identify the regulatory modules of miRNAs and genes is a challenging problem in computational biology. Recently, we have proposed a mathematical data integration framework to discover the miRNA–gene regulatory co-modules. We have applied the proposed method to integrate a set of heterogeneous data sources including the expression profiles of miRNAs and genes on 385 human ovarian cancer samples as well as miRNA–gene interactions and gene–gene interactions. The revealed co-modules show significant biological relevance and potential associations with ovarian cancers and others.

Key words Bioinformatics, MicroRNA–gene co-module, Gene regulatory network, Machine learning, Data mining, Nonnegative matrix factorization

1 Introduction

MicroRNAs (miRNAs) are a class of ~22 nt small noncoding RNAs which play crucial regulatory roles in repressing mRNA translation or mediating mRNA degradation by targeting mRNAs in a sequence-specific manner [2]. miRNAs, transcriptional factors, mRNAs, and other molecules combine to form complex biological regulatory systems, which cooperatively determine the progression of many cellular behaviors and diseases [10, 39, 52]. In the past decade, a great number of experimental and computational progresses have been made on the miRNA-related problems including identification of genes which encode miRNAs [3, 23, 24, 36], prediction of the miRNA target genes within multiple genomes [9, 27, 40, 46], and extraction of miRNA expression patterns based on microarray data [33]. Moreover, matched expression profiles of

Anastasia Malek and Oleg Tchernitsa (eds.), *Ovarian Cancer: Methods and Protocols*, Methods in Molecular Biology, vol. 1049, DOI 10.1007/978-1-62703-547-7_16, © Springer Science+Business Media New York 2013

miRNA and mRNA on the same set of samples are dramatically accumulated, which can provide a systematic and dynamical view on miRNA–mRNA regulatory mechanisms [15, 32]. However, most of miRNAs still have unknown functions and uncertain targets, and the underlying regulatory mechanisms between miRNA and genes are not yet well understood.

The combination of predicted miRNA–gene regulatory interactions and gene interaction networks or pathways provides basic resources to systematically explore the characteristics of miRNA regulatory system. There have been some exploratory studies in the literatures which attempted to decipher how miRNAs, genes, and proteins interact on a systems level. For example, global miRNA regulation in cellular networks [8, 14, 28, 48] or combinatorial miRNA regulation in cellular pathways [13, 53] have been carefully studied. Coordinated regulation between the transcriptional and miRNA layers has also been explored based on their combined regulatory networks [39, 52]. Undoubtedly, all these studies have advanced our understanding and provided insights into miRNA–gene regulation [48]. However, we are still far from fully understanding the underlying regulatory mechanisms between miRNAs and genes, and systematic studies of the regulatory networks including miRNAs are only now in their early stage.

Modular structure of biological systems has been extensively described and explored in the past. Recognizing the modular organization of biological networks has greatly advanced our understanding of complex cellular systems [12, 16, 35, 49]. However, little is known about the modular organization of the miRNA–gene regulatory systems. Describing and identifying functional miRNA–gene regulatory modules is a challenging task in computational biology due to the following reasons. Firstly, one gene can be simultaneously regulated by multiple different miRNAs, and one miRNA can regulate a large number of genes [21, 29]. Due to this multiplicity, the modular pattern has to be a miRNA–gene *co-module* which is a set of miRNAs and their corresponding co-regulated genes. Secondly, the miRNA–mRNA targeting regulations differ among tissues and conditions, which is essential to form complex biological systems. Thirdly, it is known that miRNAs physically interact with mRNAs, and miRNA regulation affects the quantities of proteins in cells rather than the quantities of mRNAs [1]. So the expression levels of miRNAs are not always anti-correlated with those of their target genes. Lastly, the genomic data are generally noisy and incomplete especially for the predicted miRNA–gene interactions.

The complicated nature of miRNA regulation poses unique challenges to the integrative analysis of heterogeneous data sources for describing miRNA regulation mechanism. In the early stage, Yoon and De Micheli [45] proposed a method to identify miRNA–gene regulatory modules based on a predicted miRNA–gene interaction network. Recently, several methods have been proposed by further taking into account coherent expression patterns between miRNAs and genes, or the (anti)-correlations measured between each pair of miRNAs and genes [17, 34, 42]. However, these methods focus only on one or two resources, and suffer from several limitations. For example, Peng et al. proposed a two-stage integrative method by enumerating maximal bi-cliques in a combined miRNA–gene network [34]. Note that this method is sensitive to noise of the data, and produces too many star structures which cannot well reveal miRNA combinatorial regulation. Furthermore, none of these methods employs the coordination of miRNA and gene regulation, or the topological organization of biological networks including the transcriptional regulation network and the protein–protein interaction network.

To conquer the problems above, we have proposed a mathematical model for identifying miRNA–gene regulatory co-modules based on the integration of multiple types of genomic data [50]. We employed three types of data including predicted miRNA–gene interactions, the expression profiles of miRNAs and genes, and the gene–gene interaction network. The predicted miRNA–gene interactions serve as fully combined static "interaction" set, while the dynamic expression profiles of miRNAs and genes are used to identify interactions that are concurrently active. This goal is enhanced by the gene/protein interaction network, since the ultimate effect of miRNA regulation is to regulate protein activities. In order to integrate the three data, we have developed a new and efficient machine learning model. By employing the matrix representation, our method integrates miRNA and gene expression profiles using multiple nonnegative matrix factorization (NMF) technique, and simultaneously integrates networked data with a regularized term. To enhance the signal–noise separation and improve the interpretability of the resulted modules, we aim to find sparse solutions of the membership functions by applying sparsity penalties. We proved that the learning and optimization model can be effectively solved by a multiplicative iterative procedure.

We have evaluated the proposed method on a group of datasets including human miRNA and gene expression profiles of TCGA ovarian cancer samples, a miRNA–gene interaction network, and a gene interaction network. We reported 49 human miRNA–gene regulatory co-modules (a miRNA module vs. a gene module). We found that the miRNA modules are significantly enriched with miRNA clusters, and that the gene modules are enriched with known functional gene classes. The overrepresented functional classes of gene modules can potentially be transferred to their corresponding miRNA modules, resulting in a functional prediction for miRNAs. Moreover, through a literature survey we found that the identified co-modules include a significant number of cancer-related genes and miRNAs. Many of them are involved with ovarian cancer as expected. The regulatory co-modules may be helpful to reconstruct gene regulatory networks, and can provide candidates of miRNA targets for further experimental validation. In this chapter, we describe the method as well as its application on real biological data. We carefully report the biological relevance of co-module with ovarian cancer and discuss its applicability to other biological problems.

2 Materials and Methods

2.1 Methods

In this section, we describe our framework for the simultaneous integration of multiple types of data to identify miRNA–gene co-modules (Fig. 1). We begin by introducing the data briefly, and then present the mathematical formulation of the problem. Next

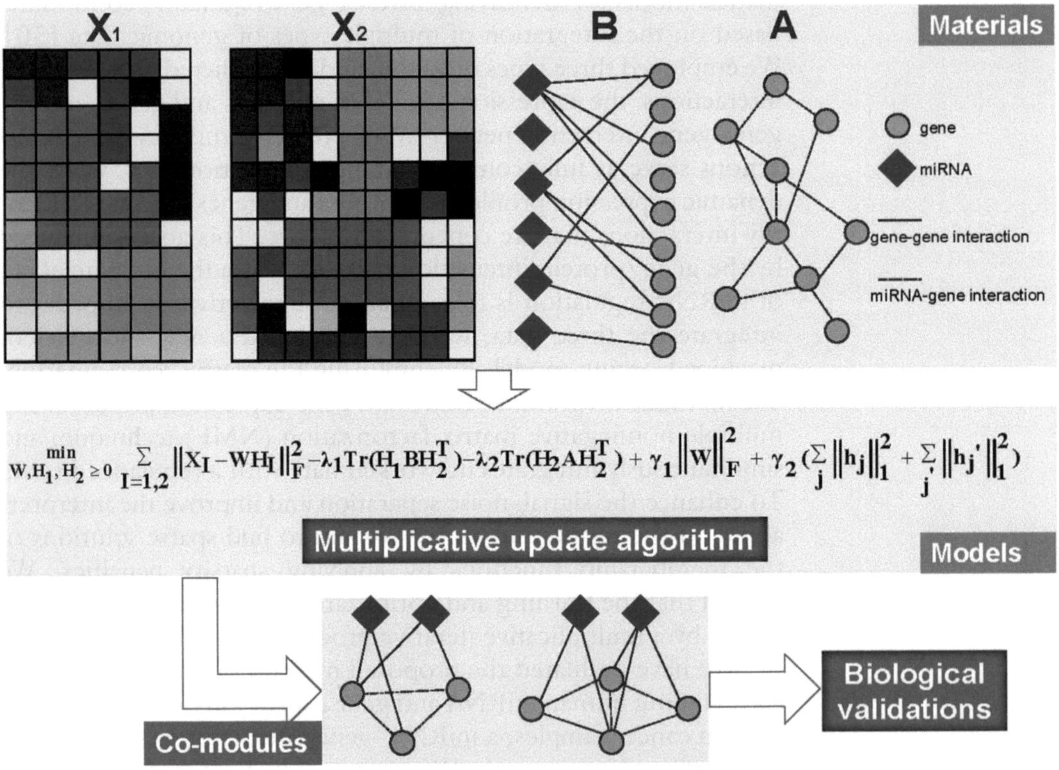

Fig. 1 Overview of the proposed method for identifying miRNA–gene regulatory co-modules. A miRNA–gene co-module is defined as the union of a set of miRNAs (a miRNA module) and a set of genes (a gene module). The inputs are (1) two sets of expression profiles (represented by the matrices X_1 and X_2) for miRNAs and genes, measured on the same set of samples; (2) a gene–gene interaction network (represented by the matrix A), including protein–protein interactions and DNA–protein interactions; and (3) a list of predicted miRNA–gene regulatory interactions (represented by the matrix B) based on sequence data. We simultaneously factor the miRNA and gene expression matrices into a common basis W and two coefficient matrices H_1 and H_2. At the same time, additional knowledge is incorporated into this framework with network-regularized constraints. Sparsity constraints are also imposed on this framework so as to obtain easily interpretable solutions. The decomposed matrix components provide information about miRNA–gene regulatory co-modules. Then the co-modules are identified based on shared components (a column in W) with significant association values in the corresponding rows of H_1 and H_2

we describe our iterative multiplicative updating algorithm. Finally, we describe various validation experiments.

2.1.1 Data Sources and Preprocessing

Due to its large number of samples and rich clinical information, we tested our method on the ovarian cancer expression data from the Cancer Genome Atlas (TCGA) Project. We downloaded miRNA and gene expression data for 385 ovarian cancer samples from the TCGA data portal (http://cancergenome.nih.gov/). We then filtered out miRNAs and genes with small absolute values and little variation across samples, obtaining a dataset with the expression profiles of 559 miRNAs and 12,456 genes. We constructed a gene–gene interaction network by combining the protein–protein interaction data used by Bossi and Lehner [4] and the DNA–protein interaction data downloaded from TRANSFAC. We filtered these data for self-interactions and genes (proteins) that were not represented in our TCGA expression data. This process resulted in a network with 31,949 gene–gene interactions. We obtained predicted miRNA–gene interactions from the MicroCosm Web site. We removed interactions involving miRNAs or genes that were not present in the expression data. The resulting miRNA–gene bipartite network has a total of 243,331 interactions.

We transform the two expression matrices into nonnegative matrices following the approach proposed by Kim and Tidor [19]. Detailed data processing can be seen in [50]. The transformed nonnegative expression matrices are our input matrices X_1 and X_2. The gene–gene interaction network and miRNA–gene bipartite network were represented with matrices B and A with consistent order of variables in X_1 and X_2.

2.1.2 Problem Formulation

To identify miRNA–gene co-modules, we designed an objective function with three components. The first is based on the nonnegative miRNA and gene expression matrices X_1 and X_2. The second considers the effects of gene–gene interactions. The last considers the effects of predicted miRNA–gene interactions. By optimizing this objective function, we obtain a joint decomposition of X_1 and X_2 that together reveals miRNA–gene regulatory modules inherent in the expression data and satisfies constraints based on prior information.

The NMF technique divides a matrix into two nonnegative matrices: a basis matrix of lower rank and a coefficient matrix [25, 33]. The squared error version of this factorization model can be defined as $\min_{W,H\geq 0} \|X - WH\|_F^2$, where W and H are the basis matrix and coefficient matrix with dimensions $s \times k$ and $k \times n$, respectively. The notation $\|\bullet\|_F$ means the Frobenius norm of a matrix. The fact that W and H are nonnegative guarantees that parts of the matrix can be combined additively to form a whole; hence, NMF is a useful technique for obtaining a part-based representation of the data. In other words, the factorization allows us to easily identify substructures in the data. However, the NMF method in its present form can only be applied to a matrix containing just one type of variable. It cannot be used to integrate multiple matrices for multiple types of variables together with prior knowledge such as networks that represent relationships among variables of the same type and/or between different types.

As our goal is to identify coordinated miRNA–gene co-modules, we assume that there is a common basis matrix W for the miRNA and gene expression matrices X_1 and X_2. The two expression matrices have dimensions $s \times m$ and $s \times n$, respectively, and will be factored into W and two coefficient matrices H_1 and H_2. This representation of the expression data can be derived by optimizing the following objective function:

$$\mathcal{F}_1(W, H_1, H_2) = \sum_{I=1,2} \|X_I - WH_I\|_F^2, \tag{1}$$

where H_1 and H_2 have dimensions $k \times m$ and $k \times n$, respectively. The parameter k is chosen prior to optimization. The solution to Eq. 1 is often not unique, and may be sensitive to noise in the expression data. Both of these limitations may confound the module discovery process. For these reasons, we will guide the optimization process toward reasonable biological solutions by incorporating prior knowledge into the objective function.

In this demonstration of our method, the prior knowledge consists of predicted miRNA–gene interactions and gene–gene interactions. The essence of our semisupervised learning method is to define constraints for the co-module identification framework such that any variables linked in these two datasets are more likely to be placed into the same co-module. In addition to improving the biological relevance of the results, such constraints can greatly facilitate the discovery of co-modules by narrowing down the large search space. Let A denote the adjacency matrix of a gene interaction network, and B denote the adjacency matrix of a bipartite miRNA–gene network. We enforce "must-link" constraints by maximizing the objective function: $\mathcal{O}_1 = \sum_{ij} a_{ij} (h_i^2)^T h_j^2 = Tr(H_2 A H_2^T)$. This term ensures that genes with known interactions have similar coefficient profiles. Similarly, the interactions between genes and miRNAs can be encoded by the following objective function: $\mathcal{O}_2 = \sum_{ij} b_{ij} (h_i^1)^T h_j^2 = Tr(H_1 B H_2^T)$.

Our inputs are the miRNA and gene expression matrices X_1 and X_2 with dimensions $s \times m$ and $s \times n$, respectively, an $m \times n$ matrix B of predicted miRNA–target interactions, and an $n \times n$ gene–gene interaction network A. To discover miRNA-gene regulatory co-modules, we combine the three objectives defined in the previous sections into a single optimization function:

$$\mathcal{F}_1(W, H_1, H_2) = \sum_{I=1,2} \|X_I - WH_I\|_F^2 - \lambda_1 Tr(H_2 A H_2^T) - \lambda_2 Tr(H_1 B H_2^T). \tag{2}$$

The parameters λ_1 and λ_2 are weights for the must-link constraints defined in A and B. The first term favors modules with miRNA and gene expression profiles that are correlated in the common basis matrix W. The second term, $Tr(H_2AH_2^T)$, summarizes all the must-link constraints in the gene–gene network. The third term, $Tr(H_1B_{12}H_2^T)$, summarizes all the must-link constraints in the miRNA–gene network.

2.1.3 Sparse Network-Regularized Multiple NMF

An important characteristic of the NMF method is that it often generates sparse representations of the data, allowing us to discover part-based patterns [25]. However, studies have shown that the NMF representation is sensitive to the quality of the data and the researcher's choice of algorithms [13]. Several approaches have been proposed to control the degree of sparseness in the W and/or H factors [13, 18]. In our network-regularized multiple NMF (NMNMF) framework, we adopt a strategy suggested by Kim and Park [18] to make the coefficient matrices H_1 and H_2 sparse. This method, denoted SNMNMF, is formulated as follows:

$$\mathcal{F}(W,H_1,H_2)=\sum_{I=1,2}\|X_I-WH_I\|_F^2-\lambda_1 Tr(H_2AH_2^T)-\lambda_2 Tr(H_1BH_2^T)$$
$$+\gamma_1\|W\|_F^2+\gamma_2\sum_j\|h_j\|_1^2+\sum_{j'}\|h_{j'}\|_1^2), \quad (3)$$

where h_j and h_j' are the jth and j'^{th} columns of H_1 and H_2, respectively. The term $\gamma_1\|W\|_F^2$ limits the growth of W, while $\gamma_2(\sum_j\|h_j\|_1^2+\sum_{j'}\|h_{j'}\|_1^2)$ encourages sparsity.

2.1.4 The SNMNMF Algorithm

In the basic NMF problem, the objective function (Eq. 3) is not convex in W, H_1, and H_2. Therefore, it is unrealistic to expect a standard optimization algorithm to find the global minimum. We have developed an algorithm that efficiently converges to a local minimum by iteratively updating the matrix decomposition. Under the rules laid out below, the objective function $\mathcal{F}$ is guaranteed not to increase when the decomposition is updated. Furthermore, the objective function remains invariant if and only if W, H_1, and H_2 are at a stationary point. This behavior can be proved in the same way as for the classical NMF algorithm [26]. Derivations of the multiplicative updating rules and proof can be seen in [50]. We note that H_1 and H_2 are updated at the same time based on their current values at each iteration. The time complexity of the proposed algorithm is $O(tk(s+m+n)^2)$, where t is the number of iterations.

2.1.5 MicroRNA–Gene Co-module Assignment

The coefficient matrices H_1 and H_2 produced by the above algorithm will be used to identify co-modules. In other NMF applications [5, 19], people have used the maximum coefficient in each column of H (or row of W) to discover patterns and determine memberships. However, this method presumes that each gene or sample can belong to one and only one pattern. In our application, some genes may be active in multiple modules and others might not participate in any module. In the former case, the gene could exert multiple functions under different conditions.

In this work we calculate a z-score for each element of the factorization based on the rows of H_1 and H_2: $z_{ij} = \frac{x_{ij} - \mu_i}{\sigma_i}$, where μ_i is the average value of miRNA j (or gene j') in H_1 (or H_2), and σ_i is the standard deviation. We assign miRNA j (gene j') to co-module i if z_{ij} (z_{ij}') is greater than a given threshold T. Note that in our approach, each miRNA/gene may be assigned to multiple co-modules, permitting the identification of multiple functionalities.

2.1.6 Assessing the Statistical Significance of a Co-module

A miRNA–gene co-module is a pair of submatrices sX_1 and sX_2 extracted from the matrices X_1 and X_2. The dimensions of the submatrices are $s \times m_1^s$ and $s \times n_1^s$, respectively. We expect that within a co-module, miRNAs and genes are highly (anti-)correlated. In order to determine whether such relations are statistically significant, we performed the following assessment. First, we define the correlation S between two matrices with the same row dimensions as the sum of the correlations between any two columns, one from each matrix, i.e., $S = \sum s_{i,j}$, where $s_{i,j} = |corr(x_i^1, x_j^2)|$, "corr" representing the Pearson's correlation coefficients. We derive the statistical significance (p-value) of the correlation between sX_1 and sX_2 by comparing it to the distribution of correlations between 1,000 random matrix pairs. Each pair is composed of two matrices with dimensions identical to sX_1 and sX_2, whose elements are extracted from randomly permuted gene and miRNA expression matrices based on X_1 and X_2. Regulatory co-modules with p-values smaller than $0.05/k$ were considered significant, where k is the number of columns in the basis matrix W.

2.1.7 Biological Significance of the Co-modules

Studies have shown that miRNAs clustered on the genome are likely to be functionally related. Accordingly, we tested each co-module for miRNA cluster enrichment. We downloaded miRNA cluster data from the miRBase Web site (http://www.mirbase.org/), with a genomic cutoff distance of 50 kb. This criterion resulted in a sample of 57 clusters containing from 2 to 49 miRNAs. The average number of members per cluster is 4.5. Most of the miRNA clusters (37 out of 57) contain only two miRNAs. We also performed a functional enrichment analysis for genes in the identified co-modules. Specifically, we looked for enrichment in Gene Ontology (GO) biological process (BP) terms and KEGG pathways. The annotations of GO (BP) terms were downloaded from http://www.geneontology.org/, and the KEGG pathways were downloaded from http://www.genome.jp/kegg/. We mapped the GO terms to NCBI gene IDs using the index file from ftp://ftp.ncbi.nlm.nih.gov/gene/. We filtered out functional sets with more than 300 genes or fewer than 5 genes, as the former are too general to be informative and the latter are too specific to be relevant. The statistical significance (*p*-value) of a module's enrichment in a functional set was calculated using Fisher's Exact Test. This statistic was transformed into a *q*-value using a false discovery rate correction [41] with respect to the number of annotation groups.

2.2 Results

We have applied this method to identify miRNA–gene co-modules by integrating multiple independent data sources. The detailed parameter setting was not discussed here (please refer [50]). We identified 49 miRNA–gene co-modules with an average of 3.8 miRNAs and 78 genes per module. Based on a distribution of correlations derived from randomized miRNA–gene co-modules, the (anti-)correlations score between miRNAs and genes is statistically significant in 69.4 % of the modules, indicating that the probability of finding similarly (anti-)correlated co-modules by chance is close to zero.

2.2.1 The Co-modules are Enriched in Genomic miRNA Clusters

Several studies have shown that miRNAs often participate in combinatorial regulation in cellular system [24, 51]. The miRNA–gene co-modules discovered by our method may shed lights on these cooperative roles. Eleven of the identified modules are significantly enriched in at least one miRNA cluster (q-value < 0.05). For example, co-module 48 contains nine miRNAs (mir-506, mir-507, mir-508-3p, mir-509-3p, mir-509-3-5p, mir-509-5p, mir-513b, mir-513c, mir-514), all of which belong to a miRNA cluster on chromosome Xq27.3.

We did comprehensive literature survey and found that spatially clustered miRNAs often have similar functions in cellular systems. A number of recent literatures support the biological significance of the co-modules [52]. For example, in co-module 10, two of the four member miRNAs (mir-449a and 449b) belong to a miRNA cluster on chromosome 5q11.2, while the other two (miR-34b* and 34c-5p) belong to a cluster on chromosome 11q23.11. In a recent study, miR-449a and 449b have been reported to have a tumor suppressing function by regulating Rb/E2F1 activity [44]. In addition, miR-34b* and 34c-5p were reported to be targeted by p53 and they cooperatively control cell proliferation in ovarian cancer [7].

To take another example, three of the seven miRNAs in module 16 (miR-96, miR-182*, miR-183) are clustered on chromosome 7q32.2 and are reported to be dysregulated in various cancers. These miRNAs (along with others) cooperatively repress FOXO1, affecting cell cycle controls and apoptotic responses in endometrial cancer [31]. The differential expressions of these miRNAs appear to depend on the mismatch repair status, a behavior characteristic of undifferentiated proliferative states in colon cancer [37]. In addition, these miRNAs were identified as important biomarkers in the detection and prognosis of prostate cancer [38]. All this evidence shows that our co-modules can indeed group miRNAs with cooperative roles and provide insights into their functional mechanisms.

2.2.2 The Co-modules are Enriched in Known Functional Sets

To evaluate the biological relevance of the 49 co-modules, we calculated their enrichment in GO biological process terms and KEGG pathways using the hypergeometric test. (This test applies only to the genes in the co-modules.) Twenty-six (53.1 %) of the gene modules have at least one overrepresented GO biological process term with an FDR-corrected q-value <0.05. Taken together, the modules are enriched in 367 different GO biological processes and 57 KEGG pathways. The most frequently enriched biological processes are nuclear division, immune system process, microtubule-based processes, inflammatory response, response to external stimulus, cell cycle, and cell adhesion. When we performed the same test on a set of random modules, only 3.0 % (2.4 %) were enriched in any GO biological process. These observations demonstrate the power of our method in grouping genes that participate in the same processes or pathways.

2.2.3 The miRNA–Gene Co-modules are Strongly Implicated in Cancer

Since our input data included the miRNA and gene expression profiles of ovarian cancer samples, we expect the identified co-modules to be related to cancer. To verify this, we used a cancer miRNA benchmark dataset of 147 miRNAs from a review article [20]. Each of these miRNAs was reported in the literature to be dysregulated in one or more cancers. Among these, 41 are relevant to ovarian cancer. Note that this dataset does not include any information from the TCGA ovarian cancer data. Our co-modules involve 117 different miRNAs, 52 of which belong to the benchmark set of cancer miRNAs. This ratio is highly significant ($p = 1.1 \times 10^{-6}$) (Fig. 2). Even more importantly, 21 of the 52 miRNAs shared by our results and the benchmark are related to ovarian cancer, with an enrichment significance of $p = 7.2 \times 10^{-6}$.

Furthermore, 69.4 % of the modules contain at least two miRNAs that are known to be cancer related. For example, module 42 has seven miRNAs, five of which belong to the benchmark. Four of them (mir-199a-5p, mir-199b-3p, mir-127-3p, mir-214) are also reported to play roles in ovarian cancer [20]. Further supporting this interpretation, the genes of this co-module are enriched in numerous cancer-related pathways such as hedgehog signaling pathway, cell differentiation, TGFβ signaling pathway, and Wnt signaling pathway.

We explored cancer gene enrichment in the gene modules using the large-scale, human-curated knowledge database of the Ingenuity Pathway Analysis (IPA) system. Most of the modules

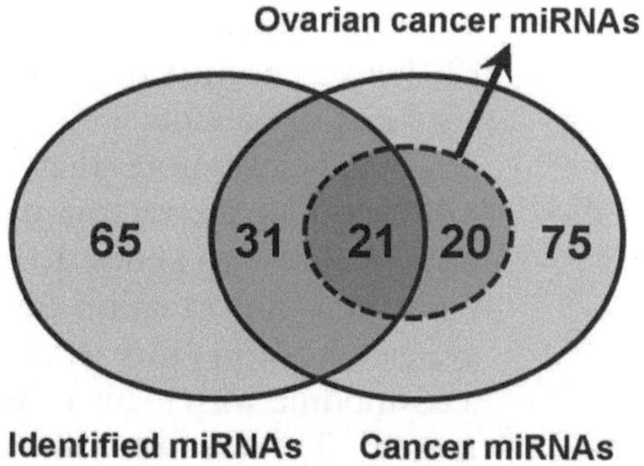

Fig. 2 About 44.4 % of the miRNAs in identified co-modules have previously been reported to be cancer related (hypergeometric test, $p = 1.1 \times 10^{-6}$). Of these, 21 miRNAs were specifically related to ovarian cancers (hypergeometric test, $p = 7.2 \times 10^{-6}$)

(63.3 %) are highly enriched in cancer genes (multiple test corrected p-value < 0.05, as reported by the IPA system). Moreover, ten of the modules are significantly enriched in ovarian cancer genes. For example, the 129 genes in module 23 include 64 cancer genes and 13 ovarian cancer genes. This module is overrepresented in several cancer-related pathways, including cell communication, TGFβ signaling pathway, and PPAR signaling pathway. These observations confirm that the miRNA–gene co-modules discovered in this study play important roles in various cancers, especially ovarian cancers.

2.2.4 Network Analysis of the Co-modules

Based on the principle of our method, the genes in a co-module are likely to function together as a network, and miRNAs in a co-module are likely to cooperatively target groups of networked genes. We found that in many of the co-modules identified by our method, the genes can be organized into highly connected networks using the IPA system and its database of molecular interactions [6]. Specifically, based on the IPA system, we found that 67.4 % of the co-modules is significantly connected to form at least one highly significant scored network with cutoff larger than 30.

We took co-module 40 as an example, and we constructed a dense network of 35 genes [50]. According to the IPA system, this network is significantly enriched with genes participating in cell death, cell cycle, tumor morphology, cellular growth and proliferation, and tissue development. Strikingly, miR-222 and miRNA-99a are anti-correlated with nineteen genes in this network (Pearson's correlation coefficients < -0.21, p-values $< 5.0 \times 10^{-5}$). This widespread anti-correlation strongly implies that the two miRNAs participate in regulating the overrepresented biological processes in the co-module. In other words, we can transfer those functions to these two miRNAs, especially to miR-222 which is anti-correlated with 17 genes. Moreover, the literature reports that both miR-222 and miR-99a are dysregulated in various cancers [20]. In a recent study, miR-222 has been implicated in the survival rate of patients with sporadic ovarian cancer [43].

Finally, we note that based on our input knowledge (the miRNA–gene interaction data), miR-222 is linked to this network through just two genes: KIF20B and STMN1. However, the complementary information on gene–gene connections and miRNA–gene expression (anti-)correlations permits us to place miR-222 in a co-module with many other genes that could be direct or indirect targets. These results, including the co-module's high level of enrichment in known cancer miRNAs, cancer genes, and cancer-related processes and interactions, shed light on a miRNA–gene regulatory circuit that plays an important functional role in ovarian cancer and possibly other cancers.

2.2.5 Comparison with Other Methods

Compared with other recent methods for miRNA–gene regulatory co-module identification [17, 34, 45], our method has several advantages: (1) it can incorporate prior knowledge such as a gene interaction network as a constraint on the solution space; to the best of our knowledge, this form of data has not been considered by any other algorithm for this task; (2) it simultaneously integrates several different types of data; (3) it provides sparse solutions that are more easily interpreted in biological contexts; and (4) it can be solved in a reasonable amount of computing time. In addition, our general framework is applicable to many other problems involving heterogeneous data sources. Due to the diversity of our data sources, it is difficult to make a fair comparison between our results and those of other methods. Nevertheless, we implemented the EBC method developed by Peng et al. [34] for comparison to show the above analysis [50].

2.3 Discussion and Conclusion

miRNAs play crucial roles in gene regulation which have been comprehensively reported in previous studies. However, little is known about the combinatorial regulatory mechanisms that frequently occur between miRNAs and genes. The large-scale availability of miRNA and gene expression profiles from the same samples, miRNA–gene interaction networks, and gene interaction networks provides an unprecedented opportunity to discover and accurately characterize miRNA–gene regulatory co-modules.

In this chapter, we describe the method developed by us recently, which can integrate these three data sources to identify miRNA–gene regulatory co-modules efficiently. We reported the biological relevance of the identified co-module on the expression profiles of ovarian cancer samples from the TCGA project. The co-modules reveal cooperation between miRNAs and genes, and provide new insights into the transcript and post-transcript regulatory organization of ovarian cancer. As genomic data sources increase in volume and diversity, our framework provides new avenues for the systematic interpretation of combinatorial regulatory mechanisms. We emphasize that our method is equally useful for many biological problems requiring the integration of multiple types of inputs. In particular, it is suitable for computational problems involving multidimensional data (data of multiple variables for the same set of samples) and independent priors identifying known relationships between the variables (e.g., miRNA–gene and gene–gene relationships). For example, Kutalik et al. explored gene–drug co-modules based on gene expression and drug response data from 60 cancer samples [22] recently. The quality of the modules obtained in that study suffered from the small number of samples and noise of input data. One could employ our framework to incorporate known gene–gene interactions, known gene–drug relationships, and drug–drug similarities to improve the module discovery. Currently, we observe a fast-increasing trend toward generating multidimensional genomic data, which are profiled on the same set of samples. Meanwhile, we are gaining more and more knowledge regarding the associations or relationships between different genomic variables. The new method described here can serve as a powerful framework for the simultaneous integration of diverse data to discover complex regulatory patterns.

Acknowledgements

This project was supported by the National Natural Science Foundation of China (No.11001256), the 'Special Presidential Prize—Scientific Research Foundation of the CAS, and the Special Foundation of President of AMSS at CAS for 'Chen Jing-Run' Future Star Program.

References

1. Baek D et al (2008) The impact of microRNAs on protein output. Nature 455:64–71
2. Bartel DP (2004) MicroRNAs: genomics, biogenesis, mechanism, and function. Cell 116: 281–297
3. Bentwich I et al (2005) Identification of hundreds of conserved and nonconserved human microRNAs. Nat Genet 37:766–770
4. Bossi A, Lehner B (2009) Tissue specificity and the human protein interaction network. Mol Syst Biol 5:260
5. Brunet JP et al (2004) Metagenes and molecular pattern discovery using matrix factorization. Proc Natl Acad Sci U S A 101: 4164–4169
6. Calvano SE et al (2005) Inflamm and host response to injury large scale collab. res. program (2005) A network-based analysis of systemic inflammation in humans. Nature 437: 1032–1037
7. Corney DC et al (2007) MicroRNA-34b and MicroRNA-34c are targets of p53 and cooperate in control of cell proliferation and adhesion-independent growth. Cancer Res 67:8433–8438
8. Cui Q et al (2006) Principles of microRNA regulation of a human cellular signaling network. Mol Syst Biol 2:46
9. Enright AJ et al (2003) MicroRNA targets in *Drosophila*. Genome Biol 5:R1
10. Garzon R et al (2006) MicroRNA expression and function in cancer. Trends Mol Med 12:580–587
11. Gusev Y et al (2007) Computational analysis of biological functions and pathways collectively targeted by co-expressed microRNAs in cancer. BMC Bioinformatics 8:S16
12. Hartwell LH et al (1999) From molecular to modular cell biology. Nature 402:C47–C52

13. Hoyer P (2004) Non-negative matrix factorization with sparseness constraints. J Mach Learn Res 5:1457–1469
14. Hsu CW et al (2008) Characterization of microRNA-regulated protein-protein interaction network. Proteomics 8:1975–1979
15. Huang JC et al (2007) Using expression profiling data to identify human microRNA targets. Nat Methods 4:1045–1049
16. Ihmels J et al (2002) Revealing modular organization in the yeast transcriptional network. Nat Genet 31:370–377
17. Joung JG et al (2007) Discovery of microRNA-mRNA modules via population-based probabilistic learning. Bioinformatics 23:1141–1147
18. Kim H, Park H (2007) Sparse non-negative matrix factorizations via alternating nonnegativity-constrained least squares for microarray data analysis. Bioinformatics 23: 1495–1502
19. Kim PM, Tidor B (2003) Subsystem identification through dimensionality reduction oflarge-scale gene expression data. Genome Res 13:1706–1718
20. Koturbash I et al (2010) Small molecules with big effects: the role of the microRNAome in cancer and carcinogenesis. Mutat Res. doi:10.1016/j.mrgentox.2010.05.006
21. Krek A et al (2005) Combinatorial microRNA target predictions. Nat Genet 37:495–500
22. Kutalik Z et al (2008) A modular approach for integrative analysis of large-scale geneexpression and drug-response data. Nat Biotechnol 26:531–539
23. Lagos-Quintana M et al (2003) New microRNAs from mouse and human. RNA 9:175–179
24. Lai EC et al (2003) Computational identification of *Drosophila* microRNA genes. Genome Biol 4:R42
25. Lee DD, Seung HS (1999) Learning the parts of objects by non-negative matrix factorization. Nature 401:788–791
26. Lee DS, Seung HS (2001) Algorithms for non-negative matrix factorization. Adv Neural Inf Process Syst 13:556–562
27. Lewis BP et al (2003) Prediction of mammalian microRNA targets. Cell 115:787–798
28. Liang H, Li WH (2007) MicroRNA regulation of human protein protein interaction network. RNA 13:1402–1408
29. Lim LP et al (2005) Microarray analysis shows that some microRNAs downregulate large numbers of target mRNAs. Nature 433: 769–773
30. Lu J et al (2005) MicroRNA expression profiles classify human cancers. Nature 435: 834–838
31. Myatt SS et al (2010) Definition of microRNAs that repress expression of the tumor suppressor gene FOXO1 in endometrial cancer. Cancer Res 70:367–377
32. Nunez-Iglesias J et al (2010) Joint genome-wide profiling of miRNA and mRNA expression in Alzheimer's disease cortex reveals altered miRNA regulation. PLoS One 5:e8898
33. Paatero P, Tapper U (1994) Positive matrix factorization: A non-negative factor model with optimal utilization of error estimates of data values. Environmetrics 5:111–126
34. Peng X et al (2009) Computational identification of hepatitis C virus associated microRNAmRNA regulatory modules in human livers. BMC Genomics 10:373
35. Qi Y, Ge H (2006) Modularity and dynamics of cellular networks. PLoS Comput Biol 2:e174
36. Rodriguez A et al (2004) Identification of mammalian microRNA host genes and transcription units. Genome Res 14:1902–1910
37. Sarver AL et al (2009) Human colon cancer profiles show differential microRNA expression depending on mismatch repair status and are characteristic of undifferentiated proliferative states. BMC Cancer 9:401
38. Schaefer A et al (2010) Diagnostic and prognostic implications of microRNA profiling in prostate carcinoma. Int J Cancer 126:1166–1176
39. Shalgi R et al (2007) Global and local architecture of the mammalian microRNAtranscription factor regulatory network. PLoS Comput Biol 3:e131
40. Stark A et al (2003) Identification of *Drosophila* microRNA targets. PLoS Biol 1:e60
41. Storey JD, Tibshirani R (2003) Statistical significance for genome-wide studies. Proc Natl Acad Sci U S A 100:9440–9445
42. Tran DH et al (2008) Finding microRNA regulatory modules in human genome using rule induction. BMC Bioinformatics 9:S5
43. Wurz K et al (2010) MiR-221 and MiR-222 alterations in sporadic ovarian carcinoma: relationship to CDKN1B, CDKNIC and overall survival. Genes Chromosomes Cancer 49:577–584
44. Yang X et al (2009) miR-449a and miR-449b are direct transcriptional targets of E2F1 and negatively regulate pRb-E2F1 activity through a feedback loop by targeting CDK6 and CDC25A. Genes Dev 23(20):2388–2393
45. Yoon S, DeMicheli G (2005) Prediction of regulatory modules comprising microRNAs and target genes. Bioinformatics 21(S2): ii93–ii100
46. Xie X et al (2005) Systematic discovery of regulatory motifs in human promoters and 3′ UTRs by comparison of several mammals. Nature 434:338–345
47. Xu J, Wong C (2008) A computational screen for mouse signaling pathways targeted by microRNA clusters. RNA 14:1276–1283

48. Yuan X et al (2009) Clustered microRNAs' coordination in regulating protein-protein interaction network. BMC Syst Biol 3:65
49. Zhang S, Jin G, Zhang XS, Chen L (2007) Discovering functions and revealing mechanisms at molecular level from biological networks. Proteomics 7:2856–2869
50. Zhang S, Li Q, Liu J, Zhou XJ (2011) A novel computational framework for simultaneous integration of multiple functional genomic data to identify microRNA-gene regulatory modules. Bioinformatics (ISMB2011) 27: i401–i409
51. Zhang X et al (2010) Synergistic effects of the GATA-4-mediated miR-144/451 cluster in protection against simulated ischemia/reperfusion-induced cardiomyocyte death. J Mol Cell Cardiol 49:841–850
52. Zhou Y et al (2007) Inter- and intra-combinatorial regulation by transcription factors and microRNAs. BMC Genomics 8:396

Part IV

Cellular Structure and Metabolism Analysis

Chapter 17

Energy Metabolism and Changes in Cellular Composition in Ovarian Cancer

Anastasia Malek

Abstract

Ovarian cancer possesses metabolic properties typical for any malignancy as well as some specific characteristics. Most of the methodological approach to study metabolism and molecular composition of the living cells are suitable for ovarian cancer research, however, might require minor modifications. The chapter reviews various laboratory techniques adapted to study ovarian cancer.

Key words Ovarian cancer, Cellular metabolism, Proteome profiling, Posttranscriptional modification

1 Cancer Cell Biology Apart from Genome Research

The basic functional characteristics of tumor cells include the following: sustaining proliferative signalling, evading growth suppressors, resisting cell death, enabling replicative immortality, inducing angiogenesis, activating invasion and metastasis, reprogramming energy metabolism, and evading immune destruction [1]. Genetic alterations are considered the primary causative factors of all of the features acquired by cells during and as the result of malignant transformation. Recent advances in high-throughput technologies in genome research have provided opportunities to further comprehend the role of genetics sources in malignant phenotype formation. However, a knowledge of the factors that may cause or/and trigger this phenotype is not sufficient. Exploring the underlying mechanisms is necessary for a clear understanding of cancer cell biology. Aberrations in cellular signalling and metabolic pathways and alterations in expression patterns and secondary modification of proteins, carbohydrates, and lipid molecules are essential for the development of cancer phenotypes. In contrast to genetic alterations, these structural changes are more complex and dynamic, which makes assessing their impacts challenging. Recent

Anastasia Malek and Oleg Tchernitsa (eds.), *Ovarian Cancer: Methods and Protocols*, Methods in Molecular Biology, vol. 1049, DOI 10.1007/978-1-62703-547-7_17,

approaches, such as the -omics scale of analysis, require advanced technical and computational support. The following chapters (from Chapters 18 to 22) describe several comprehensive methods of studying ovarian cancer cell composition on an -omics scale. This chapter provides a brief overview of relevant aspects of ovarian cancer pathogenesis.

2 Ovarian Cancer and Associated Metabolic Shifts

Development and metastatic dissemination of ovarian cancer is largely confined to the peritoneal cavity and is associated with excessive production of ascitic fluid. Cancer cells exfoliated from primary tumors can persist and proliferate suspended in ascitic fluid and colonize the peritoneum. Specific patterns of ovarian tumor spread are associated with certain metabolic characteristics. A cancer-specific metabolic shift from oxidative phosphorylation to glycolysis was described by Otto Warburg in 1923 [2], and this theory was recently supported by the discovery of "fuel" from the host cells [3]. Fundamental changes in the pathways of energy metabolism can be observed in various types of cancer, including ovarian carcinomas. In addition to these alterations, ovarian cancer cells enhance lipid catabolism and obtain energy-rich lipids from adipocytes that form visceral fat deposits in the underlying mesothelium. Human adipocytes can promote homing, migration, and invasion of ovarian cancer cells [4]. Adipocyte-ovarian cancer cells in coculture showed the direct transfer of lipids from adipocytes to ovarian cancer cells, promoting in vitro and in vivo tumor growth [4]. An increase in lipolysis-promoting activity was also detected in the ascitic fluid in patients with ovarian cancer [5]. Alterations in lipid metabolism may occur in ovarian cancer cells suspended in ascites and cells that form peritoneal metastases. Lipid metabolism and transport are promising targets for therapeutic intervention. Other metabolic alterations can be evaluated by full metabolomic profiling and may indicate new aspects regarding energy homeostasis in ovarian cancer cells. Chapter 18 presents methods based on a combination of chromatography and mass spectrometry (LC-MS and GC-MS) that allows researchers to profile the metabolome of ovarian cancer (both primary and metastatic) cells versus cells of the normal ovary. Various metabolic alterations associated with ovarian cancer progression have been evaluated using this method. For example, alterations in carbohydrate metabolism associated with metastatic processes have been shown in addition to increased fatty acid oxidation in both primary and metastatic tumors [6]. This approach can be used to evaluate metabolic changes associated with other clinically relevant parameters, such as responses to chemotherapy, disease recurrence, overall survival, and discovery of new prognostic markers or therapeutic targets. A detailed analysis focused on specific biochemical pathways may be performed using the methods described in Chapter 19. High resolution multinuclear magnetic resonance spectroscopy (MRS) allows noninvasive and simultaneous monitoring of various metabolites of interest in intact tissues or extracts from living systems. The technique exploits the magnetic properties of different nonradioactive isotopes, such as ^{1}H, ^{31}P, ^{13}C, for structural analysis and quantitative measurement of various metabolites. This approach was used to investigate phosphatidylcholine metabolism in ovarian cancer [7].

Specific metabolic reactions are generally analyzed using radio- or fluorescent-labelled tracers. These techniques are not discussed in the book, since they are well established, described elsewhere, and can be applied in ovarian cancer research without substantial modification.

3 High-Throughput Approaches in Protein Research

Intraperitoneal development of ovarian cancer is substantially influenced by cellular functionality and composition. After they detach from the primary tumor, ovarian cancer cells became resistant to anoikis, change their cellular shape and adhesive characteristics, and form multicellular aggregates (spheroids). Because anchorage- and vascular-independent three-dimensional structures can grow in suspension, the spheroids may represent a key component of chemoresistance in ovarian cancer [8]. The ability of ovarian cancer cells to penetrate the submesothelial matrix and anchor metastatic implants is mediated by enhanced motility and invasiveness [9]. Substantial changes in synthesized protein patterns provide a structural background for functional gains. Proteome profiling is the method of choice for defining global shifts in the synthetic activity of cancer cells, while assessing the repertoire of surface and secreted molecules provides a basis for developing screening and early diagnostic approaches [10]. High-throughput proteomic technology using two-dimensional liquid chromatography tandem mass spectrometry (2D-LC-MS/MS) coupled with chemical labelling by isobaric tags can be used in comparative proteomic analysis. Labelling technologies, either isobaric tags for relative and absolute quantification (iTRAQ) or tandem mass tagging (TMT), allow simultaneous analysis and relative quantification of samples. Both approaches have been applied in ovarian cancer research in patients [11] and cell culture in experimental settings [12]. Changes in the protein patterns in certain cellular compartments can be tracked after isolation of specific cell lysates. Chapter 20 describes quantitative 2D-LC-MS/MS profiling coupled with TMT labelling of the whole cell lysate, secreted proteins and a crude membrane fraction prepared from cultured ovarian cancer cells. Experimental treatment was shown to result in suppression of a tumourigenic phenotype, and proteome profiling of treated cells versus the untreated control was performed to identify the proteins implicated in the process of tumourigenic reversion based on cellular localization. The method usually yields approximately 1,000 proteins with significantly varying expression between the samples, providing material for further validation and analysis.

The analytic approach presented in Chapter 21 is recommended for high-throughput assessment of changes in expression for a select set of proteins. For example, the ability of ovarian cancer cells to attach and penetrate the peritoneum is mediated by a defined pattern of adhesive molecules and proteases [9], while epithelial–mesenchymal transition depends on the activity of certain cellular signalling cascades [13]. Reverse phase protein array (RPPA) is an optimal method for simultaneously studying selected proteins in multiple tissue or cell culture samples [14]. Because protein lysates are spotted on the same slide, this method allows direct comparison of protein expression between samples. RPPA has been used to study various signalling pathways involved in anchorage-independent survival [15] and chemoresistance in ovarian cancer cells [16], indicating a broad application of the method.

4 Assessment of Posttranslational Protein Modification

In addition to quantitative changes in the protein repertoire due to expression dysregulation, the process of posttranslational protein modification is substantially altered in cancer cells, resulting in qualitative changes in cellular composition. Important examples of posttranslational protein modification (e.g., phosphorylation, acetylation, methylation, prenylation, ubiquitination, sumoylation, and glycosylation) and their implications in cancerogenesis have been reviewed in the literature [17]. For example, aberrant phosphorylation of signal transducers and activators of the transcription (STAT3) protein are induced by lysophosphatidic acid (LPA), which stimulates cancer cell motility [18]. Because LPA is a common compound in the ascitic fluid of ovarian cancer patients, chronic LPA-induced STAT3 phosphorylation may be a target for anti-metastatic therapy. Pharmacological disturbance of the acetylation/deacetylation equilibrium reduces the chemoresistance potential of ovarian cancer. A combination of docetaxel with a histone deacetylase inhibitor has been explored as a promising strategy to increase the sensitivity of ovarian cancer to taxol-based chemotherapy [19]. Induction of the ubiquitination of proteins that mediate signalling pathways promoting cancer is another promising anti-cancer strategy [20]. Thus, pharmacological interruption of specific posttranslational protein modifications that drive oncogenic progression is a promising therapeutic approach, while exploring cancer-specific posttranslational changes in secreted proteins may offer a plethora of marker candidates for early diagnostics or therapy monitoring. However, a limiting factor in posttranslational modification research is that the technologies used to screen vast numbers of molecules for a particular type of modification are often not available or are weakly reproducible. In general, research in this area requires the study of discreet modifications in specific proteins of interest. Although ovarian cancer research does not involve specific methods of posttranslational protein modification analysis, an excellent collection of relevant protocols is available in the literature [21].

In the context of ovarian cancer research, changes in protein glycosylation are of particular importance. The 5-year survival rate drops from 93.5 to 27.6 % when comparing the time of diagnosis at stage I versus stage IV [22]. There is a critical unmet need for sensitive and specific routine screening tests for early diagnosis that can reduce the lethality of ovarian cancer by reliably detecting the disease at its earliest and most treatable stages. Specific changes in serum proteins glycosylation in ovarian cancer patients provides perspectives for diagnostic approaches, which are currently being explored [23, 24]. Chapter 22 describes the profiling of *N*-glycans from glycoproteins of ovarian carcinoma cells by high performance anion exchange chromatography with pulsed amperometric detection (HPAEC-PAD) and matrix-assisted laser desorption/ionization with time of flight mass spectrometry (MALDI-TOF MS). This complex approach allows quantitative profiling and structure elucidation of *N*-glycans released from the glycoproteins in ovarian cancer cells. Other MS-based methods of glycome profiling could be applied after consideration of related technical details [25].

The majority of methods that globally assess cellular protein patterns and composition are based on mass spectrometry approaches and are equally applicable in many areas of cancer research. Coupled with various techniques, including affinity-based enrichment, extraction methods, multidimensional separation technologies, and probe labelling, mass spectrometry provides a number of specific methods that can be used in various experimental settings to analyze different types of protein modifications. Recent developments in mass spectrometry-based approaches for systematic, qualitative, and quantitative determination of cellular composition promises to bring new insights into malignant cell structural organization and homeostasis.

References

1. Hanahan D, Weinberg RA (2011) Hallmarks of cancer: the next generation. Cell 144: 646–674
2. Warburg O (1956) On the origin of cancer cells. Science 123:309–314
3. Martinez-Outschoorn UE, Sotgia F, Lisanti MP (2012) Power surge: supporting cells "fuel" cancer cell mitochondria. Cell Metab 15:4–5
4. Nieman KM, Kenny HA, Penicka CV, Ladanyi A, Buell-Gutbrod R et al (2011) Adipocytes promote ovarian cancer metastasis and provide energy for rapid tumor growth. Nat Med 17: 1498–1503
5. Gercel-Taylor C, Doering DL, Kraemer FB, Taylor DD (1996) Aberrations in normal systemic lipid metabolism in ovarian cancer patients. Gynecol Oncol 60:35–41
6. Fong MY, McDunn J, Kakar SS (2011) Identification of metabolites in the normal ovary and their transformation in primary and metastatic ovarian cancer. PLoS One 6:e19963
7. Iorio E, Ricci A, Bagnoli M, Pisanu ME, Castellano G et al (2010) Activation of phosphatidylcholine cycle enzymes in human epithelial ovarian cancer cells. Cancer Res 70: 2126–2135
8. Shield K, Ackland ML, Ahmed N, Rice GE (2009) Multicellular spheroids in ovarian cancer metastases: biology and pathology. Gynecol Oncol 113:143–148
9. Kwon Y, Cukierman E, Godwin AK (2011) Differential expressions of adhesive molecules and proteases define mechanisms of ovarian tumor cell matrix penetration/invasion. PLoS One 6:e18872
10. Zhang Y, Xu B, Liu Y, Yao H, Lu N et al (2012) The ovarian cancer-derived secretory/releasing proteome: a repertoire of tumor markers. Proteomics 12:1883–1891
11. Wang LN, Tong SW, Hu HD, Ye F, Li SL et al (2012) Quantitative proteome analysis of ovarian cancer tissues using a iTRAQ approach. J Cell Biochem 113:3762–3772
12. Sinclair J, Metodieva G, Dafou D, Gayther SA, Timms JF (2011) Profiling signatures of ovarian cancer tumour suppression using 2D-DIGE and 2D-LC-MS/MS with tandem mass tagging. J Proteomics 74:451–465
13. Colomiere M, Ward AC, Riley C, Trenerry MK, Cameron-Smith D et al (2009) Cross talk of signals between EGFR and IL-6R through JAK2/STAT3 mediate epithelial-mesenchymal transition in ovarian carcinomas. Br J Cancer 100:134–144
14. Sheehan KM, Calvert VS, Kay EW, Lu Y, Fishman D et al (2005) Use of reverse phase protein microarrays and reference standard development for molecular network analysis of metastatic ovarian carcinoma. Mol Cell Proteomics 4:346–355
15. Irie HY, Shrestha Y, Selfors LM, Frye F, Iida N et al (2010) PTK6 regulates IGF-1-induced anchorage-independent survival. PLoS One 5:e11729
16. Carey MS, Agarwal R, Gilks B, Swenerton K, Kalloger S et al (2010) Functional proteomic analysis of advanced serous ovarian cancer using reverse phase protein array: TGF-beta pathway signaling indicates response to primary chemotherapy. Clin Cancer Res 16: 2852–2860
17. Krueger KE, Srivastava S (2006) Posttranslational protein modifications: current implications for cancer detection, prevention, and therapeutics. Mol Cell Proteomics 5:1799–1810
18. Seo JH, Jeong KJ, Oh WJ, Sul HJ, Sohn JS et al (2010) Lysophosphatidic acid induces STAT3 phosphorylation and ovarian cancer cell motility: their inhibition by curcumin. Cancer Lett 288:50–56
19. Chao H, Wang L, Hao J, Ni J, Graham PH et al (2013) Low dose histone deacetylase inhibitor, LBH589, potentiates anticancer effect of docetaxel in epithelial ovarian cancer via PI3K/Akt pathway. Cancer Lett 329(1):17–26
20. Tomek K, Wagner R, Varga F, Singer CF, Karlic H et al (2011) Blockade of fatty acid synthase induces ubiquitination and degradation of phosphoinositide-3-kinase signaling proteins in ovarian cancer. Mol Cancer Res 9:1767–1779
21. John Wiley & Sons I (2010) Post-translation modification. http://www.currentprotocols.com/WileyCDA/CurPro3Category/L1-3600,L2-3621.html
22. National Cancer Institute SFS (2011) http://seer.cancer.gov/statfacts/html/ovary.html
23. Alley WR Jr, Vasseur JA, Goetz JA, Svoboda M, Mann BF et al (2012) N-linked glycan structures and their expressions change in the blood sera of ovarian cancer patients. J Proteome Res 11:2282–2300
24. Wu J, Xie X, Liu Y, He J, Benitez R et al (2012) Identification and confirmation of differentially expressed fucosylated glycoproteins in the serum of ovarian cancer patients using a lectin array and LC-MS/MS. J Proteome Res 11:4541–4552
25. Mechref Y, Hu Y, Garcia A, Hussein A (2012) Identifying cancer biomarkers by mass spectrometry-based glycomics. Electrophoresis 33:1755–1767

Chapter 18

Metabolomic Profiling of Ovarian Carcinomas Using Mass Spectrometry

Miranda Y. Fong, Jonathan McDunn, and Sham S. Kakar

Abstract

Most of the research on tumor cell metabolism has focused on glucose utilization. However, when glucose is limited, solid tumors are forced to catabolize alternative substrates such as fatty acids and amino acids as an energy source. Measuring these alternations in tumor cell metabolism enables us to track neoplastic changes in the tissue to lead towards a more reliable diagnostic outcome. Although a very small number of elements are used in biochemistry, the metabolome is structurally diverse for the production of simple compounds such as phosphate and amino acids as well as more structurally complex compounds such as nucleotides, oligosaccharides, and complex lipids. Characterization of the metabolome, therefore, requires analytical methods that can handle a wide range of molecular structures and physicochemical properties, including solubility, polarity, and molecular weight. A further factor for consideration in the selection of technology for metabolomics is the wide range of concentrations of biochemical typically present in biological systems. MS has established itself as the high-throughput, information-rich, industrially stable approach to assess both the composition of diverse sample types as well as changes to that composition following perturbation.

Key words Ovarian cancer, Ultra performance liquid chromatography, Mass spectrometry, Metabolites, Metabolomics, Detection methods

1 Introduction

Ovarian cancer is known as "the silent killer" as the disease is largely asymptomatic until the disease has metastasized, making it the main factor for the poor prognosis of ovarian cancer patients [1]. The early warning signs of ovarian cancer are not disease specific but rather present themselves as vague abdominal discomfort, abdominal pain not dissimilar to menstrual cramps, bloating, urinary changes, and feeling full [1, 2]. However, diagnosis based off symptoms alone will detect cancer in 1 % of patients [2]. Because of vague symptoms, approximately 63 % of ovarian cancer cases are diagnosed at Stage IV, which has a 5-year survival rate of 27.6 %, making it the most lethal malignancy of the female reproductive

Anastasia Malek and Oleg Tchernitsa (eds.), *Ovarian Cancer: Methods and Protocols*, Methods in Molecular Biology, vol. 1049, DOI 10.1007/978-1-62703-547-7_18, © Springer Science+Business Media New York 2013

system and the fifth cause of cancer death in women. If ovarian cancer is diagnosed at Stage I when the carcinoma is still localized, the 5-year survival rate is 92.4 % [3]. Therefore, it is imperative that we be able to detect the carcinomas before they have metastasized. Current detection strategies include transvaginal ultrasound and blood CA-125 levels. However, both detection methods have disadvantages. With ultrasound, cancer could be mistaken for functional cysts in premenopausal women due to the dynamic nature of the ovarian surface [4]. CA-125 has a high false-positive rate [4] that can arise from a variety of conditions including endometriosis, fibroids, hemorrhagic ovarian cysts, acute pelvic inflammatory disease, menstruation, first trimester pregnancy, and several other cancer types [5]. In addition, CA-125 is often not detectable in early stage of ovarian cancer [6]. Alternative methods are being developed for patients who have normal CA-125 levels but are suspected to having recurrent disease based on clinical symptoms [7]. These methods include other potential biomarkers, the most promising being human epididymis protein 4 (HE4) [8–12], despite detection rates of 50–60 % in early-stage ovarian cancer. A comprehensive study comparing the sensitivity of ovarian cancer biomarkers to discriminate between benign and malignant masses has been described [13] as well as the role of molecular markers in prognosis and therapy reviewed [14]. It is important that suggested biomarkers have predictive value as indicated by sensitivity of 75 % or greater as well as specificity of 99.6 % to be able to detect early-stage cancer when it is the most treatable [6].

One approach to identify disease biomarkers is to use information-rich analytical tools such as omics-scale biological methods to characterize the composition of the target tissue during health and disease states. In this case, it is important to understand the biochemical alterations that are known to occur during neoplastic transformation. The energy metabolism alteration in cancer cells was first described by Otto Warburg in 1923, who showed that cancer cells shift from oxidative phosphorylation to glycolysis resulting in the generation of lactate for ATP production while their oxygen requirements remain similar to non-transformed tissues [15]. This Warburg Effect results in a net energy production loss and thus requires the cancer cells to increase their glucose uptake through the expression of several isoforms of glucose transporters (GLUT 1–9) [16] and to increase their glucose catabolism.

In 1919, Peyton Rous had begun laying the groundwork for what is now known as oncovirology. He created a cell-free tumor filtrate that he injected into healthy chickens, thus identifying a transmissible factor in chickens that could cause sarcoma formation and this became one of the earliest, highly reproducible tumor models, which he named the Rous sarcoma virus (RSV) [17]. By the mid-1920s, Carl and Gerty Cori had established themselves as experts in the field of physiologic glucose consumption. The Cori's contribution to cancer metabolism was to utilize the Rous sarcoma model to test whether Warburg's findings were merely an in vitro phenomenon or an important part of the pathophysiology of cancer. The Cori's established tumors in a single wing of a cohort of chickens and measured glucose and lactate levels in the arterial and venous blood for both the tumor-bearing wing and the contralateral wing [18]. Their findings recapitulated Warburg's observations in tissue culture and led to conceptual models of cancer as a predominantly metabolic disease.

During the decades that followed, as biochemical probes were developed to map metabolic pathways, researchers often found that tumors expressed a different suite of metabolic activities. These activities included alterations in redox homeostasis, nucleoside biosynthesis, amino acid uptake, tRNA synthesis and turnover, and fatty acid synthesis. However, it was not just biochemical probes that were found to differentiate tumors from nonneoplastic tissues. As part of the molecular biology revolution in the late 1960s, the emerging tools for dissecting gene sequence, structure, expression, and function were also applied to cancer biology systems. The increased complexity of genomic space, the generalizability of DNA-based approaches, and some early successes in this field caused a rapid expansion of investigation into the molecular biology of cancer that dwarfed the efforts in cancer metabolism at the time. Interestingly, the first oncogene that was identified was the transformative component of RSV, Src [19].

Interplay between oncogenes and metabolic alterations has been documented. For example, the Akt pathway including nuclear factor κ-B (NF-κB) and hypoxia-inducible factor 1 (HIF1) has been linked to hyperactive glycolysis [16, 20, 21]. Similarly, Myc increases expression of transporters and glycolytic enzymes – in particular GLUT, hexokinase 2, and lactate dehydrogenase [16, 22]. In addition, tumor metabolism differentially expresses glycolytic isoenzymes, such as pyruvate kinase (PKM2), which can shift between a dimer and a tetramer to adapt to the energy requirements of the cells [23, 24]. However, PKM2 can also be bypassed by the accumulation of phosphoenolpyruvate (PEP) resulting in PEP-dependent phosphorylation and activation of phosphoglycerate mutase which produces pyruvate directly from 3-phosphoglycerate [25]. However, oncogenesis can result in a diverse panel of metabolic alterations that could be tissue specific or generic across human cancers. Therefore, a comprehensive metabolic analysis of solid tumors could reveal valuable metabolites for both early diagnoses of cancer as well as to monitor disease progression and/or recurrence to inform clinical management of cancer patients. These biomarkers could conceivably be used as surrogate end points in clinical trials and could suggest new metabolic targets for cancer management as well as provide complementary targets for chemotherapy treatment.

The human metabolome is thought to be comprised of a few thousand biochemicals, although current technologies can measure approximately 350–800 compounds in a typical sample.

While a very small number of elements are used in biochemistry (predominantly carbon, hydrogen, nitrogen, oxygen, phosphorous, and sulfur), the metabolome is structurally diverse and includes simple compounds such as phosphate and amino acids as well as nucleotides, oligosaccharides, and complex lipids. Characterization of the metabolome, therefore, requires analytical methods that can handle a wide range of molecular structures and physicochemical properties, including solubility, polarity, and molecular weight. A further factor for consideration in the selection of technology for metabolomics is the wide range of concentrations of biochemicals typically present in biological systems.

Metabolomics is a systematic analytical tool used for identification of biochemical metabolites from cellular processes, a term that includes several types of analyses ranging from nuclear magnetic resonance spectroscopy (NMR), mass spectrometry (MS) and tracer-based studies to metabolic foot printing [26]. While each of these methods has unique advantages, MS has established itself as the high-throughput, information-rich, industrially stable approach to assess both the composition of diverse sample types as well as changes to that composition following perturbation.

A mass spectrometer is an analytical instrument that uses electric and/or magnetic fields to separate charged compounds, coupled to high-sensitivity electronics for the detection of those charged compounds. In order to achieve optimal coverage of a metabolome, fractionation of the biochemical extract needs to occur prior to mass spectral analysis. The current method of choice for high reproducibility biochemical fractionation is ultrahigh performance liquid chromatography (UHPLC). Traditionally, reverse phase media (such as the lipophilic C18 resin) provide excellent separation of diverse chemical structures based on their hydrophobicity.

LC-MS typically utilizes electrospray ionization to generate charged species for analysis. While this method can be optimized to detect either anions or cations depending on the buffer system used in the chromatography, there are several compounds that are not amenable to analysis by this method, specifically sterols and sugars. The preferred method for detection of these compounds is still chemical derivatization and analysis on a gas chromatography-mass spectrometry (GC-MS) system.

2 Materials

2.1 Tissue Preparation

1. Dry ice to keep tissues frozen during processing and for shipping.
2. Razor blade.
3. 70 % ethanol for cleaning the razor blade between samples.
4. Milligram scale.

5. 2-mL cryopreservation tube (Wheaton).
6. Shipping container.

2.2 Reagents

2.2.1 Simple Chemicals

1. Methanol.
2. Formic acid (LC-MS grade).
3. Ammonium bicarbonate (LC-MS grade): 6.5 mM, pH 8.
4. Bistrimethyl-silyl-trifluoroacetamide (GC-MS grade).
5. Acetonitrile (LC-MS grade).
6. Dichloromethane (LC-MS grade).
7. Cyclohexane (LC-MS grade).
8. Triethylamine (LC-MS grade).

2.2.2 Composed Solutions for Liquid Chromatography

Solvents for LC should be prepared within a week of use and can be stored:

1. 0.1 % formic acid in deionized water (18 Mohm).
2. 0.1 % formic acid in methanol.
3. mM Ammonium bicarbonate (pH 8) in deionized water (18 Mohm).
4. 6.5-mM ammonium bicarbonate (pH 8) in methanol.

2.2.3 Reconstitution Solutions for Liquid Chromatography Standardization

1. Positive ion mode LC-MS standards: d7-glucose, d3-methionine, d3-leucine, d8-phenylalanine, d5-tryptophan, bromophenylalanine, d4-tyrosine, d5-indole acetate, d9-progesterone, and d4-dioctyl phthalate.
2. Positive ion mode LC-MS standard stock solutions: Stock solutions are prepared in either water or ethanol depending on solubility at either 1 or 10 mg/ml (concentrations must be determined concentrations to optimize performance with the LC-MS system).
3. Positive ion mode LC-MS reconstitution solution: Stock solutions are combined in empirically determined ratios (from 0.25 to 5 ml) into a cocktail along with 0.1 volume equivalents of 0.1 % formic acid in water. The stock is then further diluted 1:5 with 0.1 % formic acid in water.
4. Negative ion mode standards: d7-glucose, d3-methionine, d3-leucine, d8-phenylalanine, d5-tryptophan, bromophenylalanine, d15-octanoate, d19-decanoate, d27-tetradecanoate, and d35-octadecanoate.
5. Negative ion mode LC-MS standard stock solutions: Stock solutions are prepared in either water or ethanol depending on solubility, at either 1 or 10 mg/ml (concentrations must be empirically determined to optimize performance with the LC-MS system).

6. Negative ion mode LC-MS reconstitution solution: Stock solutions are combined in empirically determined ratios (from 1 to 12 ml) into a cocktail along with 0.3 volume equivalents of ammonium bicarbonate (6.5 mM, pH 8, in water). The stock is then further diluted 1:5 with an ammonium bicarbonate solution (6.5 mM, pH 8, in water).

2.2.4 Reconstitution Solution for Gas Chromatography Standardization

1. Stock solutions of even chain length 1-phenylalkanes (C6–C18), BHT, and amyl benzene (1 mg/ml in cyclohexane) are combined in equal volumes with 0.1 volume equivalents of cyclohexane into an amber vial.
2. GC/MS reconstitution solution: Dilute GC standard cocktail 1:10 with 5 % triethylamine in dichloromethane/acetonitrile/cyclohexane (5:4:1).

2.3 Equipment and Software

1. Tissue homogenizer (Geno/Grinder 2000) or equivalent energetic tissue disaggregation system (e.g., probe sonicator).
2. Analytical drying system (N2 blower or centrivap).
3. Benchtop centrifuge capable of 1,000 × *g*.
4. Waters Acquity Ultra Performance Liquid Chromatography System (UPLC) (Waters, Milford, MA) or equivalent liquid chromatography system.
5. Thermo-Finnegan LTQ linear ion trap mass spectrometer or equivalent mass spectrometer with tandem MS capability.
6. Thermo-Finnigan Trace DSQ fast-scanning single-quadrupole mass spectrometer or equivalent.
7. Gas Chromatograph column: 20 m × 0.18 mm with 0.18-μm film phase 5 % phenyldimethyl silicone.
8. Metabolyzer™ (Metabolon, Durham, NC) or equivalent metabolite identification software package.
9. Ingenuity Pathway Analysis (IPA, Ingenuity® Systems).

3 Methods

3.1 Tissue Collection

1. Collect tissues at the time of biopsy or autopsy and snap freeze them in liquid nitrogen. They can then be stored at −80 °C for long-term storage (*see* **Note 1**).
2. With the exception of an anticoagulant such as EDTA for the preparation of plasma from whole blood, no additives should be used.

3.2 Tissue Sample Selection

1. In order to assess the tumor type as well as stage and grade, each sample should be sectioned (6 μM), stained with H&E, and analyzed by a licensed pathologist. The samples should

contain at least 70 % tumor tissue. An official pathology report can be generated that shows non-identifying patient information such as race and age. Patient history is also provided on the pathology report along with cancer type and presence or absence of metastases either in the abdominal area resulting in omental masses or in the lymph nodes.

2. Sample criteria should be established to differentiate between primary carcinomas and metastatic carcinomas and a standard set for "normal" samples. For example, nonmetastatic carcinomas of Stage I through IIIC can be considered primary carcinomas. Tumor subtypes can range from papillary serous adenocarcinoma to mucinous adenocarcinoma to better understand the alterations that occur in a cancer versus normal tissue (*see* **Note 2**). Patient age should also be considered to best represent the average patient population.
3. Metastatic ovarian cancer samples were selected based on the criteria that metastasis had occurred. In all cases, the advanced stage of the carcinomas resulted in omental masses. These masses were selected for the study. The metastatic samples can also range in subtype from adenocarcinoma to endometrioid adenocarcinoma.
4. Normal tissues should be selected based on the absence of cancer. Patients can present with benign cysts. As this is considered a "normal" condition, they are not considered disqualified. Different patients should be selected for grouping into normal, primary ovarian cancer, and metastatic ovarian cancer. For example, a patient could present with unilateral primary ovarian cancer with the other ovary absent of cancer; however, this would disqualify the other ovary for inclusion in the normal group.

3.3 Sample Preparation

1. Approximately 100 mg of material is used for each sample. A sample can be comprised of a biologic fluid or cell culture supernatant (where 100 μl are used), a packed cell pellet (where ~10,000,000 cells are used), or a piece of tissue (*see* **Note 3**). Using a clean razor blade, small 100 mg samples can be cut from the tissue while it is still frozen. The sample should then be immediately transferred to cryogenic tube and kept on dry ice as biochemical transformations are relatively rapid (*see* **Note 4**).
2. When you are ready for analysis, thaw the samples on ice, add 4 volume equivalents (approximately 0.4 ml) of water, and disaggregate the tissues by bead mill homogenization (Geno/Grinder at 1,350 strokes per minute for 5 min, or equivalent) using stainless steel and zirconium beads to increase the solvent-exposed surface area for biochemical extraction. An aliquot of each homogenate (0.1 ml) is added to cold aqueous methanol (0.45 ml of 1:4 water to methanol), capped, and agitated (Geno/Grinder at 675 strokes per minute for 2 min).

3. Separate the supernatant from insoluble material by centrifugation (5′ at 1,000 × *g*) and split the sample into three aliquots (0.11 ml each).
4. Dry these aliquots under vacuum.

3.4 Mass Spectrometry

It is critical to analyze raw and interpreted metabolomics data with experienced bioanalytical chemists due to the technical complexity of LC-MS and GC-MS data. Process controls consisting of laboratory reagents only as well as pooled control samples can improve data interpretation by identifying spectral features that are process artifacts, contaminants, and environmental interferences (*see* **Note 5**).

For tissue samples in general, including ovarian tissues and tumors, between 200 and 400 endogenous biochemicals are detected using the sample preparation method described herein. Publically available spectra-matching tools such as the NIST database for GC-MS compounds are a good starting point for biochemical identification. University core facilities and biotechnology company approaches to metabolomics typically utilize a combination of publically accessible spectral libraries as well as proprietary libraries that are built around a specific technology platform.

Oncogenic transformation profoundly alters cellular metabolism. It is common to observe that >50 % of metabolites are differentially abundant between tumor tissue and the non-transformed tissue of origin. These differences reflect the differential energetic and anabolic demands of transformed cells as well as loss of tissue-specific biochemical functions.

3.4.1 UHPLC Analysis

1. Resuspend one aliquot (aliquot 1) in 50 μl of the reconstitution solution for positive ion mode LC-MS analysis. Separate 5 μL of aliquot 1 using a Waters Acquity UPLC using gradient elution at 350 μl/min (solvent A, 0.1 % formic acid in water; solvent B, 0.1 % formic acid in methanol; 0 % solvent B to 70 % solvent B in 4 min, 70 % solvent B to 98 % solvent B in 0.5 min, and 98 % solvent B for 0.9 min). This creates an acidic sample for the analysis of metabolites that form positive ions.
2. Resuspend a second aliquot (aliquot 2) in 50 μl of the reconstitution solution for negative ion mode LC-MS analysis. Separate 5 μl of aliquot 2 using a Waters Acquity UPLC using gradient elution at 350 μl/min (solvent A, ammonium bicarbonate (6.5 mM, pH 8) in water; solvent B, ammonium bicarbonate (6.5 mM, pH 8) in methanol/water (95/5), 0 % solvent B to 70 % solvent B in 4 min, 70 % solvent B to 98 % solvent B in 0.5 min, and 98 % solvent B for 0.9 min). This creates a basic sample for the analysis of metabolites that form negative ions.

3. Used a dedicated UPLC column (2.1 mm × 100 mm Waters BEH C18 1.7 μm) for each type of sample (acidic or basic). Maintain the columns at 40 °C.
4. Instrument settings should be established to measure positive ions in aliquot 1 and negative ions in aliquot 2 in independent injections using an LTQ mass spectrometer. Instrument settings were established for this work in [27].
   - MS interface capillary: 350 °C
   - Sheath gas flow: 40 (arbitrary units)
   - Auxiliary gas flow: 5 (arbitrary units)
   - Spray voltage: 4.5 kV (positive ion mode), 3.75 (negative ion mode)
   - Mass scanning range: 99–1,000 Da
   - Scan speed: 6/s, alternating parent MS and fragmentation (MS/MS) spectra
   - Ion trap target: 2 × 104 (MS); 1 × 104 (MS/MS)
   - Ion trap fill time cutoff: 200 ms (MS); 100 ms (MS/MS)
5. MS/MS parameters:
   - Normalized collision energy: 40
   - Activation Q: 0.25
   - Activation time: 30 ms
   - Isolation window: 3 m/z
   - Dynamic exclusion time: 3.5 s

3.4.2 GC-MS Analysis

1. Resuspend a third aliquot (aliquot 3) in reconstitution solution for GC-MS analysis and combine with derivatization solution (Fluka V, Sigma-Aldrich catalog number 15238) at 60 °C for 1 h.
2. Analyze aliquot 3 by GC/MS (Thermo-Finnigan Trace DSQ fast-scanning single-quadrupole MS) at unit mass resolving power. The GC column (20 m × 0.18 mm with 0.18-μm film phase 5 % phenyldimethyl silicone) is ramped from an initial oven temperature of 60–340 °C in a 16-min period. Helium is used as the carrier gas. The GC/MS is operated using electron impact ionization with a 50–750-amu scan range (*see* **Note 6**).

3.5 Analysis of MS Data

1. Contemporary high-resolution chromatography and fast and sensitive mass spectrometers routinely identifies 300–400 endogenous compounds in blood and tissue. These compounds come from all major biochemical classes: amino acids and their catabolites, carbohydrates and organic acids, lipids and membrane-related compounds, and nucleotides and cofactors (Fig. 1). With all of the process controls in place, the system

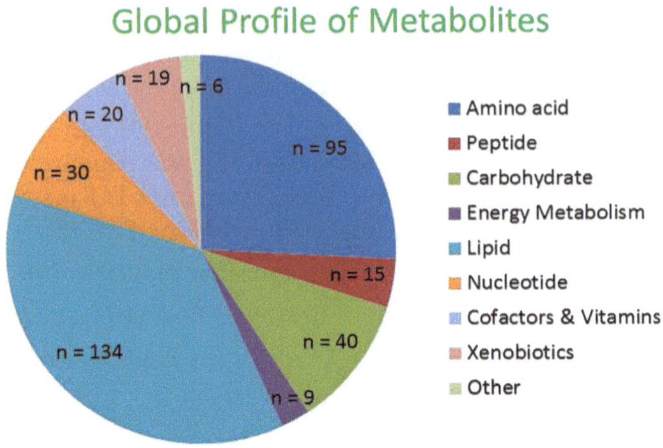

Fig. 1 Distribution of the compound classification for each molecule identified. *n* number of molecules in each class. Reproduced from ref. [29]

described above performs very reproducibly and the technical variability for all metabolites typically observed is 10–15 % (*see* **Note** 7).

2. Metabolite identification from massive libraries of mass spectra has required the development of novel data visualization and feature extraction software. One such suite of tools, Metabolyzer™, employs the rules outlined above: chromatogram and spectral alignments across a series of related samples [28]. Chromatogram alignment allows cross comparison of metabolite signals within a set of related samples which in turn improves the accuracy of metabolite identification and abundance estimation. Experimental mass spectra are compared against an in silico library of mass spectra that were generated by analyzing thousands of purified reference chemicals on the analytical platform (*see* **Note 8**). The relative abundance of each compound is calculated based on the intensity of one or more mass spectral features from each compound.

   The primary alternative approach to the library-based (chemocentric) analysis of metabolomic data has been an approach based on analysis of the raw data (ion-centric). In the ion-centric approach, high-dimensional data analysis techniques such as clustering and principal component analysis are typically used to discern trends in the data. The ion-centric approach has proved useful at describing general trends in groups of samples – generally separating metabolomic profiles of diseased from healthy tissues. However, as was found with raw spectra-based approaches to proteomics data analysis, the lack of analyte confirmation limits how the data can be used and raises the concern that any separation that tracks with groups may not be due to underlying biological differences between samples.

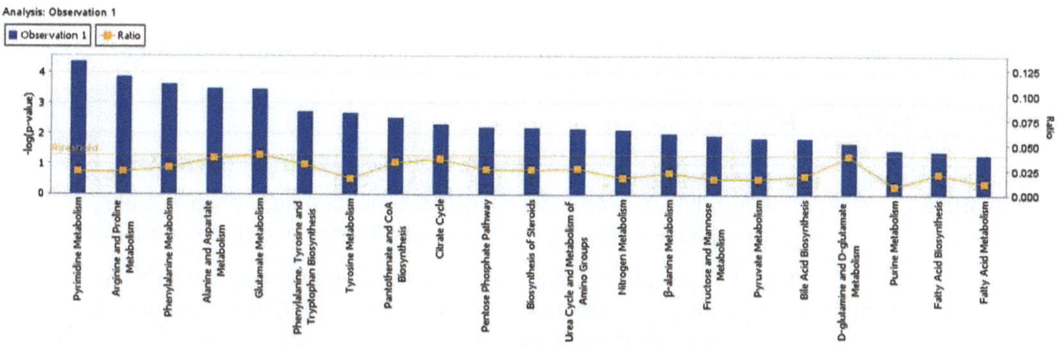

Fig. 2 Canonical pathway analysis generated using IPA software (abridged)

3. Software programs such as Ingenuity Pathway Analysis (IPA) can help you pinpoint metabolic network alterations. An Excel file without headers works well to import your data. However, unique molecule identifiers such as KEGG or HMDB are necessary for analysis as well as the fold change and p value for each compound. One of the features is a canonical pathway assembly. A representative sample can be found in Fig. 2. Based on this pathway, the metabolite interactions can be assembled (Table 1). For example, in the phenylalanine pathway, phenylalanine is converted to tyrosine by phenylalanine hydroxylase or phenylpyruvate by an aminotransferase (Fig. 3). A meticulous search of the literature can provide the metabolite conversions and the responsible enzymes.

4 Notes

1. Tissue samples can be procured from a tissue collection bank. If your local institute does not have a collection bank, there are several located around the country, including University of Alabama at Birmingham (UAB), MD Anderson Cancer Center, and the National Cancer Institute Cooperative Human Tissue Network. Most will provide tissues for a fee; however most universities preferentially select their own faculty as recipients.
2. Experimental design and sample preparation are crucial aspects of metabolomic studies. To understand ovarian cancer as a whole, different subtypes can be combined. However, serous adenocarcinomas are the most common subtype of ovarian cancer, so samples can be limited to one subtype.
3. In order to achieve the deepest coverage of the cancer metabolome, 100 mg of tissue is used and tumor tissues should be assessed histologically to ensure that they contained at least

Table 1
Top 15 canonical pathways listed in IPA for EOC versus normal with associated molecules

Canonical pathway	Molecules
Aminoacyl-tRNA biosynthesis	Glycine, L-alanine, L-aspartate, L-cysteine, L-glutamate, L-glutamine, L-histidine, L-isoleucine, L-leucine, L-methionine, L-phenylalanine, L-proline, L-serine, L-threonine, L-tryptophan, L-tyrosine, L-valine
Urea cycle and metabolism of amino groups	Citrulline, creatine, fumarate, L-aspartate, L-glutamate, L-ornithine, L-proline, *N*-(L-arginino)succinate, *N*-acetyl-L-glutamate, putrescine, sarcosine, spermidine, spermine
Arginine and proline metabolism	4-Guanidinobutanoic acid, 5-aminovaleric acid, citrulline, creatine, fumarate, GABA, L-aspartate, L-glutamate, L-ornithine, L-proline, *N*-(L-ARGININO)succinate, *N*-acetylputrescine, putrescine, pyruvate, spermidine, spermine, trans-4-hydroxy-L-proline
Glycine, serine, and threonine metabolism	Betaine, choline, creatine, D-glycerate, dimethylglycine, glycine, L-aspartate, L-cysteine, L-serine, L-threonine, phosphorylcholine, phosphorylethanolamine, pyruvate, sarcosine
Alanine and aspartate metabolism	2-Oxoglutarate, β-alanine, citrate, fumarate, L-alanine, L-asparagine, L-aspartate, N-(L-arginino)succinate, N-acetyl-L-aspartate (NAA), pyruvate, succinate
Glutamate metabolism	2-Oxoglutarate, citrate, fumarate, GABA, glutathione, glutathione disulfide, L-glutamate, L-glutamine, *N*-acetyl-D-glucosamine 6-phosphate, succinate
Nitrogen metabolism	AMP, glycine, L-asparagine, L-aspartate, L-glutamate, L-glutamine, L-histidine, L-phenylalanine, L-tryptophan, L-tyrosine
β-alanine metabolism	β-alanine, dihydrouracil, GABA, L-aspartate, L-histidine, quinolinate, spermidine, spermine, uracil
Valine, leucine, and isoleucine biosynthesis	(3S)3-Methyl-2-oxopentanoate, α-ketoisocaproic acid, L-isoleucine, L-leucine, L-valine, pyruvate
Phenylalanine, tyrosine, and tryptophan biosynthesis	L-histidine, L-phenylalanine, L-tryptophan, L-tyrosine, phenylpyruvate, phosphoenolpyruvate
Methionine metabolism	L-cysteine, L-methionine, L-serine, *N*-formylmethionine, *O*-succinylhomoserine, ribose, *S*-adenosylhomocysteine
Phenylalanine metabolism	4-Hydroxylphenylacetate, fumarate, L-phenylalanine, phenyllactate (PLA), phenylpyruvate, pyruvate, succinate
Cyanoamino metabolism	glycine, L-asparagine, L-aspartate, L-cysteine, L-glutamate, L-serine
Pantothenate and CoA biosynthesis	β-alanine, dihydrouracil, L-cystine, L-valine, pyruvate, uracil
Cysteine metabolism	3-sulfino-L-alanine, glutathione, L-alanine, L-cysteine, L-cystine, L-serine, pyruvate

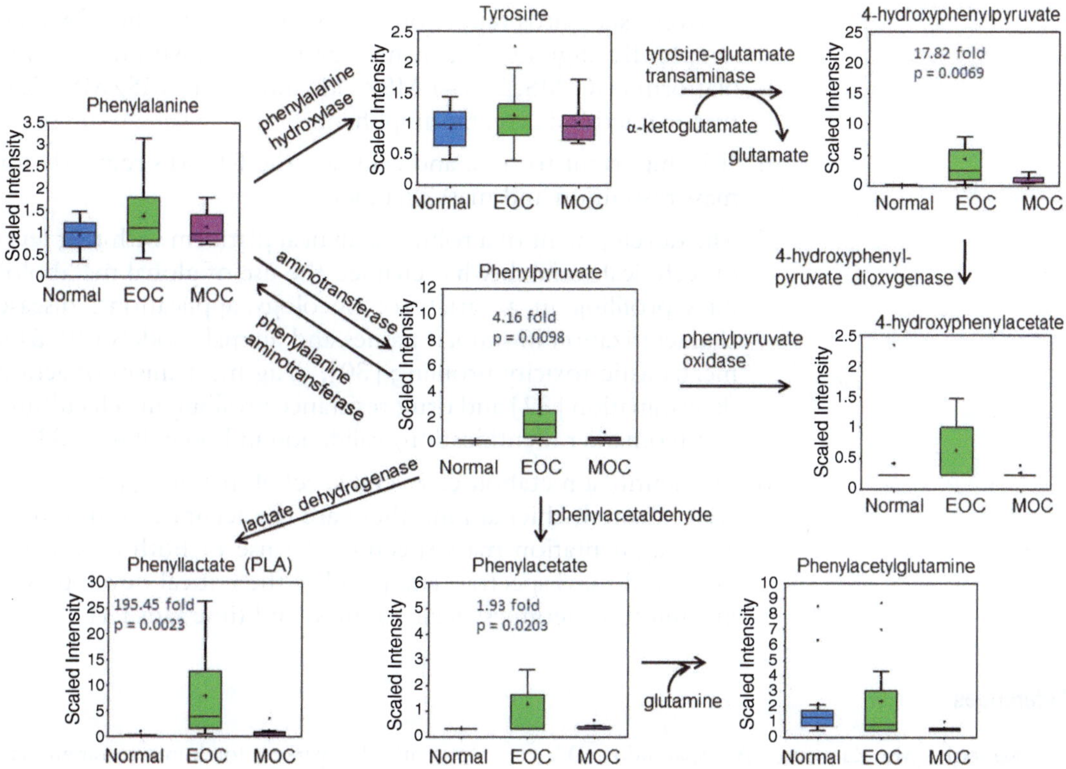

Fig. 3 Phenylalanine metabolic network with associated enzymes. Phenylalanine and tyrosine analyzed by LC/MS pos.; phenylpyruvate, phenyl acetate, phenylacetylglutamine, phenyllactate, and 4-hydroxyphenylpyruvate via LC/MS negative ion spray; 4-hydroxyphenylacetate via GC/MS. *Box legend*: + inside box represents mean value, *bar* inside box represents median value, *upper bar* represents maximum of distribution, *lower bar* represents minimum of distribution, and *circle* represents extreme data points (Reproduced from ref. [29])

70 % transformed tissue. Recent technology developments have reduced the amount of tissue required to generate a high-quality metabolomic signature while leaving tissue intact. This new technique allows parallel histopathology and metabolomic characterization of as little as 3 mg of tissue, approximately the size of a core needle biopsy. Using this approach, one simply transfers the core needle biopsies directly into a methanol solution (1.6 ml of 4:1 methanol to water) for 12 h. The tissue is then removed from the solution and can be processed for histologic assessment, including formalin fixation and paraffin embedding. The methanol solution then contains the extracted metabolites from the system and can be prepared for GC-MS and LC-MS/MS analysis.

4. Dry ice is extremely cold, −78.5 °C. Protective gloves should be used during handling to prevent burns.

5. The internal standards serve as mile posts to standardize each chromatography run for chromatogram alignment while the

recovery standards report on the extraction efficiency for each sample. By aligning all chromatography runs within the same platform (GC-MS, LC(−)-MS/MS, and LC(+)-MS/MS), feature extraction is greatly simplified.

6. It is important to tune and calibrate the GC-MS regularly for mass resolution and mass accuracy.
7. The development of a robust analytical platform with that level of technical variability has enabled the use of global metabolomics profiling in a variety of oncology applications: disease characterization in human tissues and animal models [29–31], mechanistic toxicity profiling [30], drug mechanism of action determination [32] and drug resistance profiling in cell culture, and biomarker identification/validation in bodily fluids [33].
8. To identify a metabolite, several spectral matching parameters are evaluated; chief among them are the accurate elution time and fragmentation mass spectra. The use of both chromatogram and mass spectral data parallels the critical development in clinical proteomics: accurate mass and time tags [34].

References

1. Koutsaki M, Zaravinos A, Spandidos DA (2012) Modern trends into the epidemiology and screening of ovarian cancer. Genetic substrate of the sporadic form. Pathol Oncol Res 18(2):135–148
2. Cass I, Karlan BY (2010) Ovarian cancer symptoms speak out – but what are they really saying? J Natl Cancer Inst 102:211–212
3. National Cancer Institute Stat Fact Sheet. http://seer.cancer.gov/statfacts/html/ovary.html
4. Nossov V, Amneus M, Su F, Lang J, Janco J et al (2008) The early detection of ovarian cancer: from traditional methods to proteomics. Can we really do better than serum CA-125? Am J Obstet Gynecol 199:215–223
5. Neesham D (2007) Ovarian cancer screening. Aust Fam Physician 36:126–128
6. Cesario S (2010) Advances in the early detection of ovarian cancer: how to hear the whispers early. Nurs Womens Health 14:222–234
7. Bhosale P, Peungjesada S, Wei W, Levenback CF, Schmeler K et al (2010) Clinical utility of positron emission tomography/computed tomography in the evaluation of suspected recurrent ovarian cancer in the setting of normal CA-125 levels. Int J Gynecol Cancer 20:936–944
8. Lin B, White JT, Wu J, Lele S, Old LJ et al (2009) Deep depletion of abundant serum proteins reveals low-abundant proteins as potential biomarkers for human ovarian cancer. Proteomics Clin Appl 3:853–861
9. Zhen H, Yang S, Wu H, Wang S, Lv J et al (2010) LyGDI is a promising biomarker for ovarian cancer. Int J Gynecol Cancer 20: 316–322
10. Kothandaraman N, Bajic VB, Brendan PN, Huak CY, Keow PB et al (2010) E2F5 status significantly improves malignancy diagnosis of epithelial ovarian cancer. BMC Cancer 10:64
11. Hellstrom I, Hellstrom K (2008) SMRP and HE4 as biomarkers for ovarian carcinoma when used alone and in combination with CA125 and/or each other. Adv Exp Med Biol 622:15–21
12. Lowe K, Shah C, Wallace E, Anderson G, Paley P et al (2008) Effects of personal characteristics of serum CA125, mesothelin, and HE4 levels in healthy postmenopausal women at high-risk for ovarian cancer. Cancer Epidemiol Biomarkers Prev 17:5480–5487
13. Nolen B, Velikokhatnaya L, Marrangoni A, De Geest K, Lomakin A et al (2010) Serum biomarker panels for the discrimination of benign from malignant cases in patients with an adnexal mass. Gynecol Oncol 117:440–445
14. Zagouri F, Dimopoulos MA, Bournakis E, Papadimitriou CA (2010) Molecular markers in epithelial ovarian cancer: their role in prognosis and therapy. Eur J Gynaecol Oncol 31:268–277

15. Warburg O (1956) On the origin of cancer cells. Science 123:309–314
16. Levine AJ, Puzio-Kuter AM (2010) The control of the metabolic switch in cancers by oncogenes and tumor suppressor genes. Science 330:1340–1344
17. Rous P, Robertson OH, Oliver J (1919) Experiments on the production of specific antisera for infections of unknown cause : I. Type experiments with known antigens-a bacterial hemotoxin (megatheriolysin), the pneumococcus, and poliomyelitic virus. J Exp Med 29:283–304
18. Cori CF, Cori GT (1925) The carbohydrate metabolism of tumors. J Biol Chem 65: 397–405
19. Friis RR, Schwarz RT, Schmidt MF (1977) Phenotypes of Rous sarcoma virus-transformed fibroblasts: an argument for a multifunctional Src gene product. Med Microbiol Immunol 164:155–165
20. Elstrom RL, Bauer DE, Buzzai M, Karnauskas R, Harris MH et al (2004) Akt stimulates aerobic glycolysis in cancer cells. Cancer Res 64:3892–3899
21. Kim JW, Tchernyshyov I, Semenza GL, Dang CV (2006) HIF-1-mediated expression of pyruvate dehydrogenase kinase: a metabolic switch required for cellular adaptation to hypoxia. Cell Metab 3:177–185
22. Rimpi S, Nilsson JA (2007) Metabolic enzymes regulated by the Myc oncogene are possible targets for chemotherapy or chemoprevention. Biochem Soc Trans 35:305–310
23. Mazurek S, Boschek CB, Hugo F, Eigenbrodt E (2005) Pyruvate kinase type M2 and its role in tumor growth and spreading. Semin Cancer Biol 15:300–308
24. Mazurek S, Eigenbrodt E (2003) The tumor metabolome. Anticancer Res 23:1149–1154
25. Vander Heiden MG, Locasale JW, Swanson KD, Sharfi H, Heffron GJ et al (2010) Evidence for an alternative glycolytic pathway in rapidly proliferating cells. Science 329:1492–1499
26. Spratlin JL, Serkova NJ, Eckhardt SG (2009) Clinical applications of metabolomics in oncology: a review. Clin Cancer Res 15: 431–440
27. Evans AM, DeHaven CD, Barrett T, Mitchell M, Milgram E (2009) Integrated, nontargeted ultrahigh performance liquid chromatography/electrospray ionization tandem mass spectrometry platform for the identification and relative quantification of the small-molecule complement of biological systems. Anal Chem 81:6656–6667
28. Dehaven CD, Evans AM, Dai H, Lawton KA (2010) Organization of GC/MS and LC/MS metabolomics data into chemical libraries. J Cheminform 2:9
29. Fong MY, McDunn J, Kakar SS (2011) Identification of metabolites in the normal ovary and their transformation in primary and metastatic ovarian cancer. PLoS One 6:e19963
30. Parman T, Bunin DI, Ng HH, McDunn JE, Wulff JE et al (2011) Toxicogenomics and metabolomics of pentamethylchromanol (PMCol)-induced hepatotoxicity. Toxicol Sci 124:487–501
31. Sreekumar A, Poisson LM, Rajendiran TM, Khan AP, Cao Q et al (2009) Metabolomic profiles delineate potential role for sarcosine in prostate cancer progression. Nature 457:910–914
32. Watson M, Roulston A, Belec L, Billot X, Marcellus R et al (2009) The small molecule GMX1778 is a potent inhibitor of NAD+ biosynthesis: strategy for enhanced therapy in nicotinic acid phosphoribosyltransferase 1-deficient tumors. Mol Cell Biol 29: 5872–5888
33. Ganti S, Weiss RH (2011) Urine metabolomics for kidney cancer detection and biomarker discovery. Urol Oncol 29:551–557
34. Conrads TP, Anderson GA, Veenstra TD, Pasa-Tolic L, Smith RD (2000) Utility of accurate mass tags for proteome-wide protein identification. Anal Chem 72:3349–3354

Chapter 19

Choline Metabolic Profiling by Magnetic Resonance Spectroscopy

Egidio Iorio, Alessandro Ricci, Maria Elena Pisanu, Marina Bagnoli, Franca Podo, and Silvana Canevari

Abstract

The revised version of cancer hallmarks, depicting the biological properties acquired during tumor development and progression, includes the capability to modify or reprogram cellular metabolism. High-resolution multinuclear magnetic resonance spectroscopy (MRS) provides noninvasive means of monitoring metabolites that play a central role in several pathways, measuring the rates at which reactions within the pathways take place, and investigating how these rates are controlled in such a way that a metabolic precursor and cofactors are provided according to the demand. Here we describe comprehensive methods for assaying the activity of key enzymes involved in the phosphatidylcholine metabolic pathways responsible for phosphocholine accumulation in ovarian cancer cells using high-resolution ^{1}H and ^{31}P MRS analyses of cell lysates or cytosolic preparations.

Key words Phosphatidylcholine metabolism, Choline kinase, Phospholipases C and D specific for phosphatidylcholine, Glycerophosphocholine phosphodiesterase, Magnetic resonance spectroscopy

1 Introduction

Ovarian cancer is a heterogeneous disease, but shares with the majority of solid and hematologic tumors a variety of dysregulated molecular events as outlined in the seminal classification of cancer hallmarks by Hanahan and Weinberg [1]. Subsequent accumulated evidences brought to a revised version of cancer hallmarks with the inclusion of further alterations characteristic of tumor oncogenesis and progression, such as changes in the mechanisms controlling cell bioenergetics [2, 3]. Major metabolic hallmarks of cancer cells are the well-known enhanced glucose uptake and increased metabolic fluxes through glycolysis compared with the Krebs cycle [4], as well as the more recently characterized aberrant choline phospholipid metabolism [5–8].

Anastasia Malek and Oleg Tchernitsa (eds.), *Ovarian Cancer: Methods and Protocols*, Methods in Molecular Biology, vol. 1049,
DOI 10.1007/978-1-62703-547-7_19,

At present, the evaluation of metabolic alterations mainly relies on gas chromatography, liquid chromatography-mass spectrometry (LC-MS/MS), and high-resolution multinuclear magnetic resonance spectroscopy (MRS). In the last 20 years MRS has been extensively used to investigate biochemical pathways in intact tissues and in their extracts in living systems ([9–13] and references therein).

An interesting aspect of MRS is the ability to noninvasively and simultaneously monitor various small molecules of biological importance present in cells and tissues and to highlight details of the cellular biochemistry that otherwise could not be easily detected with usual classical biochemical techniques, which include complex and potentially destructive procedures for separation and purification. Thus, MRS provides noninvasive means of monitoring metabolites that play central role in several pathways, measuring the rates at which reactions within the pathways take place in vivo, and investigating how these rates are controlled in such a way that a given metabolic precursor and its cofactors are provided according to the demand.

The technological developments of MRS methods and the use of different nonradioactive isotopes such as ^{1}H, ^{31}P, ^{13}C allowed quantitative measurements of basal levels of some metabolites in tissues of healthy subjects and detection of alterations in biochemical pathways and physiological parameters relevant to cell bioenergetics and metabolism of phospholipids, neutral lipids, amino acids, and osmolytes, as well as to the monitoring of drug uptake and kinetics, in cancer cells and extracts. Some major applications of MRS of these nuclei are summarized in Table 1.

The proton (^{1}H) is endowed with the highest NMR sensitivity and its spectra can therefore reach the highest signal-to-noise ratio levels. The protons of water generate a strong signal that is exploited in MRI, while the proton signals from other compounds are increasingly used for metabolic studies. Another nucleus that has been used most extensively for metabolic studies is ^{31}P, which is the naturally occurring phosphorus isotope. Although ^{31}P is less sensitive than ^{1}H MRS, its chemical shift range is larger, and ^{31}P MRS does not require the application of pulse sequences for strong solvent signal suppression. The ^{13}C isotope has a natural abundance of only 1.1 % and has a much lower intrinsic NMR sensitivity than ^{1}H. Therefore, in the absence of isotopic enrichment, ^{13}C signals of biological molecules are very weak. ^{13}C-labelling can be particularly useful for investigations on specific metabolic pathways such as glycolysis and choline metabolism.

MRS profiles greatly contributed since the 1990s to identify the characteristics of an altered choline phospholipid metabolism in cancer cells and tissues as a potential source of novel indicators of tumor progression and response to therapy [5–8]. At the same time, high-resolution MRS methods allowed the detection of steady-state

Table 1
Summary of the major utilized nuclei to monitor cancer cell metabolism by MRS signals

Isotope	Resonance frequency at 2.35 T (MHz)	Sensitivity relative to ^{1}H	Monitoring of metabolite levels/fluxes and physiological parameters
^{1}H	100	100	Choline phospholipid metabolism Glycolysis and products (lactate, alanine) Cr and PCr Neutral lipids metabolism (mobile lipids) Amino acids (including taurine) Inositols Tissue-specific metabolites (citrate and polyamines in prostate; *N*-acetyl aspartate in neuronal cells) Glutamine and glutamate pH (intra- and extracellular)
^{31}P	40.5	6.6	Bioenergetics (NTP, NDP, AMP, PCr, sugar phosphates, NAD^{+}) Phospholipid metabolism (PME, PDE, DPDE) Pi and pH (intra- and extracellular)
^{13}C	25.1	1.6	Flux of metabolites in biochemical pathways (glycolysis, tricarboxylic acid cycle, derivatives of phospholipid metabolism) Structure of carbohydrates

Cr Creatine, *PCr* phosphocreatine, *PME* phosphomonoesters, *PDE* phosphodiesters, *DPDE* diphosphodiesters, *NTP* nucleotide triphosphate, *NDP* nucleotide diphosphate, *AMP* adenosine-monophosphate, *Pi* inorganic phosphate

levels and fluxes of metabolites in the pathways responsible for biosynthesis and catabolism of phosphatidylcholine (PtdCho), the major phospholipid of eukaryotic cell membranes [7, 8].

Changes in the ^{1}H MRS spectral profile comprising the trimethylammonium headgroup signals of choline-containing metabolites (collectively called "total choline" or tCho resonance, centered at 3.2 ppm) reflect the altered contents and metabolic fluxes of phosphocholine (PCho), glycerophosphocholine (GPCho), and free choline (Cho) through the biosynthetic and catabolic pathways of the PtdCho-cycle (Fig. 1). In particular, an elevation of the in vivo tCho resonance is reported as a common hallmark of a large variety of cancers. Our group was the first to characterize the substantially modified ^{1}H MRS tCho spectral profile of aqueous extracts of ovarian cancer epithelial cells compared with those of non-tumoral counterparts (examples in Fig. 2) and to explore the underlying biochemical mechanisms [14, 15]. The observed increase in tCho reported in the progression from normal to cancer cells was mainly due to a substantial increase in PCho. This metabolite is either produced by choline

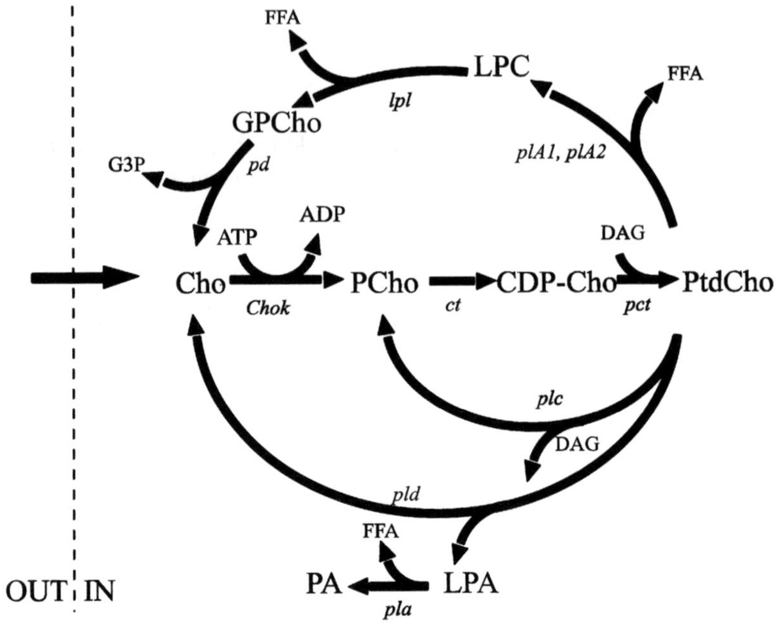

Fig. 1 Schematic representation of phosphatidylcholine (PtdCho) de novo biosynthesis and catabolism. Metabolites: *CDP-Cho* cytidine diphosphate choline, *Cho* choline, *DAG* diacylglycerol, *FFA* free fatty acid, *G3P sn*-glycerol-3-phosphate, *GPCho* glycerophosphocholine, *LPA* lysophosphatidate, *LPC* lysophosphatidylcholine, *PA* phosphatidate, *PCho* phosphocholine. Enzymes: *Chok* choline kinase (EC 2.7.1.32), *ct* cytidylyltransferase (EC 2.7.7.15), *lpl* lysophospholipase (EC 3.1.1.5), *pct* phosphocholine transferase (EC 2.7.8.2), *pd* glycerophosphocholine phosphodiesterase (EC 3.1.4.2), *pla* phospholipase A_2 (EC 3.1.1.4), and phospholipase A_1 (EC 3.1.1.32), *plc* phospholipase C (EC 3.1.4.3), *pld* phospholipase D (EC 3.1.4.4). *OUT* extracellular medium, *IN* intracellular medium

kinase (Chok) in the first reaction of the three-step biosynthetic Kennedy pathway or via phospholipase C (plc)-mediated PtdCho catabolism or by the combined action of PtdCho-specific phospholipase D (pld) and Chok. Moreover GPCho, the product of complete PtdCho deacylation, can be hydrolyzed by a specific phosphodiesterase (GPCho-pd) into glycerophosphate and choline, providing a further source of substrate to the Kennedy pathway to form PCho (Fig. 1). Through its multiple mechanisms of hydrolysis PtdCho can also generate second messengers and mitogens such as diacylglycerol (DAG), phosphatidate (PA), and lysophosphatidate (LPA) (Fig. 1). Thus, the altered level of a choline metabolite such as PCho in ovarian cancer cells results from changes in the activity of a number of different enzymes involved in both synthetic and catabolic pathways of the PtdCho-cycle, which in turn produces mitogens and second messengers under the action of a network of oncogene-driven cell signaling pathways [7, 15].

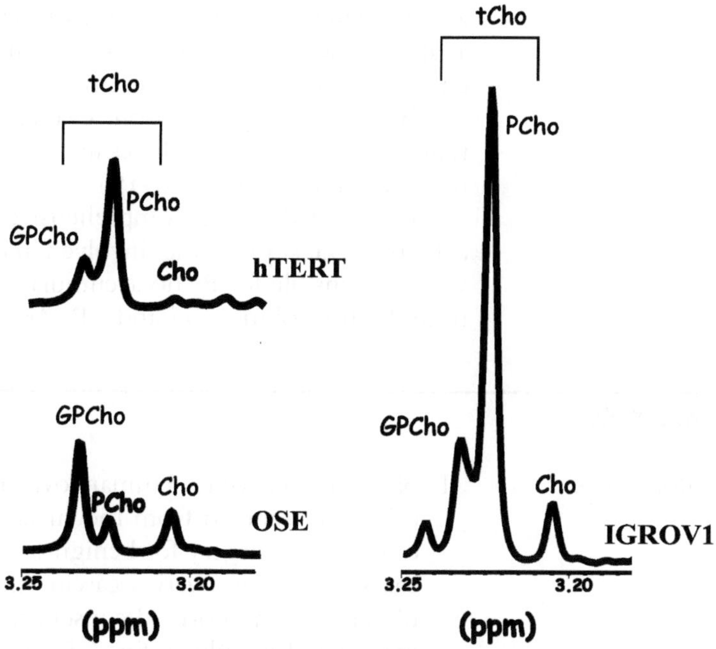

Fig. 2 Representative partial ^{1}H MRS spectra of aqueous extracts of ovary epithelial nontumor and tumor cells. Expanded ^{1}H MR spectral profiles (700 MHz) of tCho of normal ovary surface epithelial (OSE) cells, and non-tumoral immortalized hTERT cells and an ovarian carcinoma cell line (IGROV1). *Cho* choline, *GPCho* glycerophosphocholine, *PCho* phosphocholine, *tCho* total choline containing metabolites (GPCho+PCho+Cho)

Several other methods, based on the use of radiolabelled precursors and/or fluorescent dyes, have been applied to investigate the PtdCho metabolism in cancer cells. Compared to these methods, MRS has the advantages of not requiring procedures for separation and purification of metabolites, and avoiding the use of radioisotope substrates and the artifacts due to quenching of fluorescent probes.

The major limit of MRS is its low intrinsic sensitivity. Since the quality of measurements depends upon achieving an adequate signal-to-noise ratio, even ^{1}H MRS experiments may require long acquisition times with a metabolite detectability threshold which can hardly be lower than about 200 μM. While the sensitivity continues to be a limiting factor for multinuclear MRS techniques, the use of ultrahigh magnetic field strengths and emerging techniques such as dynamic nuclear polarization (DNP) are providing advances that reduce these limitations.

A peculiar advantage of MRS is the high spectral resolution and the possibility to simultaneously detect and quantify the consumption of an exogenously added substrate along with the product(s) formation. Thus, it is possible not only to measure the basal levels of intracellular metabolites present in the sample but also to determine the activities of key enzymes involved in the analyzed metabolic pathway(s). In this way, the MRS approach enables simultaneous measurements of different enzyme activities on the same cell preparation, evaluating in a snapshot the rearrangement of metabolic fluxes under different experimental conditions (examples in refs. 16–19).

Here we describe comprehensive methods for assaying the activity of the key enzymes involved in the PtdCho metabolic pathways responsible for PCho accumulation in ovarian cancer cells by using high-resolution ^{1}H and ^{31}P MRS in cell lysates.

2 Materials

2.1 Cell Culture

1. Non-tumoral cells: Human ovarian surface epithelial (OSE) cells were scraped from the surface of normal human ovaries obtained at surgery for benign or malignant gynecological diseases other than ovarian carcinoma. All human materials were obtained with informed consent from patients. OSE cells were maintained in culture for 3–5 passages in a 1:1 (v/v) ratio of MCDB-105 and M-199 culture media supplemented with 15 % fetal calf serum and their origin confirmed by immunohistochemical assay for expression of cytokeratin 8/18 and vimentin. Lifespan of short-term cultures of OSE cells was increased up to 15–16 passages by simian virus 40 (SV40) large T antigen transfection, thus obtaining IOSE cells. Stably immortalized IOSE cells were obtained by transfection with the cDNA of the catalytic subunit of the human telomerase reverse transcriptase (kindly provided by Dr. R. A. Weinberg, Whitehead Institute, Cambridge, MA), thus obtaining hTERT cells.
2. Ovarian cancer cell lines: IGROV1 cells were kindly provided by J. Bénard, Institute Gustave Roussy, Villejuif, France; OVCAR3 and SKOV3 cells were obtained from the American Type Culture Collection.
3. MCDB-105/M-199 Complete Medium: 450 mL of MCBD-105/M-199 medium, 15 % fetal bovine serum (FBS), 5 mL of 100 μg/mL gentamycin. Store medium at 4 °C and warm to 37 °C prior to use.
4. Roswell Park Memorial Institute-1640 (RPMI), 10 % FBS, 5 mL of 100× penicillin/streptomycin. Store medium at 4 °C and warm to 37 °C prior to use.
5. FBS. Dispense into 50 mL aliquots and store at −20 °C. Thaw before adding to culture medium.
6. Phosphate-buffered saline buffer (PBS): 137 mM NaCl, 2.7 mM KCl, 10 mM $Na_2HPO_4 \cdot 2\ H_2O$, 2 mM KH_2PO_4, pH 7.4. Sterilize by autoclaving.
7. Trypsin–EDTA solution: 0.05 % trypsin-0.02 % EDTA.

2.2 Buffers

Prepare all solutions using ultrapure water (prepared by purifying deionized water to attain a resistivity of 18 MΩ cm at 25 °C) and analytic grade reagents. Prepare buffers immediately before use.

1. Choline kinase buffer: 100 mM Tris–HCl, 10 mM dithiothreitol, 1 mM EDTA in H_2O, pH 8.0.
2. PtdCho-phospholipases buffer: DMG 50 mM, pH 7.4.

2.3 Chemicals

1. Adenosine 5′-triphosphate disodium salt solution (ATP).
2. Alkaline phosphatase (AP).
3. Choline chloride.
4. Deuterium oxide.
5. 1,2-Dihexanoyl-*sn*-glycero-3-phosphocholine (C6PtdCho).
6. Dimethylglutarate (DMG).
7. Dithiothreitol.
8. Ethylenediaminetetraacetic acid (EDTA).
9. l-α-Glycerophosphorylcholine.
10. Magnesium chloride.
11. Methylenediphosphonic acid.
12. Orthophosphoric acid.
13. Trimethylsilylpropionic-2,2,3,3-d4 acid sodium salt (TSP).
14. Tris(hydroxymethyl)aminomethane (Tris–HCl).

2.4 Equipment, Suppliers, and Software

1. Laminar flow bench hood and cell culture incubator.
2. Ultrasonic disintegrator.
3. Vacuum concentrator with refrigerated trap.
4. Potter-homogenizer for gentle sample disruption.
5. Centrifuge with capability to reach 20,000 × *g* at 4 °C.
6. High-resolution NMR spectrometer.

3 Methods

The here reported quantitative NMR experimental assays allowing elucidation of the aberrant PtdCho metabolism in ovarian cancer are performed at 9.4 T (Bruker AVANCE spectrometer). The individual steps necessary to perform these assays are described in this section in a schematic way so that these experiments can be adapted to different magnetic fields, regardless of the spectrometer and probes used in different laboratories.

The assays are divided into three major sections: Subheading 3.1, in which the intracellular content of soluble Cho-containing metabolites were determined; Subheading 3.2, in which Cho is exogenously added to cell lysates to measure the Chok enzymatic activity; Subheading 3.3.1, in which a short PtdCho (C6PtdCho) is exogenously added to cell lysates to measure the PtdCho-specific plc and pld enzymatic activities; Subheading 3.3.2, in which GPCho is exogenously added to cell lysates to measure the enzyme activity of GPCho-pd.

3.1 Determination of Soluble Choline-Containing Metabolites Levels in Aqueous Cell Extracts

This method allows a precise identification of the ^{1}H MRS spectral profiles in the 3.20–3.24 ppm region typical of trimethylammonium headgroups of PtdCho precursors and catabolites, as fingerprints of a specific physiopathological state of the cell/tissue analyzed.

1. Recover cells by trypsinization of culture when they reach 60–70 % confluence (*see* **Note 1**) and 24 h after culture medium change; count cells, and assess viability (should be more than 80–90 %) and membrane integrity by Trypan blue staining.
2. Wash cells twice with ice-cold physiological saline solution and resuspend pellets in 0.5 mL of ice-cold twice-distilled water.
3. Prepare cell extracts by adding 10 volumes of ethanolic solution (EtOH:H_2O, 77:23, v/v) and sonicate samples at 20 kHz by an ultrasonic disintegrator, e.g. MK2, Mk2 (exponential probe, 8 μm peak-to-peak) and centrifuge at 14,000 × *g* for 30 min (*see* **Note 2**).
4. Lyophilize supernatants twice in a RVT 4104 Savant lyophilizer, and resuspend the residue in 700 μL D_2O containing 0.1 mM 3-(trimethylsilyl)-propionic-2,2,3,3-d4 acid sodium salt (TSP) as internal standard.
5. Carry out ^{1}H MRS analyses of cell extracts using a 60° flip angle pulse, preceded by 2.00 s presaturation for water signal suppression (interpulse delay 2.00 s, acquisition time 1.70 s, spectral width 12 ppm, 16,000 data points).
6. Perform ^{31}P MRS analyses of cell extracts at 161.97 MHz using a 60° flip angle, acquisition time 0.81 s, interpulse delay 2.5 s, 4,000 transients. Determine metabolite concentrations by measuring signal areas with respect to methylendiphosphonic acid (added as internal reference). Determine correction factors to compensate for partial magnetic saturation and nuclear Overhauser effect in each set of experiments for the signals of interest by comparing the measured peak areas with those obtained at equilibrium (flip angle 90°, interpulse delay 40 s) without interpulse irradiation of coupled protons. Chemical shifts are referenced to external 85 % orthophosphoric acid [16, 17].

7. Determine metabolite concentrations (C(m)) by measuring the area (integral) of the signals of the corresponding metabolite chemical groups (I(mcg)), normalized to the number of cells and refer to the concentration of the reference standard (C(r)). Furthermore, refer each integral to the number of equivalent protons in the metabolite chemical group (N(mcg)) and in the reference standard molecule (N(r)), and apply the equation:

$$C(m) = [I(mcg)] / [I(r)] \times [N(r)] / [N(mcg)] \times [C(r)].$$

8. Measure substrate and product concentrations in MRS assays from the areas of the corresponding NMR signals corrected for the respective factors of partial saturation of the magnetization vector (*see* **Note 3**).

3.2 Choline Kinase Activity

This method allows quantification of Chok activity in aqueous extracts or directly in cell lysates in the NMR tube by evaluating the substrate and product concentrations by measuring the areas of the corresponding ^1H MRS signals.

1. Obtain cytosolic preparations from cell pellets (40×10^6 cells) homogenized in a Potter-homogenizer in the presence of 4 vol of 100 mM Tris–HCl, pH 8.0, containing 10 mM dithiothreitol and 1 mM EDTA in D_2O.
2. Disrupt the homogenate by ultrasonication, remove the particulate fraction by centrifugation at 20,000×*g* for 30 min at 4 °C by microfuge centrifuge, and introduce the supernatant (cytosolic preparation) in the NMR tube.
3. Add to the cytosolic preparation choline chloride, ATP and Mg^{2+} ions in Tris–HCl buffer (to final concentrations of 5 mM Cho, 10 mM ATP, and 10 mM $MgCl_2$) at 25 °C.
4. Perform the reaction in excess of substrate ([14, 15] and references therein) and simultaneously measure substrate and product concentrations from the areas of the corresponding NMR signals (corrected for the respective factors of partial saturation of the magnetization vector) in the linear portion (10–60 min, correlation coefficient R^2 between 0.97 and 0.99) of the curve representing the time course of PCho production (a representative example is reported in Fig. 3) (*see* **Note 4**).
5. Confirm absolute PCho quantification by MRS analyses of ethanolic extracts of the reaction mixtures at the end of the experiment [14].
6. Alternative procedures are discussed in **Notes 5** and **6**.

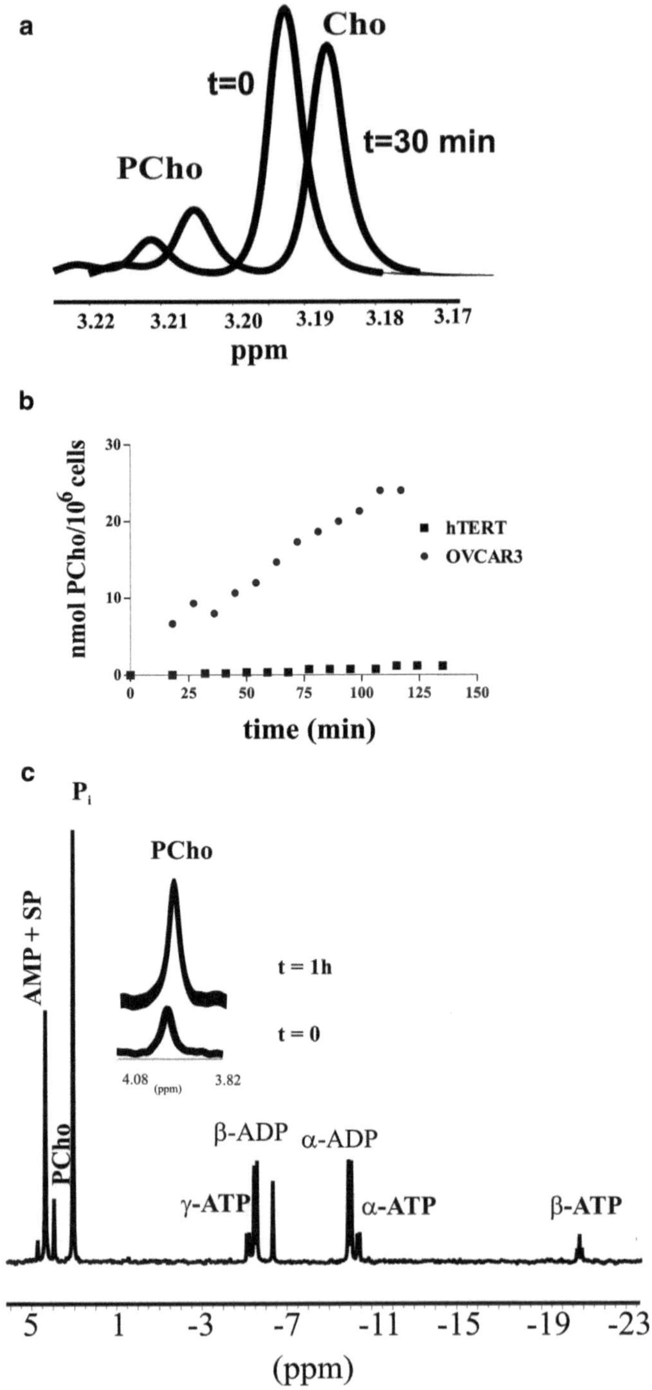

Fig. 3 Basal activity rates of Chok-mediated PCho production. (**a**) Representative ^{1}H MRS Chok assay performed on cell cytosolic preparations by measuring the increase in MRS PCho signal area at different times after addition of exogenous Cho, ATP, and $MgCl_2$, pH 8.0. (**b**) Time course of net PCho production in representative experiments using hTERT and epithelial ovarian carcinoma (EOC) samples. (**c**) ^{31}P MRS spectrum of cell extracts at time $t=0$. ^{31}P MRS analyses allow

3.3 PtdCho-Specific Phospholipases and GPCho-pd Activities

3.3.1 PtdCho-Specific Phospholipases

The activities of PtdCho-specific plc and pld are determined by measuring the Cho NMR signal either on fresh lysates in the NMR tube or on cell extracts obtained at different time points (generally 15, 30, 45, 60 min) to simulate kinetic reaction in NMR tubes. In particular, Cho formation is measured by ^{1}H MRS as product of the following catabolic pathways (*see* Fig. 4a, b for a representation of the overall reactions' scheme):
pld-mediated C6PtdCho hydrolysis.

(a) $$\text{C6PtdCho} \xrightarrow{\text{pld}} \text{Cho}$$

and

phosphodiesterase (pd)-mediated hydrolysis of GPCho formed by the combined action on C6PtdCho of pla (plA1 and plA2) and lysophospholipases (lpl).

(b) $$\text{C6PtdCho} \xrightarrow{\text{pla}} \text{lysoC6PtdCho} \xrightarrow{\text{lpl}} \text{GPCho}$$

plus

(c) $$\text{GPCho} \xrightarrow{\text{GPCho-pd}} \text{Cho}$$

The overall activity rate of Cho released by the pathways in (a) and (b) *plus* (c) is here referred to as C6PtdCho-pld*.

The PtdCho-plc activity is determined from the additional increase in Cho production in the same cell lysates as above, in the presence of exogenous alkaline phosphatase (AP), according to the reactions:

(d) $$\text{C6PtdCho} \xrightarrow{\text{plc}} \text{PCho}$$

plus

(e) $$\text{PCho} \xrightarrow{\text{AP}} \text{Cho}$$

Fig. 3 (continued) quantitative determination of Chok-mediated PCho production rates simultaneously with the time course of ATP consumption and ADP formation. The representative example shows that, although other enzymatic reactions compete with Chok for ATP utilization, the concentration of this metabolite is still maintained in excess in the time window utilized for the Chok assay. The *inset* shows the change in PCho signal area before and after ATP addition to the reaction mixture. *ADP* adenosine-diphosphate, *AMP* adenosine-monophosphate, *ATP* adenosine triphosphate, *Pi* inorganic phosphate, *SP* phosphorylated sugars

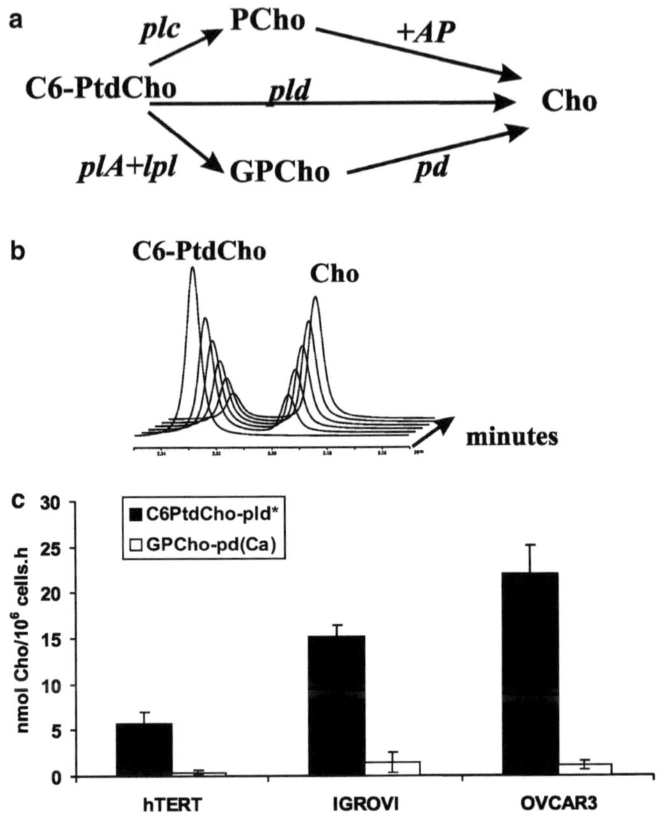

Fig. 4 (**a**) Schematic representation of PtdCho-specific phopholipases and GPCho-pd assays. (**b**) Time course of net Cho production using C6PtdCho as substrate in a representative experiment using an EOC cell line. (**c**) Net Cho production in cell lysates (DMG 50 mM, 10 mM $CaCl_2$, pH 7.2) in the presence of different substrates (C6PtdCho for pld* and GPCho for GPC-pd(Ca) activities)

1. Resuspend cell pellets ($15–20 \times 10^6$ cells) in *PtdCho-phospholipases* lysis buffer (DMG 50 mM, pH 7.4), and sonicate three times for 30 s (*see* **Note 7**); centrifugate the lysate at $20,000 \times g$ for 30 s and perform the assays on supernatants using as substrate a monomeric short-chain PtdCho, C6PtdCho, below the critical micellar concentration [20], 5.0 mM in 10 mM $CaCl_2$, pH 7.2 (*see* **Note 7**).
2. Divide each cell lysate into four aliquots (15×10^6 cells each), two prepared in the presence or absence of C6PtdCho (to determine, by subtraction, the contribution of endogenous Cho) and two in the presence or absence of AP (to determine the contributions of either pld* or PC-plc activity to the final Cho content).
3. Add GPCho as substrate instead of C6PtdCho to determine the maximum contribution of PtdCho deacylation *plus* GPCho-pd-mediated Cho production under the ionic conditions utilized in the present assay. In our EOC models this

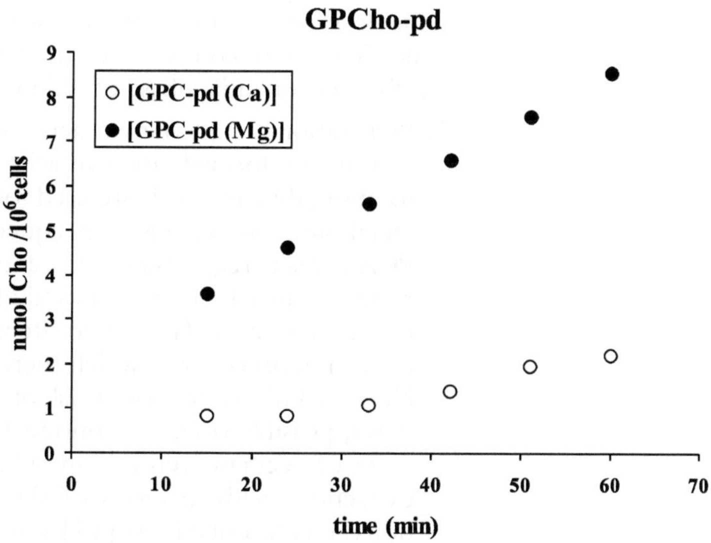

Fig. 5 Time course of net Cho production by GPCho-pd using GPCho as exogenous substrate with two different buffers: GPC-pd (Ca), in DMG 50 mM, 10 mM $CaCl_2$, pH 7.2; GPC-pd (Mg), in DMG 50 mM, 10 mM $MgCl_2$, pH 7.2

contribution is less than 10 % of that of total C6PtdCho-pld* (Fig. 4c, *see* **Note 8**).

4. Determine the C6PtdCho-plc activity from the further increase in Cho production in the cell extracts of the same sample used for measuring the pld activity by adding to the reaction mixture exogenous alkaline phosphatase (AP, 20 U/0.7 mL), according to the reactions (d) and (e) (*see* Fig. 4a).

3.3.2 GPCho-Phosphodiesterase

1. Resuspend cell pellets ($15–20 \times 10^6$ cells) in lysis buffer (DMG 50 mM, pH 7.2), and sonicate three times for 30 s; centrifugate the lysate at 20,000 × *g* for 30 s and perform the assays on supernatants using as substrate GPCho.
2. Determine GPCho-pd activity by adding exogenous GPCho (5 mmol/L) to the cell lysate, in the presence of 10 mmol/L of $MgCl_2$ (*see* ref. 18, **Note 9** and Fig. 5).
3. Measure Cho formation by ^{1}H-MRS as a product of the GPCho catabolic pathway. As reported before, also for the GPCho-pd activity, it is possible to work on cell extracts [14, 18].

4 Notes

1. The intracellular content of PtdCho metabolites and the activity of enzymes involved in the PtdCho-cycle are strictly related to the phase of cell growth (i.e., log-phase, early or late confluence). In fact, it is well known that in cell culture at confluence

the level of PCho decreases, while the content of GPCho increases when compared to the levels of these metabolites in cells at exponential phase of cell growth.

2. Preparation of aqueous extracts requires protein precipitation, typically performed either in acid (e.g., PCA) or in ethanolic solution; dual methods are used for simultaneous extraction of metabolites in organic and aqueous phases. Preparation of PCA extracts requires sample neutralization (by e.g., KOH or NaOH) and subsequent removal of salts by appropriate chelating compounds. These two steps are avoided in ethanolic extraction procedures, which therefore offer the advantages of higher simplicity and lower risk of degradation of some metabolites, possibly occurring during large pH jumps. Thus, after years of accurate verification of qualitative and quantitative extraction yields in terms of absolute metabolite concentrations and reproducibility [19], ethanolic extraction is proposed as the simplest method applicable to a variety of tissues and cells, including ovary cancer cell lines.
3. Detailed interpretation of MRS spectra relies on the ability to assign signals to specific metabolites. In addition, it is necessary to quantify the signals in terms of metabolites ratios, or better in terms of absolute concentrations.
4. Chok activity is determined by linear regression analysis of data points in the linear portion (10–60 min, *see* Fig. 3a as a representative example) of the time course curve of PCho production using graphic software. The rate of linear PCho production essentially coincides with that of Cho consumption in the same time interval, indicating that no major interference arising from other reactions competing for substrate or product utilization takes place. This aspect represents the major advantage of this method compared to conventional colorimetric/enzymatic assays on cell lysates.
5. Alternatively perform ^{31}P NMR experiments in the same cytosolic preparations [14, 17]. A representative example is shown in Fig. 3c.
6. It is also possible to perform Chok activity assay on the bench directly by using aqueous extracts protocols. Briefly, subfractionate equally the cytosolic preparation in separate vials. In each vial add all the components of mixture reaction (ATP, Mg^{2+}, and Cho) and finally stop the reaction at different time points (generally 15, 30, 45, 60 min) to simulate the kinetic reaction in NMR tubes. The basal PCho content is obtained by a single sample where all components (except choline) of reaction are added.
7. No protease inhibitors were added to cell lysates, in order to optimize the conditions of ^{1}H MR spectral analyses. We

checked that no differences in phospholipase assays were observed in cell lysates incubated in the presence or absence of protease inhibitors, indicating that Cho and PCho were not produced by protein degradation up to 120 min.

8. The activity of phospholipases could depend dramatically on the physical structure of PtdCho. We chose for our ^{1}H MRS assay in aqueous buffer the monomeric form of C6PtdCho. In this form the trimethylammonium signal of this phospholipid (3.22 ppm) does not interfere with the resonance of free Cho (3.20 ppm). Furthermore, this method has the advantage of avoiding the steps of separation of organic and polar phases needed when lecithin is used as substrate for choline-producing reactions.
9. The activity of pld could be evaluated to a sufficient level of approximation through an indirect method, by subtracting from the activity of C6PtdCho-pld* that of the maximum GPCho-pd measured in 10 mM $CaCl_2$ (GPCho-pd (Ca)). In order to estimate the Cho contribution of GPCho-pd in the pld* assay, a separate GPCho-pd assay was performed in the presence of Ca^{2+}. These experiments confirmed a very low rate of Cho production by GPCho-pd in the presence of Ca^{2+} in our experimental model.

Acknowledgments

This work was supported by AIRC 2007–2010, AIRC IG9147 (2009–2011), Special Oncology Programme RO 06.5/N.ISS/Q09, Ministry of Health, Italy and Accordo di Collaborazione Italia-USA ISS/530 F/0 F29.

References

1. Hanahan D, Weinberg RA (2000) The hallmarks of cancer. Cell 100:57–70
2. Canevari S, Gariboldi M, Reid JF et al (2006) Molecular predictors of response and outcome in ovarian cancer. Crit Rev Oncol Hematol 60:19–37
3. Hanahan D, Weinberg RA (2011) Hallmarks of cancer: the next generation. Cell 144:646–674
4. Gatenby RA, Gillies RJ (2007) Glycolysis in cancer: a potential target for therapy. Int J Biochem Cell Biol 39:1358–1366
5. Podo F (1999) Tumour phospholipid metabolism. NMR Biomed 12:413–439
6. Beloueche-Babari M, Chung YL, Al-Saffar NM et al (2010) Metabolic assessment of the action of targeted cancer therapeutics using magnetic resonance spectroscopy. Br J Cancer 102:1–7
7. Podo F, Canevari S, Canese R, Pisanu ME et al (2011) MR evaluation of response to targeted treatment in cancer cells. NMR Biomed 24: 648–672
8. Glunde K, Bhujwalla ZM, Ronen SM (2011) Choline metabolism in malignant transformation. Nat Rev Cancer 11:835–848
9. Ackerman JJ, Grove TH, Wong GG et al (1980) Mapping of metabolites in whole animals by ^{31}P NMR using surface coils. Nature 283:167–170
10. Gadian DG (1995) NMR and its applications to living systems, 2nd edn. Oxford University Press, Oxford, UK

11. Negendank W (1992) Studies of human tumors by MRS: a review. NMR Biomed 5:303–324
12. Mountford CE, Doran S, Lean CL et al (2004) Proton MRS can determine the pathology of human cancers with a high level of accuracy. Chem Rev 104:3677–3704
13. Gillies RJ, Morse DL (2005) In vivo magnetic resonance spectroscopy in cancer. Annu Rev Biomed Eng 7:287–326
14. Iorio E, Mezzanzanica D, Alberti P et al (2005) Alterations of choline phospholipid metabolism in ovarian tumor progression. Cancer Res 65:9369–9376
15. Iorio E, Ricci A, Bagnoli M et al (2010) Activation of phosphatidylcholine cycle enzymes in human epithelial ovarian cancer cell. Cancer Res 70:2126–2135
16. Granata F, Iorio E, Carpinelli G et al (2000) Phosphocholine and phosphoethanolamine during chick embryo myogenesis: a ^{31}P-NMR study. Biochim Biophys Acta 1483:334–342
17. Podo F, Ferretti A, Knijn A et al (1996) Detection of phosphatidylcholine-specific phospholipase C in NIH-3T3 fibroblasts and their H-ras transformants: NMR and immunochemical studies. Anticancer Res 16:1399–1412
18. Podo F, Carpinelli G, Ferretti A et al (1992) Activation of glycerophosphocholine phosphodiesterase in Friend leukemia cells upon in vitro-induced erythroid differentiation.^{31}P and ^{1}H NMR studies. Isr J Chem 32:47–54
19. Proietti E, Carpinelli G, Di Vito M et al (1986) ^{31}P-nuclear magnetic resonance analysis of interferon-induced alterations of phospholipid metabolites in interferon-sensitive and interferon-resistant Friend leukemia cell tumors in mice. Cancer Res 46:2849–2857
20. Hergenrother PJ, Martin SF (1997) Determination of the kinetic parameters for phospholipase C (*Bacillus cereus*) on different phospholipid substrates using a chromogenic assay based on the quantitation of inorganic phosphate. Anal Biochem 251:45–49

Chapter 20

Proteomic Profiling of Ovarian Cancer Models Using TMT-LC-MS/MS

John Sinclair and John F. Timms

Abstract

Herein, we have utilized two cellular models of epithelial ovarian cancer (EOC), where transfer of normal chromosome 18 material into the EOC cell lines TOV-112D and TOV-21G induced in vitro and in vivo suppression of tumorigenic phenotype in derived hybrid clones. Two-dimensional-liquid chromatography tandem mass spectrometry (2D-LC-MS/MS) with tandem mass tagging (TMT) was then employed to profile the whole cell, secreted and crude membrane proteomes of the parental and hybrid cell models to identify differentially expressed proteins as potential markers of ovarian tumor suppression. Protein changes of interest were confirmed by immunoblotting in additional hybrid and revertant cell lines. This method afforded quantitative coverage of around 1,000 unique proteins and is applicable to the analysis of any cell model, tissue or biofluid.

Key words Proteomic profiling, Tandem mass tags (TMT), Two-dimensional liquid chromatography, Mass spectrometry, Microcell-mediated chromosome transfer, Ovarian tumor suppression

1 Introduction

Identifying molecular markers of epithelial ovarian cancer (EOC) may provide novel approaches to screening and could enable targeted treatment and the design of novel therapies. Although blood is recognized as a highly important source of disease-related biomarkers, the complexity and dynamic range of protein abundance in body fluids has hampered proteomic biomarker discovery and alternative approaches using cell models may be more successful. In addition, profiling of relevant cell models may aid in the understanding of the molecular mechanisms associated with tumor initiation and progression.

Liquid chromatography tandem mass spectrometry (LC-MS/MS) has become the method of choice for high-coverage protein expression profiling with quantification strategies employed falling into two broad classes; those that are label-free and those which

Anastasia Malek and Oleg Tchernitsa (eds.), *Ovarian Cancer: Methods and Protocols*, Methods in Molecular Biology, vol. 1049, DOI 10.1007/978-1-62703-547-7_20, © Springer Science+Business Media New York 2013

involve differential protein or peptide labeling [1, 2]. In general terms, label-free quantitation methods involve comparison of peptide ion currents (or spectral counts) between samples and are more reliant upon chromatographic reproducibility. In contrast, labeling strategies permit the mixing of samples prior to LC-MS; in some cases upstream of any fractionation. Thus, multiple specimens can be run simultaneously with the same peptides (or proteins) being identically separated and co-eluted into the mass spectrometer with ion intensities being directly compared in the same MS or MS/MS scans. Labeling strategies thus improve throughput and quantitative accuracy.

Differential labeling falls into two categories: those which use chemical derivatization or enzymatic modification of proteins (or peptides) following sample collection and those which use incorporation of isotope-labeled amino acids in vivo. Chemical labeling approaches make use of tags with the same (isobaric labeling) or different masses (isotopic labeling). Isobaric labeling, exemplified by isobaric tags for relative and absolute quantitation (iTRAQ) [3–5] and tandem mass tags (TMT) [6–8], consist of amine-reactive peptide tags which generate specific fragment ions in MS/MS. Samples are differentially labeled (usually at the peptide level following digestion) and then combined and concurrently analyzed by LC-MS/MS, with relative quantification performed by comparison of intensities of "reporter" fragments in an ion-sparse region of the MS/MS spectra of the corresponding labeled peptides. Ratios of "reporter" ions for assigned peptides are then computed and integrated into protein ratios which are then evaluated statistically. The major advantage of these MS/MS-dependent quantification strategies is that the multiplex labeling does not increase the mass complexity of the sample and only peptides subjected to collision-induced dissociation (CID) fragmentation are quantified. In addition, higher signal-to-noise ratios can be achieved with MS/MS-based detection versus MS-mode measurements.

High proteomic coverage is essential in discovery studies and necessitates the use of multiple, orthogonal fractionation steps based on different physicochemical properties of the proteins/peptides. Typical workflows, like the one described herein, incorporate cellular fractionation, protein digestion (usually with trypsin), and two-dimensional peptide LC (e.g., strong cation exchange followed by reverse-phase LC) linked directly to MS/MS through an electrospray source. Whilst isobaric protein labeling workflows have been described [9], both iTRAQ and TMT have been optimized for peptide-based labeling, and the labeling should be applied at the earliest possible point in the workflow to minimize differences due to sample processing. There are several drawbacks to isobaric labeling that are worth mentioning. The iTRAQ/TMT reagents are expensive and only give signals when peptides are subjected to fragmentation. Thus, the strategy misses peptides not selected for MS/MS, lowering proteomic coverage. Dedicated software must be used for data analysis, although commercially available software packages (Mascot, Proteome Discoverer, and Protein Pilot) now integrate reporter ion quantification and MS/MS data search output. It is also evident that higher energy (CID) methods and careful tuning are required for optimal "reporter" fragmentation to provide highest quantitative accuracy [10–12]. The method described herein, integrates CID with higher energy collisional dissociation (HCD) for the same precursor ions on an LTQ Orbitrap XL instrument.

Tumorigenic progression is driven by an accumulation of genetic alterations, including the activation of oncogenes and inactivation of tumor suppressor genes. Previous studies using metaphase comparative genomic hybridization have identified chromosomes displaying a high incidence of deletions in ovarian tumors, and which are postulated to be potential sites of tumor suppressor genes [13]. In particular, chromosome 18 (Ch18) was identified to be genetically altered in a high percentage of tumors. In our previous work, microcell-mediated chromosomal transfer (MMCT) of normal Ch18 material into two EOC cell lines, TOV-112D and TOV-21G, generated hybrids that displayed significant suppression of proliferation, anchorage-independent growth, and invasiveness and reduced tumor growth in nude mice compared to their parental cell lines [14, 15].

The primary aim of this work was to apply a quantitative 2D-LC-MS/MS profiling strategy incorporating TMT labeling to whole cell lysate, the secreted fraction and a crude membrane preparation of these EOC cell models to identify protein changes associated with suppression of tumorigenic phenotype in order to identify candidate biomarkers and putative tumor suppressor genes. The cellular, secreted, and crude membrane proteomes were probed in order to optimize coverage of protein changes and afforded a combined quantitative coverage of around 1,000 unique proteins when combined with 2D-LC-MS/MS. Fig. 1 shows a schematic of the workflow used. Numerous proteins displaying significantly altered expression were identified that were related to suppression of tumorigenic phenotype in the two cell models [8]. The quantitative protein expression profiling method described herein is a modified version of the one reported in ref. [8] and is applicable for the comparison of any model cell lines, tissues or biofluids.

2 Materials

2.1 Cell Culture

1. Cells: EOC cell lines TOV-112D and TOV-21G obtained from ATCC and two Ch18 MMCT hybrid clones derived from each (18D22 and 18D23, 18G5 and 18G1.26, respectively) [15].

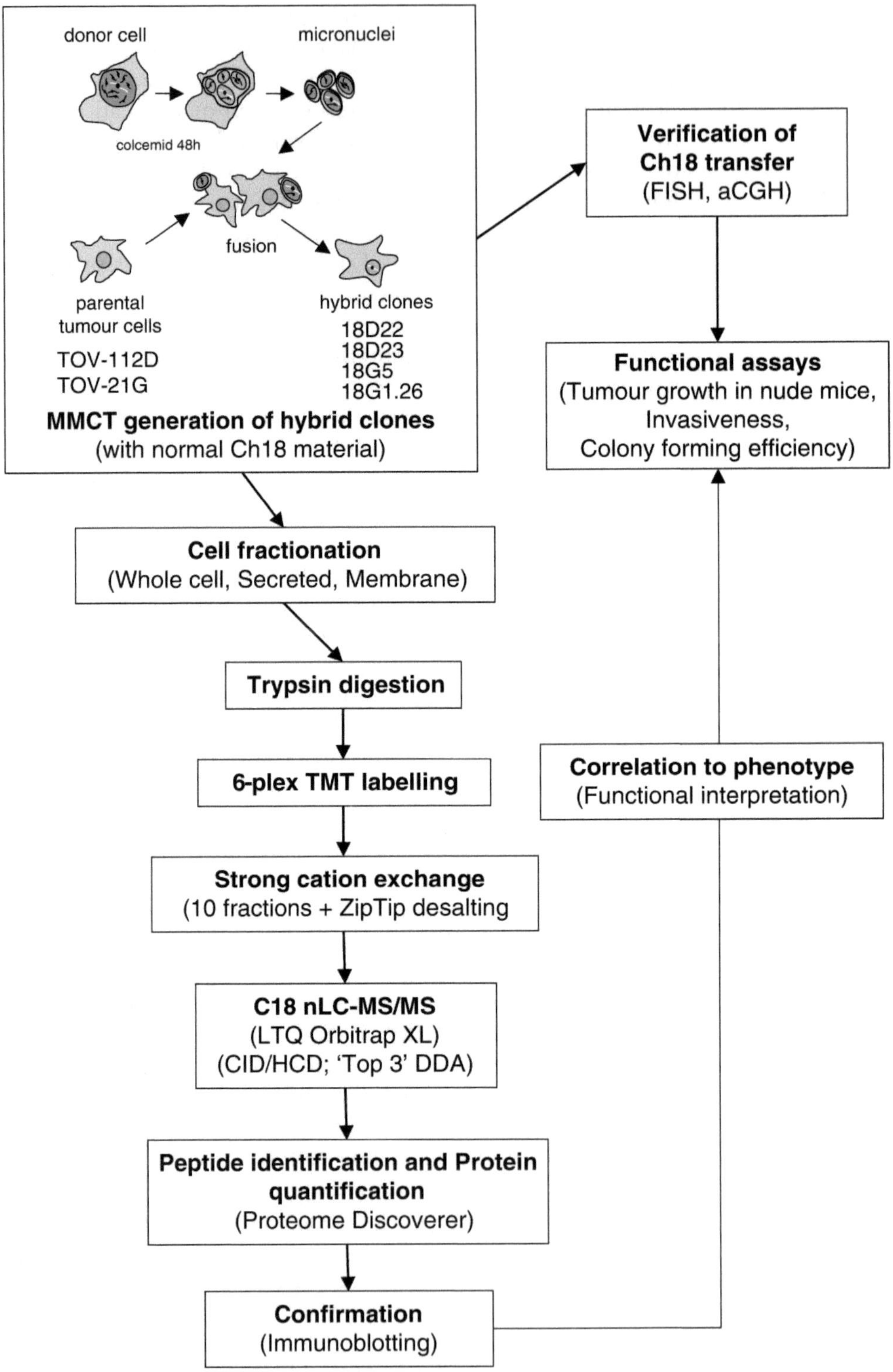

Fig. 1 Generation of cell models of ovarian tumor suppression and their proteomic characterization. A schematic of microcell-mediated chromosome transfer (MMCT) for generation of hybrid cell lines, their verification and functional characterization is shown alongside their proteomic comparison using 2D-LC-MS/MS with TMT labeling for relative quantification

2. MCB105 and 199 media (Sigma, St Louis, MO, USA) 1:1 ratio containing, 15 % (v/v) fetal calf serum (FCS), supplemented with 2 mM l-glutamine, 100 mg/mL streptomycin, 100 units/mL penicillin and with 400 U/mL hygromycin B for the hybrid clones (all from Invitrogen, Paisley, UK). Stored at 4 °C and warmed to 37 °C prior to use.
3. Trypsin–EDTA solution: 0.25 % trypsin, 1 mM EDTA (Invitrogen, Paisley, UK). Stored at4 °C.
4. Dimethyl sulfoxide (DMSO), sterile, tissue culture grade.

2.2 Preparation of Cell Fractions

1. Phosphate-buffered saline buffer (PBS): 137 mM NaCl, 2.7 mM KCl, 10 mM $Na_2HPO_4 \cdot 2\ H_2O$, 2 mM KH_2PO_4, pH 7.4. Sterilize by autoclaving.
2. 2D lysis buffer: 4 % (w/v) CHAPS, 0.5 % Nonidet-P40/ IGEPAL CA-630, 8 M urea, 2 M thiourea, 10 mM Tris–HCl (pH 8.3), 1 mM EDTA. Aliquot and store at −20 °C.
3. Protease inhibitor stocks: 42 mM 4-(2-Aminoethyl) benzenesulfonyl fluoride hydrochloride (AEBSF) in ddH_2O (100×), 0.26 mM (5 TIU/mg) aprotinin solution (100×), 10 mM leupeptin in ddH_2O (1,000×), 1.46 mM pepstatin in 100 % ethanol (1,000×). All from Sigma, St Louis, MO, USA. Store in aliquots at −20 °C, except aprotinin solution, which is stored at 4 °C.
4. Phosphatase inhibitor stocks: 5 mM bisperoxovanadium 1,10-phenanthroline (bpVphen) in ddH_2O (1,000×), 5 mM fenvalerate in 100 % ethanol (1,000×), 200 mM sodium orthovanadate in ddH_2O (100×), 1 mM okadaic acid in 100 % ethanol (1,000×). All from Sigma, St Louis, USA. Store in aliquots at −20 °C.
5. Coomassie Plus (Bradford) Protein Assay (Pierce, Rockford, IL, USA) and SpectraMax® Microplate Reader (Molecular Devices, Sunnyvale, CA, USA) or equivalent.
6. Bovine serum albumin (BSA) standards in lysis buffer.
7. Centriplus YM-3 filters: MWCO 3 kDa (Millipore Corporation, Billerica, MA, USA).
8. SpeedVac/Eppendorf Concentrator 5301 (VWR International, Lutterworth, UK).
9. Hypotonic lysis buffer: 10 mM HEPES (pH 7.4), 5 mM KCl, 5 mM $MgCl_2$. Store at −20 °C.
10. Dounce homogenizer.
11. Ultracentrifuge: Optima (Beckman Coulter UK Ltd, High Wycombe, UK) or equivalent.
12. Radio Immunoprecipitation Assay (RIPA) buffer: 150 mM NaCl, 10 mM Tris (pH 7.4), 0.1 % SDS, 1 % Nonidet-P40/

IGEPAL CA-630, 0.5 % sodium deoxycholate, 5 mM EDTA. Aliquot and store at −20 °C.

2.3 Trypsin Digestion and TMT Labeling

1. Acetone: 100 % acetone stored at −20 °C.
2. Dissolution buffer: 100 mM triethyl ammonium bicarbonate (TEAB) (pH 8.0), 0.5 % (w/v) SDS. Aliquot and store at −20 °C.
3. Reducing solution: 200 mM tris(2-carboxyethyl) phosphine in 200 mM TEAB (pH 8.0). Prepare fresh.
4. Alkylation solution: 375 mM iodoacetamide in 100 mM TEAB (pH 8.0). Prepare fresh.
5. Trypsin solution: 500 ng/μL sequencing-grade modified trypsin (Promega, Southampton, UK) in 5 mM acetic acid. Store at −20 °C.
6. SpeedVac/Eppendorf concentrator 5301 (VWR International, Lutterworth, UK).
7. Acetonitrile (ACN): 100 % HPLC grade ACN.
8. TMTsixplex Isobaric Mass Tagging Kit (Thermo Scientific, Rockford, IL, USA).
9. Quenching solution: 5 % Hydroxylamine in 200 mM TEAB (pH 8.0). Make fresh.
10. Lo-Bind eppendorf tubes (Eppendorf AG, Hamburg, Germany).

2.4 Strong Cation Exchange Chromatography

1. Buffer A: 5 % ACN (v/v) in 5 mM NaH_2PO_4 made with HPLC grade water, acidified to pH 2.0 with formic acid. Prepare fresh.
2. Buffer B: Buffer A + 1 M NaCl. Prepare fresh.
3. Polysulfoethyl column: 1 mm i.d. × 15 cm, 5 μm bead size, 300 Å pore size (PolyLC Inc., Columbia, MD, USA).
4. Ultimate 3000 LC system loading pump (Dionex Corporation, Salt Lake City, UT, USA).
5. ZipTips (Millipore Corporation, Billerica, MA, USA).
6. Acetonitrile (ACN): 50 % HPLC grade ACN in HPLC grade water.
7. Trifluoroacetic acid (TFA): 0.5 % HPLC grade TFA in HPLC grade water.
8. ACN/TFA: 50 % ACN (v/v), 0.5 % TFA (v/v).
9. Lo-Bind eppendorf tubes (Eppendorf AG, Hamburg, Germany).

2.5 LC-MS/MS

1. Ultimate 3000 nano LC system (Dionex Corporation, Salt Lake City, UT, USA) linked to a LTQ Orbitrap XL mass spectrometer (Thermo Scientific, Rockford, IL, USA) (*see* **Note 1**).

2. C18 PepMap guard column: 300 μm i.d. × 5 mm, 5 μm bead size, 100 Å pore size (Dionex Corporation, Salt Lake City, UT, USA).
3. C18 PepMap nano LC column: 75 μm i.d. × 150 mm, 3 μm bead size, 100 Å pore size (Dionex Corporation, Salt Lake City, UT, USA).
4. Solvent A: 0.1 % formic acid in HPLC grade water.
5. Solvent B: 0.1 % formic acid, 99.9 % ACN.
6. Xcalibur 2 (Thermo Scientific), Proteome Discoverer 1.3 (Thermo Scientific), and Mascot Server 2.2 (Matrix Science, London, UK) software.

3 Methods

3.1 Cell Culture

1. Culture TOV-112D and TOV-21G cell lines in 15-cm tissue culture dishes in MCB105/199 media at 37 °C in a 5 % CO_2-humidified incubator. Culture hybrid clones (18D22, 18D23, 18G5, and 18G1.26) under the same conditions with an additional 400 U/mL of hygromycin to maintain clonal selection.
2. Passage cells by trypsinization according to standard procedures when 70–80 % confluent.
3. Stocks of cells can be stored. Resuspend in 10 % DMSO and 90 % FCS, freeze slowly overnight to −80 °C in an insulated isopropanol container and submerge in liquid nitrogen for long-term storage.

3.2 Preparation of Cell Fractions

3.2.1 Preparation of Whole Cell Lysates

1. For preparation of whole cell lysates, wash cells (1 × 15-cm plate) at ~80 % confluence with ice-cold PBS and add 500 μL of 2D lysis buffer per plate. Place dishes immediately on ice.
2. Scrape cells and collect in labeled tubes.
3. Homogenize by passage through a 25-gauge needle five times. Vortex and remove insoluble material by centrifugation (13,000 × *g*, 10 min, 4 °C) and transfer supernatant to fresh tubes.
4. Determine protein concentration using the Coomassie Plus (Bradford) Protein Assay. Make a 5 mg/mL stock of BSA in 2D-lysis buffer and prepare serial dilutions of 0, 0.25, 0.5, 1.0, 2.5, and 5.0 mg/mL to make a standard curve. Use a 96-well flat-bottomed assay plate and make triplicate measurements for the BSA standards and four replicates for the experimental samples. For this, add 2 μL of sample per well and 200 μL of assay reagent and mix without introducing bubbles. Use a microplate reader at a wavelength of 595 nm and calculate protein concentrations using the standard curve (*see* **Note 2**).

3.2.2 Preparation of Secreted Protein

1. For preparation of secreted protein, wash 5 × 15-cm plates of cells at 80 % confluence twice in PBS at 37 °C. Further incubate cells for 24 h in serum-free medium.
2. Replace with 10 mL of fresh serum-free medium and collect as "conditioned media" after a further 24 h (*see* **Note 3**).
3. Remove floating cells and cellular debris from the "conditioned media" by centrifugation (10,000 × *g*, 10 min, 4 °C).
4. Add protease inhibitors AEBSF, aprotinin, leupeptin, and pepstatin from stocks to give final concentrations of 0.42 mM, 2.6 μM, 10 μM, and 1.46 μM, respectively.
5. Concentrate the samples 25-fold (to ~2 mL) and desalt by ultrafiltration through Centriplus YM-3 filters (MWCO 3 kDa).
6. Dry down samples in a SpeedVac and resuspend in 100 μL of 2D lysis buffer.
7. Determine protein concentrations as described above (Subheading 3.2.1, **step 4**).

3.2.3 Preparation of Crude Membrane Fractions

1. For preparation of crude membrane fractions, scrape 1 × 15-cm plate of 80 % confluent cells in 1 mL of chilled hypotonic lysis buffer supplemented with protease inhibitors at the final concentration indicated above.
2. Homogenize in a chilled Dounce homogenizer (at least 25 strokes).
3. Pellet the crude nuclear fraction by centrifugation (800 × *g*, 5 min, 4 °C) in a bench-top centrifuge.
4. Collect the supernatant and ultracentrifuge in appropriate tubes (100,000 × *g*, 60 min, 4 °C).
5. Wash the pellet (crude membrane fraction) in 2 mL hypotonic lysis buffer and recentrifuge. Resuspended the resulting pellet in 1 mL of chilled RIPA buffer supplemented with protease inhibitors using final concentrations described above (Subheading 3.2.2, **step 4**).
6. Remove insoluble material by centrifugation (13,000 × *g*, 10 min, 4 °C) and transfer supernatant to fresh tubes.
7. Determine protein concentrations as described above (Subheading 3.2.1, **step 4**).

3.3 Trypsin Digestion and TMT Labeling (See Note 4)

1. Acetone precipitate equal amounts of protein (100 μg) from the whole cell lysate, secreted and crude membrane fractions of each cell line by adding four times the sample volume of 100 % acetone at −20 °C. Vortex and allow to precipitate for 60 min at −20 °C. Centrifuge (13,000 × *g*, 10 min, 4 °C) and carefully decant and dispose of the supernatant. Allow the acetone to evaporate from the uncapped tube at room temperature for 30 min. Samples may be frozen for storage at this point.

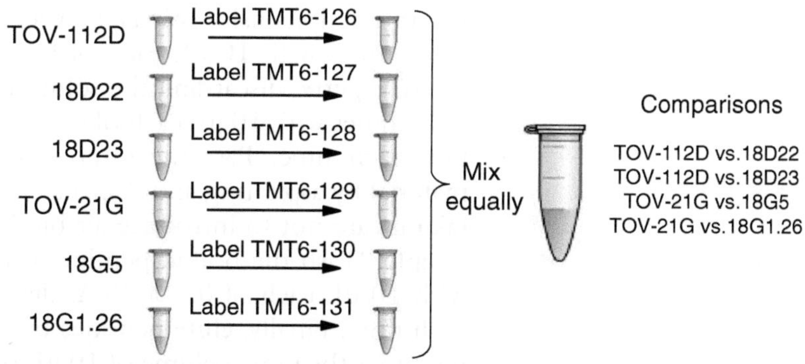

Fig. 2 Labeling strategy used for comparison of parental cell lines and hybrid clones. The parental cell line TOV-112D was labeled with TMT reagent 126 and its hybrid cell lines, 18D22 and 18D23, were labeled with reagents 127 and 128, respectively. The parental cell line TOV-21G was labeled with TMT reagent 129 and its hybrid cell lines, 18G5 and 18G1.26, were labeled with reagents 130 and 131, respectively. Samples were mixed equally prior to 2D-LC-MS/MS analysis and compared as shown

2. Resuspend the protein pellets in 100 μL of dissolution buffer.
3. Add 5 μL of reducing solution (9.5 mM final concentration of tris(2-carboxyethyl) phosphine) and incubate for 1 h at 55 °C.
4. Add 5 μL of freshly prepared alkylation solution (17 mM final concentration of iodoacetamide) and incubate for 30 min at room temperature in the dark.
5. Add 5 μL of trypsin solution (2.5 μg/100 μg protein) and incubate overnight at 37 °C.
6. Reconstitute a tube of each TMT label in 41 μL of 100 % ACN and carefully add to the appropriate sample tube (*see* Fig. 2 for labeling strategy).
7. Allow labeling reactions to proceed for 1 h at room temperature (*see* **Note 4**).
8. Quench reactions by adding 8 μL of quenching solution and incubate for 15 min at room temperature.
9. Combine samples at equal amounts and dry down in a SpeedVac. Samples can be frozen for storage at this stage.

3.4 Strong Cation Exchange Chromatography

1. Resuspend in 4 μL of buffer A.
2. Inject half (50 μg) of the sample onto a Polysulfoethyl column (pre-equilibrated for 25 min in buffer A) using an Ultimate 3000 LC system loading pump.
3. Apply a 5–55 % gradient of buffer B at 50 μL/min over 30 min using the loading pump and collect 150 μL fractions every 3 min to generate 10 fractions.

4. Desalt fractions using ZipTips: wet the C18 packing material three times with 10 μL each of 50 % ACN using a standard 10 μL pipette, discarding the solution each time. Wash the tip three times with 10 μL each of 0.5 % TFA, discarding the solution each time. Pass the sample solution over the packing material by aspirating and dispensing a minimum of ten times, taking care not to introduce air bubbles. Retain the unbound sample. Wash the bound peptides on the C18 tip three times with 10 μL each of 0.5 % TFA, discarding the wash solution each time. Finally, elute peptides by aspirating and dispensing ten times the same volume of 10 μL of 50 % ACN/0.5 % TFA, collecting into a Lo-Bind Eppendorf tube.
5. Dry fractions down in a SpeedVac. Samples can be frozen for storage at this stage.

3.5 LC-MS/MS

1. Resuspend samples in 10 μL of 0.1 % formic acid.
2. Inject 5 μL of sample from the autosampler onto the C18 PepMap guard column and wash for 3 min with 100 % solvent A at a flow rate of 25 μL/min.
3. Switch to the analytical C18 PepMap nano LC column with 10 % solvent B and apply a linear gradient of 10–50 % B over 90 min, then to 100 % B over 3 min. Continue with 100 % B for 20 min and then reduce to 10 % B over 0.5 min and continue for a further 20 min to re-equilibrate the column for the next injection.
4. Operate the mass spectrometer (LTQ Orbitrap XL) in the data-dependent mode for automated switching between MS and MS/MS acquisition. Acquire survey full scan MS spectra (from *m/z* 400–2,000) in the Orbitrap (FT) with a resolution of 60,000 at *m/z* 400. Select the "top 3" most intense ions for both CID and HCD. Select a target ion value of 1×10^6 and maximum scan time of 500 ms for the survey full scan in the FT. Select target ion values of 1×10^5 and 1×10^4 and scan time settings of 300 and 150 ms for FT-MSn (HCD) and IT-MSn (CID), respectively (*see* **Note 5**). Set resolution of fragment ion detection (in the FT) at 7,500. Acquire centroid data in both detectors.
5. Dynamically exclude ions selected for MS/MS for 60 s.
6. Enable the lock mass option for accurate mass measurement, using the polydimethylcyclosiloxane ion (*m/z* 455.120025) as an internal calibrant (*see* **Note 6**).

3.6 Data Analysis

1. Process the raw data files generated in Xcalibur using Proteome Discoverer 1.3. Set up the workflow shown in Fig. 3 using the following instructions and parameters.
2. Input RAW files in the Spectrum Files node.

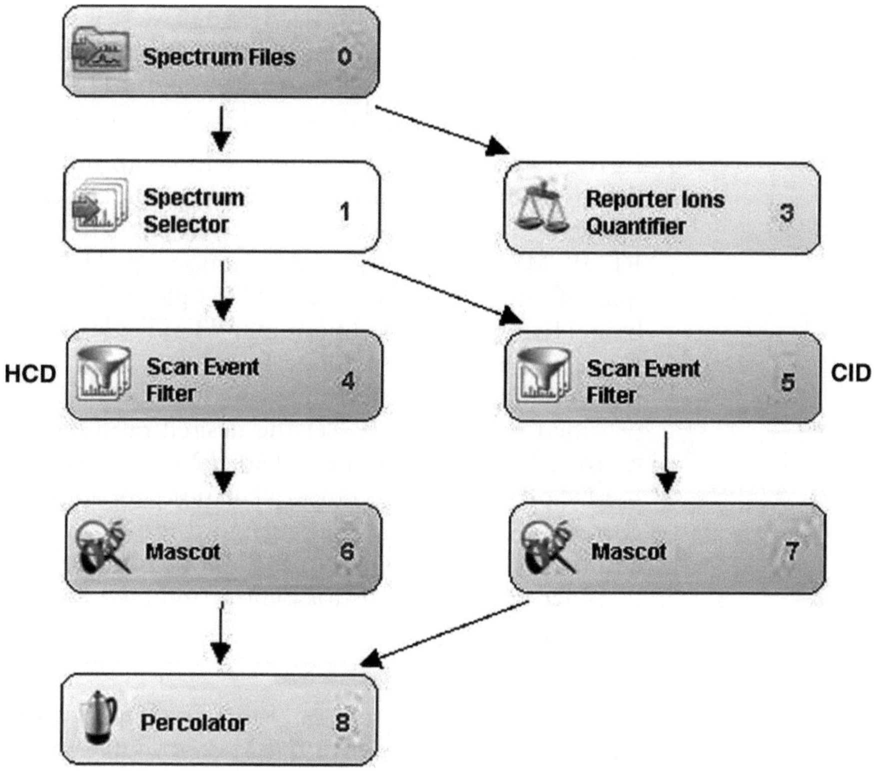

Fig. 3 Data analysis workflow in Proteome Discoverer. For instructions and settings, *see* Subheading 3.6

3. In the Spectrum Selector, use MS1 precursor, minimum precursor mass 350 Da, maximum precursor mass 6,500 Da, select MS order as MS2 and an S/N threshold as 1.5. All other settings as default or "0".
4. In the Scan Event Filter for HCD, set analyzer to FTMS, activation type to HCD and all other parameters to "Any".
5. In the Scan Event Filter for CID, set analyzer to ITMS, activation type to CID and all other parameters to "Any".
6. In the Mascot node for HCD, select the most recent version of the SwissProt database (updated in Mascot Server), select trypsin as the enzyme, number of missed cleavages as 1, instrument type as ESI-FTICR, taxonomy as human, precursor mass tolerance as 10 ppm, fragment mass tolerance as 20 mμ and do not average precursor masses. Set methionine oxidation and N-terminal acetylation as dynamic modifications and carbamidomethylation of cysteines and TMT modification of peptide N-termini and lysine residues as static modifications.
7. In the Mascot node for CID, select the parameters as described above, but using ESI-TRAP as instrument type and a fragment mass tolerance of 0.6 Da.

8. In the Percolator used for decoy database searching and estimation of false discovery rate (FDR), apply a maximum delta Cn of 0.05, a target FDR (strict) of 0.01, a target FDR (relaxed) of 0.05, and validation based on *q* value.
9. In the Reporter Ions Quantifier, choose an integration window tolerance of 10 ppm and "most confident centroid" for integration method. Set the scan event filters to mass analyzer FTMS, MS order to MS2 and activation type HCD. Set up the quantification method using TMT6plex/+229.163 Da on lysine (K) for residue modification and TMT6plex/+229.163 Da for N-terminal modification. Input masses of the tags and reporter ion isotopic distributions (this information should be provided with each kit). Set the desired ratio reporting: here ratios 127/126, 128/126, 130/129, and 131/129 were used. For reporter ion ratio calculation, apply quantity value correction and set the fold-change threshold and maximum allowed fold-change (*see* **Note** 7). For protein quantification, consider protein groups for peptide uniqueness and use only unique peptides.
10. Run the analysis (*see* **Note 8**).
11. Apply search result filters, only allowing peptides with a score >20 and equal to or above the Mascot significance threshold of $p<0.05$.
12. Accept only quantitative information for proteins with at least 2 peptide matches, using the median value of the peptide ratios and a % variability of less than 20 %.
13. Validate changes of interest by immunoblotting with specific antibodies using standard techniques. In our study, additional hybrid clones were examined, as well as revertant cell lines with a demonstrated loss of the normal Ch18 material and reversion of the tumorigenic suppression phenotype.
14. Bioinformatics analysis may also be performed to examine gene ontology enrichment (e.g., using the BINGO plug-in for Cytoscape), intracellular pathway involvement (e.g., using Ingenuity Systems Pathway Analysis), and protein–protein interactions (e.g., using the STRING database).

4 Notes

1. Other instrumentation and modes of operation can be used for peptide identification and MS/MS-based quantification using TMT isobaric tags. Fragmentation and quantification of reporter ions can be achieved using HCD/CID (as described here), MS3 [16], or proton transfer reaction (PTR)-MS [17]

on the Orbitrap Velos and by pulsed Q collision-induced dissociation/CID (PQD/CID) [10] on the LTQ Orbitrap Discovery or LTQ ion trap instruments. The TMT approach has also been successfully applied using Q-TOF [18], TOF/TOF [7], Triple Quadrupole [19, 20] instruments and those equipped with electron transfer dissociation (ETD) capability [21].

2. It is recommended that at least four replicate assays are performed for each sample for accurate protein determination. Dilute concentrated samples with lysis buffer if necessary.

3. Conditioned media is generated in this way to avoid contamination of the sample from abundant proteins present in the FBS used in the culture medium. Whilst the cells used here were tolerant to serum starvation for 48 h, this should be tested for other cell types. In addition, it is not known what effect serum starvation may have on global protein secretion.

4. Reagents and protocol are provided in the TMTsixplex Isobaric Mass Tagging Kit. Carry out all steps from this point forward using siliconized tubes. The TMT tags are *N*-hydroxysuccinimide esters of a differentially, stable isotope-labeled entity, and as such, will react with the primary amino groups of the trypsin-generated peptides (i.e., N-terminal amino and lysine side chain ε-amino groups). Whilst, isobaric for labeled peptides, the six TMTs fragment during HCD to generate six reporter ions that are unique in mass, the intensities of which are used to determine the relative amounts of peptides across the six samples.

5. Use Tune Plus V2.4 SP2 in instrument software for adjusting these parameters. For example, if the sample amount is low, then increasing the MSn scan times is advisable. Tune Plus V2.4 SP2 automatically adjusts the HCD normalized collision energy depending upon the charge state of TMT-tagged precursor ions.

6. Polydimethylcyclosiloxanes are an almost ubiquitous contaminant of laboratory air. Although they create a background signal, they can be used for internal mass calibration during the run. Here, the polydimethylcyclosiloxane ion (*m/z* 455.120025) was used as an internal calibrant.

7. A fold-change threshold of 2.0 and maximum allowed fold-change of 100 were used in this study.

8. The whole experiment should be run in triplicate and the data from each processed separately in Proteome Discoverer. The results files can then be uploaded together in Proteome Discoverer to compare the experiments and identify reproducible changes.

References

1. Cox J, Mann M (2007) Is proteomics the new genomics? Cell 130:395–398
2. Timms JF, Cutillas PR (2010) Overview of quantitative LC-MS techniques for proteomics and activitomics. Methods Mol Biol 658: 19–45
3. Ross PL, Huang YN, Marchese JN et al (2004) Multiplexed protein quantitation in Saccharomyces cerevisiae using amine-reactive isobaric tagging reagents. Mol Cell Proteomics 3:1154–1169
4. Choe L, D'Ascenzo M, Relkin NR et al (2007) 8-plex quantitation of changes in cerebrospinal fluid protein expression in subjects undergoing intravenous immunoglobulin treatment for Alzheimer's disease. Proteomics 7:3651–3660
5. Pierce A, Unwin RD, Evans CA et al (2008) Eight-channel iTRAQ enables comparison of the activity of six leukemogenic tyrosine kinases. Mol Cell Proteomics 7:853–863
6. Thompson A, Schafer J, Kuhn K et al (2003) Tandem mass tags: a novel quantification strategy for comparative analysis of complex protein mixtures by MS/MS. Anal Chem 75: 1895–1904
7. Dayon L, Hainard A, Licker V et al (2008) Relative quantification of proteins in human cerebrospinal fluids by MS/MS using 6-plex isobaric tags. Anal Chem 80:2921–2931
8. Sinclair J, Metodieva G, Dafou D et al (2011) Profiling signatures of ovarian cancer tumour suppression using 2D-DIGE and 2D-LC-MS/MS with tandem mass tagging. J Proteomics 74:451–465
9. Sinclair J, Timms JF (2011) Quantitative profiling of serum samples using TMT protein labelling, fractionation and LC-MS/MS. Methods 54:361–369
10. Bantscheff M, Boesche M, Eberhard D et al (2008) Robust and sensitive iTRAQ quantification on an LTQ Orbitrap mass spectrometer. Mol Cell Proteomics 7:1702–1713
11. Griffin TJ, Xie H, Bandhakavi S et al (2007) iTRAQ reagent-based quantitative proteomic analysis on a linear ion trap mass spectrometer. J Proteome Res 6:4200–4209
12. Guo T, Gan CS, Zhang H et al (2008) Hybridization of pulsed-Q dissociation and collision-activated dissociation in linear ion trap mass spectrometer for iTRAQ quantitation. J Proteome Res 7:4831–4840
13. Ramus SJ, Pharoah PD, Harrington P et al (2003) BRCA1/2 mutation status influences somatic genetic progression in inherited and sporadic epithelial ovarian cancer cases. Cancer Res 63:417–423
14. Dafou D, Grun B, Sinclair S et al. (2010) Microcell mediated chromosome transfer identifies EPB41L3 as a functional suppressor of epithelial ovarian cancers. Neoplasia 12:579–589
15. Dafou D, Ramus SJ, Choi K et al (2009) Chromosomes 6 and 18 induce neoplastic suppression in epithelial ovarian cancer cells. Int J Cancer 124:1037–1044
16. Ting L, Rad R, Gygi SP et al (2011) MS3 eliminates ratio distortion in isobaric multiplexed quantitative proteomics. Nat Methods 8:937–940
17. Wenger CD, Lee MV, Hebert AS et al (2011) Gas-phase purification enables accurate, multiplexed proteome quantification with isobaric tagging. Nat Methods 8:933–935
18. van Ulsen P, Kuhn K, Prinz T et al (2009) Identification of proteins of Neisseria meningitidis induced under iron-limiting conditions using the isobaric tandem mass tag (TMT) labeling approach. Proteomics 9:1771–1781
19. Stella R, Cifani P, Peggion C et al (2011) Relative quantification of membrane proteins in wild-type and prion protein (PrP)-knockout cerebellar granule neurons. J Proteome Res 11:523–536
20. Byers HL, Campbell J, van Ulsen P et al (2009) Candidate verification of iron-regulated Neisseria meningitidis proteins using isotopic versions of tandem mass tags (TMT) and single reaction monitoring. J Proteomics 73:231–239
21. Viner RI, Zhang T, Second T et al (2009) Quantification of post-translationally modified peptides of bovine alpha-crystallin using tandem mass tags and electron transfer dissociation. J Proteomics 72:874–885

Chapter 21

Characterization of Signalling Pathways by Reverse Phase Protein Arrays

Katharina Malinowsky, Claudia Wolff, Christina Schott, and Karl-Friedrich Becker

Abstract

Reverse phase protein array (RPPA) is a very suitable technique to analyze large numbers of proteins in small samples like for example tumor biopsies. Beside their small size another major hindrance for the analysis of proteins from biopsies is the extraction of proteins from formalin-fixed and paraffin-embedded (FFPE) tissues. Here we describe a protocol, allowing quantitative extraction of large numbers of proteins from FFPE tissues and their subsequent analysis by RPPA. To elucidate the role of epidermal growth factor receptor (EGFR) signalling in ovarian cancer, we analyzed 23 primary tumors and corresponding metastases for the expression of 25 proteins involved in EGFR signalling with special emphasis on epithelial–mesenchymal transition (EMT). We found a significant correlation of Snail with $EGFR^{(Tyr1086)}$ and p38 $MAPK^{(Thr180/Tyr182)}$ in primary ovarian carcinoma and with $EGFR^{(Tyr1086)}$ in their corresponding metastases. Additionally, we showed that high expression levels of the E-cadherin repressor Snail in primary tumors combined with high expression levels of the pp38 $MAPK^{(Thr180/Tyr182)}$ in metastasis lead to an increased risk for death in ovarian carcinoma patients.

Key words Reverse phase protein array (RPPA), Protein extraction, Signalling, Proteomic profiling, Formalin-fixed and paraffin-embedded tissue (FFPE)

1 Introduction

To optimize patient selection for therapy, new methods, which are able to provide information on the entire spectrum of deregulated pathways before and during treatment, are needed. The reverse phase protein array (RPPA) technology is a very potent new tool that allows simultaneous analysis of multiple proteins. Recent research demonstrates the feasibility of this technology for clinical applications [1]. With help of the RPPA approach protein networks deregulated in disease can be characterized in great detail, thus allowing the identification of new therapeutic targets and biomarkers for diagnosis. So far most of the clinical relevant studies using RPPA technology are carried out on fresh or frozen samples.

Anastasia Malek and Oleg Tchernitsa (eds.), *Ovarian Cancer: Methods and Protocols*, Methods in Molecular Biology, vol. 1049, DOI 10.1007/978-1-62703-547-7_21,

This is a major drawback as most clinical samples world wide are fixed in formalin. But as extraction of proteins from formalin-fixed and paraffin-embedded (FFPE) tissues has been a major issue, only a few extract-based studies are done on this kind of material. So far immunohistochemistry (IHC) is the gold standard to analyze proteins from FFPE tissues. Nevertheless, this method seems not very suitable for the simultaneous analysis of subtle quantitative changes in large numbers of proteins changing within tissues at the same time and may not be sensitive enough to detect for example phospho-proteins.

Over the last decades several groups developed a number of protocols allowing successful extraction of proteins from FFPE tissues and their subsequent analysis by a variety of methods, e.g., western blot and mass spectrometry [2–9]. An overview over the different extraction protocols is given in a recent publication by Berg et al. 2010 [10]. By combining proteins extracted from FFPE tissues with RPPA it is now possible to analyze complete protein signalling networks in large patient cohorts allowing the clinical relevant identification of biomarkers and therapeutic targets.

A major bottleneck for the usage of RPPA in quantitative studies is the availability of highly specific antibodies. In a typical RPPA proteins are not separated by their molecular weight; therefore, it is not possible to differentiate between "specific" and possible "unspecific" signals directly on the array. One has to be sure to use only rigorously validated antibodies when working with this method. All antibodies we use in our study are thoroughly validated by western blot analyses regarding their sensitivity and specificity and we recently suggested an algorithm for the optimized validation of antibodies for the usage in RPPAs [11]. Until today we established more than 100 antibodies for use with the RPPA technology on FFPE tissues.

Ovarian cancer is one of the leading causes of death among cancers of the female genital tract in the developed world [12]. The major problem regarding the treatment of this highly metastatic disease is its mostly late diagnosis (FIGO stages III and IV) which normally does not occur before the metastatic setting [13]. As metastasis is the main reason for therapy failure in cancer, the identification of molecules or pathways involved in this process has a high impact on the development of appropriate therapies for highly metastatic cancers. In addition to molecular characterization of primary tumors pathways changing upon metastasis should be analyzed in detail to identify possible inhibitors of tumor progression at this stage [14].

We applied the new methodology to extract proteins from FFPE tissues and their subsequent analysis by RPPA to identify proteins deregulated during the metastasis of ovarian cancer.

Epithelial to mesenchymal transition (EMT) is described as an important step during the progression of cancer to a metastatic stage and could be shown to be essential for the growth and dissemination of ovarian cancer cells [15–19]. The epidermal growth factor receptor (EGFR) is either mutated or over-expressed in a number of epithelial cancers including ovarian cancer. The cell adhesion molecule E-cadherin and its main transcriptional repressor snail are important regulators of EMT. Previous studies showed a correlation of snail expression with poorer patient survival in ovarian cancer patients [20] and an association between overexpression of snail and down-regulation of E-cadherin in this tumor type [21, 22]. Regulation of EMT by EGFR signalling could be demonstrated in cell culture [23] but studies linking deregulation of EGFR to EMT in primary ovarian cancers were missing so far. In our RPPA-based study we analyzed samples from 23 patients with advanced ovarian cancers (FIGO III or IV) for the expression of 25 proteins corresponding to EGFR signalling and EMT (Table 1) in the primary tumors and the corresponding metastases. The study provided us with three major results. First, we could demonstrate a correlation of snail with p-EGFR$^{(Tyr1086)}$ and p-p38$^{(Thr180/Tyr181)}$ in primary tumors hinting at a possible regulation of snail by deregulated EGFR signalling in primary tissues. Second, the study showed major differences in the expression and activation of signalling molecules between primary tumors and metastases as only a subset of signalling pathways detected in primary tumors were present in the corresponding metastases (Fig. 1). Only 11 of the 25 proteins analyzed correlated between primary tumor and corresponding metastasis providing evidence for the theory that determination of proteins and pathways deregulated during metastases might serve as therapeutic target inhibition in this step of cancer progression. Third, we could demonstrate co-overexpression of snail in the primary tumor and p-p38$^{(Thr180/Tyr181)}$ in the corresponding metastasis correlates significantly with poorer patient survival [24].

Our data show the high feasibility of the RPPA methodology to analyze large numbers of proteins from formalin-fixed tumor material and to quantify changes in tumor biology during metastasis. Thus RPPA is very promising tool for future studies taking into account small amounts of sample (e.g., from biopsies) and often only subtle changes in protein expression (especially phosphoproteins) when comparing different disease states or therapy settings. Here we provide detailed protocols for protein extraction from FFPE material in combination with RPPA that can be used to characterize deregulated signalling pathways in ovarian cancer patients.

Table 1
Primary antibodies used in the study of ovarian cancer by RPPA

Antibody against (provider)	Blocking	Dilution Prim. Antibody	Dilution solution
β-Actin; AC-15 (Sigma Aldrich)	5 % MP/TBST	1:5,000	5 % MP/TBST
Phospho-AKT (Ser473); #9271 (New England Biolabs)	5 % MP/TBST	1:1,000	5 % BSA/TBST
AKT; #4691 (New England Biolabs)	5 % MP/TBST	1:1,000	5 % BSA/TBST
Cytokeratin 18; #4548 (New England Biolabs)	5 % MP/TBST	1:1,000	5 % BSA/TBST
E-Cadherin; Clone 36 (AEC) (BD Biosciences)	5 % MP/TBST	1:10,000	5 % MP/TBST
Phospho-ERα (Ser118); #2511 (New England Biolabs)	5 % MP/TBST	1:1,000	5 % MP/TBST
ERα; 578–595 (Sigma Aldrich)	5 % MP/TBST	1:3,000	TBST
Phospho-EGFR (Tyr1086); ZMD.504 (Invitrogen)	5 % MP/TBST	1:5,000	5 % BSA/TBST
EGFR; #2232 (New England Biolabs)	5 % MP/TBST	1:100	5 % BSA/TBST
Phospho-ERK1/2 (Thr202/Tyr204); #9101 (New England Biolabs)	5 % MP/TBST	1:1,000	5 % BSA/TBST
ERK1/2; #9102 (New England Biolabs)	5 % MP/TBST	1:1,000	5 % BSA/TBST
Phospho-GSK3β; #9336 (New England Biolabs)	5 % MP/TBST	1:1,000	5 % BSA/TBST
GSK-3β; #9315 (New England Biolabs)	5 % MP/TBST	1:1,000	5 % BSA/TBST
Phospho-Her2 (Tyr1248); #44-900 (Invitrogen)	5 % MP/TBST	1:1,000	5 % BSA/TBST
Her2; A0485 (DakoCytomation)	5 % MP/TBST	1:1,000	TBST
Histone H3; #9715 (New England Biolabs)	5 % MP/TBST	1:5,000	5 % BSA/TBST
Phospho-HSP 27 (Ser82); #2401 (New England Biolabs)	5 % MP/TBST	1:1,000	5 % BSA/TBST
HSP 27; #2402 (New England Biolabs)	5 % MP/TBST	1:1,000	5 % MP/TBST
Phospho-p38; (Thr180/Tyr182); #4631 (New England Biolabs)	5 % MP/TBST	1:1,000	5 % BSA/TBST
p38; #9212 (New England Biolabs)	5 % MP/TBST	1:1,000	5 % BSA/TBST
Phospho-PAK1 (Thr212); PK-18 (Sigma Aldrich)	5 % MP/TBST	1:1,000	5 % MP/TBST
PAK1; #2602 (New England Biolabs)	5 % MP/TBST	1:1,000	5 % BSA/TBST
PTEN; #9552 (New England Biolabs)	5 % MP/TBST	1:1,000	5 % BSA/TBST
Snail; 9H2 (Dr. Kremmer, München, Germany [27])	5 % MP/TBST	1:2,500	5 % MP/TBST
Phospho-STAT3 (Tyr705); #9145 (New England Biolabs)	5 % MP/TBST	1:1,000	5 % BSA/TBST
STAT-3; #4904 (New England Biolabs)	5 % MP/TBST	1:1,000	5 % BSA/TBST
α-Tubulin; DM1A (Sigma Aldrich)	5 % MP/TBST	1:5,000	5 % MP/TBST
Vimentin; V9 (DakoCytomation)	5 % MP/TBST	1:1,000	5 % MP/TBST

MP milk powder, *TBST* tris buffered saline plus Tween100 (0.1 %), *BSA* bovine serum albumine

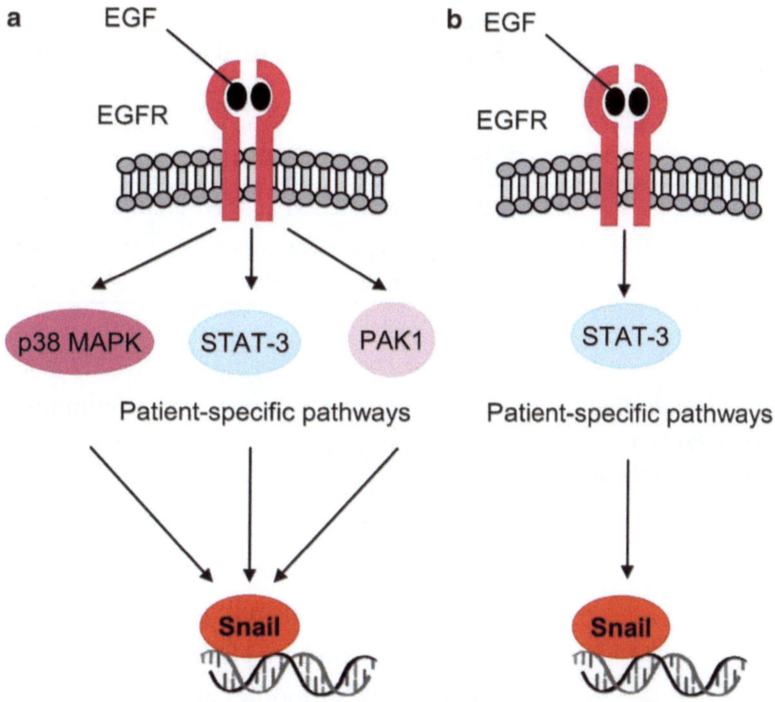

Fig. 1 Schematic overview of the deregulated pathways we found in primary tumors and metastases. EGFR dependent activation of snail in primary tumors (**a**) and metastases (**b**)

2 Materials

2.1 Deparaffinization of and Protein Extraction from Slide-Mounted FFPE Sections

1. Ethanol or isopropanol, 100 % (v/v).
2. Ethanol, 70 % (v/v).
3. Ethanol, 96 % (v/v).
4. Qproteome FFPE Tissue Kit (Qiagen, Hilden, Germany); (*see* **Note 1**).
5. Xylene.
6. Collection tube sealing clip (e.g., from Eppendorf, Hamburg, Germany).
7. Glass slides.
8. Needles or blades.
9. Parafilm.
10. Staining dishes with proper slide holders.

2.2 Reverse Phase Protein Array (RPPA)

1. Qproteome FFPE Tissue Kit buffer (Qiagen, Hilden, Germany).
2. Microtiter plates (V-bottom).
3. Nitrocellulose covered glass slides.
4. Sealing foils for microtiter plates.

Table 2
Secondary antibodies used in the study of ovarian cancer by RPPA

Secondary Ab (provider)	Dilution Sec. Ab	Dilution solution
Anti-Mouse # A931 (GE Healthcare)	1: 10,000	5 % MP/TBST
Anti-Rabbit # 7074 (New England Biolabs)	1: 2,000	5 % MP/TBST

2.3 Chemiluminescence Protein Detection on RPPA/Western Blot

1. Detection reagents for chemiluminescence.
2. TBST-buffer: 20 mM Tris–HCl, pH 7.4, 140 mM NaCl, 1 % (v/v) Tween-20.
3. Peroxidase blocking reagent (Dako, Glostrup, Denmark).
4. Blocking buffers (depending on antibodies used).
   (a) 5 % no fat milk powder in TBST (w/v).
   (b) 5 % BSA in TBST (w/v).
5. Primary antibodies against proteins of interest (for antibodies and dilution conditions *see* Table 1).
6. Reagents for film developing.
7. Secondary antibodies (for suggested secondary antibodies and dilution conditions *see* Table 2).
8. Sypro Ruby protein stain reagent.
9. 7 % acetic acid/10 % methanol in H_2O.
10. Films.
11. Sheet protector foils (clear and as thin as possible).

2.4 Equipment

1. Microtome.
2. Thermomixer.
3. Vortex mixer.
4. Shaker.
5. Water bath.
6. Centrifuge with plate-adapters.
7. Arrayer or alternative a handhold spotting device (for a detailed protocol using the latter *see* ref. [25]).
8. Autoradiography cassettes.
9. Cool room (4 °C) with shaker.
10. Darkroom with red-light.
11. Film developing machine.
12. Slide incubation chambers.

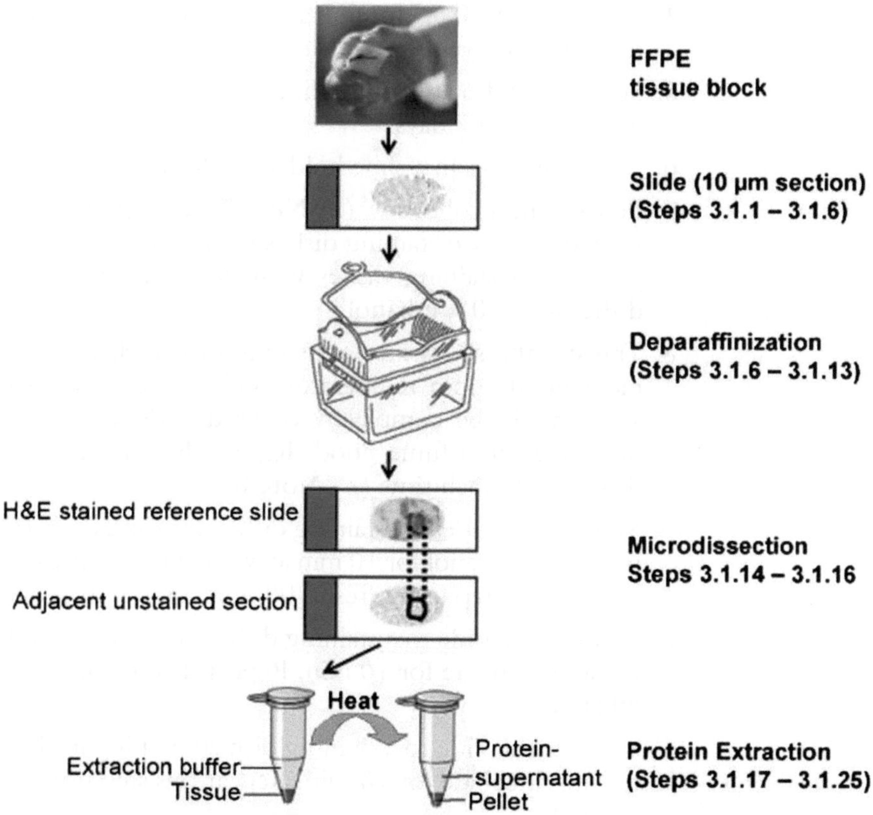

Fig. 2 Schematic overview of the extraction protocol used to prepare formalin-fixed and paraffin-embedded tissue samples of 23 patients with ovarian cancer for RPPA analysis

3 Methods

3.1 Deparaffinization of Slide-Mounted FFPE Sections and Protein Extraction

Here we provide a protocol for protein extraction from slide-mounted FFPE sections. Before starting with the actual extraction FFPE tissue blocks have to be cut, excessive paraffin has to be removed and the tissue area of interest must be transferred into the extraction buffer. Subsequently the proteins are extracted from the tissue in two heating steps. For an overview of the protein extraction procedure *see* Fig. 2.

1. Stain a 2 μm tissue section by a standard H&E protocol (*see* **Note 2**).
2. Let a pathologist identify the area of interest (*see* **Note 3**). We recommend a minimum of 85 % tumor cells to avoid measuring influences of "normal" or stroma cells.
3. Cut the number of sections you suppose to extract in 100 μl of extraction buffer using a microtome and place them on slides (*see* **Notes 4** and **5**).

4. Incubated at 50 °C for at least 4 h (you can keep them at this temperature for up to 16 h).
5. Store the slides at room temperature until further use but not for more than 7 days.
6. Place the slides in a slide holder (*see* **Note 6**).
7. Prepare the alcohol row (*see* **Note** 7). Use three staining dishes with xylene, two staining dishes with 100 % ethanol or isopropanol, two staining dishes with 96 % ethanol, two staining dishes with 70 % ethanol.
8. Transfer the slides into a staining dish with fresh xylene and incubate at room temperature (15–25 °C) for 10 min. The slide should be completely covered. Xylene washes must be performed in a fume hood. Repeat this staining twice, using fresh xylene each time (*see* **Note 8**).
9. Transfer the slide to a staining dish containing fresh 100 % ethanol or isopropanol for 10 min at room temperature (15–25 °C). Repeat this step using fresh 100 % ethanol or isopropanol.
10. Transfer the slide to a staining dish containing fresh 96 % ethanol and incubate for 10 min. Repeat this step using fresh 96 % ethanol.
11. Transfer the slide to a staining dish containing fresh 70 % ethanol and incubate for 10 min. Repeat this step using fresh 70 % ethanol.
12. Now all paraffin is removed and the slide can be transferred to a staining dish containing fresh distilled water and immerse for 30 s (Slides may stay in water for up to 3 h at RT, if protein extraction is not possible after deparaffinization).
13. Remove the first slide from water dish and eliminate excess water by tapping the slide carefully on a paper towel. Do not touch the section with the paper towel and ensure that sections do not dry out.
14. Place the corresponding HE-stained slide behind the deparaffinized slide. The sections on both slides should be arranged in the same position.
15. Excise area of interest on the deparaffinized slide according to the marked HE-stained slide. This is done best with a needle or a blade. Transfer the procured cells to a 1.5 ml collection tube containing one volume (preferably 100 μl) of chilled extraction buffer, briefly vortex and kept on ice (*see* **Note 9**).
16. Steps 13–15 must be repeated for each sample you want to extract.
17. After a final vortexing step seal the collection tube with a parafilm and with a collection tube sealing clip additionally.
18. Incubate on ice for another 15 min and mix by vortexing.

19. Cook the samples at 100 °C for 20 min (we recommend using a water bath).
20. Incubate the tube at 80 °C for 2 h with agitation at 750 rpm, using a Thermomixer.
21. Place the samples at 4 °C for 1 min and remove sealing.
22. Centrifuge at 14,000 × *g* and 4 °C for 15 min, then transfer the supernatant containing extracted proteins to a new 1.5 ml collection tube.
23. If desired, the protein concentration can be determined (*see* **Notes 10** and **11**).
24. To assure quality of the lysates we recommend testing of protein integrity in at least one sample of each extraction batch by a β-actin western blot. We usually test about 10 % of the samples in each study collective.
25. The extracted proteins can be stored at −20 °C for up to 1 week. For long-term storage, aliquot the extracted proteins and store at −80 °C (*see* **Note 12**). Avoid repeated freeze–thaw cycles.

3.2 Spotting

We normally use the BioOdyssey™ Calligrapher™ MiniArrayer (Bio-Rad, Munich, Germany) to generate our arrays, but this can also be done with more advanced arrayers (e.g., from Aushon BioSystems, Inc.) or for fewer samples by a handhold device (e.g., MicroCaster Arrayer from Whatman). For an overview of the spotting procedure with a handhold device *see* [25]. The following protocol for sample preparation and spotting is adapted to the use of an eight pin spotting device and must be adjusted if other numbers of pins are used. For an overview of the methodology *see* Fig. 3.

3.2.1 Sample Preparation

To guaranty measurement of protein amounts in the linear dynamic range of the according antibody we prepare our samples in fivefold dilution curves plus buffer spot as negative control. Additionally, we spot our samples in triplicates to account for technical variations and possible loss of single spots.

1. Thaw protein extracts on ice and mix them by vortexing.
2. To avoid saturation and unspecific artifacts, dilute the lysates in the extraction buffer (undiluted, 1:2, 1:4, 1:8, and 1:16); the final volume for spotting should be more than 5 μl in each well.
3. Arrange the lysates on a 384-well plate on ice, in a special order according to the arrangement of spotting pins in the pin-head. We place four undiluted samples next to each other in wells 1–4, then dilution 1:2 in wells 5–8, 1:4 in wells 9–12, 1:8 in wells 13–16, and 1:16 in wells 17–20. Each dilution-series ends with one well of buffer as negative control (wells 21–24).

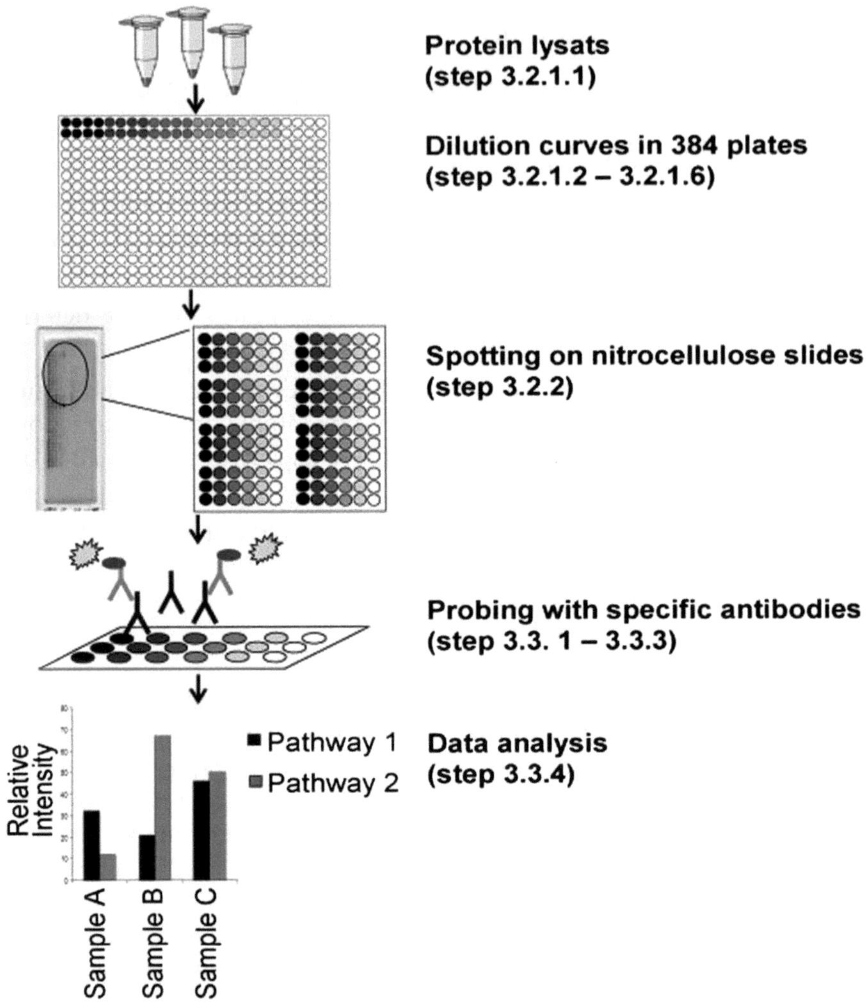

Fig. 3 Schematic overview of the spotting procedure by which samples are prepared for final analysis of protein expression. Samples are diluted in a sixfold dilution curve (undiluted, 1:2, 1:4, 1:8, 1:16, buffer spot) and blotted in three replicates onto a nitrocellulose covered glass slide

4. Seal the plate with a foil.
5. Centrifuge at 4 °C and about 900 × *g* for 1–2 min (to get rid of air bubbles).
6. Keep the plate on ice until use.

3.2.2 Spotting Procedure

Put your source plate and the desired number of nitrocellulose covered glass slides to be spotted into the machine and start program (*see* **Note 13**). Slides can be stored at 4 °C for up to 12 month. For longer storage some groups suggest to store the slides at −80 °C.

3.3 Chemiluminescence Protein Detection on RPMA

We recommend the staining of one of the spotted slides with Sypro Ruby for normalization (*see* **Notes 14** and **15**).

3.3.1 Estimation of Total Protein with Sypro Ruby Staining

1. Take slide from 4 °C storage and pre-wet it briefly in TBST-buffer.
2. After discarding the TBST-buffer, incubate the slide in a solution of 7 % acetic acid and 10 % methanol for 15 min in a staining dish with gentle agitation.
3. Wash in four changes of deionized water for 5 min each.
4. Incubate the slide in Sypro Ruby stain reagent for 10–15 min in a staining dish with gentle agitation.
5. Wash the slide four to six times for 1 min each in deionized water.
6. Visualize the staining on an imaging system and save file as .tif.
7. Analyze, e.g. with MicroVigene software (VigeneTech, Carlisle, US) according to the company instructions.

3.3.2 Incubating Slides with Antibodies

1. Take slides from 4 °C storage and pre-wet them shortly (up to RT) in TBST-buffer by gently shaking in an incubation chamber on a shaker or rocker (*see* **Notes 15** and **16**).
2. Discard the TBST-buffer and pour peroxidase blocking reagent on the slides completely covering them and shake them gently for 1 h at room temperature.
3. Wash three times with TBST-buffer for 2 min each.
4. Incubate the slides in the blocking buffer suitable for the antibody of choice (Table 1).
5. Shake gently at room temperature for at least 1 h.
6. Incubate the slides with the primary antibody at 4 °C over night (16 h), while gently shaking (Table 1).

3.3.3 Signal Detection

1. Wash three times for 10 min each in TBST-buffer at room temperature.
2. Incubate the slide with the secondary antibody for 1 h at room temperature shaking gently (Table 2).
3. Wash three times with TBST-buffer for 10 min each, while shaking at room temperature.
4. Take the slides out of the incubation chamber and remove excess TBST-buffer from the slides but be careful not to let them dry completely!
5. Place the slides on a glass plate and pour the detection reagent directly on top of the slides (app. 500 μl per slide); incubate for 5 min at room temperature (*see* **Note 17**).
6. Remove the detection reagent, cover the slides with protector foil, and put it in an autoradiography cassette.

7. Apply films for different exposure times in the dark. The optimal exposure period depends on various factors, like the antibody used, but 1 min should be a good starting time.
8. Develop the films (by hand or using a developing machine).

3.3.4 Analysis

1. Scan the slides individually on a scanner with at least 600 dpi and save them as .tif.
2. Analyze with freeware like ScionImage (Scion Corporation, Frederick, USA) or use commercial software packages, e.g., MicroVigene (VigeneTech, Carlisle, USA) according to the company instructions.
3. Normalize to total protein (Sypro Ruby detection, *see* Subheading 3.3, **step 1**).

4 Notes

1. Here we describe how to extract proteins from FFPE tissue employing the commercially available Qproteome FFPE Tissue Kit (Qiagen, Hilden, Germany). But during the last few years several protocols for protein extraction from FFPE tissue have been established. For an overview *see* ref. [10].
2. This protocol describes how to use a particular area of a tissue slide (e.g., tumor area). If you are interested in extracting proteins from the whole slide, Subheading 3.1, **step 1–2** and **14** may be skipped.
3. The size of this area will be important to determine the number of necessary slides per volume of extraction buffer. It emerged that the buffer volume should be around 100 μl to obtain highest protein yields. The amount of tissue which can be extracted is depending on various factors, like tissue type and cell density. But to give an approximate value: For an area of about 0.5 cm in diameter use 100 μl of the buffer.
4. We recommend using 10 μm sections. Paraffin may be more difficult to remove from thicker sections. Although using double amount of 5 μm sections may increase the protein yield we would recommend this only for very small areas like, e.g., biopsies because this will be more time and material consuming.
5. If you want to mark your slides, the pen has to be xylene and ethanol resistant (you may use a pencil).
6. For large amounts of slides it could save time and reagents to place the slides crisscross in the holder.

   Additionally you may mount two sections of one block on the same slide to save time.
7. The alcohol series has to be renewed after 5 cycles to guarantee correct concentrations of the reagents.

8. If processing samples containing large amounts of paraffin, repeat the xylene treatment two more times.
9. We use unstained slides as histological stains can decrease the yield of the extracted proteins. The decrease depends on the kind of dye used and on the staining time. When a 10 s hematoxylin (Mayer) staining protocol is used for example the protein yield drops to about 50 % compared to unstained tissue. You get out even less by using Fast Red and many stainings did not work at all: methyl blue, hematoxylin (Gil), for instance [26].
10. Which quantification method is best, depends on the used buffer. Before use check the compatibility of the chosen method. For Qproteome FFPE Tissue Kit buffer protein yield can be measured by the Lowry (e.g., Protein Assay Kit, Bio-Rad) or BCA method (e.g., Micro BCA Protein Assay Kit, Pierce).
11. The following reasons may account for low protein yields:
    (a) Poor quality of starting material. Samples that were fixed for over 24 h or stored for very long periods may allow only incomplete extraction of protein.
    (b) Too little starting material. Increase the amount of starting material.
    (c) Insufficient deparaffinization or too much paraffin in sample. If you are processing samples containing large amounts of paraffin, repeat the xylene treatment an additional two times. Paraffin may be more difficult to remove from thicker sections (we recommend using 10 μm sections).
12. We use 96-well FluidX-Plates for storage of our samples. These minimize evaporation effects by good sealing of the tubes (better than normal reaction tubes), it is possible to take out single samples and the plates can be put directly into our pipetting device for generation of dilution curves.
13. Comments on spotting: Humidity can be an issue during spotting. We recommend a humidity of 50–60 % to obtain optimal results. During long runs samples might evaporate so it can be helpful to split sample into smaller groups to avoid long exposure times in the spotter.
14. This slide is needed during analysis for normalization of the antibody signals. Theoretically the most adequate way of normalization would be to stain each slide with Sypro Ruby before applying the first antibody and normalize to intern total protein in every case. There are two practical reasons anyway for using only one or a few of the spotted slides. First some antibodies do not give proper signals when used on a previously Sypro Ruby stained slide and second if you have large numbers of slides the staining will get really expensive soon.

15. Sypro Ruby staining does not work in combination with some commercially available cell extraction buffers. In such cases you get very strong background staining in the buffer spots and total protein concentrations can not be evaluated. In such cases normalization to at least two house keeping proteins (e.g., b-actin and tubulin) or usage of an alternative dye for total protein (e.g., Fastgreen FCF) can be an alternative approach.
16. As an incubation chamber Heraeus Quadriperm can be used. Using this unit only 3 ml of antibody dilution and peroxidise blocking reagent are needed.
17. Mixing ECLplus and ECLadvance combines advantages of both solutions: stronger and long-lasting signals.

References

1. Mueller C, Liotta LA, Espina V (2010) Reverse phase protein microarrays advance to use in clinical trials. Mol Oncol 4(6):461–481
2. Addis MF, Tanca A, Pagnozzi D, Crobu S, Fanciulli G, Cossu-Rocca P, Uzzau S (2009) Generation of high-quality protein extracts from formalin-fixed, paraffin-embedded tissues. Proteomics 9(15):3815–3823
3. Becker KF, Schott C, Hipp S, Metzger V, Porschewski P, Beck R, Nahrig J, Becker I, Hofler H (2007) Quantitative protein analysis from formalin-fixed tissues: implications for translational clinical research and nanoscale molecular diagnosis. J Pathol 211(3): 370–378
4. Crockett DK, Lin Z, Vaughn CP, Lim MS, Elenitoba-Johnson KS (2005) Identification of proteins from formalin-fixed paraffin-embedded cells by LC-MS/MS. Lab Invest 85(11):1405–1415
5. Ikeda K, Monden T, Kanoh T, Tsujie M, Izawa H, Haba A, Ohnishi T, Sekimoto M, Tomita N, Shiozaki H, Monden M (1998) Extraction and analysis of diagnostically useful proteins from formalin-fixed, paraffin-embedded tissue sections. J Histochem Cytochem 46(3): 397–403
6. Nirmalan NJ, Harnden P, Selby PJ, Banks RE (2009) Development and validation of a novel protein extraction methodology for quantitation of protein expression in formalin-fixed paraffin-embedded tissues using western blotting. J Pathol 217(4):497–506
7. Palmer-Toy DE, Krastins B, Sarracino DA, Nadol JB Jr, Merchant SN (2005) Efficient method for the proteomic analysis of fixed and embedded tissues. J Proteome Res 4(6): 2404–2411
8. Sage L (2005) Proteomics gets out of a fix. J Proteome Res 4(6):1903–1904
9. Shi SR, Liu C, Balgley BM, Lee C, Taylor CR (2006) Protein extraction from formalin-fixed, paraffin-embedded tissue sections: quality evaluation by mass spectrometry. J Histochem Cytochem 54(6):739–743
10. Berg D, Hipp S, Malinowsky K, Bollner C, Becker KF (2010) Molecular profiling of signalling pathways in formalin-fixed and paraffin-embedded cancer tissues. Eur J Cancer 46(1):47–55
11. Schuster C, Malinowsky K, Liebmann S, Berg D, Wolff C, Tran K, Schott C, Reu S, Neumann J, Faber C, Hofler H, Kirchner T, Becker KF, Hlubek F (2012) Antibody validation by combining immunohistochemistry and protein extraction from formalin-fixed paraffin-embedded tissues. Histopathology 60(6B): E37–E50
12. Ferlay J, Shin HR, Bray F, Forman D, Mathers C, Parkin DM (2010) Estimates of worldwide burden of cancer in 2008: GLOBOCAN 2008. Int J Cancer 127(12):2893–2917
13. Vergara D, Merlot B, Lucot JP, Collinet P, Vinatier D, Fournier I, Salzet M (2010) Epithelial-mesenchymal transition in ovarian cancer. Cancer Lett 291(1):59–66
14. Sheehan KM, Calvert VS, Kay EW, Lu Y, Fishman D, Espina V, Aquino J, Speer R, Araujo R, Mills GB, Liotta LA, Petricoin EF 3rd, Wulfkuhle JD (2005) Use of reverse phase protein microarrays and reference standard development for molecular network analysis of metastatic ovarian carcinoma. Mol Cell Proteomics 4(4):346–355
15. Geho DH, Bandle RW, Clair T, Liotta LA (2005) Physiological mechanisms of tumor-cell

invasion and migration. Physiology (Bethesda) 20:194–200
16. Thompson EW, Newgreen DF, Tarin D (2005) Carcinoma invasion and metastasis: a role for epithelial-mesenchymal transition? Cancer Res 65(14):5991–5995, discussion 5
17. Ahmed N, Maines-Bandiera S, Quinn MA, Unger WG, Dedhar S, Auersperg N (2006) Molecular pathways regulating EGF-induced epithelio-mesenchymal transition in human ovarian surface epithelium. Am J Physiol Cell Physiol 290(6):C1532–C1542
18. Ahmed N, Thompson EW, Quinn MA (2007) Epithelial-mesenchymal interconversions in normal ovarian surface epithelium and ovarian carcinomas: an exception to the norm. J Cell Physiol 213(3):581–588
19. Bagnato A, Rosano L (2007) Epithelial-mesenchymal transition in ovarian cancer progression: a crucial role for the endothelin axis. Cells Tissues Organs 185(1–3):85–94
20. Blechschmidt K, Sassen S, Schmalfeldt B, Schuster T, Hofler H, Becker KF (2008) The E-cadherin repressor Snail is associated with lower overall survival of ovarian cancer patients. Br J Cancer 98(2):489–495
21. Elloul S, Silins I, Trope CG, Benshushan A, Davidson B, Reich R (2006) Expression of E-cadherin transcriptional regulators in ovarian carcinoma. Virchows Arch 449(5): 520–528
22. Imai T, Horiuchi A, Wang C, Oka K, Ohira S, Nikaido T, Konishi I (2003) Hypoxia attenuates the expression of E-cadherin via up-regulation of SNAIL in ovarian carcinoma cells. Am J Pathol 163(4):1437–1447
23. Larue L, Bellacosa A (2005) Epithelial-mesenchymal transition in development and cancer: role of phosphatidylinositol 3' kinase/AKT pathways. Oncogene 24(50): 7443–7454
24. Hipp S, Berg D, Ergin B, Schuster T, Hapfelmeier A, Walch A, Avril S, Schmalfeldt B, Hofler H, Becker KF (2010) Interaction of snail and p38 mitogen-activated protein kinase results in shorter overall survival of ovarian cancer patients. Virchows Arch 457(6):705–713
25. Wolff C, Schott C, Malinowsky K, Berg D, Becker KF (2011) Producing reverse phase protein microarrays from formalin-fixed tissues. Methods Mol Biol 785:123–140
26. Becker K, Schott C, Becker I, Höfler H (2008) Guided protein extraction from formalin-fixed tissues for quantitative multiplex analysis avoids detrimental effects of histological stains. Proteomics Clin Appl 2:737–743
27. Rosivatz E, Becker KF, Kremmer E, Schott C, Blechschmidt K, Hofler H, Sarbia M (2006) Expression and nuclear localization of snail, an E-cadherin repressor, in adenocarcinomas of the upper gastrointestinal tract. Virchows Arch 448(3):277–287

Chapter 22

N-Glycosylation Analysis by HPAEC-PAD and Mass Spectrometry

Sebastian Kandzia and Júlia Costa

Abstract

Changes in protein glycosylation are a hallmark of most types of cancer including ovarian carcinoma. The structural elucidation of glycans is technically challenging and it requires complementary chromatographic and spectroscopic techniques among others. Here, we describe the profiling of *N*-glycans from glycoproteins of SKOV3 ovarian carcinoma cells by high-performance anion exchange chromatography with pulsed amperometric detection (HPAEC-PAD) and matrix-assisted laser desorption/ionization with time-of-flight mass spectrometry (MALDI-TOF MS). Mass spectrometry as a complementary method enables precise mass determination of *N*-glycan mixtures thus corroborating data obtained from HPAEC-PAD mapping in conjunction with reference oligosaccharide structures.

Key words Ovarian carcinoma, Protein glycosylation, HPAEC-PAD, MALDI-TOF MS, Peptide *N*-glycosidase F, Complex *N*-glycans, High mannose *N*-glycans

1 Introduction

A hallmark of tumor cell phenotype consists of changes in glycosylation of cell surface glycoproteins. These changes include both the under- and overexpression of naturally occurring glycan structures, as well as neo-expression of glycans normally restricted to embryonic tissues. Ovarian carcinoma is the leading cause of death from gynecological cancers in many Western countries. At present the used biomarker is the mucin CA125 but its use is limited due to lack of sensitivity and specificity [1]. In addition, changes in glycosylation have also been found in ovarian carcinoma cells [2]. Therefore, the detailed structure analysis of glycans from glycoconjugates within the field of Glycomics constitutes a valuable strategy for the identification, characterization, and quantification of novel glycan structures associated with ovarian cancer. This knowledge may lead to the development of novel diagnostic and/or therapeutic tools.

Anastasia Malek and Oleg Tchernitsa (eds.), *Ovarian Cancer: Methods and Protocols*, Methods in Molecular Biology, vol. 1049, DOI 10.1007/978-1-62703-547-7_22, © Springer Science+Business Media New York 2013

In this chapter, we describe the following techniques: high-performance anion exchange chromatography with pulsed amperometric detection (HPAEC-PAD) and direct matrix-assisted laser desorption ionization with time-of-flight mass spectrometry (MALDI-TOF MS) applied to the profiling and structure elucidation of *N*-glycans released from glycoproteins of the human SKOV3 ovarian carcinoma cell line.

HPAEC-PAD is a high-performance liquid chromatography (HPLC) method that uses pellicular ion-exchange resins at high pH for glycan (monosaccharides and oligosaccharides) separation. Glycans are detected by an electrochemical method, the pulsed amperometric detection, at the picomole range, without the requirement of derivatization [3]. The separation of oligosaccharides is achieved at alkaline pH and under these conditions the hydroxyl groups of monosaccharide constituents are ionized to their oxyanions. Separation is based on which hydroxyl groups are ionized and their accessibility to the quaternary amine of the stationary phase. At high pH the overall acidity of reducing oligosaccharides is primarily from oxyanion formation at the anomeric hydroxyl, the 2-OH groups of pyranosides, and the 3-OH groups of the *N*-acetylglucosamine (GlcNAc) residues. The importance of accessibility is observed with fucosylated compounds, which are less retained as compared to their non-fucosylated structures [4]. Many positional isomers of *N*-glycans are well separated by high-resolution HPAEC-PAD [3].

The quantification of oligosaccharides is an important issue and can be performed using the pulsed amperometric detection. A given structure has a characteristic electrochemical response that may be calculated and used for mol% quantification of this specific structure within a mixture of oligosaccharides in conjunction with defined reference glycans analyzed in the same analytical sequence.

HPAEC-PAD is a technique that allows the rapid and sensitive mapping of N-linked oligosaccharides from glycoproteins or individual protein glycosylation sites thereof. In addition, separated glycans can be collected and digested using various specific exoglycosidases and re-analyzed and/or subjected to various mass spectrometry analysis techniques.

Mass spectrometry techniques are widely used for mass profiling and structure determination of glycans [5–7]. Matrix-assisted laser desorption ionization mass spectrometry (MALDI-MS) is a robust technique and is suitable for the analysis of molecules with large molecular masses and has a high sensitivity for neutral glycans complementing, e.g., chromatographic oligosaccharide mapping. For MALDI ionization the sample is dried in the presence of an ultraviolet absorbing matrix of low molecular weight, forming crystals containing the glycans to be analyzed [8]. The matrix absorbs radiation from a laser (e.g., nitrogen laser radiation of 337 nm) and transfers energy to the glycans, which are ionized and, in positive mode, are detected as pseudomolecular ions $[M+H]^+$, $[M+Na]^+$, or $[M+K]^+$. Addition of small amounts of sodium ions into the matrix improves the quality of spectra by suppressing the detection of multiple other alkali ion adducts than sodiated ions. Alternatively CsCl can be added whereby both $[M+Na]^+$ and $[M+K]^+$ adducts are converted into $[M+Cs]^+$ ions. MALDI sources are often linked to time-of-flight analyzers.

Since peptides and detergents interfere with the MALDI-MS analysis, careful selection of purification procedures of the glycan samples is important in order to avoid ion suppression. Oligosaccharide profiling of native glycans (as isolated after HPAEC-PAD separation) can also be performed with liquid chromatography electrospray ionization LC-ESI-MS (neutral glycans and charged forms, e.g., sialylated, sulfated or phosphorylated variants).

Mass spectrometric techniques alone or in combination with liquid chromatography techniques have been largely used to analyze protein glycosylation changes as markers of disease. For example, HPAEC-PAD in combination with MALDI-TOF MS have been used to monitor modifications in glycosylation of beta-trace protein in congenital disorder of glycosylation Ia [9]. In the context of ovarian carcinoma, this methodology allowed the identification of the LacdiNAc structure in the *N*-glycans of secreted glycoproteins from the SKOV3 ovarian carcinoma cell line. The LacdiNAc may constitute a potential novel marker of ovarian carcinoma [10].

2 Materials

Prepare all solutions using MilliQ water (18 mΩ) and analytical grade reagents. Prepare and store all reagents at room temperature (unless indicated otherwise). Wear powder-free gloves.

2.1 N-Glycan Isolation, Desialylation, and Desalting

1. 10×PNGase F (peptide *N*-glycosidase F) buffer: 0.5 M NaH_2PO_4, 0.1 M EDTA, pH 7.5.

   Weigh 39.0 g $NaH_2PO_4 \times 2\ H_2O$ and 18.6 g Na-EDTA, transfer it in a 500 mL beaker and dissolve it in water (ca. 400 mL) with stirring. Adjust to pH 7.5 by using 50 % NaOH (ca.15 mL). Transfer the solution in a 500 mL measuring flask and adjust with water to a volume of 500 mL and filter through a 0.2-μm filter into a 500 mL bottle. Store at 20 °C.

2. 1×PNGase F buffer: 50 mM NaH_2PO_4, 10 mM EDTA, pH 7.5.

   Transfer 25 mL of the 10×PNGase F buffer pH 7.5 into a 250 mL measuring cylinder. Add water (150 mL), mix, adjust to pH 7.5 using 50 mM NaH_2PO_4 (ca. 23 mL) and add water to a volume of 250 mL.

3. Ammonium acetate buffer: 100 mM ammonium acetate, pH 5.0.

   Weigh 0.771 g ammonium acetate, transfer into a 250 mL beaker, dissolve in ≈80 mL of water, adjust pH to 5.0 with 1.2 mL of the 20 % acetic acid, transfer into a 100 mL measuring flask and fill up to 100 mL with water.

4. Solution 20 % (v/v) of the acetic acid.

   Fill 30 mL water in a 50 mL measuring flask, add carefully 10 mL acetic acid by using a graduated pipette and fill up with water to a final volume of 50 mL. Store at 20 °C.

5. A working solution 5 % (v/v) of the neuraminidase from *Arthrobacter ureafaciens.*

   Dilute an appropriate amount of enzyme (Roche, Manheim, Germany; usually 0.5 μL = 5 mU per digest) with 100 mM ammonium acetate solution, pH 5.0. The working solution is stable for 24 h.

6. PNGase F (Roche).

7. Cartridge conditional solution (Subheading 3.1.4, **step 1**): 80 % (v/v) acetonitrile, 0.1 % trifluoroacetic acid.

8. Elution solution (Subheading 3.1.4, **step 3**): 40 % acetonitrile, 0.1 % trifluoroacetic acid.

9. Neutralizing solution (Subheading 3.1.4, **step 3**) NH_4OH 2.5 % in water (v/v).

10. Hypercarb tip conditional solution (Subheading 3.1.5, **step 2**): 80 % acetonitrile (Rotisolv HPLC Gradient Grade, Roth, Karlsruhe, Germany), 0.1 % TFA (Roth).

11. Elution solution (Subheading 3.1.5, **step 5**): Acetonitrile 20 % in water.

12. Benzonase (Sigma-Aldrich, Steinheim, Germany).

13. Trypsin (Merck, Darmstadt, Germany).

14. Complete protease inhibitor cocktail (Roche).

2.2 HPAEC-PAD Eluents

1. Eluent 0.1 M NaOH

   Degas 1.5 L MilliQ water, by bubbling helium, in a 2 L flask, for 10 min; add 10.5 mL 50 % NaOH (p.a., Baker, Deventer, The Netherlands); complete the 2 L volume with degassed MilliQ water; once in the eluent flask, degas for 15 min prior to use; keep at 20 °C; it is stable for a month (*see* **Note 1**).

2. Eluent 0.1 M NaOH/0.6 M sodium acetate.

   Weigh 98.4 g of sodium acetate (Sigma-Aldrich) and solubilize in 500 mL MilliQ water in a 1 L beaker; filter the solution (0.2 μm filter previously washed with MilliQ water) and transfer to a 2 L flask; add 10.5 mL 50 % NaOH; add degassed MilliQ water up to 2 L; once in the eluent flask, degas for 15 min prior to use; keep at 20 °C; it is stable for a month (*see* **Note 1**).

2.3 MALDI-TOF MS Matrix Solutions

1. Matrix preparation: Freshly prepare the 2,5-dihydroxybenzoic acid (DHB) matrix by suspending 1 mg of DHB in 0.1 mL of ethanol in ultrapure water (9:1 v/v) to produce 10 mg/mL matrix concentration.
2. Sample and matrix are mixed on the MALDI plate at a ratio of 1:1 (typically 1 μL each) and allowed to dry at room temperature.

2.4 Glycan Standards

1. Sialic acid reference standards commercially available *N*-acetylneuraminic acid and *N*-glycolylneuraminic acid (Calbiochem, Darmstadt, Germany).
2. Complex glycan standards are obtained from erythropoietin and characterized as described before [11].
3. All complex-type *N*-glycans of different antennarity including partially de-galactosylated structures and high mannose glycan standards are from TheraProteins Lda, Oeiras, Portugal (*see* **Note 2**).

2.5 Equipment, Supplies, and Software

1. SpeedVac concentrator.
2. Water bath.
3. Heating block.
4. Whatman GF/C filter.
5. Hypercarb columns.
6. Hypercarb cartridges (Thermoquest, Cat. No. 60106–304).
7. ICS-3000 ion chromatography system of Dionex Corporation (Sunnyvale, CA, USA), consisting of an AS autosampler, a DC detector/chromatography module, and a DP dual pump.
8. CarboPac PA200 guard column (3 × 50 mm, Dionex, Sunnyvale, CA, USA) and CarboPac PA200 analytical column (3 × 250 mm, Dionex, Sunnyvale, CA, USA).
9. Carbohydrate membrane desalter device (CMD 300; Dionex, Sunnyvale, CA, USA).
10. Bruker REFLEX time-of-flight (TOF) instrument equipped with a N_2-Laser (337 nm).
11. Chromeleon Chromatography Management System.
12. Bruker DataAnalysis for TOF.
13. Glyco-Peakfinder platform.

3 Methods

In Subheading 3.1, tryptic peptides of SKOV3 cells proteins are obtained (Subheading 3.1.1), and the corresponding *N*-glycans are enzymatically released with PNGase F (Subheading 3.1.2), desialylated (Subheading 3.1.3) and desalted either for HPAEC-PAD

(Subheading 3.1.4) or MALDI-TOF MS (Subheading 3.1.5) analyses. In Subheadings 3.2 and 3.3 the analyses of *N*-glycans by HPAEC-PAD and MALDI-TOF MS are described, respectively. Glycans may also be fractionated by HPAEC-PAD (Subheading 3.2) for subsequent analysis by MALDI-TOF MS.

3.1 N-Glycan Isolation, Desialylation, and Desalting

3.1.1 Tryptic Digestion of SKOV3 Glycoproteins

1. Centrifuge 4.2×10^7 cells (cell pellet from 3 T175 T-flasks) in PBS, 5 min at $500 \times g$. Add to the pellet 600 μL of 2 % NP40 in PBS pH 7.2 and 0.1 % of benzonase nuclease (200 units). Incubate 30 min at room temperature.
2. Precipitate proteins with 4 volumes of 100 % ethanol for 2 h at −20 °C.
3. Centrifuge the proteins at $10{,}000 \times g$, 10 min, and dry the pellet in a SpeedVac concentrator.
4. Dissolve the pellet in 600 μL of 0.3 M Tris–HCl pH 8.3 containing 6 M urea and 1 mM DTE and incubate for 90 min at room temperature, with occasional vortexing. Dilute to 1.4 mL with water.
5. Add 50 μg trypsin (5 μL of stock solution at 10 mg/mL; *see* **Note 3**) and 0.02 % Na-azide (2.8 μL of stock solution at 10 %). Incubate for 6–8 h at 37 °C. Add further 20 μg (2 μL) trypsin. Incubate overnight at 37 °C.
6. To inactivate the trypsin, incubate 10 min at 90 °C followed by cooling in ice. Add 28 μL of 100× Complete protease inhibitor cocktail solution and incubate for 1 h at room temperature.
7. Centrifuge at $10{,}000 \times g$, 10 min, at room temperature. Wash the pellet two more times with 400 μL of 1×cc PNGase F digestion buffer.
8. Apply the pooled supernatants over a 5 kDa vivaspin concentrator, washed previously with 1×cc PNGase F digestion buffer, and exchange the buffer to 1×cc PNGase F digestion buffer ($15{,}000 \times g$).
9. To clarify the glycopeptides, centrifuge 5 min at $10{,}000 \times g$, collect the supernatant and reextract the pellet with 200 μL 1×cc PNGase F buffer.

3.1.2 N-Glycan Release from SKOV3 Glycopeptides

1. *N*-Glycans are released with PNGase F from glycopeptides of SKOV3 cells obtained as described in Subheading 3.1.1. For that, prepare 135 μL of a glycopeptide solution (obtained from 150 μg of protein) by dilution with water and add 15 μL of 10×PNGase F buffer (*see* **Note 4**).
2. Add 5 U (5 μL) of PNGase F and incubate at 37 °C, for 2–3 h.
3. Add more 5 U (5 μL) of PNGase F.
4. After 8–14 h, add more 1.3 U (1.3 μL) of PNGase F (optional).

5. After 20 h, stop the digestion, e.g., via ethanol precipitation of the enzyme. Dry the supernatant in a SpeedVac concentrator and afterwards dissolve the glycans in water. If the oligosaccharides are to be further processed purify them with Hypercarb columns; otherwise store the sample at −20 °C until further use.

3.1.3 Desialylation of Native N-Glycans

Native *N*-glycans are desialylated either by mild acid hydrolysis (*see* **Note 5**) or by sialidase treatment. Acid hydrolysis is used for a fast preliminary analytical screening. For complete, though more time consuming, desialylation of native *N*-glycans digestion with *A. ureafaciens* neuraminidase (sialidase) is performed. It consists of the following steps:

1. Prepare the digestion mixture by combining the appropriate oligosaccharide amount (0.1–1 nmol in max. 25 μL in water) with 15 μL of the 100 mM ammonium acetate buffer pH 5.0 and 5 μL of *A. ureafaciens* neuraminidase working solution (5 %), fill up with water to a final volume of 45 μL. Then, incubate at 37 °C for 2 h in a water bath, add further 5 μL *A. ureafaciens* neuraminidase working solution (1:20), incubate at 37 °C for 2–12 h in a water bath.
2. Incubate at 95 °C for 15 min in a heating block (enzyme inactivation), incubate in an ice bath for 2 min, and centrifuge briefly (to spin down condensed water from the lid).
3. Dry in a SpeedVac concentrator (to remove a volatile interfering substance from the enzyme preparation) and resolubilize in water.
4. If required, further clean-up (removal of salts, etc.) can be achieved using Hypercarb columns as described in Subheadings 3.1.4 or 3.1.5. In this case most of the sialic acid is lost as well as sulfated and phosphorylated glycans (*See* **Note 6**).

3.1.4 Desalting/Purification of N-Glycans Before HPAEC-PAD

Before HPAEC-PAD analysis, *N*-glycans released from 100–250 μg of glycopeptides should be carefully desalted using 100 mg Hypercarb cartridges. The detailed procedure is as follows:

1. Cartridges are conditioned with 80 % (v/v) acetonitrile in 0.1 % trifluoroacetic acid and three times with water.
2. *N*-glycans solubilized in water are then loaded onto the column, followed by three washes with water.
3. The *N*-glycans from SKOV3 cells are eluted with 40 % acetonitrile in 0.1 % trifluoroacetic acid, neutralized with 2.5 % (v/v) NH_4OH and are dried in a SpeedVac concentrator.

3.1.5 Desalting/Purification of N-Glycans Before MALDI-MS

Before MALDI-MS analysis desialylated (neutral) oligosaccharides are desalted by using a micro Hypercarb-phase that removes contaminating salts and low molecular weight compounds such as peptides/detergents, which could interfere with mass spectrometric analysis or affect its reproducibility. Small amounts of samples to be analyzed by MALDI-TOF MS must be co-crystallized in the matrix, which can be impaired by impurities. In addition the presence of several cations (Na^+, K^+, Ca^{2+}) lead to detection of multiple pseudomolecular ions in spectra. Micro Hypercarb desalting enables the cleaning up of 1–100 pmol quantities of oligosaccharides. The detailed procedure is as follows:

1. 5–30 μL of the material from a Hypercarb cartridge are manually filled into a 200 μL pipette tip which contains a small piece of a Whatman GF/C filter.
2. Conditioning: 100 μL of an 80 % acetonitrile (Rotisolv HPLC Gradient Grade, Roth, Cat. No. 8825.2)/0.1 % TFA (Roth, Cat. No. P088.1) solution is filtered through the micro Hypercarb tip. Subsequently, the Hypercarb tip is washed with 3–4× each 100 μL of ultrapure water; the pH of the final wash step is checked and should be pH 4–7.
3. Sample application: the sample is applied (100 μL volume) by air pressure using an appropriate syringe.
4. The loaded micro-tip is washed 3 × with each 100 μL of water (*see* **Note 7**).
5. Oligosaccharides are eluted from a 30 μL Hypercarb micro-tip with 150 μL of 20 % acetonitrile in water (*see* **Note 8**).
6. The eluted oligosaccharides are dried in a SpeedVac concentrator and dissolved in 1–40 μL of water and can be stored at −20 °C until further analysis.

3.2 Analysis of Desialylated N-Glycans by HPAEC-PAD

1. The analysis of *N*-glycan structures through HPAEC-PAD was performed using an ICS-3000 ion chromatography system of Dionex Corporation (Sunnyvale, CA, USA), consisting of an AS autosampler, a DC detector/chromatography module, and a DP dual pump. The software used for instrument control is Chromeleon. Loop of injection is 50 μL.
2. A 20 μL sample is injected into an equilibrated CarboPac PA200 guard column (3 × 50 mm, Dionex, Sunnyvale, CA, USA) which is connected to a CarboPac PA200 column (3 × 250 mm, Dionex, Sunnyvale, CA, USA) (*see* **Note 9**).
3. Elute the *N*-glycans by using the following concentration gradient of 0.1 M sodium hydroxide (A) and 0.1 M sodium hydroxide/0.6 M sodium acetate at a constant flow rate of 0.4 mL/min and at 30 °C column temperature: $t1 = 0$ min, $A = 100$ %; $t2 = 11$ min, $A = 99.2$ %; $t3 = 22$ min, $A = 95.5$ %; $t4 = 36$ min, $A = 82$ %; $t5 = 45$ min, $A = 70$ %; $t6 = 47$ min, $A = 0$ %; $t7 = 52$ min, $A = 0$ %; $t8 = 53$ min, $A = 100$ %; and $t9 = 60$ min, $A = 100$ %.

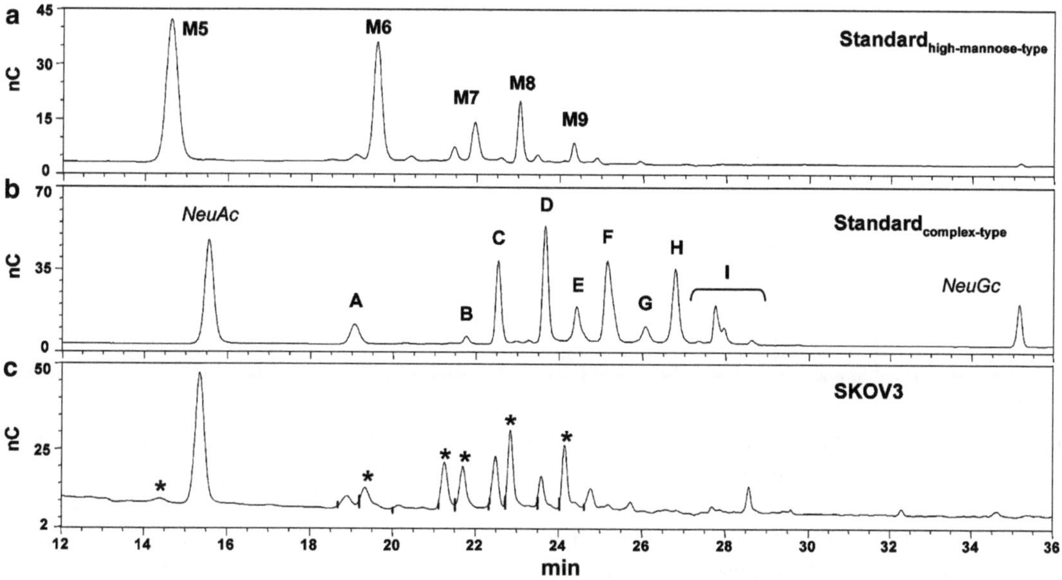

Fig. 1 HPAEC-PAD analysis of the desialylated *N*-glycans released from SKOV3 cells. (**a**) High mannose glycan standards from RNase B, structures are M5, $Man_5GlcNAc_2$; M6, $Man_6GlcNAc_2$; M7, $Man_7GlcNAc_2$; M8, $Man_8GlcNAc_2$; M9, $Man_9GlcNAc_2$. (**b**) Complex reference glycan standards from erythropoietin from CHO cells, structures (all proximally α6-fucosylated) are A, diantennary; B, 2,4-triantennary; C, 2,6-triantennary; D, tetraantennary; E, triantennary + one LacNAc repeat; F, tetraantennary + one LacNAc repeat; G, triantennary + two LacNAc repeats; H, tetraantennary + two LacNAc repeats; I, triantennary + three LacNAc repeats and tetraantennary + three LacNAc repeats. (**c**) Total *N*-glycans of SKOV3 cells. *Asterisks* indicate high mannose glycans with 5–9 mannose residues assigned based on retention time and MALDI-TOF MS analysis of the corresponding fractions collected after online desalting (reproduced from Machado with permission from Oxford University Press). GlcNAc, *N*-acetylglucosamine; Man, mannose; LacNAc, *N*-acetylactosamine

4. The electrochemical detection of the oligosaccharides is performed by application of the subsequent detection potentials (E) and durations (t): $E1 = 50$ mV, $t1 = 400$ ms; $E2 = 750$ mV, $t2 = 200$ ms; and $E3 = -150$ mV, $t3 = 400$ ms.
5. The data are collected and the sample chromatograms are acquired by using Chromeleon Chromatography Management System Version 6.8.
6. The chromatograms of 150 pmol high mannose *N*-glycans mixture, 150 pmol desialylated complex *N*-glycans mixture, and the *N*-glycans released with peptide *N*-glycosidase F from total glycoproteins of SKOV3 cells and desialylated by mild acid hydrolysis are shown in Fig. 1a–c.
7. Subsequent MS analysis of *N*-glycan fractions separated by HPAEC-PAD requires online desalting using a carbohydrate membrane desalter device (CMD 300; Dionex, Sunnyvale, CA, USA). The CMD 300 device is installed after the electrochemical cell of an ion chromatography system of the Dionex Corporation (Sunnyvale, CA, USA). *N*-glycans eluting from

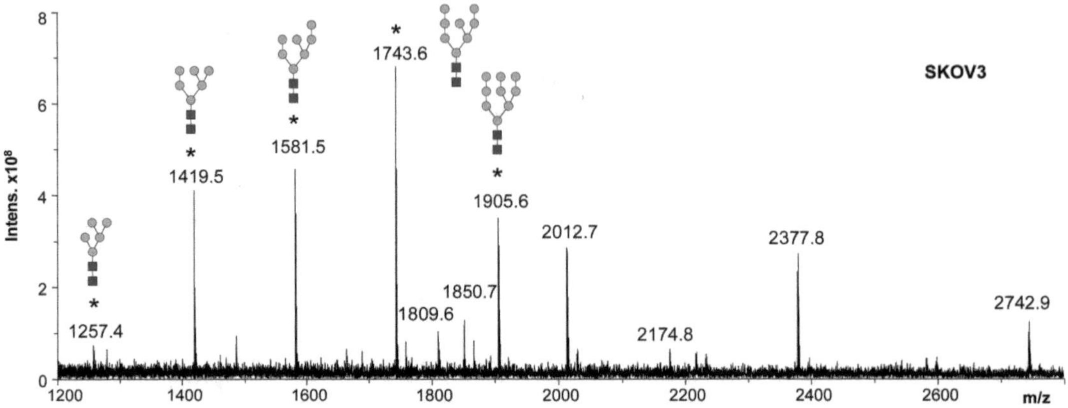

Fig. 2 MALDI-TOF MS analysis of total desialylated *N*-glycans from SKOV3 cells. *Asterisks* indicate signals corresponding to high mannose glycans $Man_5GlcNAc_2$–$Man_9GlcNAc_2$ (structures are represented on top of the peaks; *grey circles* represent Man and *black squares* represent GlcNAc). Peaks at *m*/*z* 2,012.7, 2,174.8, 2,377.8, and 2,742.9 are compatible with triantennary-Gal, triantennary, tetraantennary-Gal, and tetraantennary + one LacNAc-Gal complex glycans with proximal fucose, respectively (reproduced from Machado with permission from Oxford University Press)

CarboPac PA200 columns during HPAEC-PAD analysis are detected prior to passage through the CMD 300 and eluted from the CMD 300 in diluted acetic acid (gradient 0–180 mM). *N*-glycans are collected either manually by individual peaks or peak groups or automatically by time using a fraction collector. Prior to MS analysis the collected glycan fractions can be repurified by using Hypercarb mini-columns (pipette tips) as described in Subheading 3.1.5.

3.3 Analysis of N-Glycans by MALDI-TOF MS

Molecular mass determination is performed by MALDI-TOF MS analysis using, e.g. a Bruker REFLEX time-of-flight (TOF) instrument equipped with a N_2-Laser (337 nm) and a pulse frequency of 3 ns and 10^7–10^8 W/cm^2 intensity at a surface area 0.2 mm^2. *N*-glycans are dissolved in ultrapure water (1–10 pmol/μL) and mixed 1:1 with a solution of 10 mg/mL DHB in ethanol–water (9:1); 1 μL of the mixture solution is spotted onto a stainless steel target and air dried. Positive ion mode spectra are recorded at an accelerating potential of 28 kV; recording mass ranges for non-derivatized desialylated *N*-glycans is between *m*/*z* 800 and 7,000. Neutral glycans have only low affinity for protons, therefore Na^+ or K^+ is added to the matrix. Positive ion mass spectra are recorded by summing individual spectra obtained from 50 to 100 laser shots (Fig. 2). The detailed procedure is as follows:

1. Weigh 10 mg DHB in a 1 mL tube.
2. Add 900 μL ethanol and 100 μL of water and mix vigorously with DHB.

3. Solubilize desialylated underivatized glycans in water yielding a concentration of 10 pmol per 10 μL.
4. Prepare a 1:1 mixture of matrix and sample.
5. Pipette 1 μL aliquot onto a polished stainless steel target and dry by air.
6. Collect MALDI-TOF MS spectra data.
7. Analyze mass spectra data with, e.g., the Bruker DataAnalysis for TOF 1.5j program (Bruker Daltonics GmbH) and smooth spectra using the Savitzky Golay algorithm. Structures are tentatively assigned to various *N*-glycans based on their observed masses in comparison with the calculated masses of known *N*-glycans (considering their monosaccharide compositions) and taking into account the biosynthetic N-glycosylation pathway (*see* **Note 10**). Further annotation of *N*-glycans and database searches can also be performed using the Glyco-Peakfinder platform [12].

4 Notes

1. CO_2 reacts with NaOH yielding $NaHCO_3$ that interferes with the electrode and alters the baseline signal. Therefore, degassing of water and eluents is required, which is accomplished by bubbling helium. Flasks should be covered after degasing to minimize CO_2 solubilization.
2. TheraProteins has an extended catalogue of reference oligosaccharide standards.
3. The trypsin solution is freshly prepared in 0.01 % TFA.
4. For recombinant erythropoietin secreted by SKOV3 cells [10] *N*-glycans are released from the glycoprotein with PNGase F in similar conditions as those described in Subheading 3.1.2, **step 1**, and previous trypsin digestion is not required.
5. Desialylation by mild acid hydrolysis is an alternative approach that can be applied for a fast analytical screening of structures; however, it might cause partial defucosylation (loss of proximal α1,6-fucose) of *N*-glycans and some degalactosylation. For mild acid hydrolysis dilute the *N*-glycans in ultrapure water to a final volume of 25 μL, add 25 μL of 10 mM sulfuric acid and incubate 90 min at 80 °C. Neutralize with 10 μL of 50 mM sodium hydroxide, check pH with pH strips and dry by SpeedVac concentration.
6. Under the described conditions without Hypercarb purification, good baselines and no influence of retention times are observed in HPAEC-PAD analysis.
7. The Hypercarb micro-tip should not get dry.

8. The procedure of elution is as follows: the first 50 μL of the 150 μL of eluting solvent is collected in a 500 μL Eppendorf vial, the micro-tip is left for 2 min and the remaining eluting solvent is slowly ejected by using air pressure from a syringe into the collecting vial.
9. Use of a guard column is optional.
10. For confirmation of the structure MS/MS or digestion with exoglycosidases is performed.

Acknowledgements

We acknowledge Fundação para a Ciência e a Tecnologia, Portugal, projects PTDC/SAU-NEU/100724/2008 and PIC/IC/82765/2007.

References

1. Kulasingam V, Pavlou MP, Diamandis EP (2010) Integrating high-throughput technologies in the quest for effective biomarkers for ovarian cancer. Nat Rev Cancer 10:371–378
2. Abbott KL, Nairn AV, Hall EM et al (2008) Focused glycomic analysis of the N-linked glycan biosynthetic pathway in ovarian cancer. Proteomics 8:3210–3220
3. Townsend RR, Hardy MR, Lee YC (1989) Separation of oligosaccharides using high-performance anion-exchange chromatography with pulsed amperometric detection. Methods Enzymol 179:65–76
4. Montreuil J, Bouquelet S, Debray H et al (2003) Glycoproteins. In: Chaplin MF, Kennedy JF (eds) Carbohydrate analysis - a practical approach, 2nd edn. Oxford, Oxford University Press, pp 181–293
5. Morelle W, Michalski JC (2005) The mass spectrometric analysis of glycoproteins and their glycan structures. Curr Anal Chem 1:29–57
6. Sutton-Smith M, Dell A (2006) Analysis of carbohydrates/glycoproteins by mass spectrometry. In: Celis JE, Carter N, Simons K, Small JV, Hunter T, Shotton D (eds) Cell biology, volume 4, 3rd edn. Burlington, San Diego, London, Elsevier Science, p 415–425
7. Harvey DJ (2011) Analysis of carbohydrates and glycoconjugates by matrix-assisted laser desorption/ionization mass spectrometry: an update for the period 2005–2006. Mass Spectrom Rev 30:1–100
8. Hillenkamp F, Karas M (1990) Mass spectrometry of peptides and proteins by matrix-assisted ultraviolet laser desorption/ionization. Methods Enzymol 193:280–295
9. Pohl S, Hoffmann A, Rudiger A et al (1997) Hypoglycosylation of a brain glycoprotein (beta-trace protein) in CDG syndromes due to phosphomannomutase deficiency and N-acetylglucosaminyl-transferase II deficiency. Glycobiology 7:1077–1084
10. Machado E, Kandzia S, Carilho R et al (2011) N-Glycosylation of total cellular glycoproteins from the human ovarian carcinoma SKOV3 cell line and of recombinantly expressed human erythropoietin. Glycobiology 21:376–386
11. Brito C, Kandzia S, Graca T et al (2008) Human fucosyltransferase IX: specificity towards N-linked glycoproteins and relevance of the cytoplasmic domain in intra-Golgi localization. Biochimie 90:1279–1290
12. Maass K, Ranzinger R, Geyer H et al (2007) "Glyco-peakfinder"–de novo composition analysis of glycoconjugates. Proteomics 7:4435–4444

Part V

In Vitro Assays in Ovarian Cancer Research

Chapter 23

In Vivo and In Vitro Properties of Ovarian Cancer Cells

Anastasia Malek

Abstract

Specific biological properties of ovarian cancer cells can be modeled and studied using in vitro experiments. Any experimental setting can closely reflect some aspects of the native conditions; however, parameters that differ from in vivo aspects must be considered. Familiarity with existing and well-established, as well as new, cell culture techniques provides a basis for correct experimental design and production of reliable scientific results. This chapter presents a short comparative review of the techniques used for cell culture establishment and maintenance of ovarian cancer cells, as well as laboratory methods used to characterize malignant features of these cells, including the epithelial–mesechymal transition, cell motility and invasiveness, resistance to detachment-induced apoptosis, and stem cell content.

Key words Ovarian cancer, Primary cell culture, Cancer stem cells, Anoikis, Cell motility, EMT

1 Advantages and Drawbacks of Cell Culture Techniques

Many of the specific biological properties of ovarian cancer cells, such as the ability to survive in suspension, formation of multicellular complexes (spheroids), equilibrium between epithelial and mesenchymal phenotypes, and the ability to modify surrounding tissues, have been successfully explored in in vitro experiments. Primary and established ovarian cancer cell cultures are essential tools for fundamental and preclinical research. Cell cultures are easily manipulated and far less expensive to maintain compared to laboratory animals. However, little is known about how culture conditions alter cell biology and if properly isolated cells reflect the properties of intact tissues. Comparing various native growth conditions of ovarian cancer cells may provide relevant observations and assumptions. Significant differences in gene expression profiles between primary tumors and omental metastases were demonstrated in early studies [1, 2]. Several invasion-related genes (e.g., matrix metalloproteinase, growth factors, and cell surface adhesion molecules) are highly overexpressed in the cells of secondary lesions, reflecting the pathophysiological needs of metastatic tissues.

Anastasia Malek and Oleg Tchernitsa (eds.), *Ovarian Cancer: Methods and Protocols*, Methods in Molecular Biology, vol. 1049, DOI 10.1007/978-1-62703-547-7_23, © Springer Science+Business Media New York 2013

A recent analysis of site-dependent expression of relevant molecules in primary ovarian tumors, effusion, and solid metastases revealed significant differences [3]. These data indicate the genetic plasticity of ovarian cancer cells and their ability to react to environmental stimuli. Moreover, the genetic variability of cells within the tumor maintains selective proliferation of cells with optimal properties. Cell lines established from tumor tissues are cultured ex vivo for extended periods of time and are supposed to be genetically uniform. However, the cell line may not infinitely maintain the properties of the original tissue. For instance, correlations between the expression patterns of genes implicated in multidrug resistance in clinical ovarian cancer samples and established cell lines have not been observed [4]. In order to reduce impact of in vitro culturing, preclinical studies are often performed using material obtained directly from patients and maintained ex vivo for as short a time period as possible [5].

2 Ovarian Tissue Xenografts and Primary Cell Culture

The functional properties of ovarian cancer cells obtained after surgery can be analyzed using several approaches. Pieces of solid tissue can be implanted subcutaneously (s.c.) in the mammary fat pad or under the subrenal capsule in immune-compromised animals [6, 7]. Xenografts closely reflect the original tissue in terms of gene expression, histochemistry, and morphology and can be used for preclinical research or personalized analysis of the patient. However, establishing successful tissue xenografts depends on the length of time between tissue removal from the patient and implantation into immune-deficient mice. In addition, this technique requires surgical skills.

Tumor tissue can be mechanically dissociated to collect cell aggregates that are approximately 200–300 μm and contain all of the necessary components, including tumor cells, fibroblasts, endothelial cells, lymphocytes, and the extracellular matrix. A suspension of these tumor-derived cell aggregates can be injected intraperitoneally (i.p.) into immune-deficient animals to model i.p.-disseminated ovarian cancer [8]. Tumor progression can closely mimic many of the events that are observed in ovarian cancer patients, including consistent development of peritoneal carcinomatosis, malignant ascites, increase in serum CA125 levels, and distant metastasis. Intraperitoneal dissemination may also be modeled using malignant cells obtained from ascetic effusion.

Tumor tissue can be transferred into primary cell cultures. This approach is quite labor intensive and assumes changes in conditions from in vivo to in vitro. However, several advantages justify broad application of primary cell culture. During the initial passages, ovarian cancer cells can be isolated from the cellular mixture and used as monocultures in subsequent experiments, which ensures their comparative characters. If a cancer cell/fibroblast coculture is required, the cells can be mixed in the necessary ratio. Importantly, cells can be frozen at or after the first passage. The stored material provides an opportunity to use the same cell culture in various experiments. It is still unclear how similar the primary cell cultures are to the cells from the initial tumor, although it seems to be based on the length of time in culture. In one study, the expression patterns from 2-week primary cell cultures that were directly profiled and compared to the original flash-frozen tumor tissue showed a high correlation [9]. Only 0.35 % of the genes were differentially expressed between the groups. Another study that used fresh and cultured ovarian cancer cells obtained from ascitic fluid showed similar results [10]. However, in vitro culturing ultimately induces adoptive genetic alterations, triggers selection and results in cell senescence. The empirical recommendation for inexperienced scientists is to complete the experiments within 6–8 passages.

Chapter 24 discusses establishment of primary cell cultures from tumor tissues and ascetic effusion. The technical details of mechanical tissue dissociation are provided with supportive illustrations. The alternative approaches of enzymatic tissue disaggregation using trypsin or collagenase are described in Chapters 25 and 27.

3 Ovarian Cancer Stem Cells

Although the cancer stem cell hypothesis has become very popular in recent years, it is still debatable [11]. The hypothesis postulates that malignant tumors are initiated and maintained by a small population of tumor cells that share similar biological properties with normal embryonic and adult stem cells. Cancer stem cells (CSCs) or cancer-initiating cells (CICs) have been identified in several types of cancer, including breast, pancreas, colon, prostate, and ovarian cancer [12, 13]. CSCs from different tumor types exhibit similar functional and morphologic properties and appear to define tumor malignancy. In addition, CSCs are specifically resistant to radiation and chemotherapy. In the case of ovarian cancer, a threefold increase in CSCs was observed in metastatic compared to primary tumors, and CSCs were considerably more resistant to chemotherapy than the total population of cancer cells [14]. The current data suggest that unique and specific survival mechanisms allow CSCs to escape from therapeutic intervention and drive tumor growth, progression, and recurrence. According to this model, estimating the number of CSCs present in tumors could define patient prognoses and focus treatment on the CSC population to achieve complete tumor eradication. Because CSCs will be the focus of intensive research for some time, a method of ovarian CSC enrichment is described in Chapter 25.

4 Assessment of Anoikis

Anoikis is a specialized form of apoptosis that is triggered by a lack of attachment to other cells or the extracellular matrix. Malignant transformation of epithelial cells is often associated with suppression of anoikis in that cancer cells become able to detach from the primary tumor, survive in the lymph or bloodstream and form distant metastasis [15]. In most solid tumors, anchorage-independent survival is limited by the passage of time from the primary tumor to the secondary location. In contrast, ovarian cancer cells persist in the peritoneal fluid over long period of time and interact with other cellular and noncellular components of ascetic effusion to actively proliferate. The peritoneal cavity is considered a specific compartment for ovarian cancer growth rather than solely a pathway of dissemination. The mechanisms of anoikis that overcome and resist treatment should be constantly activated in the ovarian cancer cells that float in the ascetic effusion. Anoikis is evaded by restoring intercellular interactions and formation of multicellular complexes (spheroids). This phenomenon can be assayed in a gyratory shaker culture. Various speeds of gyration (from 60 to 200 RPM) can be applied to induce or reduce intracellular interactions [16]. In this assay, depleted medium is optimally used to minimize the confounding effects of serum-derived extracellular matrix components. The molecular pathways involved in regulating anoikis are often altered in ovarian cancer cells. Overexpression of the anti-apoptotic factor Bcl-xl in ovarian cancer has been demonstrated [17], while the role of the HGF/Met [18], VEGFA/VEGFR2 [19], and TrkB [20] signalling cascades in anoikis inhibition was recently explored. Active research in this area has been encouraged by the possibility of functional links between tolerance to anoikis and chemoresistance. Evaluation of crosstalk between anoikis- and chemoresistance mechanisms may reveal potential approaches to overcoming the latter. However, the currently published data are inconsistent [21]. The specific biological properties of floating cancer cells and their influence on the progression and chemoresistance of ovarian cancer will require further investigation. Chapter 26 discusses the MTT-based colorimetric assay for estimating cell resistance to anoikis, with Trypan blue staining and flow cytometry as alternative methods.

5 Ovarian Cancer Cell Motility

Increased motility and invasiveness are the basic properties of cancer cells and are essential in the metastatic process. Several in vitro assays have been well established and are broadly used to evaluate the movement capacity of cancer cells. The ability to move on adherent surfaces are being analyzed using cell spreading [16] or wound healing ("scratch") [22] (see also Chapter 31) assays. Both techniques can be combined with imaging live cells during migration to monitor and quantify cell movement. The trans-well migration (Boyden chamber) assay allows analysis of cell motility in a three-dimensional space and estimates the effects of various soluble regulatory factors. None of the methods used in cancer research precisely reflect the specificity of ovarian cancer movement during colonization of the peritoneal cavity. Interactions between cancer cells and the mesothelial cell layer that lines the peritoneal cavity present a particular phenomenon in recruiting various adhesion, signalling, and enzymatic molecules [23]. Peritoneally localized patterns of metastatic spread suggest the presence of specific microenvironmental factors that provide homing cues to guide malignant cells to receptive niches that permit the growth of secondary lesions. Coculturing ovarian cancer and mesothelial cells provides a model to study the adhesive properties of ovarian cancer in close-to-real conditions [24]. Invasive behavior and matrix remodeling properties of ovarian cancer cells can be studied using a three-dimensional model of the submesothelial extracellular matrix, which consists of polyethylene glycol, collagen, and various matrix components [25, 26]. Sophisticated three-dimensional models containing human [27] or mouse [28] extracellular and cellular components allow maintenance of an in vitro structure that closely mimics the peritoneum. After adding ovarian cancer cells, these models reflect the complex process of developing ovarian cancer metastases and can be investigated in detail.

6 Epithelial–Mesenchymal Transition

Emerging evidence suggests that the epithelial–mesenchymal transition (EMT) plays a crucial role in aggressive epithelial ovarian cancer, including increased migration and invasion abilities that contribute to chemoresistance and CSC populations. EMT is a global process that interferes with cellular homeostasis and alters many signalling pathways, such as epidermal growth factor (EGF), fibroblast growth factor (FGF), platelet-derived growth factor (PDGF), insulin-like growth factor (IGF), vascular endothelial growth factor (VEGF), hepatocyte growth factor (HGF), transforming growth factor-β (TGF-β), stem cell factor (SCF), bone morphogenetic proteins (BMP), the Wnt-signalling pathway, integrins, Notch transcription factors, prostaglandin E2 (PGE2), cyclooxygenase-2 (COX-2), parathyroid hormone (PTH), and estrogens [29]. Specific aspects of EMT in ovarian cancer and implementation in disease progression have been recently discussed [30, 31]. Chapter 27 describes EMT assessment in ovarian cancer cell culture and tissue samples using flow cytometry and immunohistochemistry. The chapter also contains a list of antibodies that can be used to detect epithelial and mesenchymal markers in ovarian cancer cells.

Part V of the book does not cover all of the existing in vitro techniques used to study ovarian cancer. The techniques described are aimed at mimicking several of the characteristics of ovarian cancer. The commonly used approaches that have been modified for ovarian cancer research are presented rather than specific methods. We encourage the modification of well established or newly developed methods to study ovarian cancer, while considering the specific biological properties of this malignancy.

References

1. Lancaster JM, Dressman HK, Clarke JP, Sayer RA, Martino MA et al (2006) Identification of genes associated with ovarian cancer metastasis using microarray expression analysis. Int J Gynecol Cancer 16:1733–1745
2. Bignotti E, Tassi RA, Calza S, Ravaggi A, Bandiera E et al (2007) Gene expression profile of ovarian serous papillary carcinomas: identification of metastasis-associated genes. Am J Obstet Gynecol 196:245.e1–245.e11
3. Davidson B (2007) Anatomic site-related expression of cancer-associated molecules in ovarian carcinoma. Curr Cancer Drug Targets 7:109–120
4. Gillet JP, Calcagno AM, Varma S, Marino M, Green LJ et al (2011) Redefining the relevance of established cancer cell lines to the study of mechanisms of clinical anti-cancer drug resistance. Proc Natl Acad Sci USA 108: 18708–18713
5. Haglund C, Aleskog A, Nygren P, Gullbo J, Hoglund M et al (2012) In vitro evaluation of clinical activity and toxicity of anticancer drugs using tumor cells from patients and cells representing normal tissues. Cancer Chemother Pharmacol 69:697–707
6. Zachary C, Dobbin AAK, Angela Ziebarth, Monjri Shah, Adam D Steg, Ronald David Alvarez, Michael G Conner, Charles N Landen; University of Alabama at Birmingham, Birmingham, AL (2012) Use of an optimized primary ovarian cancer xenograft model to mimic patient tumor biology and heterogeneity. 2012 ASCO Annual Meeting (Poster Discussion Session) Abstract 5036
7. Lee CH, Xue H, Sutcliffe M, Gout PW, Huntsman DG et al (2005) Establishment of subrenal capsule xenografts of primary human ovarian tumors in SCID mice: potential models. Gynecol Oncol 96:48–55
8. Bankert RB, Balu-Iyer SV, Odunsi K, Shultz LD, Kelleher RJ Jr et al (2011) Humanized mouse model of ovarian cancer recapitulates patient solid tumor progression, ascites formation, and metastasis. PLoS One 6:e24420
9. Bignotti E, Tassi RA, Calza S, Ravaggi A, Romani C et al (2006) Differential gene expression profiles between tumor biopsies and short-term primary cultures of ovarian serous carcinomas: identification of novel molecular biomarkers for early diagnosis and therapy. Gynecol Oncol 103:405–416
10. Provencher DM, Finstad CL, Saigo PE, Rubin SC, Hoskins WJ et al (1993) Comparison of antigen expression on fresh and cultured ascites cells and on solid tumors of patients with epithelial ovarian cancer. Gynecol Oncol 50:78–83
11. Alison MR, Lin WR, Lim SM, Nicholson LJ (2012) Cancer stem cells: in the line of fire. Cancer Treat Rev 38:589–598
12. Pan Y, Huang X (2008) Epithelial ovarian cancer stem cells-a review. Int J Clin Exp Med 1:260–266
13. Zhang S, Balch C, Chan MW, Lai HC, Matei D et al (2008) Identification and characterization of ovarian cancer-initiating cells from primary human tumors. Cancer Res 68:4311–4320
14. Alvero AB, Chen R, Fu HH, Montagna M, Schwartz PE et al (2009) Molecular phenotyping of human ovarian cancer stem cells unravels the mechanisms for repair and chemoresistance. Cell Cycle 8:158–166
15. Guadamillas MC, Cerezo A, Del Pozo MA (2011) Overcoming anoikis–pathways to anchorage-independent growth in cancer. J Cell Sci 124:3189–3197
16. Klausen C, Leung PC, Auersperg N (2009) Cell motility and spreading are suppressed by HOXA4 in ovarian cancer cells: possible involvement of beta1 integrin. Mol Cancer Res 7:1425–1437
17. Frankel A, Buckman R, Kerbel RS (1997) Abrogation of taxol-induced G2-M arrest and apoptosis in human ovarian cancer cells grown as multicellular tumor spheroids. Cancer Res 57:2388–2393
18. Tang MK, Zhou HY, Yam JW, Wong AS (2010) c-Met overexpression contributes to

the acquired apoptotic resistance of nonadherent ovarian cancer cells through a cross talk mediated by phosphatidylinositol 3-kinase and extracellular signal-regulated kinase 1/2. Neoplasia 12:128–138
19. Sher I, Adham SA, Petrik J, Coomber BL (2009) Autocrine VEGF-A/KDR loop protects epithelial ovarian carcinoma cells from anoikis. Int J Cancer 124:553–561
20. Yu X, Liu L, Cai B, He Y, Wan X (2008) Suppression of anoikis by the neurotrophic receptor TrkB in human ovarian cancer. Cancer Sci 99:543–552
21. Brigulova K, Cervinka M, Tosner J, Sedlakova I (2010) Chemoresistance testing of human ovarian cancer cells and its in vitro model. Toxicol In Vitro 24:2108–2115
22. Liang CC, Park AY, Guan JL (2007) In vitro scratch assay: a convenient and inexpensive method for analysis of cell migration in vitro. Nat Protoc 2:329–333
23. Sodek KL, Murphy KJ, Brown TJ, Ringuette MJ (2012) Cell-cell and cell-matrix dynamics in intraperitoneal cancer metastasis. Cancer Metastasis Rev 31:397–414
24. Watanabe T, Hashimoto T, Sugino T, Soeda S, Nishiyama H et al (2012) Production of IL1-beta by ovarian cancer cells induces mesothelial cell beta1-integrin expression facilitating peritoneal dissemination. J Ovarian Res 5:7
25. Barbolina MV, Adley BP, Kelly DL, Shepard J, Fought AJ et al (2009) Downregulation of connective tissue growth factor by three-dimensional matrix enhances ovarian carcinoma cell invasion. Int J Cancer 125:816–825
26. Barbolina MV, Adley BP, Kelly DL, Fought AJ, Scholtens DM et al (2008) Motility-related actinin alpha-4 is associated with advanced and metastatic ovarian carcinoma. Lab Invest 88: 602–614
27. Kenny HA, Dogan S, Zillhardt M, Mitra A, Yamada SD, Krausz T, Lengyel E (2009) Organotypic models of metastasis: a three-dimensional culture mimicking the human peritoneum and omentum for the study of the early steps of ovarian cancer metastasis. Cancer Treat Res 149:335–351
28. Khan SM, Funk HM, Thiolloy S, Lotan TL, Hickson J et al (2010) In vitro metastatic colonization of human ovarian cancer cells to the omentum. Clin Exp Metastasis 27:185–196
29. Thiery JP, Acloque H, Huang RY, Nieto MA (2009) Epithelial-mesenchymal transitions in development and disease. Cell 139:871–890
30. Davidson B, Trope CG, Reich R (2012) Epithelial-mesenchymal transition in ovarian carcinoma. Front Oncol 2:33
31. Nakayama K, Nakayama N, Katagiri H, Miyazaki K (2012) Mechanisms of ovarian cancer metastasis: biochemical pathways. Int J Mol Sci 13:11705–11717

Chapter 24

Establishment of Primary Cultures from Ovarian Tumor Tissue and Ascites Fluid

Brigitte L. Thériault, Lise Portelance, Anne-Marie Mes-Masson, and Mark W. Nachtigal

Abstract

We have refined the technique for isolating and propagating cultures of primary epithelial ovarian cancer (EOC) cells derived from solid tumors and ascites. Both protocols involve a simple yet rapid method for the growth and propagation of EOC tumor and ascites cells in a basal culture medium without the addition of growth factors. Isolation of tumor EOC cells involves the mechanical disruption of the tumor tissue with the help of a cell scraper, while ascites-derived EOC cells are mixed with growth medium and placed directly into culture with very little manipulation. We further describe a partial trypsinization method to eliminate fibroblast contamination from primary EOC cells derived from solid tumors. These methods allow for the direct application of many molecular, cellular, and functional analyses within a few weeks of initial isolation, with the added potential of retrospective analyses of archived cells and tissues. Thus, we have included steps for long-term cryopreservation of early-passage EOC cells. Initial isolation of EOC cells can be completed within 1 h, and primary cells are further expanded in culture for several weeks.

Key words Epithelial ovarian cancer, Tumor tissue, Primary culture, Ascites, Ovary, Immunocytochemistry

1 Introduction

Epithelial ovarian cancer (EOC) remains the most lethal of the gynecological malignancies, due to the lack of distinct symptoms during the early course of the disease and insidious peritoneal spread at later stages [1]. Much knowledge is being uncovered into the molecular pathways driving the progression and metastatic spread of EOC tumors [2–5]. The majority of this information is being revealed through the study of either EOC primary tumor sections and/or established, immortalized EOC cell lines [6–8]. To this end, many groups have developed EOC cell lines to provide useful tools to study the functional implications of EOC development and progression. Although established cell lines are easy to culture and maintain for prolonged periods, a well-known

Anastasia Malek and Oleg Tchernitsa (eds.), *Ovarian Cancer: Methods and Protocols*, Methods in Molecular Biology, vol. 1049, DOI 10.1007/978-1-62703-547-7_24, © Springer Science+Business Media New York 2013

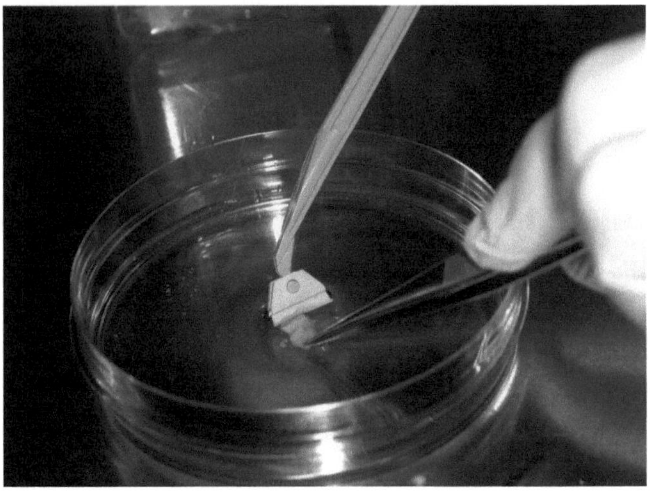

Fig. 1 Isolation of primary EOC cells from tumor tissue with the help of a cell scraper

caveat of these EOC cell lines is that they possess genetic and biochemical abnormalities driven by immortalized growth. Researchers must keep in mind when using established cell lines that inherent genetic abnormalities may misrepresent crucial pathways regulating tumorigenesis and that cell lines may demonstrate altered responses to targeted therapies.

With the development of more precise and efficient analysis platforms such as next-generation sequencing or expression arrays (RNA, protein) that require small amounts of starting material, many research groups are now opting to establish short-term cultures of freshly isolated EOC tumor or ascites for their studies [9–12]. The ability to culture and characterize freshly isolated EOC cells from either solid tumors or ascites offers an important experimental system that resembles the patient situation more closely, providing a better tool to develop potential interventions with higher therapeutic applicability.

Several methods have been described for the primary culture of EOC cells from solid tumors or from the ascites of ovarian cancer patients [13–17]. For the isolation and culturing of solid tumor EOC cells, we have employed three different methods: (1) enzymatic dissociation with collagenase [18], (2) mechanical tissue disruption via a cell scraper, and (3) derivation of EOC cells via explant cultures. These three methods are all suitable for isolation and culture of EOC tumor cells; however, the mechanical disruption of EOC cells with the use of a cell scraper has proven the quickest and most efficient method to date and will be described in detail in this protocol (Fig. 1). Once isolated, the cells are maintained in an ovarian surface epithelial (OSE) culture environment to which we have added serum and an antifungal and antibiotic to

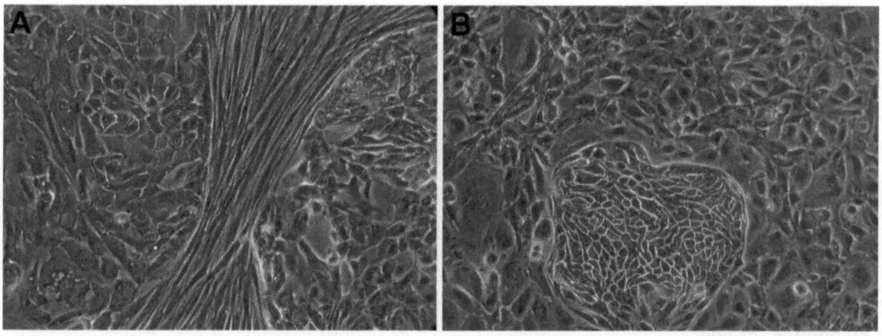

Fig. 2 Representative images of primary cultures 1 week post-isolation. (**a**) Fibroblasts cells are elongated cells, while epithelial cells have a cobblestone shape. (**b**) Epithelial cell nests embedded in a group of larger epithelial cells. Immunocytochemistry analysis should be done to confirm the cell types

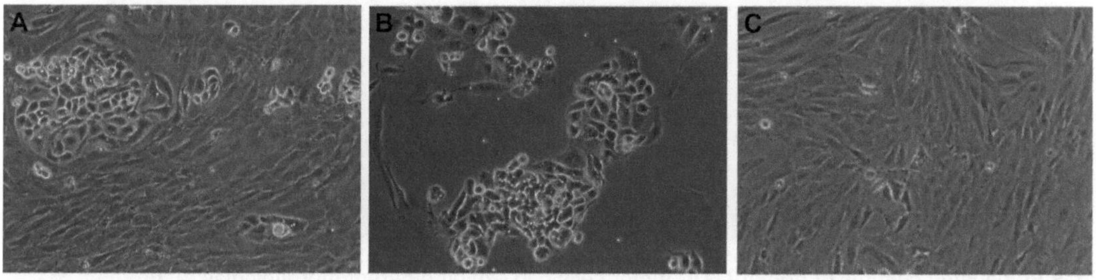

Fig. 3 Partial trypsinization of primary EOC tumor cell cultures. (**a**) Confluent cell layer of epithelial and non-epithelial cells at passage-0. (**b**) Adherent epithelial cells that did not lift during partial trypsinization. (**c**) Mixed cell types sensitive to partial trypsinization that were replated into a new culture dish

eliminate the risk of microbial contamination. It is possible to add growth factors and hormones to this culture medium (epidermal growth factor (EGF), bovine pituitary extract (BPE), insulin, hydrocortisone, beta-estradiol, progesterone); however, the addition of supplements can alter the growth and epithelial morphology of EOC cells [19, 20]. For both EOC solid tumor and ascites cultures, we have opted for a basal culture medium that reduces the growth of normal stromal cells while favoring the growth of EOC cells which are more self-sufficient. Cells are grown at 37 °C with 5 % CO_2 and 5–7 % O_2 to reproduce in vivo conditions as closely as possible.

Once isolated, EOC tumor tissue cells adhere very rapidly (within 24 h) to the culture dish. Primary EOC cells will have generally reached confluence within a week of culture (Fig. 2). A major concern regarding the isolation of EOC cells directly from solid tumors is the presence of multiple cell types, namely, fibroblasts. This is why we perform a partial trypsinization to separate these major cell types (Figs. 3 and 4). Fibroblasts are less adherent than epithelial cell types and will detach more rapidly from the culture

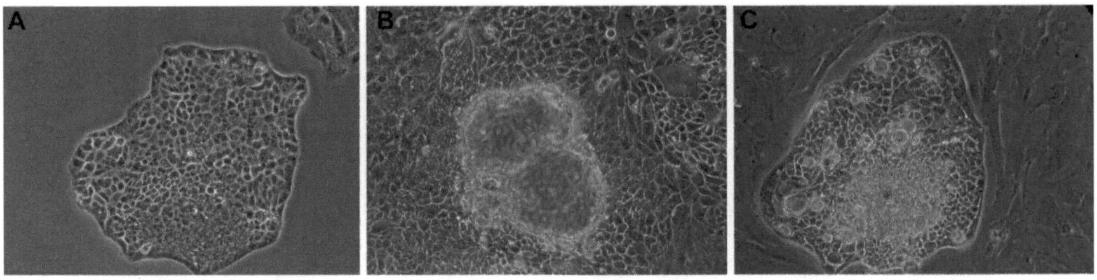

Fig. 4 Growth of trypsin-resistant cells. (**a**) Trypsin-resistant cell foci. (**b**) Formation of multilayer foci. (**c**) Foci surrounded by senescent cells

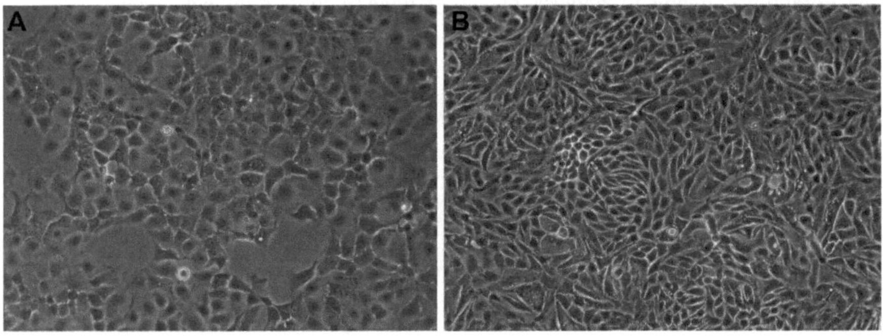

Fig. 5 Propagated cultures of primary EOC tumor cells can exhibit different morphologies (**a, b**)

dish. Once the fibroblast contaminants have been removed from the epithelial cells, both cell types can be amplified separately and successfully placed in cryogenic storage (epithelial cultures depicted in Fig. 5).

When cells have reached confluence, they must be trypsinized and split into new culture dishes for continuous culture. The ratio and frequency at which the cells will be split depends on the growth rate of the cells. It is very important with these cultures to maintain an adequate cell density, as cells that are too sparse will have much more difficulty to grow and multiply and may undergo premature senescence. As a general rule, primary tumor EOC cells are split at a 1:2 ratio every 3 or 4 days. Most EOC cell culture will senesce or die after 2–3 months in culture; however, some cultures will grow for longer periods, up to 8 weeks in average, and a minority may become cell lines. Proliferating cultures can then be frozen with DMSO and stored for years in long-term cryostorage (liquid nitrogen or ultra-low −150 °C freezer). Epithelial cell cultures can be confirmed by immunocytochemistry with antibodies towards cytokeratins 7, 8, 18, and 19 [18, 21].

For the isolation and culture of EOC cells from ascites, we employ a relatively simple and rapid method, which avoids the timely and costly purification of EOC cells from other cell

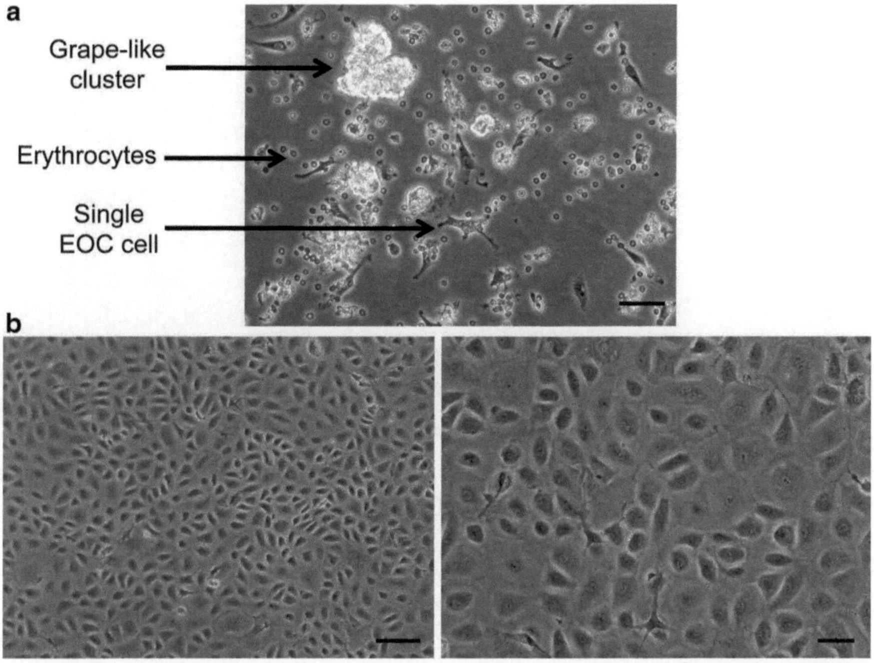

Fig. 6 Primary cultures of human EOC cells from patient ascites. (**a**) Cells 1 day after initial seeding. Note the mixture of cells in the culture including adherent epithelial cells, grapelike clusters of EOC cells that will attach and from which adherent epithelial cells will migrate, and erythrocytes. Bar = 100 μm (**b**) Confluent monolayer of primary human EOC cells illustrating epithelial cobblestone morphology. *Left panel* bar = 100 μm, *right panel* bar = 400 μm

types present in the ascites, namely, erythrocytes (Fig. 6a) [22]. As mentioned previously, to avoid the addition of extraneous growth factors that could induce altered cellular characteristics such as an epithelial to mesenchymal transition [20], we have opted for a basal media composed of two types of culture media, supplemented with serum and antibiotics. We find that although many erythrocytes are present at initial plating, most of these are removed after the first media change (as they are nonadherent), leaving the adherent EOC cells (Fig. 6b). Fibroblast contamination of ascites-derived EOC cells has rarely been observed; however, growth of fibroblasts was not supported in long-term cultures when cells were maintained in EOC culture medium [22]. As with primary tumor EOC cell cultures, cytokeratin immunostaining can confirm the presence of epithelial cells.

As ascites fluid is usually abundant in many ovarian cancer patients (~200 mL, but in our experience ranges from 50 mL to 7 L), a much larger starting yield (several million EOC cells) is obtained as opposed to primary tumor isolations. This yield can then be expanded greatly depending on the initial volume of ascites received and processed. Primary EOC cells isolated from ascites will typically reach confluence by 3–7 days, at which time the majority

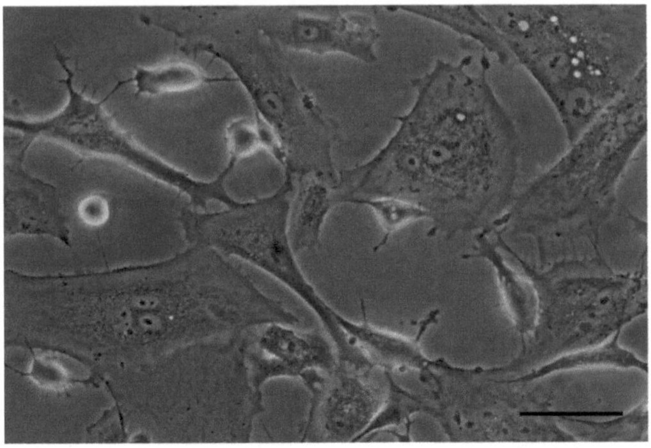

Fig. 7 Primary culture of a recurrent, chemoresistant Stage 3c serous ovarian adenocarcinoma. Bar = 100 μm

of cells should be frozen as passage-0 stocks; the remaining cells can thus be rapidly expanded for immediate experimental use. Maintenance of an adequate cell density is also important in the culture of healthy EOC cells derived from ascites. Cells are split at a 1:2 ratio (maximum of 1:3 dilution) every 3–4 days as to avoid premature senescence. Cultures can be propagated for several passages, but most will inevitably senesce (around 12–15 passages). To ensure a healthy and proliferative starting material, we typically perform experiments on primary EOC cells within passages 2–6.

Human EOC consists of several different histological subtypes, and we receive samples that reflect the expected prevalence observed in patients. Serous, mucinous, clear cell, and poorly differentiated EOC cells have been successfully cultured and archived. Very few endometrioid samples have been grown, as this histotype occurs rarely and infrequently develops ascites. The majority of primary EOC cells derived from ascites display a similar epithelial cobblestone morphology (Fig. 6b) and growth rate regardless of histotype when using the culture conditions described in this chapter.

The most significant factor that affects the ability to isolate and culture EOC from patient ascites is the effect of chemotherapy. We have had less success growing EOC cells from patients who have recently undergone neoadjuvant chemotherapy treatment for their disease. As the standard of ovarian cancer patient treatment evolves to the administration of neoadjuvant chemotherapies [23], this may impact the amount and/or the viability of tumor or ascites fluid that can be collected. The collection of chemotherapy-naïve ascites fluid is important to the successful isolation and culture of EOC cells for subsequent functional studies. It should be noted that previous chemotherapy has not precluded developing short-term EOC cell cultures from patients that later present with drug-resistant disease (Fig. 7).

The protocols described in this chapter allow for the rapid and simple isolation and successful establishment of EOC cells from both primary tumors and ascites. The material obtained from these short-term cultures allows for a multitude of subsequent investigative techniques. For example, assays involving spheroid culture systems can be established [22], in addition to xenograft models where short-term cultured EOC cells can be manipulated and tested for in vivo tumorigenic capacity [17]. Furthermore, tumor-initiating cells have been successfully isolated from either primary EOC tumors or ascites and cultured for expression and functional analyses [17, 24].

2 Materials

2.1 Material and Reagents

Prepare all solutions using deionized, ultrapure water dH_2O (18 MΩ cm at 25 °C) and tissue culture grade reagents. All reagents and solutions must be sterile. Unless otherwise indicated, store reagents at room temperature.

1. Fresh ovarian tumor tissue samples or ascites (*see* **Notes 1** and **2**).
2. OSE Medium 1× (Wisent Multicell #316-090-CL, Wisent Bioproducts, St-Bruno, QC, Canada). Store at 4 °C (*see* **Note 3**).
3. OSE Complete Medium: 450 mL of OSE Medium 1×, 50 mL fetal bovine serum (FBS; final 10 % v/v), amphotericin B 2.5 μg/mL, gentamicin 50 μg/mL. Store medium at 4 °C and warm to 37 °C before use.
4. Fetal bovine serum (FBS): Dispense into 50 mL aliquots, and store at −20 °C. Thaw before adding to culture medium.
5. Phosphate-buffered saline buffer (PBS): 137 mM NaCl, 2.7 mM KCl, 10 mM $Na_2HPO_4{\cdot}2H_2O$, 2 mM KH_2PO_4, pH 7.4.
6. Liquid nitrogen.
7. Isopropanol, ACS reagent grade.
8. Ethylenedinitrilo-tetraacetic acid (EDTA), 0.5 M, pH 8.0.
9. Dimethyl sulfoxide (DMSO), sterile, tissue culture grade.
10. Trypsin–EDTA solution: 0.05 % v/v trypsin/0.53 mM EDTA. Filter-sterilize with 0.22 μm filter. Store at 4 °C and pre-warm to room temperature (20–24 °C) prior to use.
11. Gentamicin solution, 1,000×, liquid (50 mg/mL). Store at 4 °C.
12. Amphotericin B (antifungal), 100×, solubilized (250 μg/mL). Store at 4 °C.
13. Penicillin–streptomycin, 100×, liquid (10,000 U/mL penicillin, 10,000 μg/mL streptomycin). Dispense into 5 mL aliquots, and store at −20 °C. Thaw before adding to culture medium.

14. EOC tumor cell culture freezing medium: 90 % v/v FBS, 10 % v/v DMSO, store indefinitely in a non-frost-free freezer at −20 °C (*see* **Note 4**).
15. EOC ascites cell culture freezing medium: 70 % v/v OSE medium, 20 % v/v FBS, 10 % v/v DMSO, store indefinitely in a non-frost-free freezer at −20 °C (*see* **Note 4**).

2.2 Equipment

1. Cell culture-treated dishes, 100 mm.
2. Tissue culture-treated flasks with 0.2 μm vented cap, T75.
3. Tissue culture-treated dish 6-well.
4. Cell scrapers with flexible rubber blade, sterile.
5. Nalgene cryo 1 °C freezing container.
6. Glass coverslips, sterile.

3 Methods

Carry out all procedures at room temperature unless otherwise specified. Ensure all the reagents and apparatus are sterile.

3.1 Epithelial Ovarian Cancer Cells from Primary Tumor Samples

3.1.1 Isolation of EOC Cells from Tumor Tissue

1. The ovarian tumor specimens must be collected aseptically and transported to the laboratory on ice (*see* **Notes 1** and **2**).
2. Pre-warm the OSE complete medium in a 37 °C water bath (*see* **Note 3**).
3. Working in a tissue culture biosafety cabinet and with sterile forceps, transfer the tumor tissue (0.5–1 cm^2) into 100 mm culture dish with 8 mL of pre-warmed complete OSE culture medium.
4. While holding the piece of tumor tissue with the forceps, gently dissociate cells from the tissue with a sterile cell scraper (Fig. 1).
5. Incubate the dissociated cells overnight in a tissue culture incubator (37 °C, 5 % CO_2, 95 % air).
6. The next day, remove the medium with a sterile Pasteur pipette fixed to a vacuum and waste receptacle system.
7. With a sterile disposable serological pipette, add 8 mL of pre-warmed, fresh OSE complete medium (*see* **Note 5**).
8. Tumor-derived EOC cells can be characterized for the presence of epithelial and other contaminating cell types via immunocytochemistry (*see* **Note 6**).

3.1.2 Propagation and Freezing of EOC Tumor Cells

1. When the culture is confluent (may take 7 days or more, Fig. 2), rinse the cell layer with 4 mL of 1× PBS.
2. Perform a partial trypsinization by dissociating the cells with 1 mL of 0.05 % trypsin/EDTA and incubate 3–5 min at 37 °C to activate the trypsin (*see* **Note 7**, Fig. 3).

3. Add 4 mL of complete OSE medium to the dissociated cells and resuspend with a sterile disposable serological pipette.
4. Split the resuspended cells 1:2 into two new 100 mm culture dishes (2.5 mL of resuspended cells/dish). Add 5 mL of OSE complete medium to these new dishes.
5. Add 8 mL of OSE complete medium to the initial dish containing the remaining cells that did not detach from the trypsin treatment (*see* **Note 8**, Fig. 3).
6. Change culture medium every 3 days with 8 mL of pre-warmed, fresh complete OSE culture medium.
7. When the cultured cells are confluent, repeat **steps 1–4** (*see* **Note 9**).
8. To freeze primary EOC tumor cells, trypsinize two 100 mm dishes as in **steps 1–3** when the culture is confluent.
9. Transfer the EOC cell suspension to a sterile 15 mL conical tube.
10. Centrifuge for 5 min at 2,500 ×*g* at room temperature.
11. Carefully remove supernatant.
12. Resuspend the cell pellet in 1 mL of EOC tumor cell culture freezing medium.
13. Using a 1 mL sterile serological pipette, transfer the resuspended cells into a labelled, sterile cryogenic vial.
14. Place the vial in a Nalgene cryo 1 °C freezing container at −80 °C for a minimum of 4 h.
15. Transfer vial in liquid nitrogen or in −150 °C ultra-low freezer for long-term storage.
16. To thaw a vial of frozen primary tumor EOC cells, place in 37 °C water bath until just thawed, and while working in a tissue culture biosafety cabinet, aseptically transfer to a sterile 15 mL conical centrifuge tube.
17. Dilute cells and freezing medium with maximum volume of complete OSE culture medium (13–14 mL) and centrifuge between 1,500 and 2,500 ×*g* for 5 min at room temperature.
18. Carefully aspirate supernatant, gently resuspend cells with 8 mL fresh complete OSE culture medium, and transfer to a sterile 100 mm tissue culture dish. Culture cells according to **steps 1–6**.

3.2 Epithelial Ovarian Cancer Cells from Ascites Fluid

3.2.1 Isolation of Ascites-Derived EOC Cells

1. Freshly isolated ascites should be obtained in a sterile vacuum container or evacuated bottle(s) (Fig. 8a) (*see* **Notes 1** and **2**).
2. Use a tissue culture biosafety cabinet to aseptically transfer 25 mL of ascites to T-75 cm^2 tissue culture flasks (we typically seed ten flasks) with 0.2 μm vented caps (Fig. 8b). Add an equal volume (25 mL) of complete OSE medium to each flask.

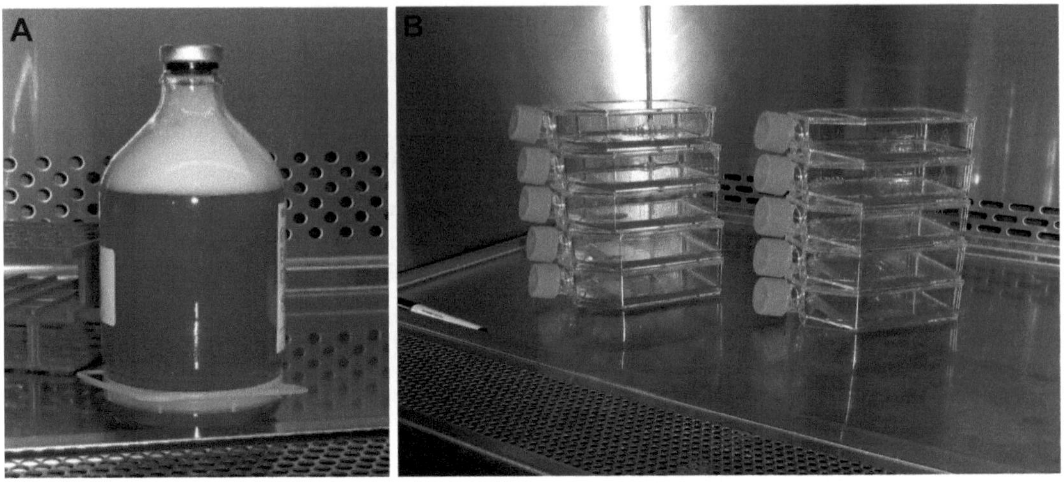

Fig. 8 Isolation and culture of primary ovarian cancer cells. (**a**) Patient ascites fluid delivered to the laboratory. (**b**) T-75 flasks containing 25 mL patient ascites and 25 mL complete OSE medium

3. Place in an incubator undisturbed for 3–4 days prior to first change of complete medium (*see* **Note 10**).
4. Additional ascites can be added to sterile tubes and clarified at 3,200 × *g* for 10 min at 4 °C. Transfer the clarified ascites (supernatant) to multiple tubes/vials and freeze at −80 °C for archival purposes (*see* **Note 11**).
5. For immediate cytological analyses, EOC cells can be separated from the ascites fluid via cytospin (*see* **Note 12**) [22].
6. As with tumor-derived EOC cells, ascites-derived EOC cultures can be characterized via immunocytochemistry for the presence of epithelial and other contaminating cell types (*see* **Note 6**).

3.2.2 Expansion and Freezing of Ascites-Derived EOC Cells

1. Medium should be replaced after approximately 3–4 days; continue to change media every 2–3 days until the flasks are confluent (Fig. 6). To passage EOC cells, wash cells once with PBS then trypsinize using a minimal volume of trypsin–EDTA solution for 5 min at 37 °C. Dilute with complete OSE medium and transfer cells to new T-75 cm^2 flasks (*see* **Note 13**).
2. To freeze stocks of primary EOC cells, wash cells once with sterile PBS then trypsinize using a minimal volume of trypsin–EDTA solution for 5 min at 37 °C.
3. Add complete OSE medium and transfer cells to sterile 15 mL conical centrifuge tubes.
4. Centrifuge at 1,500 × *g* for 5 min at room temperature.
5. Discard the supernatant and resuspend cells with appropriate volume of EOC ascites cell culture freezing medium (i.e., 1.5 mL per T-75 flask).

6. Transfer cells to sterile cryovials and place in a Nalgene cryo 1 °C freezing container (according to manufacturer's instructions). Place into a −80 °C freezer for a minimum of 4 h prior to transferring indefinitely to liquid nitrogen or a −150 °C freezer (*see* **Note 14**).
7. To thaw primary ascites EOC cells, place the vial at 37 °C until just thawed, and aseptically transfer to a sterile 15 mL conical centrifuge tube.
8. Dilute cells and freezing medium with maximum volume of complete OSE medium and centrifuge 1,500 × *g* for 5 min at room temperature.
9. Aspirate supernatant, gently resuspend cells with complete OSE medium, and transfer to a sterile T-75 tissue culture flask. Culture cells according to **step 1**.

4 Notes

1. Institutional informed patient consent and appropriate biohazard authorization is required for experimentation with human tissue.
2. Depending upon institutional screening procedures, patient samples should be treated as potentially positive for contagious pathogenic viruses (e.g., HIV or hepatitis viruses), as well as methicillin-resistant *Staphylococcus aureus* (MRSA)-positive bacteria in rare circumstances.
3. A mixture of MCDB 105 and M199 media (1:1) can be used as an alternative to OSE medium. Both media are supplied as powder for 1 L of medium. Make equal volumes of each medium separately from the powder. Measure out 90 % of required volume of water. Water temperature should be 15–20 °C. While gently stirring the water, add the powdered medium, and stir until dissolved. Do not heat. Then combine both media together with gentle stirring, and pH to 7.2 with 1 N HCl, to give pH 7.4 after filter sterilization (0.22 μm filter). Adjust volume to 1 L with sterile water. Store at 4 °C and protect from light. Prepare complete culture medium for growth of EOC cells (Subheading 2.1, **step 3**).
4. When thawed, mix thoroughly by inversion.
5. The cells will adhere rapidly onto the cell culture dish. It is important to observe the cells every day through a phase contrast microscope. If the media still contains a large amount of cellular debris and/or blood cells after 48 h post-isolation, a full media change can be performed. In general, cells will have reached confluence within a week of culture (Fig. 2).
6. The presence of epithelial cells can be confirmed upon positive immunocytochemical staining with antibodies towards cytokeratins 7, 8, 18, and 19 [18, 21].

7. One week post-isolation, different cell types may be apparent in the culture dish (Fig. 2). We have noticed that these cell types display different adherence characteristics. We can therefore attempt to separate these cell types by performing a partial trypsinization. Fibroblasts are more sensitive to trypsin and will lift first, while most epithelial cells still remain adherent. We incubate the confluent culture with 0.05 % trypsin–EDTA for a few seconds to a few minutes at 37 °C. As soon as some cells lift, discard the trypsin solution and add fresh media on the remaining adherent cells in the culture dish (Fig. 3a).
8. After several days in culture, the cells that were originally lifted after the first trypsinization are composed mainly of fibroblasts and epithelial cells (Fig. 3c). The more adherent cells left in the original dish now have more space to propagate (Fig. 3b). This partial trypsinization can be repeated after a few days if necessary to ensure that the culture contains a majority of epithelial cells.
9. After many weeks or even months, the initial trypsin-resistant, adherent cultures (*see* **Note** 7) kept in the original culture dish will form "foci" (Fig. 4). However, the time that it takes to form these foci is variable from one cell preparation to the next. Determining factors include the number of starting cells at initial plating, in addition to the capacity of these cells to adapt to tissue culture conditions. Once the "foci" are numerous and occupy the majority of the culture surface, trypsinization and amplification can be attempted. At this initial split, massive apoptosis occurs, most likely due to their reduced capacity to proliferate when dispersed. Some cultures will overcome this massive cell death and form immortalized tumor lines (Fig. 5).
10. The amount of erythrocytes and the viscosity of the fluid will vary tremendously from patient to patient, but additional processing steps (such as the removal of the erythrocytes by centrifugation over a Percoll cushion [22] or hypotonic lysis) are not necessary. The EOC cells will eventually bind to the tissue culture plastic, though it may not be clearly visible, and the erythrocytes will be removed after the first set of medium changes (Fig. 6). Furthermore, the complete OSE medium used to propagate EOC cells does not support the growth of hematopoietic cell contaminants.
11. Centrifugation of the ascites fluid can be performed to isolate clarified ascites, containing supportive growth factors and signalling molecules secreted both from the tumor cells and microenvironment within the peritoneal cavity that can be analyzed via protein identification and/or quantification methods (ELISA, immunoblot, HPLC). Analyses of ascitic fluid may provide insights into putative EOC biomarkers.

12. Separation of EOC cells using cytospin allows for characterization of metastatic EOC cells isolated directly from patients without the effects of adaptation to culture. Furthermore, the cytospin slides can be archived at 4 °C for months and easily amenable to immunocytochemical staining.
13. Split cells at a 1:2 dilution and no more than 1:3 for maintaining adequate growth of the cells over time. It should be noted that primary EOC cells have a reduced growth rate as compared with established EOC cell lines [22]. We typically split one flask of passage-0 cells at a 1:2 dilution and monitor over the next 24–48 h to observe seeding efficiency, growth, and general morphology of the cells (Fig. 6). Based on these observations, we then choose whether to proceed with freezing numerous vials of passage-0 cells for archival purposes.
14. A slow cooling rate of ~1 °C/min increases the viability of the cells. Freeze as many passage-0 cells as possible and store indefinitely in liquid nitrogen or a −150 °C freezer. Higher passage number cells can be frozen as well, but be aware that recovery and lifespan of experimentally serviceable EOC cells will be compromised (especially for EOC cells ≥passage-4). Experiments are typically performed using cells at passage-2 through passage-6, because many cell samples will stop growing, or senesce, shortly thereafter. It is unknown what the upper storage time limit might be, but cells have been successfully regrown 5 years after initial cryopreservation.

Acknowledgments

Dr. Cécile Le Page for helpful suggestions. This work was supported by the banque de tissus et de données of the Fonds de Recherche Santé Québec (FRQS) and the Manitoba Ovarian Biobank Program (MOBP) through the Manitoba Tumor Bank and CancerCare Manitoba.

References

1. Siegel R, Ward E, Brawley O, Jemal A (2011) Cancer statistics, 2011: the impact of eliminating socioeconomic and racial disparities on premature cancer deaths. CA Cancer J Clin 61: 212–236
2. Weberpals JI, Koti M, Squire JA (2011) Targeting genetic and epigenetic alterations in the treatment of serous ovarian cancer. Cancer Genet 204:525–535
3. Saad AF, Hu W, Sood AK (2010) Microenvironment and pathogenesis of epithelial ovarian cancer. Horm Cancer 1: 277–290
4. Asadollahi R, Hyde CA, Zhong XY (2010) Epigenetics of ovarian cancer: from the lab to the clinic. Gynecol Oncol 118:81–87
5. Yoshida S, Furukawa N, Haruta S, Tanase Y, Kanayama S, Noguchi T, Sakata M, Yamada Y, Oi H, Kobayashi H (2009) Expression profiles of genes involved in poor prognosis of epithelial ovarian carcinoma: a review. Int J Gynecol Cancer 19:992–997

6. Sheng Q, Liu J (2011) The therapeutic potential of targeting the EGFR family in epithelial ovarian cancer. Br J Cancer 104:1241–1245
7. Eckstein N (2011) Platinum resistance in breast and ovarian cancer cell lines. J Exp ClinCancer 30:91
8. van Jaarsveld MT, Helleman J, Berns EM, Wiemer EA (2010) MicroRNAs in ovarian cancer biology and therapy resistance. Int J Biochem Cell Biol 42:1282–1290
9. Grun B, Benjamin E, Sinclair J, Timms JF, Jacobs IJ, Gayther SA, Dafou D (2009) Three-dimensional in vitro cell biology models of ovarian and endometrial cancer. Cell Prolif 42:219–228
10. Theriault BL, Shepherd TG, Mujoomdar ML, Nachtigal MW (2007) BMP4 induces EMT and Rho GTPase activation in human ovarian cancer cells. Carcinogenesis 28:1153–1162
11. Matsumura N, Huang Z, Mori S, Baba T, Fujii S, Konishi I, Iversen ES, Berchuck A, Murphy SK (2011) Epigenetic suppression of the TGF-beta pathway revealed by transcriptome profiling in ovarian cancer. Genome Res 21:74–82
12. Ouellet V, Provencher DM, Maugard CM, Le Page C, Ren F, Lussier C, Novak J, Ge B, Hudson TJ, Tonin PN, Mes-Masson AM (2005) Discrimination between serous low malignant potential and invasive epithelial ovarian tumors using molecular profiling. Oncogene 24:4672–4687
13. Evangelou A, Jindal SK, Brown TJ, Letarte M (2000) Down-regulation of transforming growth factor beta receptors by androgen in ovarian cancer cells. Cancer Res 60:929–935
14. Hirte HW, Clark DA, Mazurka J, O'Connell G, Rusthoven J (1992) A rapid and simple method for the purification of tumor cells from ascitic fluid of ovarian carcinoma. Gynecol Oncol 44:223–226
15. Kruk PA, Maines-Bandiera SL, Auersperg N (1990) A simplified method to culture human ovarian surface epithelium. Lab Invest 63: 132–136
16. Lawrenson K, Benjamin E, Turmaine M, Jacobs I, Gayther S, Dafou D (2009) In vitro three-dimensional modelling of human ovarian surface epithelial cells. Cell Prolif 42:385–393
17. Liu T, Cheng W, Lai D, Huang Y, Guo L (2010) Characterization of primary ovarian cancer cells in different culture systems. Oncol Rep 23:1277–1284
18. Lounis H, Provencher D, Godbout C, Fink D, Milot MJ, Mes-Masson AM (1994) Primary cultures of normal and tumoral human ovarian epithelium: a powerful tool for basic molecular studies. Exp Cell Res 215:303–309
19. Auersperg N, Maines-Bandiera SL, Dyck HG, Kruk PA (1994) Characterization of cultured human ovarian surface epithelial cells: phenotypic plasticity and premalignant changes. Lab Invest 71:510–518
20. Salamanca CM, Maines-Bandiera SL, Leung PC, Hu YL, Auersperg N (2004) Effects of epidermal growth factor/hydrocortisone on the growth and differentiation of human ovarian surface epithelium. J Soc Gynecol Investig 11:241–251
21. Ouellet V, Zietarska M, Portelance L, Lafontaine J, Madore J, Puiffe ML, Arcand SL, Shen Z, Hebert J, Tonin PN, Provencher DM, Mes-Masson AM (2008) Characterization of three new serous epithelial ovarian cancer cell lines. BMC Cancer 8:152
22. Shepherd TG, Theriault BL, Campbell EJ, Nachtigal MW (2006) Primary culture of ovarian surface epithelial cells and ascites-derived ovarian cancer cells from patients. Nat Protoc 1:2643–2649
23. Onda T, Yoshikawa H (2011) Neoadjuvant chemotherapy for advanced ovarian cancer: overview of outcomes and unanswered questions. Expert Rev Anticancer Ther 11:1053–1067
24. Stewart JM, Shaw PA, Gedye C, Bernardini MQ, Neel BG, Ailles LE (2011) Phenotypic heterogeneity and instability of human ovarian tumor-initiating cells. Proc Natl Acad Sci U S A 108:6468–6473

Chapter 25

Ovarian Cancer Stem Cells Enrichment

Lijuan Yang and Dongmei Lai

Abstract

The concept of cancer stem cells (CSCs) provides a new paradigm for understanding cancer biology. Cancer stem cells are defined as a minority of cancer cells with stem cell properties responsible for maintenance and growth of tumors. The targeting of CSCs is a potential therapeutic strategy to combat ovarian cancer. Ovarian epithelial cancer cells cultured in serum-free medium can form sphere cells. These sphere cells may be enriched for cancer stem cells (CSCs). The isolation of sphere cells from solid tumors is an important technique in studying cancer cell biology. Here we describe the isolation of sphere cells from primary ovarian cancer tissue, ascites fluid, and the cancer cell line SKOV3 with stem cell selection medium.

Key words Ovarian epithelial cancer, Cancer stem cells, Sphere cells, Cell suspension culture

1 Introduction

Ovarian cancer is one of the leading causes of death among gynecologic malignancies. Optimal cytoreductive surgery followed by systemic chemotherapy with paclitaxel and cisplatin is the current standard therapy for metastatic ovarian cancer at diagnosis, with a reported response rate of over 70 %. However, the overall 5-year survival rate is only 30–40 % [1, 2]. One of the most important causes of failure in ovarian cancer treatment is the development of resistance to paclitaxel and platinum-based chemotherapy [3]. One emerging model for the development of drug-resistant tumors invokes a pool of self-renewing malignant progenitors known as cancer stem cells (CSCs) or cancer-initiating cells (CIC). According to the CSC hypothesis, cancer stem cells are defined as a rare cell population in cancer that acts like stem cells. CSCs are inherently resistant to chemotherapy because of their stem cell properties, mainly their quiescence and the expression of drug membrane transporters (e.g., ABCG2). Therefore, CSCs may survive therapy and regenerate the tumor [4–6].

Anastasia Malek and Oleg Tchernitsa (eds.), *Ovarian Cancer: Methods and Protocols*, Methods in Molecular Biology, vol. 1049, DOI 10.1007/978-1-62703-547-7_25, © Springer Science+Business Media New York 2013

The concept of cancer stem cells (CSC) provides a new paradigm for understanding cancer biology. In order to elucidate the cancer stem cell biology, we must first isolate this cell population from the cancer tissue. For identifying and isolating CSCs, three methods may be selected: (a) isolation on the basis of a side population (SP) phenotype – stem cells have been isolated by their ability to efflux Hoechst 33342 dye and are referred to as the "side population" (SP) [7]; (b) using relevant surface markers (such as CD133, CD117, or CD44) to isolate potential CSCs by fluorescence-activated cell sorting (FACS) or magnetic-activated cell sorting (MACS) [8]; and (c) culturing of sphere-like cellular aggregates in serum-free medium (SFM) containing epidermal growth factor (EGF) and basic fibroblast growth factor (bFGF) [9, 10]. This method was derived from the culturing of neural stem/progenitor cells (NSCs) [11, 12]. All established laboratory cell lines (like most other cancer cell lines) are grown in media containing serum, whereas NSCs are grown in serum-free media, since serum causes irreversible differentiation of NSCs [13, 14]. All of this method is double-edged swords: (a) Although cancer progenitor cells can be isolated using side population, the dye Hoechst 33342 is harmful to cancer cells and could decrease the cell clonogenicity [15]. Moreover, the amount of the stem cells obtained from SP cell sorting is too small for the further analysis. (b) Cell surface markers such as CD133 and CD44 in combination with flow cytometry have identified subpopulations in colon cancer and glioblastoma [16, 17]; however, the marker of ovarian cancer stem cells is still not well characterized. (c) Sphere cells formed in serum-free medium may develop a necrotic center due to diffusion limits of nutrients and oxygen, and the spheroids may also contain differentiated cells and dead cells [18]. Nevertheless, we found that under serum-free stem cell selective culture condition, primary cancer cells from ovarian cancer specimens can form nonadherent sphere and display remarkable stem cell properties, drug resistance, and propagation of their original tumor phenotype with the properties expected for CSCs. We suggest that the sphere cell subpopulation may be a more reliable model than differentiated cells grown in the presence of serum (cells adhere to plates and form compact clusters of relatively cobble-like uniform) for understanding the biology of ovarian cancer [9, 10]. Since the sphere cells can be frozen, stored, and produced in consistently large numbers, they may be a more reliable model system for understanding the biology of primary human tumors, for screening new therapeutic agents, and ultimately for guiding clinical personalized tumor therapy.

Here, we describe our methods of isolating sphere cells from primary ovarian cancer tissue, ascites fluid, and an ovarian cancer cell line.

2 Materials

Prepare all solution using ultrapure water (prepared by purifying deionized water to attain a resistivity f 18 M Ω cm at 25 °C) and analytical grade reagents. Prepare and store all reagents at 4 °C (unless the context indicates otherwise). Diligently follow all waste disposal regulations when disposing waste material.

2.1 Tissue and Cells

1. Collecting ovarian cancer tissues and ascites (*see* **Notes 1** and **2**).
2. Ovarian cancer cell line SKOV3.

2.2 Separating Medium

1. 80 mesh stainless screen filter.
2. Phosphate-Buffered Saline buffer (PBS): 137 mM NaCl, 2.7 mM KCl, 10 mM $Na_2HPO_4{\cdot}2H_2O$, 2 mM KH_2PO_4, pH 7.4 Sterilize by autoclaving.
3. Separation reagent Percoll Plus (GE Healthcare Life Science).

   Prepare 90 % and 45 % (v/v) solutions of Percoll Plus in PBS (*see* **Note 3**). Prepare a fresh dilution of Percoll each time.
4. 15 and 50 ml centrifuge tube (Axygen, USA).

2.3 Cell Culture Reagents

1. $NaHCO_3$ ×100. Dissolve 2 g $NaHCO_3$ in 10 ml of PBS ×1.
2. Trypsin–EDTA (Ethylenedinitrilo–tetraacetic acid, EDTA) solution. 0.25 %-trypsin/0.53 mM EDTA (*see* **Note 4**).
3. McCoy's 5A medium. Mix contains of one bottle of the powder, 11.9 g (Sigma-Aldrich, USA), 100 ml fetal bovine serum (FBS), 10 ml penicillin–streptomycin solution (100×), and 2.3 g $NaHCO_3$, and add water up to 1 l. Filter through 0.22 μm pore filter and make aliquot, and then store at 4 °C.
4. DMEM/F12 medium.
5. Stem cell selection medium. Include 500 ml of the serum-free DMEM/F12 medium, 10 % Knockout (KO) serum, 1 % sodium pyruvate 100×, 1 % GlutaMAX 100×, 1 % β-mercaptoethanol 100×, 1 % MEM NEAA 100×, 0.4 % basic fibroblast growth factor (bFGF) 100×, 1 % penicillin–streptomycin solution 100×, and add NaHCO3 100× up to 600 ml of final volume. Filter solutions through a 0.22 μm pore filter and store at 4 °C (*see* **Note 5**).
6. Dimethyl sulfoxide (DMSO), sterile, tissue culture grade.
7. Cryopreservation reagent. DMSO 10 %, McCoy's 5A medium 90 %. Prepare a fresh dilution of Percoll each time (*see* **Note 3**).
8. 100 and 60 mm cell culture plates (Corning, USA).
9. Poly-HEMA (2-hydroxyethyl methacrylate) (*see* **Note 6**).

3 Methods

Carry out all procedures on a super-clean culture hood. Make sure all the reagents and apparatus sterilized.

3.1 Primary Ovarian Cancer Tissues

3.1.1 Isolation of Primary Ovarian Cancer Cells from Primary Ovarian Cancer Tissue

1. Rinse about 10 g ovarian cancer tissue with PBS at least three times (*see* **Note 7**).
2. Put the tissue into a 50 ml centrifuge tube.
3. Cut the sample into 1–2 mm segments with scissors.
4. Add 20 ml 0.25 % trypsin into the tube to submerge the tissue. Screw on the cap loosely.
5. Incubate at 37 °C (*see* **Note 8**) in a humidified atmosphere containing 5 % CO_2 for 30–40 min (*see* **Note 9**).
6. Shake the tube to disaggregate the cells as much as possible without making the suspension frothy.
7. Pipette the mixture up and down several times during digestion. Check the suspension under a microscope until most of the cells are dispersed.
8. Add 20 ml the McCoy's 5A medium to neutralize the further effect of trypsin (*see* **Note 10**).
9. The mixture is then filtered by the screen filter, and the filtrate is transferred to the 15 ml centrifuge tube (*see* **Note 11**).
10. Centrifuge the tubes at 1,000 × *g* for 5 min at 4 °C.
11. Remove supernatant and resuspend the cells in 4 ml of the McCoy's 5A medium.
12. Separate cells by centrifugation in Percoll Plus at 1,500 × *g* for 30 min at 4 °C (*see* **Note 12**) (*see* Fig. 1).
13. Gently transfer the middle layer which contains the cancer cells into another tube (*see* **Note 13**), and add three times volumes of the McCoy's 5A medium containing 10 % FBS to the tube.
14. Centrifuge the tube at 1,000 × *g* for 5 min at 4 °C, remove supernatant, and resuspend in fresh McCoy's 5A medium.
15. Repeat **step 14** twice (*see* **Note 14**).
16. Transfer cells to the culture plates (*see* **Note 15**).

3.1.2 Cell Culture of Primary Ovarian Cancer

1. Culture cells in 10 cm culture plates at 37 °C in a humidified atmosphere containing 5 % CO_2 overnight.
2. Change the medium and replace with fresh culture medium after the cells are attached. Subsequently, change the medium every 2–3 days depending on the cell growth rate (*see* **Note 16**).
3. These cells grow as attached cobblestone-like monolayer epithelial cancer cells (Fig. 2a).

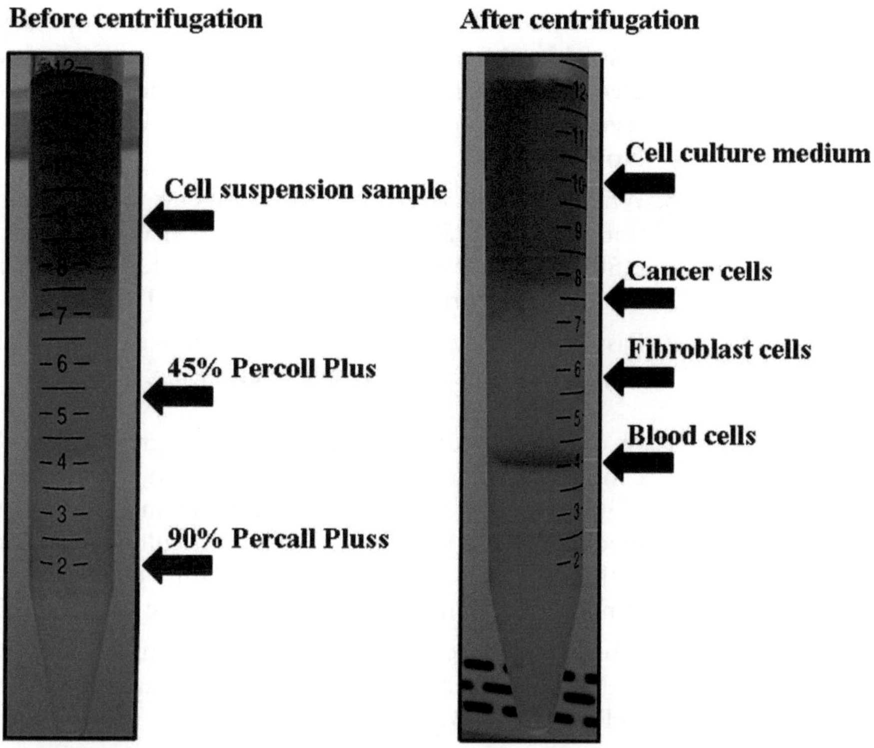

Fig. 1 Separation the cells isolated from ovarian cancer tissue by centrifugation in Percoll Plus. Cells will separate into three layers indicated

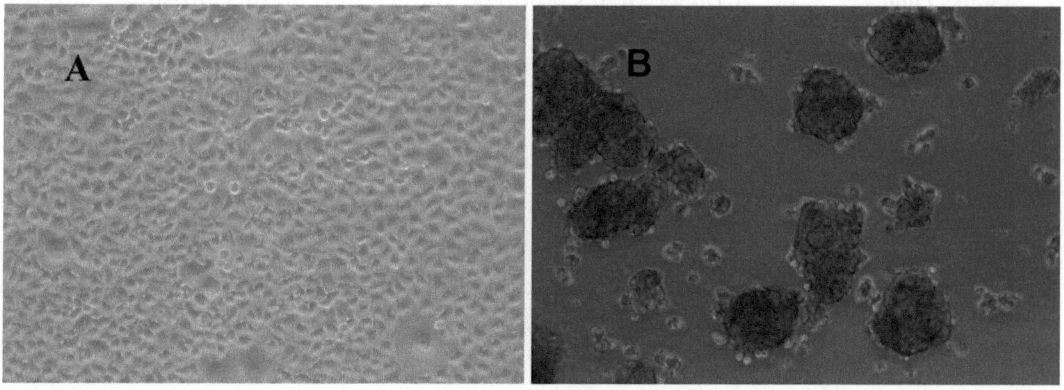

Fig. 2 Cell culture of primary ovarian cancer. (**a**) Upon adherent conditions the cells grow as attached cobblestone-like monolayer epithelial cancer cells, (**b**) After culturing upon nonadherent conditions, the cells can form spheroids or sphere cells

4. When the cells grow to 80–90 % confluence, passage the cells with 0.25 % trypsin. Since cells become round and detached, stop digestion by adding the McCoy's 5A medium. Centrifuge cells at 1,500 rpm for 5 min. Remove supernatant and resuspend cells in the McCoy's medium and distribute them into three 10 cm culture plates (*see* **Note 17**).

5. If you want to freeze the cells, the process is the same as cell passaging. After cell centrifugation, resuspend the cells with cryopreservation reagent, and then distribute them into several cryogenic vials. Store those in liquid nitrogen or −80 °C (*see* **Note 18**).
6. When you thaw cells, place the cryogenic vials (Corning®) in a water bath at 37–42 °C until just thawed. Centrifuge at 1,500 rpm for 5 min. Discard supernatant, resuspend cells, and place into culturing condition (*see* **Note 19**).
7. Passage primary cancer cells until you get enough cells to do the experiments, such as sphere culturing.

3.1.3 Sphere Cells Culture of Primary Ovarian Cancer

1. As described above (Subheading 3.1.2), grow cells to 80–90 % confluence, digest with 0.25 % trypsin, centrifuge cells at 1,500 rpm for 5 min, and resuspend in stem cell selection medium. Then transfer the cells to a culture plate pretreated with Poly-HEMA (*see* **Note 20**). Culture conditions are maintained at 37 °C in a humidified atmosphere containing 5 % CO_2.
2. Observe the cells each day. Change medium every 2 or 3 days, according to the cell growth rate and the medium pH (*see* **Note 21**).
3. These cells can form nonadherent spheroids or sphere cells; there should be almost no attached cells (Fig. 2b) (*see* **Note 22**).

3.2 Ascites Fluid of Primary Ovarian Cancer

3.2.1 Isolation of Cancer Cells from Primary Ovarian Cancer Ascites Fluid

1. Collect ascites fluid and aliquot into 50 ml centrifuge tube and centrifuge at 1,000 × *g* for 5 min. Resuspend the cell pellets in McCoy's 5A medium.
2. Then go through **steps 9–16** of Subheading 3.1.1.

3.2.2 Sphere Cell Culture from Ascites Fluid

1. Resuspend the cells directly in stem cell selection medium, and transfer the cells to a culture plate pretreated with Poly-HEMA (*see* **Notes 6, 12, 13** and **15**). Culture conditions are maintained at 37 °C in a humidified atmosphere containing 5 % CO_2.
2. Observe the cells each day. Change medium every 2 or 3 days, according to the cell growth rate and the medium pH (*see* **Note 21**).
3. The cells begin to form aggregates after 2 or 3 days culturing and become nonadherent spheroids or spheres after about a week. There should be almost no attached cells.

3.3 Ovarian Cancer Cell Line SKOV3 (Spheres Formation)

1. Thaw cells (*see* **step 6** of Subheading 3.1.2) and follow the cell culture procedures.

2. The exponential-phase attached cells are digested and further cultured in stem cell selection medium in Poly-HEMA-coated plates (*see* **steps 1–3** of Subheading 3.1.3).
3. Cells can form nonadherent spheres (*see* Fig. 2 and **Note 22**).

4 Notes

1. Institutional informed patient consent and appropriate biohazard authorization is required for experimentation with human tissue. Patient samples should be treated as potentially positive for contagious pathogens.
2. Cancer samples should be collected at the time of surgery under sterile conditions. The amount of the tissue and the volume of ascetic fluid depend on the condition of patient. Generally, we get 5–10 g of tissue or 50 ml of ascetic liquid. Store the samples on ice and transfer them to the laboratory within 20 min.
3. Separating reagent (Percoll Plus) and cryopreservation reagent (DMSO) stock solutions should be stored at room temperature away from light.
4. The trypsin can be store at −20 °C. If you use it frequently, you can store at 4 °C.
5. We prepare stem cell selection medium except bFGF first and then aliquot 50 ml medium into tubes and store at −20 °C. Thaw it at 4 °C and add 200 μl bFGF (100×) into each tube before use. Because the stem cell selection medium includes many growth factors, fresh preparation is suggested. If stored at 4 °C for a long time, the growth factors may be degraded. Moreover, contamination might easily occur at 4 °C. Of course, if you use it frequently, you can store it at 4 °C less than a week preferably.
6. Dissolve 2.4 g of Poly-HEMA in 20 ml 95 % ethyl alcohol(ETOH) by rotating for 8 h and then dilute 1:10 in 95 % ETOH (final conc. = 12 mg/ml). Store it at room temperature. Coat plates with Poly-HEMA by 4 ml/100 mm dish or 1.5 ml/60 mm dish.
7. You can also wash more than three times until the tissue is free of blood or foreign material.
8. Mix the tube up and down during the digestion in order to digest completely to obtain more cells.
9. Time period is according to the size of the tissue; more tissue needs a longer time.
10. You can also stop digestion with medium containing 10 % FBS. The amount of the medium should be equivalent to the volume of 0.25 % trypsin.

11. We filter the mixture through an 80 mesh stainless screen. Prevent the tissue leaking outside as well as you can.
12. Density gradients are often used for separation, purifications of cells, and removing of blood cells. Take two 15 ml Falcon tube, fill it with 4 ml of 90 % Percoll Plus first, and then fill up carefully with 4 ml of 45 % Percoll Plus. There is a visible line between them. You can drop a few drops of the McCoy's medium into 90 % Percoll Plus to help you to distinguish them. Then apply 2 ml of the mixture of cells and medium to the top gently. The volume of the Percoll Plus and the mixture of cells and medium depend on your own habit, but the volume of 90 % Percoll Plus and 45 % Percoll Plus must be the same. The density of the top band of the gradient of Percoll Plus is 45 % and the bottom layer is 90 %.
13. After centrifugation, there are several layers. Usually the culture medium is layered on top of the gradient and epithelial ovarian cancer cells remain in the layer above the 45 % gradient, and this layer can be removed with a pipette. An additional layer may contain fibroblast cells and red blood cells. The cell type of each layer is related to tumor sample, and we recommend that you transfer and culture each of them and then observe them carefully.
14. This step is mainly to remove the Percoll completely, because it is harmful to the cells.
15. If the number of cells exceed to 2×10^6, you should put cells into two or more 100 mm dishes. Too many cells in one dish can prevent cells from attaching to the culture dishes.
16. Usually the cancer cells grow as attached cells by the next day, and you can easily change the medium. If not, you should let the cells grow for another day. The cells might grow very quickly, and you need to change the medium according to the medium pH (the red medium changes to be yellow). If bacterial contamination occurs in the cell culture, discard the cells immediately.
17. Because the primary ovarian cancer cells are very vulnerable, trypsin is not recommended to digest the cells in the first week if the cells grow too confluent; try to pipette the cells mechanically to passage the cells.
18. Cells of each 10 cm culture plate can be aliquoted by 500 μl into 4–6 cryogenic vials.
19. You should freeze cells at a slow rate and melt cells at a fast rate.
20. Add the Poly-HEMA solution to the culture plate (4 ml to 10 cm or 1.5 ml to 6 cm) and then incubate at 37 °C in a humidified atmosphere containing 5 % CO_2 for 4 h. Remove the liquid and incubate for another 3 days. Before you culture cells, you should wash the plates with PBS three times and UV irradiate them for at least 30 min.

21. The method of changing medium of sphere cells is to centrifuge at 1,000 × *g* for 5 min and then resuspend the cells and culture them.
22. The cells begin to form aggregates after 2 or 3 days culturing and become spheres after about a week, and then you can detect the stem cell markers. The time when you use it for experiments and when you passage it depends on the cell conditions. We often start to do experiment after 2 or 3 weeks culturing.

Acknowledgments

This work was supported by the Science and Technology Commission of Shanghai Municipality 2007 Shanghai Pujiang project (to D.L. 07pj14090), the Science and Technology Commission of Shanghai Municipality 2009 YIXUEYINGDAO project (to D.L. 09411968300), and the Key Project Fund of Shanghai Municipal Health Bureau (to D.L. 2010011), Shanghai, China.

References

1. Ozols RF (2005) Treatment goals in ovarian cancer. Int J Gynecol Cancer 15:3–11
2. Cannistra SA (2004) Cancer of the ovary. N Engl J Med 351:2519–2529
3. Thigpen JT, Aghajanian CA, Alberts DS et al (2005) Role of pegylated liposomal doxorubicin in ovarian cancer. Gynecol Oncol 96:10–18
4. Dean M, Fojo T, Bates S (2005) Tumour stem cells and drug resistance. Nat Rev Cancer 5:275–284
5. Dalerba P, Cho RW, Clarke MF (2007) Cancer stem cells: models and concepts. Annu Rev Med 58:267–284
6. Reya T, Morrison SJ, Clarke MF et al (2001) Stem cells, cancer, and cancer stem cells. Nature 414:105–111
7. Szotek PP, Pieretti-Vanmarcke R, Masiakos PT et al (2006) Ovarian cancer side population defines cells with stem cell-like characteristics and mullerian inhibiting substance responsiveness. Proc Natl Acad Sci USA 103:11154–11159
8. Zhang S, Balch C, Chan MW et al (2008) Identification and characterization of ovarian cancer-initiating cells from primary human tumors. Cancer Res 68:4311–4320
9. Liu T, Cheng W, Lai D et al (2010) Characterization of primary ovarian cancer cells in different culture system. Oncol Rep 23:1277–1284
10. Ma L, Lai D, Liu T et al (2010) Cancer stem-like cells can be isolated with drug selection in human ovarian cancer cell line SKOV3. Acta Biochim Biophysy Sin (Shanghai) 42: 593–602
11. Uchida N, Buck DW, He D et al (2000) Direct isolation of central nervous system stem cells. Proc Natl Acad Sci USA 97:14720–14725
12. Kondo T, Setoguchi T, Taga T (2004) Persistence of a small subpopulation of cancer stem-like cells in the C6 glioma cell line. Proc Natl Acad Sci USA 101:781–786
13. Gage FH, Ray J, Fisher LJ (1995) Isolation, characterization and use of stem cells from the CNS. Annu Rev Neurosci 18:159–192
14. McKay R (1997) Stem cells in the central nervous system. Science 276:66–671
15. Zhong Y, Zhou C, Ma W et al (2007) Most MCF7 and SKVO3 cells were deprived of their stem nature by Hoechst 33342. Biochem Biophys Res Commun 364:338–343
16. Dirks PB (2008) Brain tumor stem cells: bringing order to the chaos of brain cancer. J Clin Oncol 26:2916–2924
17. Boman BM, Huang E (2008) Human colon cancer stem cells: a new paradigm in gastrointestinal oncology. J Clin Oncol 26:2828–2838
18. Ehrhart F, Schulz JC, Katsen-Globa A et al (2009) A comparative study of freezing single cells and spheroids: towards a new model system for optimizing freezing protocols for cryobanking of human tumours. Cryobiology 58:119–127

Chapter 26

Assessment of Resistance to Anoikis in Ovarian Cancer

Xiaoping He, Jeremy Chien, and Viji Shridhar

Abstract

Anoikis, a form of programmed cell death that occurs due to cell detachment from the extracellular matrix, is a critical mechanism in preventing ectopic cell growth. Acquisition of resistance to anoikis is a prerequisite for epithelial ovarian cancer cells to survive in ascitic fluids before forming metastatic foci. Here we describe a colorimetric method for monitoring the resistance of anoikis of ovarian cancer cells in vitro.

Key words Anoikis, Ovarian cancer, Tumor metastasis, Apoptosis, Autophagy

1 Introduction

"Anoikis" is a Greek word for "homelessness." It was first described by Steven M. Frisch in 1994 [1]. Normal epithelial cells are dependent on interactions with specific extracellular matrix (ECM) components for survival, proliferation, and differentiation functions. Upon loss of contact with ECM, epithelial cells normally undergo cell death, by a process termed "anoikis." Therefore, anoikis acts as a critical physiological barrier to metastasis [2]. Resistance to anoikis may allow survival of cancer cells during systemic circulation or in ascites, thereby facilitating secondary tumor formation in distant organs. Induction or suppression of anoikis has been shown to inhibit or promote, correspondently, metastasis of various tumors including ovarian cancer [3–9].

Apoptosis has long been recognized as a critical pathway for cell death during anoikis [2]. However recently, autophagy has emerged as a novel pathway for detachment-induced cell death, because in certain circumstances, suppression of apoptosis is insufficient to abrogate cell death via anoikis and autophagy acts as an alternative to apoptosis [10–12]. Autophagic cell death (ACD) is believed to be a result of persistent autophagic stimuli in which, ultimately, cells are depleted of organelles and critical proteins, leading to a caspase-independent form of cell death, although doubts have also been shed on the existence of true autophagic cell

Anastasia Malek and Oleg Tchernitsa (eds.), *Ovarian Cancer: Methods and Protocols*, Methods in Molecular Biology, vol. 1049, DOI 10.1007/978-1-62703-547-7_26, © Springer Science+Business Media New York 2013

death in the mammalian system [13]. When cells undergo apoptosis, there is only one outcome—the orderly elimination of the cell via activation of its suicidal molecular programs [14]. In contrast, autophagy may act as either a cytoprotective or lethal effector, all depending on the target being degraded and the extent of autophagy that is allowed to occur [15]. Moreover, autophagy is reversible [16]. Growing evidence suggests an extensive cross talk between the two killing modes [14, 15]. Beclin 1, ROS, ERK, and DAPK may be key molecules responsible for integrating autophagy and apoptosis [14].

Resistance to anoikis can be conferred by diverse molecular mechanisms in ovarian cancer, including amplification of small GTPase RAB25 [6], constitutive activation of FAK [7], epidermal growth factor receptor (EGFR) activation [8], autocrine VEGF-A/KDR loop [17], and c-Met overexpression [18]. Detailed dissection of anoikis mechanisms has potential importance regarding the development of novel antitumor therapies with the aim of restoring anoikis and inhibiting metastasis.

In this chapter, we will describe a colorimetric method for monitoring the resistance to anoikis of cancer cells in vitro. Anoikis is induced by culturing cells in suspension in ultralow attachment plates. The surface of ultralow attachment plate is a covalently bound hydrogel layer that is hydrophilic and neutrally charged. Since proteins and other biomolecules passively adsorb to polystyrene surfaces through either hydrophobic or ionic interactions, this hydrogel surface naturally inhibits nonspecific immobilization via these forces, thus inhibiting subsequent cell attachment. After a certain time of suspension culture in ultralow attachment plates, cells are replated back into regular adhesive cell culture plates to allow live cells to reattach and be detected with 3-(4,5-dimethylthiazol-2-yl)-2,5-diphenyl tetrasodium bromide (MTT). MTT is a pale yellow chemical that is cleaved by living cells to yield a dark blue formazan product which can be solubilized and quantified by spectrophotometric means. The limitation of this method may come from the influence of cell proliferation after cell reattachment, so optimal time for MTT staining is within 24 h after allowing cell to reattach to regular culture dish.

Trypan blue staining and flow cytometry assay are two alternative methods for qualifying cell resistance to anoikis other than MTT assay. Trypan blue is a vital stain used to selectively color dead cells blue, because viable cells can repel the dye and will be bright. The prodidium iodide (PI) staining may be used in flow cytometry assay to determine dead and alive cells. PI is a fluorescent vital dye that stains DNA. It does not cross the plasma membrane (PM) of cells that are viable or in the early stages of apoptosis. In contrast those cells in the late stages of apoptosis or already dead have lost PM integrity and are permeable to PI. PI is detected in the orange range of the spectrum using a 562–588 nm band-pass filter. The major limitation of both trypan blue staining and flow cytometry assay for anoikis assessment is due to the formation of cell clusters during suspension culture in which dead and live cells are overlapped. The formation of cell clusters makes it difficult to count cells under microscope or to undergo flow cytometry analysis for which single cell suspension is usually required. In this case, trypsin can be used to digest cell clusters and make them become single cells. However, trypsin treatment may further destroy the membrane structure of some dead cells, resulting in cell rupture and a false increased ratio of live/dead cells. By allowing suspended cells to reattach to regular plates, the colorimetric method using MTT successfully avoids this problem.

2 Materials

Prepare all solutions using deionized, ultrapure water dH_2O (18 MΩ cm at 25 °C) and tissue culture grade reagents. All reagents and solutions must be sterile. Unless otherwise indicated, store reagents at room temperature.

2.1 Cell Culture

1. Cell lines.
2. Phosphate-buffered saline buffer (PBS): 137 mM NaCl, 2.7 mM KCl, 10 mM $Na_2HPO_4 \cdot 2H_2O$, 2 mM KH_2PO_4, pH 7.4. Sterilize by autoclaving.
3. Ethylenedinitrilo-tetraacetic acid (EDTA), 0.5 M, pH 8.0.
4. Trypsin–EDTA solution: 0.05 % and 0.25 % trypsin/0.53 mM EDTA, pH 8.0. Filter-sterilize with 0.22 μm filter, and store at 4 °C.
5. Fetal bovine serum (FBS). Dispense into 50 ml aliquots, and store at −20 °C. Thaw before adding to culture medium.
6. Penicillin–streptomycin 100×, liquid (10,000 U/ml penicillin, 10,000 μg/ml streptomycin). Dispense into 5 ml aliquots, and store at −20 °C. Thaw before adding to culture medium.
7. Cell culture medium completed. Mix 450 ml of cell culture medium, 10 % fetal bovine serum (FBS), and 5 ml of 100× penicillin–streptomycin. Store medium at 4 °C and warm to 37 °C prior to use.
8. Ethanol 95 % (for poly-hema).
9. Poly-hema.
10. MTT (3-(4,5-dimethylthiazol-2-yl)-2,5-diphenyl tetrasodium bromide).
11. Dimethyl sulfoxide (DMSO), sterile, tissue culture grade.

2.2 Equipment

1. Tissue culture plates, dishes, or flasks (6- and 96-well flat-bottomed plate, 60 mm dishes).
2. Multichannel pipette.
3. Serological pipettes.
4. Sterile pipette tips.
5. Sterile tubes (1.5 and 5 ml).
6. Orbital shaker.
7. Bright-Line Hemacytometer.
8. Inverted light microscope.
9. Microtiter plate reader with 650 and 570 nm filters.

3 Methods

Carry out all procedures on a superclean culture hood. Make sure all the reagents, supplies, and apparatus are sterilized. Anoikis is induced by culture cells in poly-hema-coated plates that prevent cell adhesion and allow only anchorage-independent proliferation. For determining cell signaling during anoikis, cell lysates can be collected for western blot analysis without replating cells to regular attachment plates. For assessment of cell viability it be carried out using MTT colorimetric assay after replating cells to regular plates and allowing them to reattach. To evaluate effects of anoikis enhancing or inhibiting reagents, reagents can be added into medium right after cells are seeded into low attachment plates. Do not forget to set parallel untreated controls for each time points. Protocol below is considered to assay one cell line under one culture condition.

3.1 Poly-Hema Plate Preparation (See Notes 1 and 2)

Poly-hema-coated plates can be performed according to the method of Frisch and Francis [19, 20]. For each well of a 6-well plate, you will need 0.5–1.0 ml of poly-hema with final concentration 20 mg/ml. The following protocol will help to make 10 poly-hema-coated 6-well plates. Weighing poly-hema directly into a sterile flask and using stir bars that have been autoclaved will help ensure the sterility of your poly-hema plates.

1. Dissolve 1.2 g poly-hema in 60 ml 95 % ethanol to equal 20 mg/ml poly-hema solution.
2. Stir vigorously on a hot plate (at 65 °C) until dissolved.
3. In tissue culture hood, pipette 0.8 ml of poly-hema solution into each well of 6-well plate.
4. Let plates sit, partially covered with lid, until ethanol evaporates and the poly-hema has solidified (approximately 1–2 h). Periodically rock plates by hand to help ensure even coating.

5. Add remaining poly-hema solution to plates (this helps fill in any gaps in the first coat), and let sit as above. Plates can be left to dry overnight.

3.2 Cell Preparation

1. Culture cells in usual condition (37 °C, 5 % CO_2) until 70–80 % confluence.
2. Harvest the cells by trypsinization followed by PBS washing.
3. Stain 80 μl cell suspension with 20 μl of trypan blue.
4. Fill 20 μl at the hemacytometer chamber and leave undisturbed for 2 min.
5. Determine whether the cells have greater than 90 % viability.
6. Determine viable cell count and resuspend 1.3×10^7 cells in 26 ml of media to produce the cell density of 0.5×10^6 cells/ml (*see* **Note 3**).
7. Among the 26 ml of suspended cells, 2 ml is destined to be replated into regular plate immediately followed by MTT assay to obtain the absorbance value representing initial 1×10^6 cells at the beginning time point (d0). The rest 24 ml are destined to be plated into low attachment plates for monitoring cell number changes after suspension for different time points, such as 1, 3, 5, and 7 days. So 6 ml of cell suspension are plated for each time point as triplicate (2 ml/sample) and further processing is supposed to deal with always the same initial cell quantity (1×10^6cells/sample). Mix well cell suspension and proceed with cell seeding as described below.

3.3 Assessment of Resistance to Anoikis by MTT Colorimetric Assay

3.3.1 Setting the Control of d0

1. Add 1 ml of media into a 60 mm dish.
2. Pipette 2 ml of suspended cells into the 60 mm dish marked as d0.
3. Incubate in 37 °C, 5 % CO_2 overnight.
4. On the next day, make MTT solution at 5 mg/ml in PBS (*see* **Note 4**).
5. Add 1 ml of MTT reagent into the 60 mm dish.
6. Return plate to cell culture incubator (37 °C, 5 % CO_2) for 2–4 h until purple precipitate is visible (*see* **Note 5**).
7. Carefully remove and discard the media.
8. Add 2 ml of DMSO.
9. Cover the plate to protect it from light and leave plate on a shaking table for 5 min at room temperature to thoroughly mix the formazan into the solvent.
10. Remove plate cover and aliquot 2 ml of DMSO mixed solution from **step 9** into a 96-well plate (200 μl/well × 10 wells) marked as d0.

11. Add pure DMSO solution into 96-well plate in triplicate (200 μl/well, three wells) as blank controls.
12. Measure the absorbance in each well, including the blank controls, at 570 nm using a plate reader.
13. Determine the average values from readings and subtract the average value for the blank.
14. The average OD value represents cell amount of initial 1×10^6 cells at time point d0.

3.3.2 Induction of Anoikis and MTT Colorimetric Detection

1. Plate the suspended cells (1.2×10^7 cells in 24 ml) into two 6-well ultralow attachment plates (2 ml/well × 12 wells) (*see* **Notes 6** and 7).
2. Incubate in 37 °C, 5 % CO_2 for 1, 3, 5, and 7 days (*see* **Note 8**).
3. Harvest cells in triplicate on each time point (d1, d3, d5, d7): after suspension culture, gently pipette cells to break up cell clusters, and then plate 2 ml of suspension cells collected from each well into one 60 mm dish (2 ml/dish × 3 dishes).
4. Incubate at 37 °C, 5 % CO_2 overnight (*see* **Note 9**).
5. Proceed with MTT colorimetric detection as described in Subheading 3.3.1: Briefly, carefully remove and discard the media, add 2 ml of DMSO into each dish, cover the dishes, and leave them on a shaking table for 5 min at room temperature. Remove dish cover and aliquot 2 ml of DMSO mixed solution collected from each sample into a 96-well plate (for each sample, 200 μl/well × 10 wells) marked as dx (x = 1, 3, 5, or 7) (*see* **Note 10**).
6. Add 200 μl of pure DMSO solution into the same 96-well plate in triplicate (200 μl/well, three wells) as blank controls.
7. Measure the absorbance in each well, including the control blanks, at 570 nm using a plate reader.
8. Determine the average values from readings and subtract the average value for the blanks.
9. The average OD values represent cell amount of live cells with resistance to anoikis on dx (x = 1, 3, 5, or 7).
10. The percentages of cell survival are calculated using the formula: percent cell survival on d[x] = (OD value of d[x]/OD value of d0) × 100 %.

4 Notes

1. Plates need to be made at least 1 day in advance, as they will need to dry overnight. Actually, they can be made in advance and stored, wrapped in parafilm, in the 4° fridge, until needed.

2. For quality purpose, purchasing ultralow attachment plates from companies is recommended.
3. The density of suspended cells is recommended in the range of $0.5–1.0 \times 10^6$ cells/ml.
4. Once prepared, the MTT solution can be stored for 4 weeks at 4 °C protected from light. However, if the MTT reagent is bluish green, do not use.
5. From now on, keep same MTT incubation time for the following experiments.
6. If homemade poly-hema-coated plates are used, wash plates twice with 1× PBS to remove residual ethanol.
7. The suspension time and culture conditions will depend on the cell line examined.
8. Whenever changes of growth media are required, collect the cells, and centrifuge at 200 × *g* for 5 min to spin down the cells. Carefully remove the old medium and replace it with fresh medium. Gently pipette cells to resuspend them and put back into the ultralow attachment plate.
9. Time sufficient to allow the cells to attach is typically 8–12 h or overnight.
10. Keep the same MTT incubation time on different time point as on d0.

Acknowledgments

This work was supported by NIH Training Grant CA148073-02 (to X.H.), the Ovarian Cancer Research Fund PEO/MC/01.08 (to X. H.), National Cancer Institute grant CA12340 (to V.S. and J.C.), and the Mayo Clinic College of Medicine (to V.S.).

References

1. Frisch SM, Francis H (1994) Disruption of epithelial cell-matrix interactions induces apoptosis. J Cell Biol 124:619–626
2. Simpson CD, Anyiwe K, Schimmer AD (2008) Anoikis resistance and tumor metastasis. Cancer Lett 272:177–185
3. Lee YS et al (2008) The cytoplasmic deacetylase HDAC6 is required for efficient oncogenic tumorigenesis. Cancer Res 68:7561–7569
4. Frankel A et al (2001) Induction of anoikis and suppression of human ovarian tumor growth in vivo by down-regulation of Bcl-X(L). Cancer Res 61:4837–4841
5. Douma S et al (2004) Suppression of anoikis and induction of metastasis by the neurotrophic receptor TrkB. Nature 430:1034–1039
6. Cheng KW et al (2004) The RAB25 small GTPase determines aggressiveness of ovarian and breast cancers. Nat Med 10:1251–1256
7. Sood AK et al (2010) Adrenergic modulation of focal adhesion kinase protects human ovarian cancer cells from anoikis. J Clin Invest 120:1515–1523
8. He X et al (2010) Downregulation of HtrA1 promotes resistance to anoikis and peritoneal dissemination of ovarian cancer cells. Cancer Res 70:3109–3118
9. Yu X et al (2008) Suppression of anoikis by the neurotrophic receptor TrkB in human ovarian cancer. Cancer Sci 99:543–552

10. Mailleux AA et al (2007) BIM regulates apoptosis during mammary ductal morphogenesis, and its absence reveals alternative cell death mechanisms. Dev Cell 12:221–234
11. Gottlieb E (2009) Cancer: the fat and the furious. Nature 461:44–45
12. Schafer ZT et al (2009) Antioxidant and oncogene rescue of metabolic defects caused by loss of matrix attachment. Nature 461:109–113
13. Shen S et al (2011) Association and dissociation of autophagy, apoptosis and necrosis by systematic chemical study. Oncogene 30:4544–4556
14. Horbinski C, Mojesky C, Kyprianou N (2010) Live free or die: tales of homeless (cells) in cancer. Am J Pathol 177:1044–1052
15. Kenific CM, Thorburn A, Debnath J (2010) Autophagy and metastasis: another double-edged sword. Curr Opin Cell Biol 22:241–245
16. Coates JM, Galante JM, Bold RJ (2010) Cancer therapy beyond apoptosis: autophagy and anoikis as mechanisms of cell death. J Surg Res 164:301–308
17. Sher I et al (2009) Autocrine VEGF-A/KDR loop protects epithelial ovarian carcinoma cells from anoikis. Int J Cancer 124:553–561
18. Tang MK et al (2010) c-Met overexpression contributes to the acquired apoptotic resistance of nonadherent ovarian cancer cells through a cross talk mediated by phosphatidylinositol 3-kinase and extracellular signal-regulated kinase 1/2. Neoplasia 12:128–138
19. Frisch SM, Francis H (1994 Feb) Disruption of epithelial cell-matrix interactions induces apoptosis. J Cell Biol 124(4):619–626
20. Fung C, Lock R, Gao S, Salas E, Debnath J (2008 Mar) Induction of autophagy during extracellular matrix detachment promotes cell survival. Mol Biol Cell 19(3):797–806

Chapter 27

Analysis of EMT by Flow Cytometry and Immunohistochemistry

Robert Strauss, Jiri Bartek, and André Lieber

Abstract

Ovarian cancer stem cells (OCSCs) are in a transitional phase between epithelial and mesenchymal cell stages. Consequently, OCSCs possess a high degree of plasticity that complicates their identification and characterization. However, we recently demonstrated that the combined assessment of key antigens associated with cancer stem cells and the epithelial-mesenchymal transition can distinguish the phenotype of OCSCs from more differentiated cells. In this chapter we describe in detail an appropriate sample preparation for the analysis of epithelial, mesenchymal, and cancer stem cell markers by flow cytometry and immunohistochemistry in ovarian cancer. Furthermore, we provide methods for the establishment of primary ovarian cancer cultures from solid tumors.

Key words EMT, Ovarian cancer, Ovarian cancer stem cells, Flow cytometry, Immunohistochemistry, E-cadherin

1 Introduction

Cancers of epithelial origin, such as ovarian cancer, feature two distinct cell stages: epithelial and mesenchymal phenotypes. The epithelial cell shape is defined by an apicobasal polarization of cell membranes and the cytoskeleton, which leads to characteristic adherens and tight junctions that connect adjacent cells [1, 2]. In contrast, mesenchymal cells possess an irregular shape that is based on unpolarized cytoskeletons and membranes. Further mesenchymal features include increased motility, invasiveness, and the deposition of extracellular matrix components [3]. Transitions between epithelial and mesenchymal phenotypes, namely epithelial-mesenchymal transition (EMT) and mesenchymal-epithelial transition (MET), are reversible and have been accredited pivotal roles during a number of processes including embryonic development, tissue repair, cancer progression, as well as the acquisition of stem cell properties [3, 4]. Importantly, EMT and MET occur gradually,

Anastasia Malek and Oleg Tchernitsa (eds.), *Ovarian Cancer: Methods and Protocols*, Methods in Molecular Biology, vol. 1049, DOI 10.1007/978-1-62703-547-7_27, © Springer Science+Business Media New York 2013

which leads to a wide range of intermediate stages. In order to link the transitional stages between epithelial and mesenchymal phenotypes of ovarian cancer cells to cancer stem cell properties, we monitored a multitude of epithelial and mesenchymal markers by flow cytometry and immunohistochemistry [5]. Flow cytometry classically focuses on the quantitative, simultaneous analysis of multiple cell surface proteins, which allows for sorting experiments on viable cells. Moreover, the combined assessment of epithelial (e.g., E-cadherin or EpCAM) and mesenchymal antigens (e.g., CD44 or vimentin) together with a marker that selects for tumor formation in immunocompromised mice (e.g., CD133) identifies the phenotype of ovarian cancer stem cells. This technique is applicable to both, cell suspensions derived from solid tumors and adherent cultures. However, the quality of flow cytometry experiments highly depends on the sample preparation, as specific antigens might require special techniques. An example here is the major epithelial molecule E-cadherin, which contributes to "cell stickiness" due to its strong, calcium-based intercellular adhesion. Consequently, E-cadherin is targeted by peptidases commonly used for cell dissociation. Whereas treatment with Accutase, trypsin, or papain dramatically reduces E-cadherin levels on the cell surface, the detection of other molecules, such as cancer stem cell marker CD133, remains unaffected (Fig. 1). It is therefore critical to know the properties of the antigen of interest for appropriate sample preparation. In the case of E-cadherin, the use of calcium-chelating agents, such as Versene, is advisory. The analysis of intracellular antigens (e.g., vimentin) by flow cytometry requires cell fixation and permeabilization. When combined with cell surface protein staining, which is performed prior to fixation, the use of the cross-linking fixative formaldehyde is crucial. Fixation with organic solvents, such as methanol or ethanol, would lead to loss of surface antigen staining. In contrast to flow cytometry, which analyzes the presence of antigens, immunohistochemistry analysis reveals their localization within the cell. Most importantly here is the choice of suitable antibodies for meaningful analysis. As an example, the cytoplasmic domain of E-cadherin is cleaved during EMT and translocates to the cytoplasm, where it can be retained [6, 7]. The use of an antibody targeting the extracellular domain of E-cadherin might therefore underestimate the population of cells with epithelial features. Furthermore, immunohistochemistry analysis allows for the detection of secreted antigens, such as the extracellular matrix components fibronectin and laminin. The combined targeting of such epithelial or mesenchymal antigens together with a marker for tumor-initiating cells (e.g., CD133) can therefore reveal additional features of ovarian cancer stem cells that are not assessable by flow cytometry.

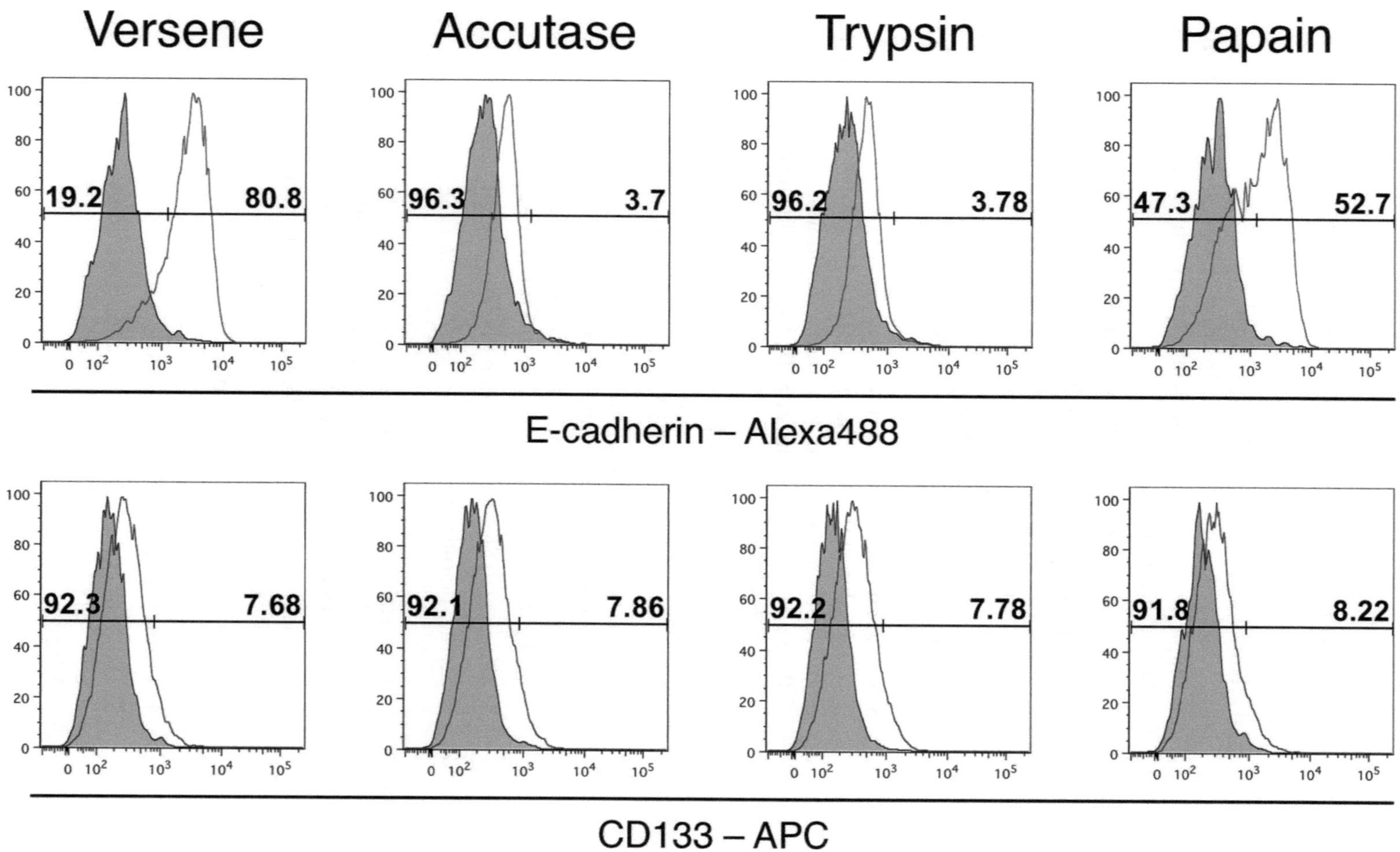

Fig. 1 Impact of cell dissociation reagents on the presence of E-cadherin and CD133. Low-passage ovarian cancer cells were treated with Versene for 60 min or peptidases (Accutase, trypsin, papain) for 15 min. The use of peptidases dramatically reduces the amount of E-cadherin on the cell surface, whereas CD133 levels are not significantly changed

2 Material

All reagents are stored at room temperature, unless otherwise indicated.

2.1 Cell Isolation from Solid Tumors

1. Tumor storage medium.
   Roswell Park Memorial Institute medium (RPMI-1640) supplemented with 1× penicillin/streptomycin and 1 μg/mL fungizone, store at 4 °C.
2. Fetal bovine serum (FBS), store at 4 °C.
3. Complete RPMI-1640 medium.
   RPMI-1640, supplemented with 10 % FBS, 1 % penicillin/streptomycin, and 1 μg/mL fungizone, store at 4 °C.
4. Phosphate-buffered saline (PBS): 137 mM NaCl, 2.7 mM KCl, 10 mM $Na_2HPO_4 \cdot 2H_2O$, 2 mM KH_2PO_4, pH 7.4. Sterilize by autoclaving.
5. Collagenase D solution 10 mg/mL.
   Dissolve 100 mg Collagenase D in 10 mL PBS. Centrifuge at 1,000 × *g* for 5 min to remove insolubles, pass through a 0.45 μM filter, and store as 500 μl aliquots in sterile Eppendorf tubes at −20 °C.
6. $CaCl_2$ solution 100 mM.
   Dissolve 147 mg $CaCl_2$ (dihydrate, FW 147.0) in 10 mL PBS, pass through a 0.2 μM filter, and store at −20 °C.
7. DNase solution 10 mg/mL.
   Dissolve 100 mg DNase I that is suitable for tissue culture purposes in 10 mL PBS, pass through a 0.2 μM filter, and store 500 μl aliquots in sterile Eppendorf tubes at −20 °C.
8. Versene, EDTA-based calcium-chelating agent, store at 4 °C.
9. Sterile, deionized water.

2.2 Flow Cytometry

1. Flow staining/wash buffer.
   Sterile phosphate-buffered saline (PBS) without magnesium/calcium supplemented with 1 % FBS, prepare fresh.
2. Formaldehyde solution 4 %. Either freshly prepared or stored at −20 °C.
3. Triton solution 0.1 %. Dissolve 50 μL Triton X-100 in 50 mL PBS.
4. Primary antibodies (*see* Table 1).
5. Dead cell exclusion dye: e.g., 7-amino-actinomycin D (7-AAD), e.g., LIVE/DEAD Fixable Red Dead Cell Stain or Fixable Viability Dye eFluor 780.

Table 1
Suggested antibodies for assessment of EMT/MET

Antibody	Species	Clone	Distributor	Dilution
Flow cytometry/cell sorting: epithelial markers				
E-cadherin-Alexa488	Mouse	67A4	Biolegend, San Diego, USA	1:50
EpCAM-FITC	Mouse	VU-1D9	STEMCELL Technologies, Vancouver, Canada	1:25
Flow cytometry/cell sorting: mesenchymal markers				
CD44-PE	Mouse	G44-26	BD Pharmingen, Franklin Lakes, USA	1:20
Vimentin-PE (intracellular)	Mouse	VI-RE/1	Abcam, Cambridge, USA	1:20
Flow cytometry/cell sorting: cancer stem cell marker				
CD133/1-APC	Mouse	AC133	Miltenyi Biotec, Bergisch Gladbach, Germany	1:10
IHC: epithelial markers				
E-cadherin-FITC	Mouse	36	BD Transduction Laboratories, Franklin Lakes, USA	1:400
EpCAM	Mouse	VU-1D9	STEMCELL Technologies, Vancouver, Canada	1:200
Claudin 7	Rabbit	Polyclonal	Abcam, Cambridge, USA	1:200
IHC: mesenchymal markers				
Fibronectin	Rabbit	Polyclonal	Abcam, Cambridge, USA	1:400
Laminin	Rabbit	Polyclonal	DAKO, Glostrup, Denmark	1:400
Vimentin	Goat	Polyclonal	Sigma, St. Louis, USA	1:100
IHC: cancer stem cell marker				
CD133	Rabbit	Polyclonal	Abcam, Cambridge, USA	1:100

2.3 Immunohistochemistry

1. Optimum cutting temperature (OCT) compound.
2. Acetone.
3. Phosphate-buffered saline (PBS).
4. Fixation solution.

   Mix 50 % acetone with 50 % methanol under fume hood, store at –20 °C.
5. Blocking solution: 2 % milk powder in PBS, freshly made.
6. Primary antibodies (*see* Table 1).
7. Fluorophore-labeled secondary antibodies (e.g., Alexa488, Alexa568).
8. VECTASHIELD with or without DAPI (Vector Labs).
9. Clear nail polish.

2.4 Equipment and Supplies

1. Laminar flow bench and cell culture incubator.
2. 6-well tissue culture plates.
3. Flow cytometer equipped with at least two lasers (488 and 633 nm).
4. Cryostat.
5. 70 μM nylon cell strainer.
6. 5 mL polystyrene round-bottom flow cytometry tubes with cell-strainer cap (35 μm nylon mesh) or alternative cell strainers (35–70 μm, nylon mesh).
7. Cryomolds, size 25 × 20 × 5 mm.
8. Superfrost slides.
9. Small paint brush.
10. 8-well chamber glass slides.
11. Cover slips, size 24 × 50 mm.
12. Glass Coplin jars or alternative glass containers that fits glass slides.
13. Humid chamber (*see* **Note 1**).

3 Methods

3.1 Flow Cytometry Analysis and Cell Sorting

Cell suspensions obtained from dissociated tumor tissue as well as from adherently growing cell cultures can be subjected to flow cytometry and cell sorting. Two corresponding methods of cells preparation followed by flow cytometry analysis are described in this section.

3.1.1 Preparation of Cell Suspensions from Solid Tumors

The method here described is suitable for cell analysis by flow cytometry, cell sorting for surface proteins, as well as for establishment of ovarian cancer cultures. Xenograft tumors or patient specimens should be stored in a 50 mL conical tube containing tumor storage medium, immediately placed on ice, and processed as soon as possible. All steps described below are carried out in a sterile laminar flow bench. Use a sterile scalpel or razor blade for tumor tissue dissection.

1. Transfer tumor tissue into a 10 cm plastic dish containing 2 mL tumor storage buffer.
2. Angle plastic dish pointing downwards from you in a way that the tumor tissue is covered by the medium. Cut the tissue into about 4 mm pieces (*see* **Note 2**).
3. Transfer medium containing tumor pieces into a 15 mL conical tube using a 5 mL pipette (*see* **Note 3**).

4. Rinse plastic dish with 2.5 mL tumor storage medium using a 5 mL pipette and transfer all remaining tumor pieces into the 15 mL conical tube.
5. Add 500 μl of 10 mg/mL Collagenase D solution resulting in a total of 5 mL containing 1 mg/mL Collagenase D.
6. Add 5 μl of 100 mM $CaCl_2$ solution, close tube, and incubate for 120 min at 37 °C. Pipette up and down every 20 min for about 2 min in order to accelerate the digestion process (*see* **Note 4**).
7. Add an equal volume (5 mL) of Versene and incubate for 60 min at 37 °C. Pipette cell suspension up and down every 20 min for about 2 min. At the end of this process, tumor pieces should be almost completely dissolved (*see* **Note 5**).
8. Add 1 mL FBS and invert tube twice.
9. Mount cell strainer on a 50 mL conical tube and pass cell suspension through cell strainer. Dissolve remaining tumor pieces in the cell strainer using a plunger of a 5 mL syringe and wash cell strainer with 25 mL complete RPMI-1640 medium.
10. Centrifuge flow-through at 300×*g* for 5 min at room temperature.
11. Optional: If large amounts of erythrocytes are observed, resuspend pellet in 3 mL sterile deionized water and immediately centrifuge at 300×*g* for 3 min at room temperature. Immediately remove water from pellet (*see* **Note 6**).
12. Resuspend pellet in 4.5 mL complete RPMI-1640 medium, transfer to a new 15 mL conical tube, and add 500 μl of 10 mg/mL DNase I. Invert tube several times and incubate for up to 30 min at 37 °C (*see* **Note 7**).
13. Add 10 mL complete RPMI-1640 medium and spin at 300×*g* for 5 min at room temperature.
14. Resuspend pellet in desired medium for tissue culturing or proceed to Subheading 3.1.3 (*see* **Note 8**).

3.1.2 Preparation of Cell Suspensions from Ovarian Cancer Cell Cultures

Culture ovarian cancer cells in 6-well plates using 2.5 mL culture medium per well. This typically results in $0.5–1 \times 10^6$ cells per well, when cells reach 90–100 % confluence.

1. Cultivate tumor cells in appropriate medium until they reach 90–100 % of confluence.
2. Wash adherent cells with PBS and detach using Versene for 30–60 min at 37 °C (*see* **Note 9**).
3. Transfer cell suspension into 15 mL conical tube containing 10 mL RPMI-1640 supplemented with 10 % FBS, spin at 300×*g* for 5 min at 4 °C, and aspirate supernatant.

3.1.3 Flow Cytometry or Cell Sorting

The following method is designed for flow cytometers equipped with at least two lasers (488 and 633 nm). Staining for surface antigens is performed prior to cell fixation on viable cells. In order to block membrane trafficking and subsequent internalization of bound antibodies, it is therefore critical to carry out the outlined steps at low temperatures. If possible, use directly fluorochrome-labeled antibodies to minimize incubation steps. In addition to the actual sample that combines all antibodies, control samples must be prepared for a combination of matching isotype control antibodies (background assessment) and for each used antibody alone (needed for color compensation). The use of a dead cell exclusion dye minimizes artifact stainings that can arise due to unspecific antibody binding to nonviable cells. For multicolor flow cytometry analysis, which often focuses on small subpopulations, it is recommended to collect at least 50,000 events of the viable cell population.

Duration of sample preparation until flow cytometry: ca. 90 min.

1. Resuspend pellet in ice-cold flow staining/wash buffer and aliquot 2.5×10^5 cells in 100 μL per sample into appropriately labeled 5 mL round-bottom flow cytometry tubes. If cell numbers are increased for cell-sorting experiments, keep this cell/volume ratio. Place samples on ice.
2. Add desired antibodies and appropriate dead cell exclusion dye depending on application. Mix by shaking the tube and incubate for 45 min on ice in the dark (*see* **Note 10**).
3. Wash samples with 3 mL flow staining/wash buffer and spin at 300 × *g* for 5 min at 4 °C. Wash fluid can be removed by simple inversion of the tube. The remaining fluid (typically 100–200 μL) can be used to resuspend the cell pellet by tapping the tube on the bench. Optional: Repeat wash step to reduce unspecific antibody binding and excessive DNA dye.
4. For direct flow cytometry analysis or cell sorting, proceed to **step 12**. For intracellular antigen staining (e.g., vimentin-PE) or fixation of flow samples, add 400 μL 4 % formaldehyde to resuspended samples. Mix sample by pipetting to avoid cell clumping. Incubate 15 min on ice in the dark.
5. Wash samples with 3 mL flow staining/wash buffer and spin at 300 × *g* for 5 min at 4 °C. Invert tube to discard supernatant and resuspend by tapping the tube on the bench.
6. Add 200 μL 0.1 % Triton solution, mix by pipetting, and incubate for 15 min at room temperature in the dark. This step permeabilizes cell membranes, which allows for access to intracellular antigens.
7. Wash samples with 3 mL flow staining/wash buffer and spin at 300 × *g* for 5 min at 4 °C. Invert tube to discard supernatant and resuspend by tapping the tube on the bench.

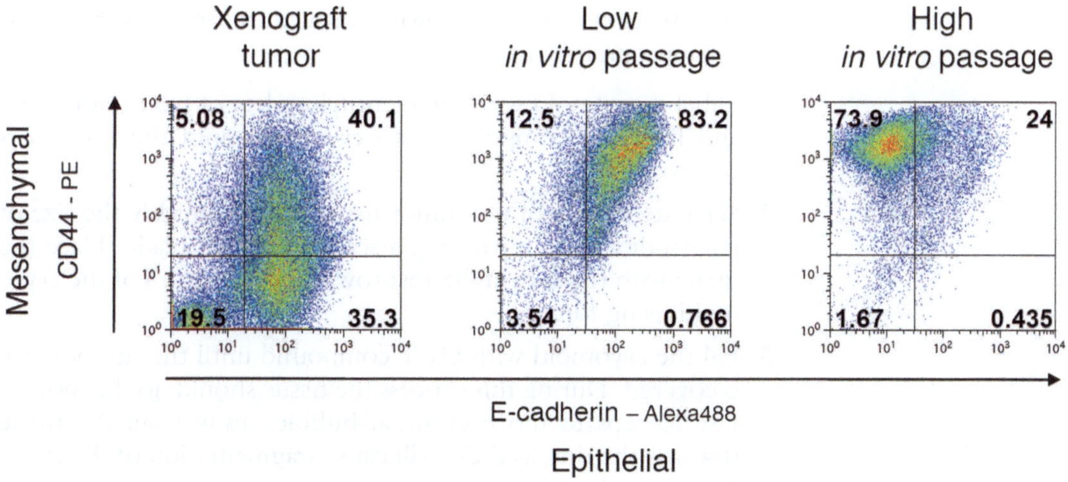

Fig. 2 Assessment of EMT during passaging in vitro by flow cytometry. Ovarian cancer xenografts contain mostly cells with an epithelial phenotype (E-cadherin positive), with a large number of cells that stain also positive for mesenchymal marker CD44 (*left panel*). Of these, only epithelial/mesenchymal hybrid cells adapt to cell culture conditions (*middle panel*). During passaging, cultures undergo EMT and enrich in E-cadherin negative/CD44 positive cells (*right panel*)

8. Add desired antibodies for intracellular antigens and incubate for 30 min on ice in the dark (*see* **Note 11**).
9. Wash samples with 3 mL flow staining/wash buffer and spin at $300 \times g$ for 5 min at 4 °C. Invert tube to discard supernatant and resuspend by tapping the tube on the bench. Optional: Repeat wash step to reduce unspecific antibody binding.
10. Add appropriate amount of flow staining/wash buffer (typically 400 μL) and mix by pipetting. Pass sample through cell-strainer cap or alternative cell strainer and subject to flow cytometry analysis (*see* **Note 12**).
11. For cell-sorting experiments, run samples at a concentration of not more than 5×10^6 cells/mL on low sample flow rate for high sorting purity. Collect cell fractions in ice-chilled receptacles containing tissue culture medium. Confirm purity of sorted cell fractions on a different flow cytometer (*see* **Note 13** and Fig. 2).

3.2 Immunohistochemistry

The following methods allow for the assessment of epithelial and mesenchymal features of ovarian cancer cells within solid tumors and adherent cultures. Immunohistochemistry analyzes for the localization of antigens, which can reveal features as cell polarization and deposition of extracellular matrix components.

3.2.1 Preparation of Frozen Tissue from Solid Tumors

Xenograft tumors or patient specimens should be stored in a 50 mL conical tube containing tumor storage medium, immediately placed on ice, and processed as soon as possible. Due to increased occurrence of artifacts and loss of antigens, it is not advisory to perform the following procedure on tissue that had been inappropriately frozen before.

1. Label a cryomold with the identifying data of the tumor tissue and fill OCT compound into cryomold until the bottom is covered.
2. Separate a piece of the tumor tissue (approximately the size of your index finger tip) using a scalpel or razor blade. Place the tissue with the side of interest towards the bottom of the cryomold using forceps.
3. Fill the cryomold with OCT compound until the tumor piece is covered. During this process the tissue should not be moved. Use forceps to move eventual bubbles away from the tissue towards the rim, as these will cause fragmentation of the tissue during sectioning.
4. Fill an ice bucket with dry ice and place cryomold onto dry ice in an even position until OCT compound is completely frozen.
5. Store cryomold at −80 °C.

3.2.2 Analysis of Frozen Tumor Tissue by Immunohistochemistry

Frozen sections often contain autofluorescent artifacts, which can lead to false-positive interpretation of results. It is therefore critical to include negative controls, using no antibodies or only secondary antibodies. The specificity of uncharacterized antibodies should be validated using various dilutions for optimal results (e.g., 1:50, 1:100, 1:200, 1:400, 1:800).

1. Equilibrate OCT compound-embedded tissues at −20 °C for at least 1 h prior to sectioning and precool cryostat to −20 °C for 20 min.
2. Remove tissue in OCT compound from cryomold and glue the back of the OCT compound block onto a cold cryostat chuck using fresh OCT compound. Place chuck appropriately into cryostat and set sectioning size to 8 μm.
3. Discard sections until tumor tissue is reached and transfer tumor tissue sections onto superfrost slides using a paint brush. Label superfrost slides using a pencil. Superfrost slides can be stored at −20 °C (*see* **Note 14**).
4. Equilibrate slide to room temperature and fix by placing into a Coplin jar filled with acetone at −20 °C for 10 min.
5. Wash slides in two consecutive Coplin jars filled with PBS at room temperature for 3 min each.
6. Prepare a parafilm screen sparing the tissue areas and place on top of the slide (*see* **Note 15**).
7. Block slide with 500 μL blocking solution on tissue area. Incubate for 20 min at room temperature.

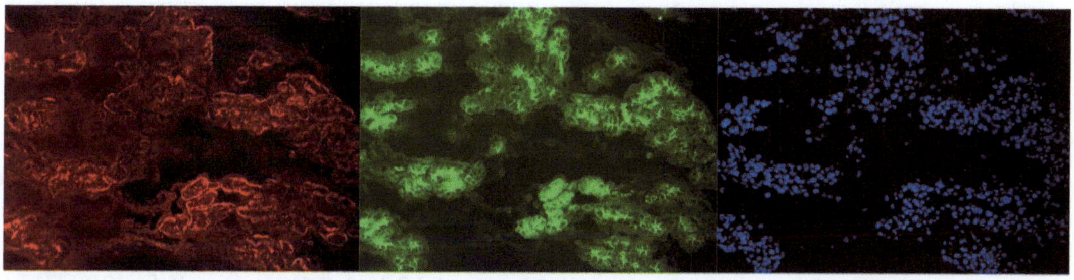

Fig. 3 Immunofluorescence analysis of EMT markers in ovarian tumors. Ovarian tumor specimen analyzed for extracellular matrix protein laminin (*left panel*), epithelial marker E-cadherin (*center panel*), and nuclei (*right panel*). The majority of tumor cells contain high amounts of E-cadherin, which is located to cellular membranes. E-cadherin-positive tumor cell nests are surrounded by laminin

8. Prepare primary antibody dilutions in a total volume of 200 μL PBS per sample, remove blocking solution, and apply antibody dilutions on top of tissue area. Incubate slide in a humid chamber at 37 °C for 90 min or at 4 °C overnight.
9. Remove antibody dilution with a pipette and wash glass slide by placing into three consecutive Coplin jars filled with PBS for 3 min each.
10. Prepare secondary antibody dilutions directed against the appropriate hosts in a total volume of 200 μL PBS per sample and apply on top of tissue area. Incubate slides in a humid chamber for 30 min at room temperature in the dark (*see* **Note 16**).
11. Remove antibody dilution with a pipette and wash glass slides by placing into three consecutive Coplin jars filled with PBS for 3 min each.
12. Let slide dry, apply VECTASHIELD (as desired with or without DAPI), and mount cover slip. Remove excessive mounting fluid using tissue paper. Seal sides of the cover slip with nail polish.
13. Analyze slides using a fluorescence microscope (Fig. 3). Slides can be stored at 4 °C for several days. For long-term storage freeze at −20 °C.

3.2.3 Analysis of Adherent Cultures by Immunohistochemistry

The initiation and maintenance of epithelial junctions between adjacent cells requires high cell densities. To adequately assess the phenotype of cells, it is advisory to fix ovarian cancer cultures, when cells reach 100 % confluency, as low cell densities can lead to reversible increases in numbers of mesenchymal cells.

1. Seed 1×10^5 cells into each well of a 8-well chamber glass slide and incubate at 37 °C in a tissue culture incubator until cells reach 100 % confluency.

2. Aspirate medium and wash with 500 μL PBS. Do not let the slide dry out throughout the consequent steps.
3. Aspirate and fix with 250 μL fixation solution for 15 min at 4 °C.
4. Aspirate and wash twice with 500 μL PBS.
5. Apply blocking solution and incubate for 20 min at room temperature.
6. Aspirate blocking solution and apply primary antibody dilutions in a total volume of 100 μL PBS per well for 90 min at 37 °C or at 4 °C overnight. Change pipette tips for each individual well from this point on to avoid cross-contamination of antibodies.
7. Aspirate antibody dilutions and wash three times with 500 μL PBS.
8. Prepare secondary antibody dilutions directed against the appropriate hosts in a total volume of 100 μL PBS per well and incubate for 30 min at room temperature in the dark (*see* **Note 16**).
9. Aspirate antibody dilutions and wash three times with 500 μL PBS.
10. Place slide on soft ground (e.g., tissue papers) and remove chambers using the chamber removal tool supplied with chamber slides.
11. Let slide dry, apply VECTASHIELD (as desired with or without DAPI), and mount cover slip (*see* **Note 17**). Remove excessive mounting fluid using tissue paper. Seal sides of the cover slip with nail polish.
12. Analyze slide using a fluorescence microscope (Fig. 4). Slides can be stored in a slide folder at 4 °C for several days. For long-term storage freeze slides at −20 °C.

4 Notes

1. A plastic box with lid can be used as a humid chamber. Put three layers of moist paper towels in the bottom of the plastic box and place a glass plate on top.
2. Start cutting by trapping the tumor at the rim of the culture dish. After initial careful sectioning, cutting speed can be rapidly increased. Avoid placing your fingers close to the cutting area.
3. It is likely that several tumor pieces remain partly connected and cannot be taken up by pipetting. Transfer while these pieces remain attached to the pipette opening when aspirating.
4. During the first pipetting step, it is mostly necessary to press tumor pieces to the bottom of the tube in a hammering-like process. Pipetting will ease with subsequent repeats.

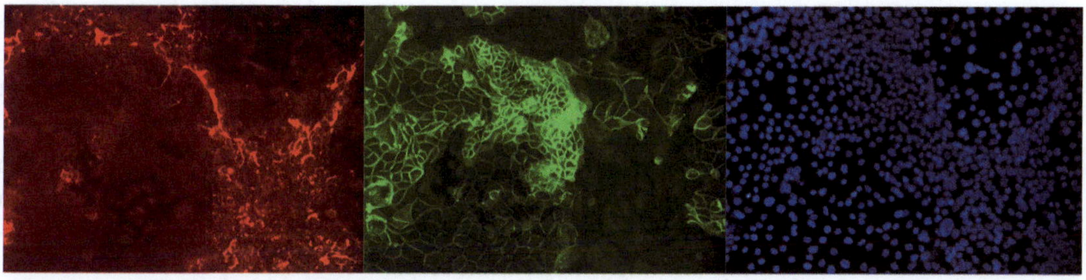

Fig. 4 Immunofluorescence analysis of EMT in adherent ovarian cancer culture. Ovarian cancer culture analyzed for extracellular matrix protein laminin (*left panel*), epithelial marker E-cadherin (*center panel*), and nuclei (*right panel*). Ovarian cancer cultures contain cells with different amounts of E-cadherin. Cells with high levels of membrane E-cadherin are small, whereas cells with lower amounts of membrane E-cadherin posses a larger cell size. Cells negative for membrane E-cadherin stain positive for mesenchymal marker laminin

5. As mentioned in the introduction, Versene can be replaced with peptidases such as trypsin, pepsin, or Accutase, if compatible with surface antigens of interest. Incubation time can be reduced to 20 min in these cases.
6. Extended exposure of tumor cells to water will drastically decrease the amount of viable cells.
7. DNase treatment dissolves cell clumps that occur due to free DNA released from dead cells.
8. It is also possible to freeze cell aliquots at −80 °C for later analysis by flow cytometry at this point. We use 40 % cell culture medium, 50 % FBS, and 10 % DMSO for this purpose.
9. It is advisory to incubate epithelial (E-cadherin positive) cell types for 60 min to obtain high amounts of single cells. Be aware that extended use of Versene (>90 min) leads to internalization of cell surface antigens.
10. The choice of the dead cell exclusion dye highly depends on already used fluorochromes conjugated to the chosen antibodies. 7-AAD (excited by 488 nm laser, emission >630 nm) can be used for immediate analysis in combination with FITC/Alexa488, PE, and APC. If formaldehyde fixation of samples is performed, a fixable DNA dye is critically needed. Conventional DNA dyes, as 7-AAD, are sensitive to fixation and must therefore be replaced by, e.g., "LIVE/DEAD Fixable Red Dead Cell Stain" (excited by 488 nm laser, emission at 630 nm) or "Fixable Viability Dye eFluor 780" (excited by 633 nm laser, emission at 780 nm).
11. If antibodies selected here are not directly fluorochrome labeled, secondary antibody detection is necessary. This is only applicable to unique antibody species.
12. Fixed samples can be stored at 4 °C in the dark for up to 5 days before analysis.

13. Due to low calcium levels in the sample fluid, which affects cell viability, sample preparation steps should be carried out as quickly as possible. Furthermore, the use of a 100 μm nozzle instead of 70 μm significantly enhances cell survival during sorting.
14. The use of a pencil is critical, as subsequent acetone fixation will remove standard pen labeling. Do not place more than three sections on one slide to avoid cross-contamination during antibody incubation steps.
15. Alternatively, tissue areas can be surround using a liquid-blocking PAP pen.
16. Place humid chamber/glass slide in a drawer or cabinet for this incubation step.
17. To avoid air bubbles during the mounting process, apply one large drop VECTASHIELD on each well and one small drop on each cross of the grid. Place cover slip vertically on one side of the wells and slowly lower the other side by moving the index finger over the cover slip applying gentle pressure.

Acknowledgements

This work was supported by the Danish Cancer Society, NIH grants R01 CA080192, R01 HLA078836, and the Pacific Ovarian Cancer Research Consortium/Specialized Program of Research Excellence in Ovarian Cancer Grant P50 CA83636.

References

1. Turksen K, Tc T (2004) Barriers built on claudins. J Cell Sci 117:2435–2447
2. Gumbiner BM (2005) Regulation of cadherin-mediated adhesion in morphogenesis. Nat Rev Mol Cell Biol 6:622–634
3. Thiery JP, Acloque H, Huang RY, Nieto MA (2009) Epithelial-mesenchymal transitions in development and disease. Cell 139:871–890
4. Strauss R, Hamerlik P, Lieber A, Bartek J (2012) Regulation of stem cell plasticity: mechanisms and relevance to tissue biology and cancer. Mol Ther 20(5):887–897
5. Strauss R, Li ZY, Liu Y, Beyer I, Persson J, Sova P et al (2011) Analysis of epithelial and mesenchymal markers in ovarian cancer reveals phenotypic heterogeneity and plasticity. PLoS One 6:e16186
6. Van Roy F, Berx G (2008) The cell-cell adhesion molecule E-cadherin. Cell Mol Life Sci 65:3756–3788
7. Ferber EC, Kajita M, Wadlow A, Tobiansky L, Niessen C, Ariga H et al (2008) A role for the cleaved cytoplasmic domain of E-cadherin in the nucleus. J Biol Chem 283:12691–12700

Part VI

Models of Ovarian Carcinogenesis

Chapter 28

Challenges in Experimental Modeling of Ovarian Cancerogenesis

Jim J. Petrik

Abstract

Ovarian cancer is a complex disease, with unclear origins, complicated, multistep tumorigenesis, and variable outcomes. As such, generating experimental models to study the disease and treatment efficacies has proven to be extremely challenging. A number of studies have utilized monolayer in vitro experiments to decipher the cellular changes in ovarian cancer and responses to different treatment approaches. Others have generated three-dimensional spheroid cultures to evaluate cellular function in an environment with more physiological contact with other cells and their matrices. Lastly, a variety of in vivo models have been used to investigate the onset and progression of ovarian cancer and how tumors respond to treatments in an intact physiological environment. This chapter discusses a number of different experimental approaches to study the etiology, biology, and pathology of ovarian tumors and their response to different anticancer therapies.

Key words Ovarian cancer, Immortalization, Transformation, Syngeneic model, Orthotopic model

Ovarian cancer is the most common gynecologic cancer and is the sixth leading cause of cancer mortality in women [1]. Due to lack of early detection tools and detection at advanced stage, ovarian cancer has a high mortality rate, with 5-year survival rates at approximately 45 % where current treatment protocols have limited effectiveness.

Ovarian cancer consists of a complex, heterogeneous group of invasive cancers that originate from different tissues. The majority of mucinous tumors originate from other tissues such as the colon or stomach and metastasize to the ovary. Endometrioid and clear-cell ovarian cancer originate from endometrial tissue and are associated with endometriosis. High-grade serous ovarian cancers originate from surface epithelial cells of the ovary or distal fallopian tube. Of these different subtypes, epithelial ovarian cancer (EOC) comprises 90 % of all ovarian cancers. The complexity of the disease of ovarian cancer leads to numerous challenges in developing in vitro and in vivo experimental models to understand the biology of the disease and to test the effectiveness of targeted therapies.

Anastasia Malek and Oleg Tchernitsa (eds.), *Ovarian Cancer: Methods and Protocols*, Methods in Molecular Biology, vol. 1049, DOI 10.1007/978-1-62703-547-7_28, © Springer Science+Business Media New York 2013

EOC is characterized by growth of the primary tumor on the ovary and initial direct extension into other organs such as the distal fallopian tubes, uterus, and adnexa. This disease is also often associated with early dissemination of tumor cells into the peritoneal cavity by way of transcoelomic metastasis [2]. Transcoelomic metastasis of ovarian tumor cells is likely responsible for a good deal of the morbidity associated with this disease due to the array of vital organs that are usually affected by this type of disease spread. This metastatic spread of disease is associated with a number of complex cellular processes that provide challenges to model with in vitro and in vivo systems. In order for this transcoelomic metastasis to occur, cells must first reduce their attachment to neighboring cells and the extracellular matrix of the primary ovarian tumor. This loss of attachment requires changes in affinity and reliance on cell–cell contact and the ECM for viability and proliferative signals.

Peritoneal disease caused by transcoelomic metastasis is associated with the formation of malignant ascites, which can cause morbidities such as abdominal distention, intestinal perforation or blockage, restricted flow of lymphatic vessels, and altered organ function. The cells that slough from the primary tumor must develop mechanisms to thrive in the peritoneal space, away from their local tumor microenvironment and supportive cellular matrix. It has been proposed that these cells adopt different characteristics from their native ovarian tumor cell counterparts, but studying these cell populations has proven to be quite difficult. An initial challenge was the isolation and propagation of both normal ovarian surface epithelial cells and ovarian tumor cells. Shepherd et al. [3] devised an elegant protocol to mechanically select OSE cells from ovarian biopsies and to isolated tumorigenic ovarian epithelial cells from the ascites of women with high-grade serous adenocarcinoma. These protocols have been very important in allowing us to conduct studies on the transformation and alteration of normal OSE cells into aggressive epithelial cells of ovarian carcinoma.

Typically, normal epithelial cells undergo a form of programmed cell death termed anoikis when they detach from the extracellular matrix, although transformed epithelial cells generally do not [4]. As cells detach and slough from the primary tumor, they must initiate mechanisms to maintain viability during their passage through the peritoneal cavity. Epithelial cells typically are reliant upon their ECM for anchorage-dependent viability. Malignant ovarian epithelial cells must avoid anoikis, the programmed cell death induced in anchorage-dependent cells following detachment from their ECM. Studies have shown that tumor cells circulating within the peritoneal environment upregulate autocrine signaling mechanism to avoid anoikis and maintain viability [5]. The study of cells in anchorage-free conditions can be difficult due to the inherent drive for cells to attach to each other and to some substrate. In order to study anoikis, cells must be cultured in attachment-free conditions, typically through the use of ultralow attachment culture plates that have a hydrophilic coating and neutral charge [6]. Following detachment, traditional apoptosis assays can be used to determine the incidence of anoikis. Assays commonly used to study anoikis include flow cytometry following propidium iodide staining [6], TUNEL analysis, or colorimetric assays that measure dye uptake through damaged cell membranes.

In addition to escaping anoikis, circulating ovarian tumor cells within the peritoneal cavity have enhanced chemotactic and migratory characteristics and are able to form multicellular spheroids, which appears to improve their survival. The ability of cells to thrive in a nutrient-poor environment is also a hallmark of ovarian cancer cells that must exist within the peritoneal space. Liu et al. [7] has shown that the proportion of tumor-initiating cancer stem cells expanded in spheroid culture is enhanced in serum-free culture conditions and that the cell populations that adapt to the nutrient-poor conditions ultimately become more tumorigenic. There are a number of approaches to the study of spheroid-forming capacity of cells. Colony- or spheroid-forming assays in soft agar are often used to predict and infer the tumorigenic potential of a specific cell population.

Circulation spheroids of transformed epithelial cells are thought to be important in the peritoneal dissemination of disease. Within the abdomen, spheroids will adhere to mesothelial layers and ECM, at which time they disaggregate and may become invasive [8–11]. Aside from the spheroid-forming experiments which utilize soft agar colonization assays, other protocols designed to assess the chemotactic, migratory, and invasive properties of ovarian tumor cells include the Boyden chamber assay and gel invasion and contraction assays.

The use of human ovarian epithelial cells for in vitro experimentation has proved to be extremely difficult. Spontaneous immortalization of primary human ovarian tumor cells rarely occurs, compared to the relatively easy transformation of rodent cancer cells. As opposed to the acquisition of an immortalized phenotype of rodent ovarian epithelial cells in vitro, human cells typically undergo senescence and require some genetic manipulation to induce transformation. Some success has been obtained by the use of viral oncogenes to disrupt cell cycle regulation and generate cultures of numerous population doublings, but these cells had difficulty in generating tumors in vivo [12]. Others have used transfection with SV40 antigen to inactivate the p53 and pRb pathways, combined with introduction of hTERT or HRAS to extend the number of population doublings and induced tumorigenicity of human ovarian surface epithelial cells [7]. Combined inactivation of p53, with transduction of Kras, c-myc, and bcl-2 in human EOC cells has also been shown to induce tumor formation in xenograft models of human ovarian cancer [13]. The malignant transformation of murine ovarian surface epithelial cells was elegantly studied by Roberts et al. [14] in which they utilized numerous in vitro and in vivo techniques to generate transformed MOSE cells representative of early, intermediate, and late stage EOC. These studies utilized a syngeneic approach that allowed for intraperitoneal implantation of transformed MOSE cells into immunocompetent mice. Greenaway et al. [15] worked further in this area with orthotopic implantation of transformed MOSE cell under the ovarian bursa in their attempt to determine the importance of interaction between the epithelial cells and the ovarian stroma in the progression of ovarian cancer. Although the rodent OSE cells are useful as they do spontaneously transform, they have limitations in similarity to human OSE cells and to inducing disease that replicates human EOC well. The species variability between easily transformed rodent OSE cells and human cancer is a limitation in our ability to accurately and effectively model the disease, as is the difficulty encountered with working with human OSE cells.

An impediment to a greater understanding of the pathogenesis of ovarian cancer is the lack of a specific causal genetic alteration. EOC arises from the spontaneous transformation of epithelial cells of the female reproductive tract. To date, no reliable inducer of OSE cell or oviductal surface epithelial cell transformation has been identified which has made it difficult to study the etiology of spontaneous EOC. Because of this issue, many researchers induce genetic alterations in ovarian epithelial cells and then reimplant the cells intraperitoneally, subcutaneously, or orthotopically within the ovarian bursal space. In an attempt to induce spontaneous transformation of ovarian epithelial cells, Connolly et al. [16] targeted the SV40 T antigen (SV40 Tag) to surface ovarian epithelial cells with the Müllerian Inhibitory Substance Type II Receptor (MISIIR) promoter. With this approach, approximately 50 % of mice develop an aggressive, bilateral ovarian serous adenocarcinoma, and while the SV40 Tag is not known to contribute to the pathogenesis of ovarian cancer in women, this model has effectively been used to generate transgenic lines for the study of EOC [17, 18]. In addition to transformation and genetic alteration, others have manipulated the culture environment to attempt to push human ovarian surface epithelial cells towards a tumorigenic phenotype. One attempt has been the use of 3-dimensional culture of human OSE to allow the cells to develop multicellular spheroids with the thought that the interaction between cells and the developing extracellular matrix would more closely model the neoplastic transformation that occurs in ovarian cancer [19]. Although these spheroids contained cells that more closely replicated surface epithelial cells in the human ovary, the ability to replicate the spontaneous transformation remained elusive. Another manipulation of the tumorigenic epithelial cells in vitro has been the introduction of plasmids or viruses that are conjugated to a fluorescent protein to allow for visualization of tumors in vivo. Through sequential fluorescence imaging, tumor growth can be monitored and measured longitudinally within each mouse and removes the necessity to sacrifice animals at various time points to examine tumor progression. A limitation of this technique has been the ability to detect and visualize fluorescence emission from within the peritoneal space, and has led some researchers to use subcutaneous implantation sites to make the tumors more accessible for imaging [20, 21]. However, recently, Nunez-Cruz et al. [22] have developed a technique using a red fluorescent protein mutant encoded within a lentiviral vector that is transduced into MOV1 ovarian cancer cells. These cancer cells are orthotopically implanted in the ovary and the researchers demonstrate the ability to detect fluorescence signal from within the peritoneal space. This approach provides the ability to orthotopically insert tumor cells into their normal tumor microenvironment and to visualize tumor growth and its natural dissemination throughout the peritoneal cavity.

Although there has been the development of a number of in vitro and in vivo models generated to study ovarian cancer in women, the perfect model has yet to be developed. We have the capability of modeling a number of events and processes that occur during the onset, development, and progression of ovarian cancer but have yet to identify the specific initiating event that gives rise to the disease. As we continue to develop more sophisticated cell- and animal-based research tools, our understanding of ovarian cancer grows, but we still have the challenge of developing better models.

References

1. Siegel R, Naishadham D, Jemal A (2012) Cancer statistics, 2012. CA Cancer J Clin 62:10–29
2. Tan DS, Agarwal R, Kaye SB (2006) Mechanisms of transcoelomic metastasis in ovarian cancer. Lancet Oncol 7:925–934
3. Shepherd TG, Theriault BL, Campbell EJ, Nachtigal EW (2006) Primary culture of ovarian surface epithelial cells and ascites-derived ovarian cancer cells from patients. Nat Protoc 1:2643–2649
4. Frankel A, Rosen K, Filmus J, Kerbel RS (2001) Induction of anoikis and suppression of human ovarian tumor growth in vivo y down-regulation of Bcl-XL1. Cancer Res 61: 4837–4841
5. Sher I, Adham SA, Petrik J, Coomber BL (2009) Autocrine VEGF-A/KDR loop protects epithelial ovarian carcinoma cells from anoikis. Int J Cancer 124:553–561
6. He X, Ota T, Liu P, Su C, Chien J, Shridhar V (2010) Downregulation of HtrA1 promotes resistance to anoikis and peritoneal dissemination of ovarian cancer cells. Cancer Res 70: 3108–3118
7. Liu J, Yang G, Thompson-Lanza JA, Glassman A, Hayes K, Patterson A, Marquez RT, Auersperg N, Yu Y, Hahn WC, Mills GB, Bast RC Jr (2004) A genetically defined model for human cancer. Cancer Res 64:1655–1663
8. Burleson KM, Casey RC, Skubitz KM, Pambuccian SE, Oegema TR Jr, Skubitz AP (2004) Ovarian carcinoma spheroids adhere to extracellular matrix components and mesothelial cell monolayers. Gynecol Oncol 93:170–181
9. Burleson KM, Hansen LK, Skubitz AP (2004) Ovarian carcinoma spheroids disaggregate on type I collagen and invade live human mesothelial cell monolayers. Clin Exp Metastasis 21:685–697

10. Ahmed N, Thompson EW, Quinn MA (2007) Epithelial-mesenchymal inter-conversions in normal ovarian surface epithelium and ovarian carcinomas: an exception to the norm. J Cell Physiol 213:581–588
11. Sodek KL, Ringuette MJ, Brown TJ (2009) Compact spheroid formation by ovarian cancer cells is associated with contractile behavior and an invasive phenotype. Int J Cancer 124: 2060–2070
12. Gregoire L, Rabah R, Schmelz EM, Munkarah A, Roberts PC, Lancaster WD (2001) Spontaneous malignant transformation of human ovarian surface epithelial cells in vitro. Clin Cancer Res 7:4280–4287
13. Sasaki R, Narisawa-Saito M, Yugawa T, Fujita M, Tashiro H, Katabuchi H, Kiyono T (2008) Oncogenic transformation of human ovarian surface epithelial cells with defined cellular oncogenes. Carcinogenesis 30:423–431
14. Roberts PC, Motitillo EP, Baxa AC, Heng HHQ, Doyon-Reale N, Gregoire L, Lancaster WD, Rabah R, Schmelz EM (2005) Sequential molecular and cellular events during neoplastic progression: a mouse syngeneic ovarian cancer model. Neoplasia 7:944–956
15. Greenaway J, Moorehead R, Shaw P, Petrik J (2008) Epithelial-stromal interaction increases cell proliferation, survival and tumorigenicity in a mouse model of human epithelial ovarian cancer. Gynecol Oncol 108:385–394
16. Connolly DC, Bao R, Nikitin AY, Stephens KC, Poole TW, Hua X, Harris SS, Vanderhyden BC, Hamilton TC (2003) Female mice chimeric for expression of the simian virus 40 Tag under control of the MISIIR promoter develop epithelial ovarian cancer. Cancer Res 63: 1389–1397
17. Hensley H, Quinn BA, Wolf RL, Litwin SL, Mabuchi S, Williams SJ, Williams C, Hamilton TC, Connolly DC (2007) Magnetic resonance imaging for detection and determination of tumor volume in a genetically engineered mouse model of ovarian cancer. Caner Biol Ther 6:1717–1725
18. Mabuchi S, Altomare DA, Connolly DC, Klein-Szanto A, Litwin S, Hoelzle MK, Hensley HH, Hamilton TC, Testa JR (2007) RAD001 (Everolimus) delays tumor onset and progression in a transgenic mouse model of ovarian cancer. Cancer Res 67:2408–2413
19. Lawrenson K, Benjamin E, Turmaine M, Jacobs I, Gayther S, Dafou D (2009) In vitro three-dimensional modeling of human ovarian surface epithelial cells. Cell Prolif 42:385–393
20. Jin ZH, Josserand V, Razkin J, Garanger E, Boturyn D, Favrot MC, Dumy P, Coll JL (2006) Noninvasive optical imaging of ovarian metastases using Cy5-labeled RAFT-c(-RGDfk-)4. Mol Imaging 5:188–197
21. Granot D, Kunz-Schughart LA, Neeman M (2005) Labeling fibroblasts with biotin-BSA-GdDTPA-FAM for tracking of tumor associated stroma by fluorescence and MR imaging. Magn Reson Med 54:789–797
22. Nunez-Cruz S, Connolly DC, Scholler N (2010) An orthotopic model of serous ovarian cancer in immunocompetent mice for in vivo tumor imaging and monitoring of tumor responses. J Visual Exp 45:1–4

Chapter 29

Transformation of the Human Ovarian Surface Epithelium with Genetically Defined Elements

Weiwei Shan and Jinsong Liu

Abstract

Success in in vitro transformation of primary cells from the human ovarian surface epithelium (OSE) has provided significant insight to the study of human ovarian cancer. Here, we describe the method used to immortalize and transform OSE by serial introduction of viral and nonviral genetic elements as well as to test the tumorigenicity of hence established cell lines in appropriate animal models. Successful transformation of OSE cells in the laboratory is of critical significance to the study of ovarian cancer. It not only allows for testing the roles of numerous potential oncogenes in initiating and promoting human ovarian cancer but provides a convenient tool to comprehensively dissect ovarian tumorigenesis in the laboratory.

Key words Ovarian surface epithelium (OSE), Immortalization, Transformation, Retrovirus, Oncogene

1 Introduction

In 1999, Hahn et al. successfully transformed human kidney epithelial cells (HEK) and foreskin fibroblasts (BJ) by retrovirus-mediated ectopic expression of the human telomerase catalytic subunit (hTERT), the simian virus 40 (SV40) large-T (LT) antigen, and the oncogenic allele of H-RAS [1], piloting genetic transformation in vitro. This groundbreaking experiment maximized the potentials of these genetic elements while minimizing the genes required, creating a self-sufficient, labor-efficient model to transform human cells in culture. It is the specialized functions of these individual genes (the ability of hTERT to overcome cellular senescence caused by telomere erosion [2], of SV40 LT to inactivate p53 [3–5] and pRb [6, 7] to achieve immortalization, and of oncogenic H-RAS to confer proliferative advantages), the synergistic efforts orchestrated by these genes, as well as the precise order in which they were introduced that enabled the cells to acquire tumorigenicity. It was later determined that the SV40 small T antigen (ST) also plays a critical role in facilitating transformation by binding to and inactivating protein phosphatase 2A (PP2A) [8].

Anastasia Malek and Oleg Tchernitsa (eds.), *Ovarian Cancer: Methods and Protocols*, Methods in Molecular Biology, vol. 1049, DOI 10.1007/978-1-62703-547-7_29, © Springer Science+Business Media New York 2013

The strategy to combine hTERT, SV40 T/t antigens, and oncogenic RAS has hence been utilized to successfully transform numerous human cell types and has proven tremendously valuable in our understanding of carcinogenesis.

Epithelial ovarian cancer (EOC) is the most lethal gynecological cancer type in the United States with an estimated 21,990 new cases of EOC arising and more than 15,460 women dying of this fatal disease in the year 2011 [9]. Five histological types of EOC have been identified so far, namely, high-grade serous, low-grade serous, endometrioid, clear cell, and mucinous carcinomas [10]. Currently, the obstacle in treating and eliminating EOC resides in the difficulty to spot the disease at its curable stages, the paucity of sensitive and specific markers, and the lack of faithful models to relive disease progression in vitro. In 2004, our group successfully transformed ovarian surface epithelial (OSE) cells following the protocol established by Hahn et al., i.e., with the combination of retrovirally delivered SV40 early region, hTERT, and oncongenic H- or K-RAS, creating the first transformation model to study ovarian epithelial tumorigenesis in the laboratory [11]. H-RAS-transformed OSE cells are immortalized, clonogenic on semisolid agarose media, and rapidly tumor forming when inoculated into immunocompromised mice [11]. Furthermore, the resulting tumors were histopathologically identified to be undifferentiated carcinoma with papillary growth, stained positive for the serous marker Wilm's Tumor 1 (WT-1), invaded the omentum and liver, and generated ascites fluid [11]. Their features are reminiscent of the biological and clinical behavior of human EOC. Our model has since been applied by numerous groups to their studies and has contributed significantly to ovarian cancer research. In this chapter, we describe to the readers detailed, step-by-step procedures to achieve immortalization and transformation of OSE.

2 Materials

Prepare all solutions using deionized, ultrapure water dH_2O_2 (18 MΩ cm at 25 °C) and tissue culture grade reagents. All reagents and solutions must be sterile. Unless otherwise indicated, store reagents at room temperature and warm to 37 °C prior to apply for cell cultures.

2.1 Tissue Samples and Cell Cultures

1. Surgical specimens of human ovaries. All patients have been properly consented prior to the collection of tissue specimens. Specimens of normal, non-pathological ovarian tissues are obtained during surgical procedures. Approximately 500 mg ovarian tissue is removed and kept in a sterile 10 cm Petri dish and immediately stored at 4 °C. The Petri dish is then promptly

(within 30 min) transported to a cell culture facility where isolation of OSE cells will be performed immediately.

2. SKOV-3 (ATCC # HTB-77™).

2.2 Cell Culture

1. Phosphate-buffered saline buffer (PBS), sterile, Ca/Mg free.
2. PBS buffer supplemented with penicillin 100 U/mL and streptomycin 100 ng/mL.
3. Trypsin-EDTA solutions: 0.25 %-trypsin/0.53 mM-EDTA.
4. Dimethyl sulfoxide (DMSO), sterile, tissue culture grad. Store at 4 °C.
5. Basic medium. Dissolve Media 199 and Media 105 (Sigma-Aldrich), each, and 2.2 g of sodium bicarbonate in 1,800 mL of autoclaved double-deionized water (ddH_2O). Upon formation of uniform solvent, adjust pH of media to 7.50–7.60 using 10 M NaOH. Make up to 2 L in ddH_2O (*see* **Note 1**). Filter media through a 0.22 μM sterile filter and aliquot into 450 mL. Supplement with fetal bovine serum (FBS) 10 % (*see* **Note 2**), penicillin 100 U/mL, and streptomycin 100 ng/mL. Store in dark at 4 °C.
6. NOE (*n*ormal *o*varian *e*pithelium) medium. Supplement basic medium with epidermal growth factor (EGF) 10 ng/mL.
7. DMEM complete medium. Supplement Dulbecco's Modified Eagle Medium (DMEM) with FBS 10 % (*see* **Note 2**), penicillin 100 U/mL, and streptomycin 100 ng/mL.
8. RPMI 1640 complete medium. Supplement RPMI 1640 Medium with FBS 10 % (*see* **Note 2**), penicillin 100 U/mL, and streptomycin 100 ng/mL.
9. Tissue culture dishes (60 and 100 mm diameter).
10. Tissue culture flasks (T25, T75, T175, and T225).
11. Serological pipettes, sterile 1, 2, 5, 10, and 25 mL.
12. Autoclaved Pasteur (glass) pipettes.
13. Silicone high-vacuum grease cloning cylinders.

2.3 Cell Transfection

1. Retroviral vectors: pBabe-neo-SV40, pBabe-hygro-hTERT, pBabe-HRAS^{V12}-puro, and pBabe-eGFP-*neo* (*see* **Note 3**).
2. Phoenix Ampho packaging cells (*see* **Note 4**).
3. Transfection reagent: 2.5 M $CaCl_2$. Weigh 18.37 g $CaCl_2$ dehydrate ($2H_2O$) and dissolve in ddH_2O to make up to 50 mL. Filter sterilize through a 0.22 μm syringe filter. Store at −20 °C in 5 ml aliquots. Avoid repeated freeze-thaw cycles.
4. HEPES-buffered saline HeBS ×2: 280 mM NaCl, 50 mM HEPES, 1.5 mM Na_2HPO_4, 10 mM KCl, and 12 mM dextrose. Dissolve 16.4 g of NaCl, 11.9 g of HEPES, 0.21 g of Na_2HPO_4, 0.74 g of KCl, and 2.16 g of dextrose in 800 mL of

ddH_2O. Adjust pH to 6.95–7.05 with 5 M NaOH then make up to 1 L. Filter sterilize through a 0.22 μm syringe filter. Store at −20 °C in 50 ml aliquots. Avoid repeated freeze-thaw cycles.

5. Chloroquine stock solution 25 mM: dissolve 79.9 g powder chemical in PBS and adjust final volume to 10 mL. Filter sterilize through a 0.22 μm syringe filter. Store at −20 °C in 1 mL aliquots. Avoid repeated freeze-thaw cycles. Suggested working concentration is 25 μM chloroquine/mL media used. Polybrene stock solution 10 mg/mL. Working concentration is 8 μg polybrene/mL media used. Store at −20 °C.
6. Selection reagents. Stock solutions of Zeocin™ (100 mg/mL), puromycin HCl (10 mg/mL), Geneticin/neomycin/G418 (50 mg/mL), and hygromycin B (50 mg/mL), stored at −20 °C. Suggested working concentrations for mammalian cells are Zeocin™ 100–750 μg/mL; puromycin HCl 1–100 μg/mL; Geneticin 100–1,000 μg/mL; and hygromycin B 50–1,000 μg/mL (*see* **Note 5**).

2.4 Western Blotting

1. Radio immunoprecipitation assay buffer (RIPA): 50 mM Tris–HCl, 150 mM NaCl, 0.1 % SDS, 0.5 % Na deoxycholate, 1 % Triton X 100, and any commercially available protease inhibitor in according to the manufacturer's guide.
2. Protein lysis buffer. Dissolve protease inhibitor cocktail in 10 mL 1× RIPA buffer to make 1× lysis buffer with protease inhibitors. Store at 4 °C and avoid direct exposure to light. Use within 30 days.
3. Protein quantification assay kit colorimetric 96-well plate reader.
4. Mini PROTEAN® 3 System gel-casting apparatus (Bio-Rad).
5. 30 % acrylamide/bis-acrylamide solutions, mixing ratio 29:1 *N,N,N′,N′*-tetramethylethylenediamine solution (TEMED).
6. Resolving gel buffer: 1.5 M Tris–HCl, pH 8.8. Store at 4 °C.
7. Stacking gel buffer: 0.5 M Tris–HCl, pH 6.8. Store at 4 °C.
8. Tris-glycine SDS-polyacrylamide gel running buffer ×10. Dilute in ddH_2O prior to use.
9. Ammonium persulfate solution 10 %. Weigh 100 mg of ammonium persulfate powder and dissolve in 1 mL ddH_2O. Prepare fresh and use immediately.
10. Prestained protein ladder.
11. Mini Trans-Blot® electrophoresis gel transfer apparatus (Bio-Rad).
12. Western blot transfer buffer ×10 Transfer buffer. Mix 100 mL of Pierce® Western blot transfer buffer 10×, 700 mL of water and 200 mL of 100 % methanol. Mix well and store at 4 °C.

13. PVDF transfer membranes blotting papers.
14. Tris-buffered saline (TBS): 1.5 M NaCl, 0.1 M Tris–HCl, pH 7.5.
15. Tween-20.
16. TBS containing Tween-20 (TBS-T): 0.1 % Tween-20 in TBS.
17. TBS-T (0.1 %): Add 1 mL of Tween-20 to 1 L of TBS ×1.
18. Nonfat dry milk.
19. Blocking buffer: 5 % nonfat dry milk in TBS-T (0.1 %).
20. Antibody diluent: 1 % nonfat dry milk in TBS-T (0.1 %).
21. Western blotting detection reagents.
22. 8′ × 11′ autoradiography films, films development, and imaging equipment.

2.5 Immunohistochemical Staining

1. Tissue-Tek® cassettes.
2. Formalin 10 %.
3. Xylene.
4. Ethanol 100 %.
5. Decloaking chamber ecloaker solution.
6. Peroxide solution (0.3 %).
7. Blocking solution (*see* **Note 6**).
8. Primary and secondary antibody diluents (*see* **Note 7**).
9. Horseradish peroxidase (HRP) solution 3,3′-diaminobenzidine (DAB) solution.
10. Hematoxylin.
11. Permount.

2.6 Antibodies

Quality of antibodies from indicated suppliers was approved experimentally; however, antibodies from any other producers can be used as well.

2.7 Test Kits

1. Pierce® BCA Protein Assay Kit (Thermo Scientific).
2. TRAPeze® Telomerase Detection Kit (Millipore/Chemicon International).

3 Methods

3.1 Primary Culture of Ovarian Surface Epithelial Cells

3.1.1 Establishment of Primary Culture from Surgical Specimens

1. Surgical specimens of human ovaries should be washed twice in ice-cold PBS supplemented with penicillin 100 U/mL and streptomycin 100 ng/mL, then blotted against sterile surgical gauze. Prompt processing of surgical specimens is a key to the success of isolation OSE cells (*see* **Note 3**).
2. Prepare two to three 100 mm culture dishes with 10 mL complete NOE culture media added to each. Use a sterile surgical

scalpel and steady force to gently scrape the surface layer of specimen of ovary into culture media. After ~20 strokes, transfer the remaining tissue specimen to a new 100 mm with medium; repeat the scraping procedure as needed. It is not necessary to remove pieces of broken tissue specimen from the culture dishes. Return dishes to 37 °C incubator.

3. Remove media no sooner than 7 days of initial culture (passage0, p0) (*see* **Note 8**). Wash cells with 1× PBS and replace with 10 mL fresh NOE. After that, replenish with fresh NOE medium every 3–4 days or as needed.

3.1.2 Purification of OSE by Differentiated Trypsinization

This method takes advantage of the fact that fibroblasts are more sensitive to trypsinization and hence easier to detach from the plates by trypsin when compared to epithelial cells.

1. Examine established culture under a phase-contract light microscope. Whereas p0 primary OSE cells appear to be compact, forming a classic cobblestone pattern [12], stromal fibroblasts exhibit typical mesenchymal, elongated morphology in culture. It is critical to start experiments with a passage number of primary OSE cells as early as experimentally possible (*see* **Note 9**).
2. Remove culture media, rinse cells with PBS Ca/Ma.
3. Add 1 mL 0.05 % trypsin-EDTA to the 100 mm dish. Incubate at 37 °C for 1 min.
4. Remove dish from the incubator, gently tilt the dish, and examine under the microscope.
5. Upon viewing of sheets of floating cells, promptly add media to neutralize trypsin.
6. Discard media by aspiration.
7. Gently wash the remaining adherent cells with 1× PBS twice.
8. Replenish with 10 mL NOE. The remaining adherent cells are treated as OSE cells. Repeat this process 2–3 times as needed (*see* **Note 10**).

3.1.3 Purification of OSE by Cloning

Cloning with the help of cloning cylinders ensures a relatively pure population of OSE cells (*see* **Note 11**).

1. Examine established culture under a phase-contrast microscope considering criteria described in **step 1** of Subheading 3.1.2.
2. Before getting started, put a pea-sized amount of silicone grease in 60 mm or 100 mm culture dish and UV-irradiate for 30 min to sterilize. Autoclave cloning cylinders. If not autoclavable, UV-irradiate the cloning cylinders to sterilize.
3. Under a light microscope, pick 5–10 colonies consisting solely of OSE cells based on the morphological features of epithelial cells. Circle the colonies with a marker pen at the bottom of the dish.

4. Remove culture media.
5. Wash cells with PBS. Completely aspirate PBS.
6. With a sterile pair of forceps, pick a cloning cylinder (*see* **Note 12**) and gently grease the bottom rim against the silicone grease. Make sure the entire circumference of the rim is evenly greased.
7. With a pair of forceps, dock the greased side of the cloning cylinder over the colony marked. Gently rub the cylinder against the bottom of the plate to ensure sealing. Repeat this step for the number of colonies picked.
8. Add 50 μL 0.25 % trypsin-EDTA to each cloning cylinder. No leakage should occur if the cylinder has been greased and placed properly. Return the plate back into the incubator for 3 min, approximately.
9. Examine the detachment of cells in each cloning cylinder under the light microscope. Gently shake or tilt the dish to facilitate trypsinization.
10. Neutralize trypsin by adding 200 μL of NOE.
11. Transfer content from the cloning cylinder to one well of a 6-well plate and label. Repeat this step for the number of colonies picked.
12. Expand culture from 6-well plates to a 60 mm then 100 mm dishes when cells reach confluence.

3.2 Creation of Stable OSE Cell Lines with Retroviral SV40 T/t Antigens

Readers are suggested to create stable cell lines with the earliest passage number of OSE cells available, since primary OSE cells promptly undergo replicative senescence in culture upon continuous passaging beyond 6–8 times.

3.2.1 Transfection

1. Grow Phoenix Ampho cells in complete DMEM medium. The day before transfection, plate 2.5×10^6 Phoenix Ampho cells in a 60 mm culture dish to reach 80–90 % confluence the next day.
2. On the day of transfection, add 5 μL of 25 mM chloroquine into 5 mL of DMEM to achieve final concentration of 25 μM chloroquine/mL media (*see* **Note 13**). Replace DMEM with media containing chloroquine on Phoenix cells. Return plates to 37 °C until ready.
3. Prepare transfection cocktail as follows. Dilute 10–15 μg pBabe-neo-SV40 plasmid in ddH_2O to make up to 450 μL; add 50 μL 2 M $CaCl_2$ and 500 μL HeBS ×2 buffer. Vortex well.
4. Immediately (in 1–2 min) add the transfection complex to Phoenix cells in a dropwise fashion. Gently swirl plates to mix. Return plates back into incubator.
5. Remove transfection complex and media in 8–12 h (*see* **Note 14**). Replace with complete NOE.

3.2.2 Harvest Virus

1. First collection: 48–72 h post-transfection. Collect media from producer cells into 15 mL conical tubes (*see* **Note 15**). Combine media if replicate dishes of producer cells are used. Spin at 500×*g* for 15 min to remove cells from the viral supernatant.
2. Filter the supernatant through a 0.45 μM syringe filter (*see* **Note 16**) into a new 15 mL conical tube (~4.5 mL final supernatant).
3. Use immediately or store viral supernatant in −80 °C freezers in 1 mL aliquots.
4. If multiple collection of virus is desired, feed the producer cells with 5 mL fresh complete DMEM.
5. Harvest virus in another 48–72 h. Repeat the above steps.

3.2.3 Infection of Target Cells

1. Plate primary OSE cells (the earliest passage available) on desired culture vessels to reach 50–60 % confluence the next day. Another aliquot of NOE cells will be infected with the empty viral vector tagged with enhanced green fluorescence protein (pBabe-eGFP-neo) as a control.
2. Thaw out one vial (1 mL) of viral supernatant promptly at 37 °C and add to 4 mL of NOE media (1:4 v/v) to each T25 flask or 60 mm culture dish.
3. Add 4 μL of 10 mg/mL polybrene to 5 mL of media with viral particles to achieve final concentration of 8 μg/mL media used (*see* **Note 17**).
4. Return plates to the 37 °C incubator for 48 h.
5. Begin selection with antibiotics or infect the cells another time by repeating **steps 2–4** (*see* **Note 18**).

3.2.4 Selection with Antibiotics and Creation of Stable Cell Lines

1. Make sure that cell density reaches 60–70 % confluence prior to antibiotic selection.
2. Begin selection with antibiotics, in this case neomycin/G418/Geneticin, at 250 μg/mL concentration. Adequate amount of cell death should be visible in 2–3 days (*see* **Note 19**). If too little cell death is observed, increase the concentration of selection agent in small increments (e.g., for neomycin, in increments of 250 μg/mL).
3. Apply fresh antibiotics every 2–3 days. If cells reach confluence, split cells at a desired ratio (usually 1:3–1:4 for OSE cells) and continue selection until no overt cell death occurs any further (in 2–3 weeks). By this time NOE cells infected with pBabe-eGFP-neomycin control viral particles should appear uniformly and intensely fluorescent (>90 % eGFP positivity) when examined under a fluorescent microscope. Always remember to cryopreserve partially selected cells during each step as a backup stock.

3.2.5 Confirmation of the Expression of Virally Introduced SV40 with Western Blotting Analysis

1. Grow NOE-SV40 and NOE-eGFP cells on desired culture vessels to >90 % confluence.
2. Wash cells with PBS ×1. The following steps are performed on ice.
3. Add 1 mL RIPA ×1 buffer supplemented with protease inhibitors per 100 mm dish or 0.5 mL RIPA buffer per 60 mm dish full of cells.
4. Gently scrape the cells off the plate with a prechilled cell scraper. Collect cells in a 1.5 mL microcentrifuge tube.
5. Vortex for 10 s then place tubes on ice for 30 min. Vortex for 10 s every 10 min during the incubation.
6. Spin down cell debris at maximum speed (>6,000 × *g*) for 5 min at 4 °C.
7. Transfer supernatant to a new 1.5 mL microcentrifuge tube. Proceed to determination of protein concentration. Procedures following the Pierce® BCA Protein Assay Kit (Thermo Scientific) will be illustrated as an example here.
8. In order to measure protein concentration by BCA assay, add 10 μL of BCA blank (RIPA buffer) and standards in a 96-well plate, in duplicates. The standards are prepared according to the manufacturer's suggested protocol and will not be described here.
9. Add 2 μL of protein samples into the sample wells in duplicate. Make up the volume to 10 μL with 8 μL of RIPA buffer.
10. Prepare working reagent by mixing 1 part of reagent B and 50 parts of reagent A as suggested by protocol supplied with Pierce® BCA Protein Assay Kit. Add 200 μL to each well of blanks, standards, and samples.
11. Seal the plate with an adhesive sticker. Incubate the microplate at 37 °C for 30 min.
12. Read color changes on a plate reader at 562 nm wavelength.
13. Plot concentration against readings at 562 nm and calculate concentration of samples using standards as a reference.
14. Load 40 μg of NOE-SV40 and NOE-eGFP cells onto a 10 % SDS-acrylamide gel. Separate the proteins by electrophoresis at 150 V for approximately 1 h or until the lower molecular dye in the protein marker reaches the bottom of the gel box.
15. Transfer the gel in a wet sandwich at 100 V for 1 h onto PVDF membranes.
16. Block nonspecific binding sites with 5 % nonfat dry milk prepare in TBS-T (0.1 %) with gentle rocking for 1 h at room temperature or overnight at 4 °C.
17. Incubate the membrane with primary antibody against SV40 T diluted in 1 % nonfat dry milk in TBS-T at 4 °C overnight with gentle shaking.

18. Wash the membrane with TBS-T for three times, 10 min each.
19. Incubate the membrane with secondary antibody diluted 1:4,000 in 1 % nonfat dry milk in TBS-T for 1 h at room temperature.
20. Repeat washes in TBS-T as at **step 18**.
21. Gently blot membranes and lay on a piece of Saran wrap on bench-top with the protein side facing up.
22. Prepare enhanced ECL solution according to manufacturer's suggested protocol.
23. Apply 1.5–2 mL ECL solution to evenly cover each membrane.
24. Incubate at room temperature for 5 min.
25. Drain excessive ECL solution off the membrane on a piece of blotting paper.
26. Carefully wrap the membrane in a clean piece of Saran wrap and avoid bubbles trapped inside. Proceed to film development in a dark room.
27. Confirm that the expression of virally introduced SV40 T antigen is only present in the SV40 T/t-transduced cell line but not in the eGFP-transduced control cells.

3.3 Immortalization of NOE-SV40 Cell Culture with hTERT

3.3.1 Transduction with Vector and Selection

The transfection of Phoenix Ampho cells, production of hTERT virus, transduction of NOE-SV40 cells, and subsequent antibiotic selection with hygromycin B are followed by the procedures outlined in Subheadings 3.2.1–3.2.4 and hereby will not be reiterated.

3.3.2 Measurement of Telomerase Activity in NOE-SV40 Cells Transducted with hTERT

Telomerase detection assay is performed using the TRAPeze® Telomerase Detection Kit (Millipore/Chemicon International). This assay is highly sensitive in detecting telomerase activity. When telomerase activity is present, the telomerase adds a 6-nucleotide repeat sequence to the 3′ of a substrate, which then is amplified through PCR during the next step. The final PCR product is a ladder of products with 6 base increments starting at 50 nucleotides: 50, 56, 62, 68, etc.

1. Harvest 1×10^6 parent NOE-SV40 and derivative NOE-SV40 cells transducted with hTERT (denoted as NOE-SV40-hT) cells by trypsinization.
2. Wash pellets with PBS twice.
3. Resuspend pellets and a control pellet provided by the TRAPeze® Telomerase Detection Kit with 200 μL 1× CHAPS lysis buffer supplemented with 100 U/mL RNase inhibitor.

4. Incubate on ice for 30 min.
5. Spin samples at 6,000 × *g* for 20 min at 4 °C.
6. Transfer 160 μL supernatant to a fresh 1.5 mL microcentrifuge tube.
7. Determine protein concentration with the Pierce® BCA Protein Assay Kit as described previously.
8. Aliquot and store at −80 °C. Avoid frequent thaw-freeze cycles.
9. Dilute the control cell extracts 1:20 with 1× CHAPS buffer (from TRAPeze® Telomerase Detection Kit). Use 2 μL of this diluted lysate in each assay.
10. Aliquot 10 μL supernatant from each sample into a new tube. Heat samples at 85 °C for 10 min. Heating is going to inactive telomerase, and heated protein extracts will serve as negative controls for their respective samples.
11. Prepare a master mix of these assay components (count per reaction): 5.0 μL of 10× TRAP reaction buffer, 1.0 μL of 50× dNTP mix, 1.0 μL of TS Primer, 1.0 μL of TRAP Primer mix, 0.4 μL of *Taq* polymerase (5 U/μL), and 39.6 μL of ddH_2O (total volume is 50 μL).
12. Aliquot 48 μL master mix into 200 μL PCR tubes containing 2 μL test/positive control/negative control lysates.
13. Incubate tubes at 30 °C for 30 min.
14. Perform a 3-step PCR as follows: 1 denaturation step—94 °C/30″, 2 annealing step 59 °C/30″, and extension step 72 °C/60″, for 30 cycles.
15. Separate 25 μL PCR product on a 10 % non-denaturing (SDS-free) polyacrylamide gel in 0.5× TBE buffer for 1.5 h at 400 V or until the xylene cyanol dye front runs 75 % the length of the gel plate.
16. Stain the gel in 1 μg/mL ethidium bromide for 30 min.
17. Visualize the bands with a UV imager.
18. Data interpretation: telomerase activity, evidenced by a laddering of bands six nucleotides apart on the image of the gel, should only be present in NOE-SV40-hT cell extracts but not in parent NOE-SV40 or heat-inactivated NOE-SV40-hT extracts (Fig. 1).

3.3.3 Confirmation of Immortalization in NOE-SV40-hT Cells

Continue passaging parent NOE-SV40 and derivative NOE-SV40-hT cells in culture. Whereas NOE-SV40 cells are expected to reach senescence within 30 days in culture, NOE-SV40-hT cells should keep proliferating past 200 days without exhibiting gross abnormalities in morphology (Fig. 2).

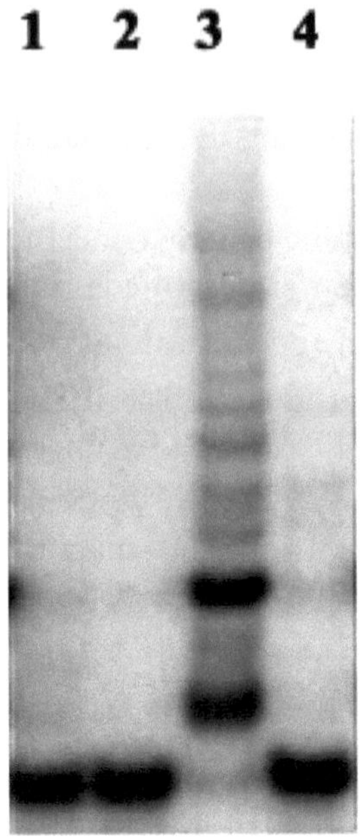

Fig. 1 Telomerase activity in SV40 T/t-transformed human ovarian surface epithelial cells (NOE-SV40) and cells containing both SV40 T/t and hTERT (NOE-SV40-hT) assayed by PCR. *Lane 1* protein abstracts from NOE-SV40 cells; *Lane 2* protein abstracts from heat-inactivated NOE-SV40 cells; *Lane 3* protein abstracts from NOE-SV40-hT exhibiting telomerase activities; *Lane 4* when protein abstracts from NOE-SV40-hT cells were heat inactivated, and no telomerase activity was detected

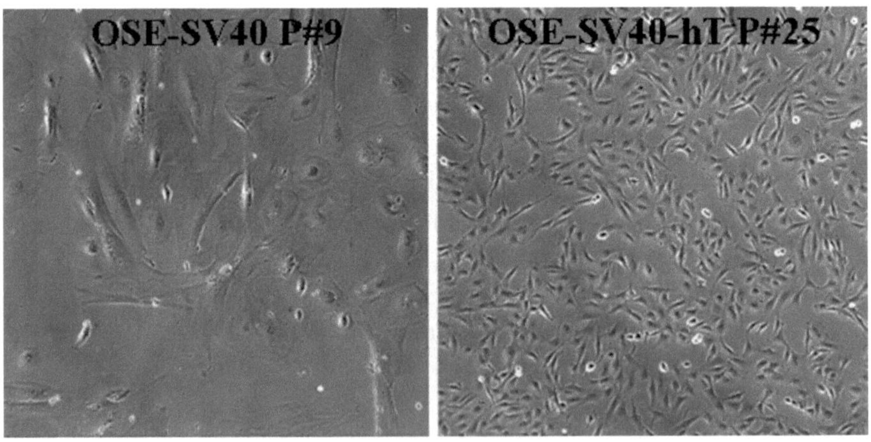

Fig. 2 Morphology of OSE-SV40 and OSE-SV40-hT upon continued passaging in culture. As shown to the *left*, OSE-SV40 cells showed clear signs of senescence at passage 9 in culture, including significantly enlarged, elongated, or fried-egg-like shapes, prominent nuclei, and stalled growth in culture for over 30 days. In comparison, OSE-SV40-hT cells were still highly proliferative in culture at passage 25 and retained typical compact, cobblestone epithelial features. Magnification: 40×

3.4 Transformation of NOE-SV40-hT Cells by Oncogenic HRAS^{V12}

3.4.1 Transduction with Vector and Selection

The transfection of Phoenix Ampho cells, production of H-ras virus, transduction of NOE-SV40-hT cells, and subsequent antibiotic selection with puromycin·HCl are followed by the procedures described previously in Subheadings 3.2.1–3.2.4 and hereby will not be reiterated.

3.4.2 Examination of the Expression of H-ras by Western Blotting

For a detailed protocol for Western blotting, refer to previous Subheading 3.2.5. The resulting cell line carrying viral SV40, hTERT, and H-ras is denoted NOE-SV40-hT-Ras.

4 Notes

1. Use a starting volume of 1,800 mL ddH$_2$O to dissolve powers, leaving sufficient space for the volume of 10 M NaOH to adjust pH. Upon reaching desired steady pH value of the media, adjust total volume to 2 L with autoclaved ddH$_2$O.
2. Prior to preparing complete media, serum needs to be heat inactivated at 65 °C for 30 min. The purpose of heat inactivation is to inactivate the ingredient "complement" in the serum that will interfere with the production or introduction of virus.
3. The pBabe-neo-SV40, pBabe-hygro-hTERT, pBabe-HRASV12-puro, and pBbabe-eGFP-*neo* vectors can be purchased from www.addgene.org. Alternatively, readers can purchase the backbone pBabe vector (from www.addgene.org or other suppliers such as www.cellbiolabs.com) and insert the rest of the fragments (e.g., SV40 early region, hygromycin resistance gene) into the vector by standard molecular cloning.
4. The Phoenix cell lines were developed by Dr. Nolan's laboratory at the Stanford University Medical Center. According to the developers, "Phoenix Ampho cells is a second-generation retrovirus producer lines for the generation of helper-free ecotropic and amphotropic retroviruses. The lines are based on the 293T cell line (a human embryonic kidney line transformed with adenovirus E1a and carrying a temperature-sensitive T antigen co-selected with neomycin). The lines were created by placing into 293T cells constructs capable of producing gag-pol, and envelope protein for ecotropic and amphotropic viruses. The lines offered advantages over previous stable systems in that virus can be produced in just a few days." (For detailed description of the Phoenix Ampho system, readers are encouraged to explore http://www.stanford.edu/group/nolan/retroviral_systems/phx.html.)
5. Final concentrations of antibiotics used for selection mammalian cells vary tremendously depending on the cell lines examined. Primary cells are likely more sensitive to antibiotics, and

the readers are suggested to start the selection process with low a concentration of antibiotics, which then can be gradually increased as the cells adapt.

6. Blocking can be performed in 3–5 % bovine serum albumin (BSA), 5–10 % normal serum, or a blocking solution commercially available, such as the Rodent Block M from Biocare Medical, Concord, CA.
7. Primary and secondary antibodies can be diluted in PBS with 1 % BSA or commercially available diluents, such as the daVinci Green solution from Biocare Medical, Concord, CA.
8. Although in general it takes about 4–6 h for adherent cells to attach the bottom of dishes/plates, it can take days for primary cells to adhere and differentiate. Therefore, it is critical to leave newly established culture of OSE cells in the initial medium undisturbed for at least 7 days to allow formation of monolayer cells.
9. When trying to obtain a relative pure population of OSE cells free of stromal cells, it is critical to start with p0-1 cells. This is because upon continued culturing, OSE cells undergo epithelial–mesenchymal transition and lose the epithelial-like features in vitro [12], making them indiscernible to mesenchymal fibroblasts in morphology when viewed under a light microscopy as well as in nature when examined by immunohistochemical methods.
10. As the determination of adequate trypsinization is highly subjective to the operator's experience, the effectiveness of this method varies tremendously and usually does not result in the removal of all the contaminating stromal cells. It is not unusual that remaining fibroblasts in the culture dish gradually outgrow the OSE population and eventually take over the entire dish. If the experimenter is new to this technique, it is suggested that a more experienced personnel offers consultation at times of needs.
11. Cloning can sometimes be integrated with differential tripsinization to achieve a highly purified population of OSE cells in the culture.
12. Cloning cylinders come in 3 sizes: small (6 mm × 8 mm), medium (8 mm × 8 mm), and large (10 mm × 10 mm). Depending on the size of the colony of cells, users can choose the desired size of cloning cylinders accordingly.
13. The addition of chloroquine presumably increases viral titer by twofold. This is thought to occur by lysosomal neutralizing activity of the chloroquine [13].
14. It is vital to remove media containing chloroquine no later than 12 h after transfection, as prolonged incubation in chloroquine will lead to cytotoxicity [13].

15. Harvest, collection, and purification of virus should be performed in a BL2 facility. It is recommended to wear PPE (personal protective equipment) including gown, shoe covers, hair bonnet, safety goggles, respiratory mask, and gloves. All materials coming into contact with virus need to be soaked in 10 % bleach for 10–15 min before disposal into biohazard containers.
16. Using filters with pore size smaller than 0.45 μM (such as 0.22 or 0.20 μM) will result in shearing of the viral envelop and inactivation of the viral particles.
17. Polybrene is a cationic molecule that binds to the surface of the cell membrane and facilitates binding of viral glycoproteins to receptors on the membrane.
18. Retrovirus particles do not infect nonproliferative cells and are generally considered less efficient in comparison with lentivirus-mediated infections. Since primary cells typically grow at a low rate and are less tranducible than immortalized or cancerous cell lines, our laboratory routinely performs two consecutive retroviral infections before starting the selection process. However, if the reader is working with a highly transducible cell line, only one infection may be sufficient to transducer the cells.
19. Always be conservative of the starting dose of antibiotics administered. It is very important to use a dose at the lower range of concentration, then gradually increase the concentration as the selection process continues. After 2–3 days into selection, cell death evidenced by floating cells should be prominent. The adequate but not excessive amount of cell death should be determined empirically by the operator based on past experience. In this case, infection rate of virus carrying pBabe-eGFP-neomycin can be visually determined under a fluorescent microscope and can serve as a reference to that of the retrovirus carrying SV40.

References

1. Hahn WC, Counter CM, Lundberg AS et al (1999) Creation of human tumour cells with defined genetic elements. Nature 400:464–468
2. Bodnar AG, Ouellette M, Frolkis M et al (1998) Extension of life-span by introduction of telomerase into normal human cells. Science 279:349–352
3. Kress M, May E, Cassingena R et al (1979) Simian virus 40-transformed cells express new species of proteins precipitable by anti-simian virus 40 tumor serum. J Virol 31:472–483
4. Lane DP, Crawford LV (1979) T antigen is bound to a host protein in SV40-transformed cells. Nature 278:261–263
5. Linzer DI, Levine AJ (1979) Characterization of a 54K dalton cellular SV40 tumor antigen present in SV40-transformed cells and uninfected embryonal carcinoma cells. Cell 17:43–52
6. Stubdal H, Zalvide J, Campbell KS et al (1997) Inactivation of pRB-related proteins p130 and p107 mediated by the J domain of simian virus 40 large T antigen. Mol Cell Biol 17:4979–4990
7. Zalvide J, DeCaprio JA (1995) Role of pRb-related proteins in simian virus 40 large-T-antigen-mediated transformation. Mol Cell Biol 15:5800–5810
8. Hahn WC, Dessain SK, Brooks MW et al (2002) Enumeration of the simian virus 40

early region elements necessary for human cell transformation. Mol Cell Biol 22:2111–2123
9. Siegel R, Ward E, Brawley O et al (2011) Cancer statistics, 2011: the impact of eliminating socio-economic and racial disparities on premature cancer deaths. CA Cancer J Clin 61:212–236
10. Tavassoli FA, Devilee P (2003) Pathology and genetics of tumors of the breast and female genital organs. IARC, Lyon, pp 113–145
11. Liu J, Yang G, Thompson-Lanza JA et al (2004) A genetically defined model for human ovarian cancer. Cancer Res 64:1655–1663
12. Auersperg N, Maines-Bandiera SL, Dyck HG et al (1994) Characterization of cultured human ovarian surface epithelial cells: phenotypic plasticity and premalignant changes. Lab Invest 71:510–518
13. Pear WS, Nolan GP, Scott ML, Baltimore D (1993) Production of high-titer helper-free retroviruses by transient transfection. Proc Natl Acad Sci 90:8392–8396

Chapter 30

In Vitro Model of Spontaneous Mouse OSE Transformation

Paul C. Roberts and Eva M. Schmelz

Abstract

An in vitro syngeneic model of neoplastic progression of murine ovarian surface epithelial (MOSE) cells represents a valid and significant model that allows for investigations into early mechanisms that impact tumorigenesis. Importantly, MOSE cells representing different stages of neoplastic transformation can be implanted back into immunocompetent mice to investigate host microenvironmental interactions that impact peritoneal dissemination and suppress immune surveillance mechanisms. Here we describe the isolation of MOSE cells that undergo spontaneous transformation upon repeated passage in cell culture. We also provide detailed in vitro assays for 3-D culturing of MOSE cells for characterizing anchorage-independent and invasive growth properties of these cells. Cell lines derived from this model have provided numerous insights into genetic, epigenetic, and biomechanical changes associated with neoplastic progression, as well as the immune responses associated with peritoneal dissemination of ovarian cancer cells.

Key words Mouse ovarian surface epithelial cells (MOSE), Neoplastic progression model, Organotypic culture, 3-D spheroid culture, Immunofluorescence microscopy

1 Introduction

Ovarian cancer is a deadly cancer with a 5-year survival rate of less than 30 % [1]. While the survival of women can be drastically improved to more than 94 % when the disease is still confined to the ovaries at time of diagnosis [2], molecular markers or events that allow for the identification of early disease have not been well established. Most ovarian cancers follow the cancer progression scheme that has been proposed by Vogelstein [3]: initiated tumor cells acquire consecutive genetic changes that allow for their expansion, progression, and metastatic outgrowth. The progression of ovarian cancer begins with primary tumor growth on the ovaries followed by shedding of malignant cells into the peritoneal cavity. Exfoliated cells can subsequently aggregate into spheroids that are disseminated throughout the abdomen by ascites, which forms as a result of fluid influx due to increased concentration of proteins and other factors secreted by tumor cells [4, 5]. Tumor spheroids in the ascites can grow and develop, eventually engrafting onto the

Anastasia Malek and Oleg Tchernitsa (eds.), *Ovarian Cancer: Methods and Protocols*, Methods in Molecular Biology, vol. 1049, DOI 10.1007/978-1-62703-547-7_30, © Springer Science+Business Media New York 2013

omentum [6], mesenteric lining, or other organs in the peritoneal cavity, where metastatic outgrowth ensues. Hence, ascites serves as both a vehicle for dissemination and contains cells and molecules that promote growth, angiogenesis, adhesion, invasion, and prevent apoptosis [4, 5]. Thus, to establish molecular markers or events that allow for diagnosis of early disease and the design of targeted prevention and treatment strategies and that increase the survival of women with ovarian cancer, a transitional model that recapitulates these aspects of ovarian progression is critical.

To study ovarian cancer, several animal models are available ranging from carcinogen-induced ovarian cancer via intra-ovarian application of DMBA ([7], oral cavity injections of dibenzopyrene [8], or targeted approaches using intrabursal silencing of *p53* and R*b1* [9], or transgenic mice (MISRIIR [10]). Interestingly, a new transgenic model for fallopian tube cancer carrying a deletion of both *Dicer* and *Pten* has recently been developed [11]. More commonly used are cell models for in vitro studies or in vivo injections into nude mice. Primary human ovarian surface epithelial were transfected with SV40 [12–15], human papillomavirus E6/E7 [12], Ras [16, 17], hTERT [16], a combination of cyclin D1, cdk4, and hTERT overexpression [18], depleted of p53 with subsequent c-Myc and k-Ras overexpression [19], or ß-hCG overexpression [20] among others to induce an immortal or transformed phenotype. Numerous established human ovarian cancer cell lines are available for investigation, but they represent mostly late-stage ovarian cancer and cannot be used in immunocompetent mice. The early precursor cell types are lacking.

Here we describe the isolation of mouse ovarian surface epithelial cells, which spontaneously transform upon serial in vitro passaging in culture. These cells recapitulate the transitional stages of ovarian cancer and can be used in both in vitro and in vivo applications in immunocompetent mice. We have shown that the progression of these cells is associated with a reduced cell size, an increased growth rate, and the increasing capacity to stratify, invade collagen, grow in 3-D cultures, and form tumors in vivo in immunocompetent C57BL/6 mice [21]. The progression of the MOSE cells is accompanied by distinct changes in gene expression; microarray analysis revealed prominent genetic changes in the functional categories proliferation, cell metabolism, and cytoskeleton [21, 22]. The observed progressive changes in cytoskeleton organization and architecture have also been described in the human disease and represent a prerequisite for the epithelial–mesenchymal transition of ovarian cancer cells [23]. Interestingly, we have recently reported a direct correlation of these aberrant cytoskeleton organizational events with changes in the biomechanical properties of the MOSE cell lines that are stage specific. Using atomic force microscopy, we were able to demonstrate that as cells progress to more malignant phenotype, the elasticity and viscosity of cells decreases, resulting in softer, more deformable cells [24]. This correlates well with the progressive dysregulated actin cytoskeletal changes [25] we observed in the different stages of MOSE cell progression [21, 22].

As noted, one of the major advantages of the cell lines derived from the in vitro spontaneous transformation of MOSE cells is that they can be transplanted back into syngeneic C57BL/B mice. Hence, tumor formation and peritoneal dissemination occur within a fully immune competent in vivo setting. Of note, the MOSE-derived ID8 clonal variant described by Roby et al. [26] has been used in several studies to characterize immune responses and immune-associated cells as a consequence of peritoneal dissemination of ovarian cancer cells [27–32]. These studies have provided significant insights into how the immune system is suppressed during peritoneal dissemination of ovarian cancer. Importantly, aggressive cell types derived from MOSE cells have been used for preclinical assessment of novel immunotherapeutic or immunomodulatory therapies designed to limit peritoneal dissemination of ovarian cancer [28, 31].

In conclusion, this model reflects critical phenotypical, genotypical, and biomechanic changes and properties of the human disease and is as such an excellent model to study ovarian cancer progression, prevention, and treatment.

2 Materials

Prepare all solutions using deionized, ultrapure water dH_2O (18 M Ω cm at 25 °C) and tissue culture grade reagents. All reagents and solutions for tissue harvest and cell culture must be sterile. Unless otherwise indicated, store reagents at 4 °C and warm to 37 °C prior to use for cell culture.

2.1 MOSE Isolation

1. Mice (female, C57BL/6J, 10–12 months old), at least 10 per experiment.
2. CO_2 incubator.
3. Surgical instruments (sharp surgical scissors, forceps).
4. Ethanol 70 %, in spray bottle.
5. Trypsin and trypsin inhibitor solutions. Prepare 0.2 % trypsin in serum-free DMEM and sterile filter (0.25 μm syringe filter). Use immediately. The trypsin inhibitor solution is aliquoted and stored at −20 °C.
6. Antibiotic–antimycotic solution (ABMS) ×100. Aliquot and store at −20 °C. Prepare a 1× dilution in sterile dH_2O for immediate use.

2.2 2-D Cell Culture

1. Deionized, sterile water (dH_2O).
2. Phosphate-buffered saline buffer (PBS), sterile, with and without Ca^{2+}/Mg^{2}.
3. Dulbecco's Modified Eagles Media (DMEM).
4. Complete growth media. Supplement Dulbecco's Modified Eagles Media (DMEM) with 4 % fetal bovine serum (FBS), murine epidermal growth factor (mEGF) 2 ng/ml, hydrocortisone 0.5 μg/ml, and ITS 1× (5 μg/ml insulin, 5 μg/ml transferrin, and 5 ng/ml sodium selenite), streptomycin 100 μg/ml and penicillin 100 U/ml (*see* **Note 1**).
5. Trypsin-EDTA solutions: 0.25 % trypsin/0.5 3mM EDTA.
6. Tissue culture treated plates (6-well, 24-well, 96-well half surface area plates).
7. Tissue culture treated flasks (T25, T75).
8. Sterile pipettes and pipette tips.

2.3 3-D Cell Culture

1. Low-adhesion 6- or 12-well cell culture plates.
2. Transwell inserts and companion plates 0.45 μm.
3. Sterile filters 0.22 and 0.4 μm.
4. DMEM (10×). Dissolve DMEM powder into 0.1 volume of deionized water to make the 10× solution. Sterile filter through a 0.22 μm vacuum filter and pellet residual precipitate. Aliquot and store at −20 °C (*see* **Note 2**).
5. BD Matrigel™ Matrix: Stored at −20 °C. Prior to use, thaw overnight at 4 °C and keep on ice.
6. Rat tail collagen type I. Use according to the product insert for coating plasticware or making collagen plugs.
7. NaOH 1 N.
8. Cell strainers 70 μm.
9. 10 % buffered formalin.

2.4 Immuno-fluorescent Staining

1. Round glass coverslips: no. 1 thickness, 12 mm diameter, cleaned, and sterile.
2. Humidity chamber: square petri dish, Parafilm®, and Whatman 1.5 mm blotting paper.
3. Paraformaldehyde fixative, 3 and 6 %. Dissolve 3 g (6 g) of paraformaldehyde in 60 ml of deionized water, add 3–4 drops (50 μl) of 1 N NaOH to adjust pH 7.3, and heat with constant stirring at 56 °C in a water bath until solubilized. Add 25 ml of 1 M HEPES, pH 7.4 and equilibrate to 100 ml with deionized water. Filter sterilize (0.4 μm), aliquot and store at −20 °C (*see* **Note 3**).
4. Permeabilization solution: 0.25 % Triton™ X-100 in PBS, pH 7.4.

5. Methanol. Stored at −20 °C.
6. Quenching solution: 50 mM glycine. Dissolve 0.375 g of glycine in 100 ml PBS to make a 50 mM solution; filter sterilize (0.2 μm) and store at 4 °C (*see* **Note 4**).
7. IFA blocking buffer: 2 % chicken serum in PBS. Filter sterilize (0.2 μm) and store at 4 °C (*see* **Note 5**).
8. PBS-Tween 20: 0.05 % Tween 20 in PBS, pH 7.4.
9. Mounting solution with antifade component such as ProLong® Gold antifade with and without DAPI.
10. Curved forceps.
11. Cleaned microscopy glass slides.

2.5 Immunohistochemistry on Paraffin-Embedded Tissue

1. 4–5 μm sections of the embedded spheroids, or plugs.
2. Xylene.
3. 100, 95, 80, 50, and 30 % ethanol.
4. PBS.
5. Coplin jars, slide holders (glass or plastic), rectangular staining dish, staining tray (or very flat pyrex containers), and glass coverslips (22 × 22 or 24 × 40 mm).
6. Vegetable steamer.
7. 10 mM citrate buffer, pH 6 or 10 as required for your antibody of choice (or commercially available 100× antigen retrieval solution).
8. Blocking solution (1 % BSA, 1 % FCS in PBS or as required by the specific antibody).
9. ABC and DAB kit (commercially available), hematoxylin counterstain solution.
10. Mounting solution (water soluble or permanent).
11. Permanent markers (such as Statmark®, not sharpies!!), or pencil.

3 Methods

The ovarian surface epithelium is isolated from the ovaries of adult female mice (C57BL/6; MHC-I H2-K^b/D^b) using standard aseptic harvesting techniques under a laminar flow hood following the guidelines described by Roby et al. [26] with modifications [21]. This procedure routinely generates immortalized cells which spontaneously progress over 30–100 passages. Of note, this procedure is also amenable to isolation of fallopian tube surface epithelium.

3.1 Isolation, Culture, and Spontaneous Transformation of Mouse Ovarian Surface Epithelial Cells

1. Euthanize mice (a minimum of 10 mice) via CO_2 inhalation (*see* **Note 6**).
2. Thoroughly saturate the skin with 70 % EtOH.
3. Make a small incision in the skin on the dorsal side and gently pull in both an anterior and posterior direction to separate skin from the body and pull back over the legs and arms and head.
4. Place animals on their backs, again liberally applying 70 % EtOH to maintain sterility as much as possible.
5. Make a ventral incision along the midline from the groin area towards the diaphragm, followed by lateral incisions at both ends to reflect back the peritoneal lining. Reflect the intestines to one side to expose the uterus. The ovaries are often buried in fat and are encased by a clear thin ovarian bursal membrane.
6. Gently resect the ovaries from the fat and fallopian tubes, making sure to reflect back the ovarian bursal membrane and place all 20 ovaries in PBS containing 1× antibiotic–antimycotic solution (PBS-ABMS) together in a sterile 60 mm cell culture plate. The collection should not take more than 20–30 min. Keep ovaries on ice bathed in PBS until ready for digestion.
7. Incubate ovaries in about 5 ml serum-free DMEM containing 0.2 % trypsin, freshly prepared, for 30 min in a CO_2 incubator at 37 °C (*see* **Note 7**).
8. Add 3 volumes of trypsin inhibitor and filter the entire solution with digested ovaries over a 70 μm sterile filter and collect the flow through. Wash with 2 volumes of trypsin inhibitor solution to recover any single cells adhering to the filter (*see* **Note 8**).
9. Pellet the epithelial cells recovered in the flow through (300 × *g*, 10 min, at RT) and wash the epithelial cell pellets twice with DMEM containing 4 % FBS.
10. Resuspend washed epithelial cells in 2–4 ml of complete growth media and transfer to 1–2 wells of a collagen-coated, 6-well tissue culture dish (ca. 100,000 cells/dish) and place in a humified 5 % CO_2 incubator at 37 °C (*see* **Note 9**).
11. Cells are subcultured at 80 % confluency using standard trypsin–EDTA cell dissociation solutions (*see* **Note 10**).
12. Every 5–10 passages, determine the cells growth rate and monitor whether they have lost contact inhibition of growth and gained the capacity for 3-D growth in soft agar or as multicellular spheroid growth under low-attachment culture conditions (*see* Subheading 3.2.1 below) (*see* **Notes 11–13**).
13. When the cells exhibit enhanced growth in soft agar, inject 1×10^6 trypsinized single cells in 100–200 μl of sterile PBS intraperitoneally into syngeneic C57BL/6 female mice and monitor tumor formation over time to confirm in vitro transformation and aggressiveness with actual in vivo tumorigenicity (*see* **Note 14**).

3.2 3-D Cultures Systems for Characterization of MOSE Cells

Frequently during neoplastic progression, cancer cells acquire resistance to anoikis and acquire the capacity to invade extracellular matrices. Soft agar assays and spheroid collagen and Matrigel organotypic cultures represent several well-established 3-D culture microenvironments that can be employed to more closely mimic in vivo microenvironments encountered by ovarian cancer cells and as such may be necessary to confirm tumorigenicity, response to treatment targeting ascites, or for coculture studies. We have found that as MOSE cells are serially passaged, they gradually acquire a resistance to anoikis and survive under nonattached culture conditions as large multicellular aggregates or spheroids.

3.2.1 3-D Spheroid Cultures

1. Trypsinize and seed 1×10^5 cells per well in low-adhesion 12-well culture dishes. Gently manually agitate dishes during the first few days of culture to prevent any nonspecific adherence of spheroids to the culture dishes (*see* **Note 15**).
2. Gently remove half of the medium from the top every 3–4 days and add the same amount of fresh medium. The compounds of choice can be added to the medium to monitor assembly, survival, or architecture of the spheroid in response to the treatment.
3. At different time points following seeding, observe formation of multicellular spheroids and make digital micrographs depicting morphology of spheroids and note any signs of cell death. Spheroid growth and survival should be monitored over a 10–21 day period as many early passage cultures will form initial spheroids which subsequently die within 5–15 days (*see* **Note 16** and Fig. 1).

3.2.2 3-D Organotypic Collagen Raft Cultures

In these cultures, cells are grown on top of a collagen raft under an air–liquid interface for 14–21 days. This allows one to monitor when MOSE cultures acquire the capacity to invade collagen and grow as multilayers in organotypic raft cultures, indicative of progression to a malignant phenotype. Collagen rafts are prepared in Transwell filter inserts, which creates a two-chamber culture system (*see* Fig. 2).

1. Prepare a neutralized 2 mg/ml collagen solution according to the product guidelines. The collagen solution is maintained on ice until it is to be distributed in the Transwell inserts. It is important to mix thoroughly without introducing air bubbles.
2. Using prechilled pipette tips, gently place 250 μl of the neutralized 2 mg/ml collagen solution into each prechilled 12-well Transwell insert housed in its corresponding companion plate. After every 3–4 wells, gently tap each side of the culture plate to evenly disperse the collagen solution. Allow the collagen gel to polymerize for at least 45–60 min at 37 °C in the incubator, prior to seeding cells (*see* **Note 17**).

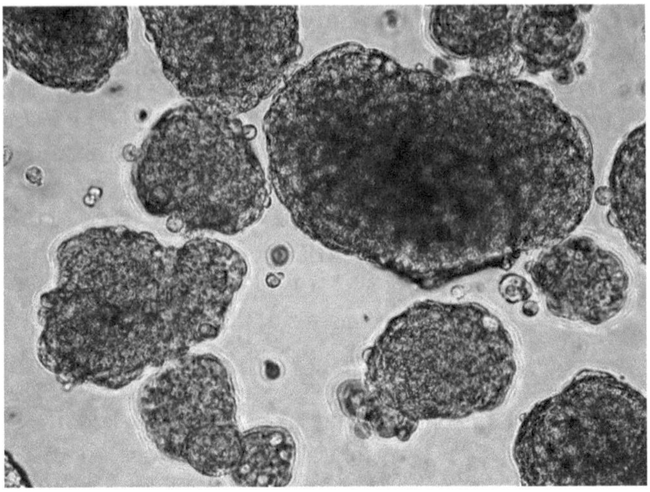

Fig. 1 MOSE spheroids (passage 180) after 2 days in culture

3. Seed cells in complete growth media at a density of 5×10^4 cells/well by adding cell suspension (ca. 200–300 μl) to the top chamber. Following seeding of cells, add media to the lower chamber and incubate overnight at 37 °C in the incubator under 5 % CO_2.
4. Once the cells have reached confluency, grow the cultures at an air–liquid interface, by removing the media in the top chamber and returning the cultures to the incubator. Media in the lower chamber is replaced every 2–3 days (*see* **Note 18**).
5. Overlay the 14–21 day old cultures with 2 % agarose, fix overnight in 10 % buffered formalin, embed in paraffin, and process for routine histopathology (*see* **Note 19**) to determine the changes in tissue architecture that correspond to the increasing aggressiveness of the cells. Early passage, benign cells typically form a monolayer on top of the collagen plug, whereas cells at later passages begin to grow as multilayers and gain the capacity to invade the collagen. For histochemical analysis of the raft cultures, follow procedure under Subheading 3.4.

3.2.3 Collagen I Embedded Cultures

Similar to the organotypic collagen raft cultures, MOSE cells can be directly embedded into collagen type I plugs and monitored for their growth and invasive properties. These cultures (also called tumorspheres) provide insights into the type of motility that MOSE cells display when encountering extracellular matrices.

1. Trypsinize cells and make a cell suspension in complete growth media containing 1×10^5 cells/ml.
2. Prepare on ice a 2 mg/ml collagen I solution by mixing 109 μl of 3.63 mg/ml of collagen I stock solution with 2.5 μl 1 N NaOH, 20 μl of 10× DMEM, 18 μl of deionized sterile water,

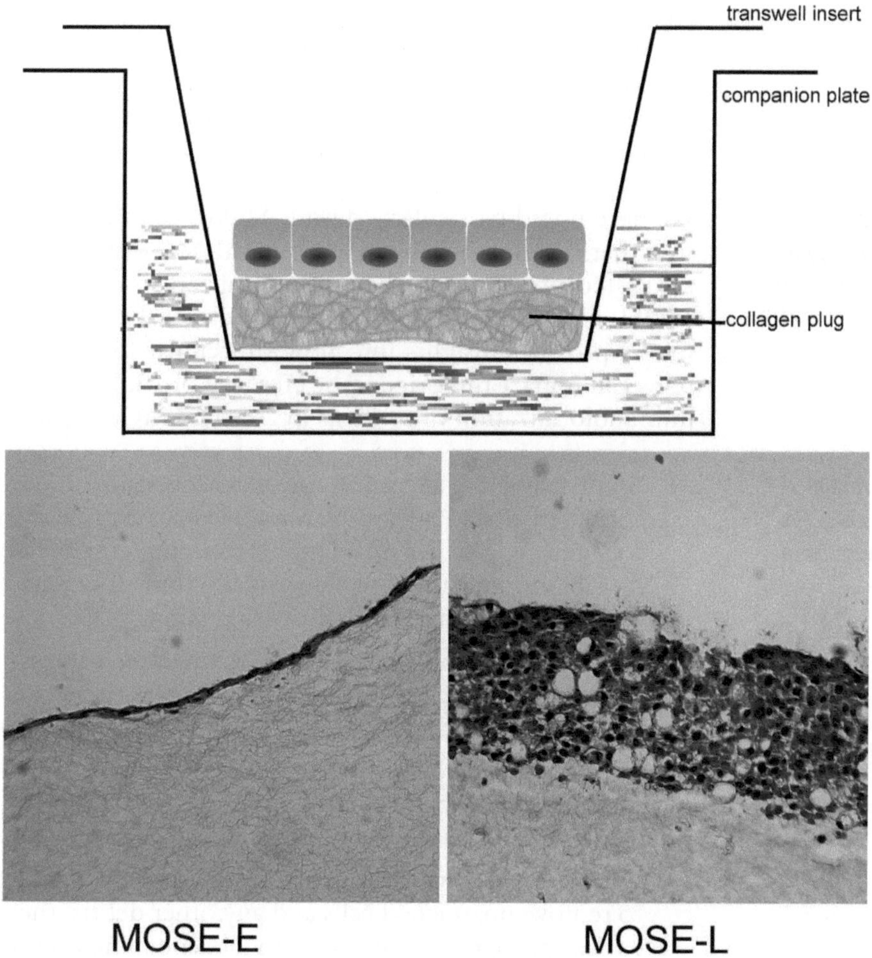

Fig. 2 Schematic of the organotypic raft culture system using Transwell filter inserts (*top*). Histochemistry of early passage (*left*) and late passage MOSE cells (*right*) cultured for 15 days on Transwell filter inserts under an air–liquid interface (*bottom*)

and 50 μl of cell suspension (5,000 cells). This is enough for seeding 6 wells of a 96-well half surface area plate. This can be scaled up according to demand. Mix thoroughly minimizing generation of air bubbles (*see* **Note 20**).

3. Pipette 28 μl/well of collagen-cell suspension to a prechilled 96-well half surface area plate, gently tapping each side of the plate after every 4–5 wells to evenly disperse collagen within the wells. Transfer the culture plate to a 37 °C 5 % CO_2 incubator to allow collagen to polymerize.
4. After 45 min, overlay collagen-embedded cell plugs with complete growth media and place the plate back into the incubator. Media is changed every 2–3 days.
5. Monitor and record growth every 2–3 days by digital microscopy.

6. Typically, embedded cultures are monitored for up 14 days, at which time the collagen cultures are fixed overnight in 10 % formalin or 3 % paraformaldehyde fixative, embedded in paraffin and sectioned for routine histochemistry or immunohistochemistry as described in Subheading 3.4 (*see* **Note 21**).

3.3 Immunofluorescent Staining of Cultured MOSE Cells

We have noted particularly during MOSE cell neoplastic progression that despite unchanged levels in mRNA, distinct cytoskeleton associated proteins are aberrantly localized in different stages of MOSE cells [21, 22]. Hence, the in vitro MOSE transformation model provides insights into how subcellular localization of proteins can impact tumorigenesis. Here we provide our protocol for immunolocalization of proteins in attached MOSE cells.

3.3.1 Growth and Fixation of MOSE Cells on Glass Coverslips

1. Aseptically place a clean, sterile glass coverslip into each well of a 24-well tissue culture plate. Coverslips can be coated with collagen type I, poly-l-lysine, fibronectin, or other basement membrane substrate to investigate differences in substrate attachment during neoplastic progression.
2. Seed cells in complete or defined growth media at 5×10^4 cells per coverslip. Press down on each coverslip to prevent air bubbles forming underneath the coverslip.
3. Monitor attached cells at 1 h post-seeding and if necessary, rinse off unattached cells and replace media. Cells can be fixed at anytime following seeding (*see* **Note 22**).
4. Prior to fixation of cells, gently wash coverslips twice with PBS to remove unattached cells and any other debris, then proceed to the appropriate fixation protocol depending on the needs of your study.
5. For methanol fixation, wash cells twice with PBS, aspirate and cover cells with methanol (−20 °C), and let sit on ice for 3 min. Aspirate off methanol and rinse the cells at least 3 times with PBS. Cells can be stored covered in PBS at 4 °C until staining with appropriate antibodies for up to 2 weeks.
6. For identification of surface proteins, wash cells twice with PBS, aspirate and cover the cells with 3 % paraformaldehyde fixative, and let sit for 10 min at RT. Remove the fixative and quench residual fixative using 50 mM glycine for 10 min. Aspirate off the quench solution and wash twice with PBS.
7. For identification of intracellular proteins, permeabilize cells following paraformaldehyde fixation by incubating cells prior to **item 8** (blocking) for an additional 10–15 min in permeabilization solution, and wash 3 times with PBS to remove residual detergent.
8. Aspirate off PBS and incubate cells overnight at 4 °C in IFA blocking buffer. Remove blocking buffer and store cells covered in PBS at 4 °C (*see* also **Note 5**).

3.3.2 Indirect Immunostaining Procedure

All staining procedures are performed using inverted coverslips (cell side down) placed on drops of prediluted antibody and incubated for various time points within a humidity chamber. The humidity chambers minimize evaporation of antibody solutions and allow for long-term incubation periods.

1. Prepare a humidity chamber by placing a precut square of Whatman paper on the inside lid of a square petri dish. Thoroughly saturate the Whatman paper with deionized water, then place a precut piece of parafilm on top of the Whatman paper, avoiding bubbles. The shallow lid allows for easy access to the chamber and coverslips. The deep portion of the petri dish will now serve as the lid, creating a well-humidified chamber.
2. For immunostaining, place 18–20 μl of prediluted primary antibody solution as a drop on the parafilm within the humidity chamber. Continue placing as many drops of antibody as required.
3. Gently remove coverslips from 24-well plate using curved forceps, remove excess liquid by blotting one end onto a paper towel, and gently lower the coverslip (cell side down) onto the antibody drop. Incubate for 20 min (RT) or up to 24 h (4 °C).
4. To recover coverslip for washing, gently pipette 75 μl of PBS-Tween 20 underneath the coverslip so that it raises up and can be easily recovered. Place coverslips cell side up into a 12-well plate for washing.
5. Wash coverslips at least 3 times for 5 min with an excess of PBS-Tween 20.
6. Repeat **steps 2–5** using appropriate fluorophore-conjugated secondary antibodies.
7. Repeat **steps 2–5** using primary antibodies derived from different species and appropriate fluorophore-conjugated secondary antibodies as needed for multi-protein detection. Importantly, place humidity chamber in the dark during incubations with fluorophores.
8. Coverslips are mounted cell side down onto a drop of ProLong® Gold antifade reagent (10–12 μl) with or without DAPI on a clean glass slide and allowed to polymerize for a minimum of 60 min prior to epifluorescent or confocal microscopy.

3.4 Histopathological Analysis of 3-D Culture of MOSE

For immunohistochemical determination of tissue architecture, protein expression, and localization that are associated with MOSE progression, typically 4–5 μm slides cut from paraffin-embedded tissues are used that allow for the staining of specific proteins. While one can use fluorochrome-conjugated secondary antibodies similar to Subheading 3.3.2, staining with HRP-biotin (ABC) systems and DAB will provide more information of tissue architecture, and cell morphology. The ABC kits (commercially available from various sources) are very specific and offer several alternatives for either highly expressed proteins or allowing for the enhancement of signals from low expressed proteins.

1. Label all slides clearly with a permanent marker or a pencil.
2. Place slides into plastic slide holder and dry at 56 °C for about 1 h in glass slide holders (may overheat in metal holder).
3. Deparaffinize and rehydrate as follows: place slides in glass slide holders of the rectangular staining dish, fill the dish with xylene, and let the slides sit for 5 min. Repeat 2 more times with fresh xylene. Line up dishes with 100, 95, 80, 50, and 30 % ethanol. Lift the slides in the slide holder from the last xylene bath, briefly touch a paper towel to remove excess xylene from the slide holder and place into the container with the 100 % ethanol for 5 min. Repeat procedure with 95, 80, 50, and 30 % ethanol. Place slides in holder in PBS for 5–15 min.
4. If your protein of choice needs antigen unmasking as indicated by the manufacturer of your antibody, fill a Coplin jar with antigen retrieval solution, place it into the basket of a vegetable steamer that is filled with water, and warm up solution. Submerge slides in the hot antigen retrieval solution, steam for 20 min and then allow to cool at room temperature for about 20 min by removing the unmasking container with the slide holder—do not take the slides out (*see* **Note 23**).
5. Add water to the bottom of the staining tray and place sections on the rubber-coated ridges—make sure they do not dry out during any of the following steps!
6. Add about 300–500 μl of blocking solution onto each slide using a plastic transfer pipette—avoid placing the solutions directly onto the sections, as they may become loose—and incubate for 1 h in the closed staining chamber.
7. Add 50–100 μl of antibody solution to the slide, cover with a 24 × 40 mm coverslip, close lid, and incubate for 1 h at room temperature or up to 24 h at 4 °C (*see* **Note 24**).
8. Remove coverslip by dipping slide upright into PBS. Place in Coplin jar and rinse 3 times with PBS for 5 min each.
9. Use the ABC and DAB kits as to the manufacturer's instructions; always be careful to prevent drying of the sections.
10. For counterstaining, add a couple of drops hematoxylin solution to the slides for a couple seconds, place into Coplin jar, and rinse gently 3 times with dH_2O until the red stain is removed.
11. For permanent mounting, place slide in slide holder of staining dishes, place into 95 % ethanol for 2 min, then twice in 100 % ethanol. Briefly remove excess ethanol from the slide holder by

touching a paper towel, then place slide holder into fresh xylene for 2 min; repeat twice.

12. Add about 50 μl of the permanent mounting solution on the slide, and cover with glass coverslip without bubbles by letting the outside of the coverslip touch the mounting solution which is gently lowered onto the section. Let dry for 2–4 h or overnight prior to light microscopic analyses (*see* **Note 25**).

4 Notes

1. Only during the early passage of cells (passage 1–10) are mEGF and hydrocortisone supplements in the medium necessary, and their use can be discontinued. Collagen-coated plates and flasks, although not required, tend to aide in initial attachment and can be discontinued after 5–10 passages. We also recommend the use of antibiotic–antimycotic solution and even ciprofloxacin during early cultures to prevent mycoplasma and fungal contamination.
2. When thawing 10× aliquots of DMEM, you will notice that it does not completely go into solution. Simply pellet out the precipitate and use the supernatant.
3. Paraformaldehyde does not readily go into solution unless heated and pH adjusted towards 7.4.
4. Alternatively, free aldehyde groups can be quenched with 50 mM NH_4Cl in PBS.
5. Typically, cells are blocked with either BSA or in diluted serum derived from the species of your secondary antibodies. Our laboratory has found that chicken-derived secondary antibodies result in less nonspecific binding. Chicken serum can be obtained from numerous commercial sources.
6. We have found that retired female breeder mice (10–12 months of age) typically have larger ovaries with expanded surface areas, which can result in better yields of epithelial cells during the initial harvesting of cells.
7. Avoid excessive agitation of ovaries during the trypsinization steps to reduce unwanted contamination from stromal cell types.
8. It is recommended to fix samples of ovaries both prior to trypsin digestion as well as immediately after to monitor for complete separation and isolation of the surface epithelium. Pancytokeratin staining can be used to confirm localization or absence (following digest) of the ovarian surface epithelium.
9. The yield of surface epithelial cells is generally low ($1–2 \times 10^5$ cells per 10 ovaries), and it is recommended to start with more mice to obtain sufficient numbers of cells.

10. Early passaged cells (1–10) are split only every 2–3 weeks at a ratio of 1:2–1:3. After passage 10, cells can generally be split at a 1:5 ratio.
11. We have found that maintaining cells as a heterogeneous population of cells instead of early subcloning as described by Roby et al. [26] allows for maintenance of heterogeneous cell lines that represent distinct stages of transformed phenotypes culminating in the establishment of aggressive late-stage variants with continued passaging (>90). This tends to delay the acquisition of more aggressive phenotypes, allowing for characterization of more subtle and gradual changes during neoplastic transformation. However, clonal variants can be established at any time point during the entire culture process by limiting dilution culture. We routinely use flow cytometric sorting to sort single cells into 96-well plates to obtain 10–15 single cell clonal variants.
12. We routinely freeze back cells every 10 passages and prepare RNA or DNA for gene expression analysis or DNA promoter methylation status.
13. We have noted that ITS can have subtle effects on gene expression and typically culture cells without ITS for 2–3 passages prior to any experimental assessment of gene expression. Removal of ITS does not have any adverse effects on growth rate, colony formation in soft agar, or on spheroid growth.
14. MOSE cells depending upon their passage number display different in vivo tumor initiating capacities. In our hands, I.P. implantation of 5×10^6 early passage MOSE cells (up to passage 30) does not induce tumor formation in C57BL/6 female mice even after 100 days. In contrast, 5×10^6 late passage cells, results in widespread peritoneal dissemination of tumors within 5–6 weeks. To extend the lifespan of the animals, lower implanted cell numbers can be used.
15. Alternatively, 12-well tissue culture treated plates can be coated with a layer of 1 % agarose to prevent attachment of cells.
16. Spheroids can also be collected and processed at any time point for further biochemical, molecular, or immunohistochemical characterization. For immunohistochemical analyses, place spheroids into an Eppendorf tube and embed spheroids in 2 % collagen or agarose. After polymerization of collagen or agarose, fix samples overnight in 10 % formalin before embedding in paraffin; alternatively, rinse spheroids with PBS, and embed directly in OCT for cryosectioning.
17. We typically prepare the collagen plugs 24 h prior to cell seeding and let them equilibrate in complete media overnight. Media is applied to both chambers and aspirated before seeding of the cells.

18. Maintain the media level in the bottom chamber such that it is level with the collagen plug.
19. To remove plug from insert, cut along the bottom with a scalpel releasing the entire plug with the membrane from the insert. The membrane can be processed along with the collagen plug.
20. The concentration of the stock collagen I solution may vary significantly depending on the lot number. Adjust as necessary to prepare a 2 mg/ml working solution.
21. Alternatively, if the interaction of tumor cells with a complex matrix is of interest or necessary to support the growth of the tumor cells, cells are embedded into Matrigel™, a complex protein mixture of solubilized basement membrane components. A growth factor reduced formulation can be substituted to define soluble factors that contribute to growth. Specific growth or differentiating factors can be added to the media overlay. Mix 50 μl of cell suspension (1×10^5 cells/ml) with 150 μl of phenol red-free Matrigel™ and plate 28 μl of this cell-Matrigel™ suspension per well in a prechilled 96-well half surface area plate. Transfer the plate to an incubator at 37 °C for 45–60 min to allow polymerization, overlay with fresh complete media and return to the incubator. Proceed as described for the collagen-embedded cultures. RNA, DNA, and protein can be directly recovered from plugs for further analysis.
22. Strong attachment to non-coated coverslips often requires at least 24 h and several rounds of replication of the cells. These cells will secrete their own basement membrane proteins. If earlier time points are important, we recommend coating the coverslips with poly-l-lysine or collagen.
23. The antibody data sheet will tell you if other methods of antigen retrieval such as microwaving are more appropriate.
24. Make sure the staining tray is level so the coverslips do not slide off the sections; this may result in drying of the sections and unspecific staining.
25. Alternatively, the dehydrating steps can be omitted if water-soluble mounting media are used. To prevent the drying of the sections during storage until analysis, use nail polish to seal the sides of the coverslips.

Acknowledgements

This work was supported by NIH grant CA118846 (E.M.S., P.C.R.) and The Fralin Research Institute Initiative for Cancer Biology at Virginia Tech (P.C.R., E.M.S.).

References

1. Howlader N et al (2011) SEER cancer statistics review, 1975–2008, National Cancer Institute, Bethesda, MD, http://seer.cancer.gov/csr/1975_2008/
2. Jemal A et al (2010) Cancer statistics, 2010. CA Cancer J Clin 60:277–300
3. Vogelstein B, Kinzler KW (1993) The multistep nature of cancer. Trends Genet 9:138–141
4. Kuk C et al (2009) Mining the ovarian cancer ascites proteome for potential ovarian cancer biomarkers. Mol Cell Proteomics 8:661–669
5. Shield K et al (2009) Multicellular spheroids in ovarian cancer metastases: biology and pathology. Gynecol Oncol 113:143–148
6. Steinberg JJ, Demopoulos RI, Bigelow B (1986) The evaluation of the omentum in ovarian cancer. Gynecol Oncol 24:327–330
7. Nishida T et al (1986) Histologic origin of rat ovarian cancer induced by direct application of 7,12-dimethylbenz(a)anthracene. Nihon Sanka Fujinka Gakkai Zasshi 38:570–574
8. Chen KM et al (2012) Induction of ovarian cancer and DNA adducts by dibenzo[a, l] pyrene in the mouse. Chem Res Toxicol 25:374–380
9. Flesken-Nikitin A et al (2003) Induction of carcinogenesis by concurrent inactivation of p53 and Rb1 in the mouse ovarian surface epithelium. Cancer Res 63:3459–3463
10. Connolly DC et al (2003) Female mice chimeric for expression of the simian virus 40 TAg under control of the MISIIR promoter develop epithelial ovarian cancer. Cancer Res 63:1389–1397
11. Kim J et al (2012) High-grade serous ovarian cancer arises from fallopian tube in a mouse model. Proc Natl Acad Sci USA 109:3921–3926
12. Gregoire L et al (2001) Spontaneous malignant transformation of human ovarian surface epithelial cells in vitro. Clin Cancer Res 7:4280–4287
13. Maines-Bandiera SL, Kruk PA, Auersperg N (1992) Simian virus 40-transformed human ovarian surface epithelial cells escape normal growth controls but retain morphogenetic responses to extracellular matrix. Am J Obstet Gynecol 16:729–735
14. Nitta M et al (2001) Characterization and tumorigenicity of human ovarian surface epithelial cells immortalized by SV40 large T antigen. Gynecol Oncol 81:10–17
15. Leung EH, Leung PC, Auersperg N (2001) Differentiation and growth potential of human ovarian surface epithelial cells expressing temperature-sensitive SV40 T antigen. In Vitro Cell Dev Biol Anim 37:515–521
16. Liu J et al (2004) A genetically defined model for human ovarian cancer. Cancer Res 64: 1655–1663
17. Adams AT, Auersperg N (1981) Transformation of cultured rat ovarian surface epithelial cells by Kirsten murine sarcoma virus. Cancer Res 41:2063–2072
18. Bono Y et al (2012) Creation of immortalised epithelial cells from ovarian endometrioma. Br J Cancer 106:1205–1213
19. Motohara T et al (2011) Transient depletion of p53 followed by transduction of c-Myc and K-Ras converts ovarian stem-like cells into tumor-initiating cells. Carcinogenesis 32:1597–1606
20. Guo X et al (2011) Overexpression of the beta subunit of human chorionic gonadotropin promotes the transformation of human ovarian epithelial cells and ovarian tumorigenesis. Am J Pathol 179:1385–1393
21. Roberts PC et al (2005) Sequential molecular and cellular events during neoplastic progression: a mouse syngeneic ovarian cancer model. Neoplasia 7:944–956
22. Creekmore AL et al (2011) Changes in gene expression and cellular architecture in an ovarian cancer progression model. PLoS One 6:e17676
23. Lee JM et al (2006) The epithelial-mesenchymal transition: new insights in signaling, development, and disease. J Cell Biol 172:973–981
24. Ketene AN et al (2012) The effects of cancer progression on the viscoelasticity of ovarian cell cytoskeleton structures. Nanomedicine 8:93–102
25. Ketene AN et al (2012) Actin filaments play primary role for structural integrity and viscoelastic response in cells. Integr Biol 4:540–549. doi 10.1039/C2IB00168C
26. Roby KF et al (2000) Development of a syngeneic mouse model for events related to ovarian cancer. Carcinogenesis 21:585–591
27. Bak SP et al (2008) Murine ovarian cancer vascular leukocytes require arginase-1 activity for T cell suppression. Mol Immunol 46:258–268
28. Hagemann T et al (2008) "Re-educating" tumor-associated macrophages by targeting NF-kappaB. J Exp Med 205:1261–1268
29. Hagemann T et al (2006) Ovarian cancer cells polarize macrophages toward a tumor-associated phenotype. J Immunol 176:5023–5032
30. Huarte E et al (2008) Depletion of dendritic cells delays ovarian cancer progression by boosting antitumor immunity. Cancer Res 68: 7684–7691
31. Tomihara K et al (2010) Antigen-specific immunity and cross-priming by epithelial ovarian carcinoma-induced CD11b(+)Gr-1(+) cells. J Immunol 184:6151–6160
32. Zhang L et al (2002) Generation of a syngeneic mouse model to study the effects of vascular endothelial growth factor in ovarian carcinoma. Am J Pathol 161:2295–2309

Chapter 31

Orthotopic, Syngeneic Mouse Model to Study the Effects of Epithelial–Stromal Interaction

James B. Greenaway and Jim J. Petrik

Abstract

One of the difficulties in studying ovarian cancer historically has been the lack of a suitable animal model that replicates the human disease. Mouse models that utilize intraperitoneal implantation of tumorigenic cells lack interaction between the transformed ovarian epithelial cells and the ovarian stroma, which we have shown to be an integral component in replicating the etiology seen in human epithelial ovarian cancer (Greenaway, Gynecol Oncol 108:385–394, 2008). Xenograft models generally require the use of immunocompromised hosts, which then eliminates the influence of the immune system in disease progression, which also has been shown to be an important part of the progression of epithelial ovarian cancer (EOC). In this chapter, we describe the generation and optimization of an orthotopic, syngeneic mouse model and illustrate the importance of facilitating epithelial–stromal cell interaction to more closely replicate human EOC.

Key words Epithelial ovarian cancer, Mouse model, Orthotopic, Syngeneic, Tumorigenesis, Epithelial-stromal

1 Introduction

Epithelial ovarian cancer is the most lethal gynecologic malignancy and is a complex disease with vague symptomology that typically leads to late detection and poor survival. We have a relatively poor understanding of the disease. Even the cell of origin of EOC is under debate, with some believing that the initial transformation occurs in the single layer of epithelial cells that line the surface of the ovary, while others contend that epithelial cells of the oviduct are the site of transformation that give rise to EOC. One of the reasons we know relatively little about this particular form of ovarian cancer is the difficulty in generating an animal model that accurately replicates the numerous characteristics of human EOC.

A number of approaches have been taken to generate experimental models to study ovarian cancer. Some models involve the use of transgenic mice to alter gene expression specifically in OSE cells to determine the potential roles of various oncogenic genes

Anastasia Malek and Oleg Tchernitsa (eds.), *Ovarian Cancer: Methods and Protocols*, Methods in Molecular Biology, vol. 1049, DOI 10.1007/978-1-62703-547-7_31, © Springer Science+Business Media New York 2013

(reviewed by Vanderhyden [1]). Other approaches involve the injection of xenograft cancer cells or OSE cells that have been transformed in vitro. Typically, these cells have been injected intraperitoneally or subcutaneously into immunocompromised murine hosts to test novel therapeutics [2–4]. Other xenograft models involve the injection of tumorigenic cells directly under the ovarian bursa in mice, which allows the tumors to develop in their normal microenvironment [5, 6], but these models lack an intact immune system, now known to be an important regulator of ovarian tumorigenesis [7–9]. To facilitate the study of ovarian cancer development in an immunocompetent mouse, a syngeneic mouse model has been developed where murine ovarian surface epithelial cells derived from C57BL-6 mice were allowed to spontaneously transform in vitro [10]. These cells were then injected back into syngeneic mice where they formed ovarian tumors.

There is evidence to suggest that the interaction between the ovarian surface epithelial (OSE) cells and the stromal compartment is important in facilitating the onset and progression of EOC. OSE cells are believed to participate in the ovulatory process by releasing proteolytic enzymes to degrade the basement membrane and follicle wall [11]. After ovulation, the OSE cells are in contact with the ovarian stromal compartment and are exposed to the growth factor-, cytokine-, and steroid-rich environment that exists there. The formation of inclusion cysts, where OSE cells become trapped within the ovarian stroma, following ovulation causes further exposure to this environment. Women with a hereditary risk of EOC have an increased incidence of inclusion cysts, lending support to this hypothesis and the importance of the epithelial–stromal interaction in EOC [12].

Selection of an appropriate mouse model to study ovarian cancer is dependent upon the central research question. If the focus of the study is on the biology or response to intervention in human ovarian cancer cells specifically, then the use of immunocompromised mice is necessary and appropriate. If the central focus is not on human versus mouse tumors, then the use of a syngeneic model with an intact immune system may be desirable. The use of an immunocompetent mouse would be essential if the focus of the study was on the development of immune-based cancer therapies, studying the role of inflammation on ovarian cancer development or development of vaccines.

The site of implantation of cells in vivo also requires careful selection, based on the goal of the study. Typical implantation sites for the study of ovarian cancer include the peritoneum, subcutaneous area, or intrabursal space, and these different sites have been shown to yield different results in ovarian tumor development and progression [13]. Subcutaneous injection of ovarian cancer cells generates tumors near the surface which may be more optimal for luminescent or fluorescent monitoring [14], which can be difficult in tumors seated within the peritoneum. Intrabursal injection of cells allows for interaction with the normal tumor microenvironment and communication with the ovarian stromal environment, which may be an important part of the tumorigenic process in ovarian cancer [5, 15, 16]. In this case, orthotopic placement of the tumorigenic epithelial cells may result in the best approximation of disease in women with epithelial ovarian cancer and allows for the epithelial–stromal interaction that we hypothesize is an important event in EOC progression.

In this chapter, we generated samples in which spontaneously transformed murine ovarian surface epithelial cells (S/T-OSE) were placed under the ovarian bursa and allowed to interact with the ovarian stroma. At advanced stage disease, we collected abdominal ascites, which contained numerous cells that had sloughed from the primary tumor following epithelial–stromal interaction and formation of a large ovarian tumor. We named these cells 28-2 cells. As a control, we injected cells directly into the peritoneum so that they could exist in the peritoneal environment without previously contacting the ovarian stroma. These were labeled IP cells. A number of functional assays were used (as described below) to evaluate the role of epithelial–stromal interaction in the pathogenesis of EOC.

2 Materials

Prepare all solutions in sterile conditions under a laminar/vertical hood, using deionized, ultrapure water dH_2O_2 (18 MΩ cm at 25 °C) and tissue culture grade reagents. All reagents and solutions must be sterile. Unless otherwise indicated, store reagents at room temperature.

2.1 Cell Culture

1. Spontaneously transformed murine ovarian surface epithelial cells, derived from C57Bl-6 mice (S/T-OSE) (*see* **Note 1**).
2. Dulbecco's Modified Eagles Media (DMEM).
3. DMEM complete medium. Supplement Dulbecco's Modified Eagles Media DMEM with 10 % fetal bovine serum (FBS), penicillin 100 U/mL, and streptomycin 100 ng/mL. Store at 4 °C.
4. Phosphate-buffered saline buffer (PBS), 1×, sterile, Ca/Mg free.
5. Trypsin-EDTA solutions: 0.25 %-trypsin/0.53 mM-EDTA. Store at 4 °C.
6. Tissue culture flasks (T75).
7. Tissue culture dishes 6-well.
8. Sterile pipettes and pipette tips.

2.2 Orthotopic/Syngeneic Mouse Model

1. C57BL-6 mice, syngeneic with the murine ovarian surface epithelial cells (60 days old).
2. Hamilton syringe, 30 G needles (Fisher Scientific).
3. Buprenorphine hydrochloride.
4. Isoflurane anesthesia system.
5. Microsurgical equipment, skin staples.
6. Hamilton syringe 0.5 mL.
7. Needle 30 G.

2.3 Immunofluorescence

1. Superfrost Plus 22 × 50 mm glass slides (Fisher Scientific).
2. 22 × 22 mm glass coverslips (Fisher Scientific).
3. Formalin 10 %, buffered with sodium phosphate (Fisher Scientific). Store at RT.
4. Permeabilization solution: 0.2 % Triton X-100 in PBS. Prepare fresh and use immediately.
5. Bovine serum albumin (BSA), powder.
6. Sodium azide, powder.
7. Blocking solution: 0.01 M PBS, 5 % BSA, 0.02 % sodium azide. Store at 4 °C.
8. Antibody diluting solution: 0.01 M PBS, 1 % BSA, 0.02 % sodium azide. Store at 4 °C.
9. 4′,6-Diamidino-2-phenylindole (DAPI) (Sigma).
10. ProLong Gold antifade (Invitrogen).

2.4 Immunoblotting

1. RIPA buffer: 50 mM Tris–HCl, 150 mM NaCl, 0.1 % SDS, 0.5 % Na. Deoxycholate, 1 % Triton X-100, pH 8.0. Supply with any commercially available protease inhibitor in concentration indicated by producer. Store at 4 °C.
2. Protein Quantification Assay.
3. 30 % Acrylamide/Bis-acrylamide stock solutions, 29:1.
4. Sodium dodecyl sulfate solution (SDS), 10 % (w/v) in ddH_2O.
5. Resolving gel buffer: 1.5 M Tris–HCl, pH 8.8.
6. Stacking gel buffer: 0.5 M Tris–HCl, pH 6.8.
7. *N,N,N′,N′*-Tetramethylethylenediamine solution (TEMED).
8. Ammonium persulfate, 10 % (w/v) in ddH_2O. Prepare fresh and use immediately.
9. Gel running buffer: 25 mM Tris-HCl, 192 mM Glycine, 0.1 % (w/v) SDS, pH 8.3. Almost always prepared from a commercial 10× solution. Dilute in ddH_2O and use immediately.
10. PVDF transfer membranes (Amersham).

11. Western blot transfer buffer: 0.025 M Tris–HCl, 0.186 M glycine, 20 % methanol, pH 8.0.
12. Mini Protean Western blot apparatus (Bio-Rad).
13. Whatmann paper (VWR).
14. Molecular weight marker (Precision Plus, Bio-Rad).
15. Tris-buffered saline (TBS): 1.5 M NaCl, 0.1 M Tris–HCl, pH 7.4.
16. Tween-20.
17. TBS containing Tween-20 (TBS-T): 0.1 % Tween-20 in TBS.
18. Nonfat dry milk.
19. Blocking solution: 5 % nonfat dry milk in TBS. Prepare fresh and use immediately.
20. Antibody dilution solution: 5 % BSA in TBS. Prepare fresh and use immediately.
21. Autoradiography films, film development, and imaging equipment.

2.5 Scratch Assay

1. Tissue cell culture plates, 6-well (Corning).
2. Glass slides, 22 × 22 mm (Fisher Scientific).
3. Pipette tip.
4. Olympus BX-61 inverted microscope (Olympus).

3 Methods

3.1 Generation of Tumor Models

C57BL6 mice are used for all experiments (*see* **Note 1**). Appropriate preoperative and postoperative care of animals in accordance with established veterinary medical and nursing practices is required.

3.1.1 Orthotopic Model

Knowledge in mouse anatomy and experience in mouse surgery is required before perform any survival surgery. All survival surgery must be performed with aseptic procedures, including sterile gloves, masks, sterile instruments, and aseptic techniques.

1. Culture S/T-OSE cells in DMEM complete medium in usual conditions (humified 5 % CO_2 incubator at 37 °C) up to confluence. Approximately 1 T-75 flask per 5 mice is necessary to generate sufficient cell yield.
2. Harvest S/T-OSE cells by trypsinization, wash twice with warmed PBS and suspend—$1 \times 10^6/5$ μL in PBS (*see* **Note 2**).
3. Prior to anesthesia, inject mice subcutaneously with 0.3 mg/kg buprenorphine to provide postsurgical analgesia.
4. Mice are anesthetized with isoflurane (3 %) inhalation until surgical plane is reached.

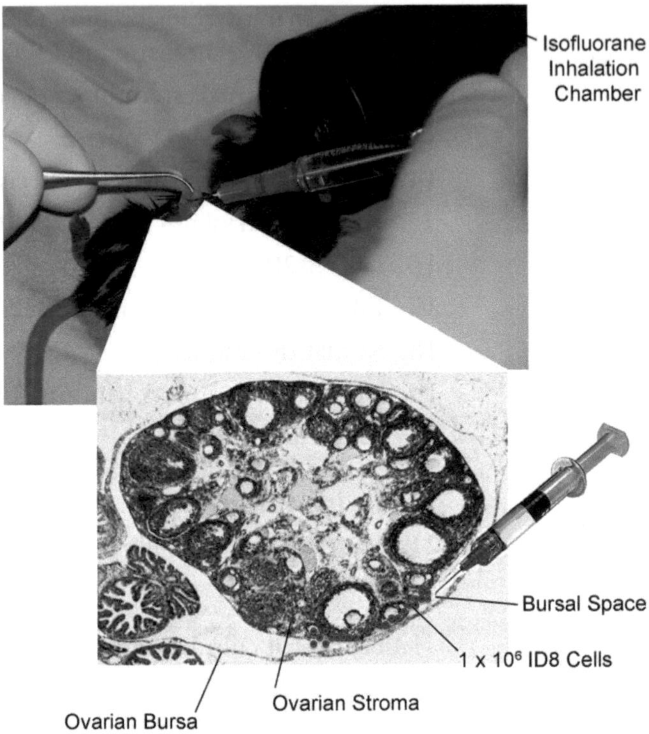

Fig. 1 Generation of an orthotopic, syngeneic mouse model of epithelial ovarian cancer. 1×10^6 spontaneously transformed murine ovarian surface epithelial cells in 5 μL PBS are injected through the ovarian bursa into the bursal space. The cells then invade through the basement membrane and interact with the ovarian stroma

5. Made dorsal midline incision and exteriorize the left ovary through the incision site (*see* **Note 3**).
6. Load 1×10^6 S/T-OSE cells in 5 μL PBS in a Hamilton syringe connected to a 30 G needle.
7. While holding the base of the ovary with forceps, advance the 30 G needle just until the ovarian bursa is penetrated (Fig. 1).
8. The plunger of the Hamilton syringe is slowly depressed until the cell solution is released into the bursal space (5 μL of cell suspension per mouse) (*see* **Note 4**).
9. After injection, return the ovary to its normal space in vivo.
10. Locate the right ovary and bring to the incision site.
11. Inject 5 μL PBS as vehicle control (*see* **Note 5**).
12. Replace the ovary and close the incision with 2 skin staples at which time the mouse is allowed to recover and monitored closely postoperatively. Mice are allowed to return to normal housing until euthanasia for tumor removal (*see* **Note 6**).

3.1.2 Intraperitoneal Model

Cells are cultured and harvested as described in previous section. Mice are housed and treated similarly to the mice used for the orthotopic model.

1. Harvest, wash, and suspend 1×10^6 S/T-OSE cells in 200 μL PBS.
2. Restrain mice manually and inject the cell suspension into the intraperitoneal space.
3. Mice are returned to normal housing until euthanasia for ascites collection and tumor removal.

3.2 Cell Collection from Cell Lines In Vivo

At 90 days post tumor induction (PTI), tumor bearing mice have large primary tumors, numerous metastatic peritoneal tumors, and the formation of abdominal ascites which contains many cells. This stage of disease replicates approximately Stage III disease in women, which is the most common stage at which the disease is initially detected. Mice that had cells injected directly into the peritoneum (IP model), without interaction with the ovarian microenvironment typically exhibit peritoneal lesions and early stages of ascites formation at 90d PTI. Explant cultures are initiated in vitro by the removal of a primary tumor at 90d PTI and placement of this tissue in growth media. With this model, we collect epithelial tumor cells that have had interaction with the ovarian microenvironment, but not the peritoneal environment.

3.2.1 28-2 Cell Line

1. At 90 days post tumor induction (PTI) in the orthotopic tumor model, ascites fluid was aspirated just prior to euthanasia for tumor removal.
2. Ascites aspirate was centrifuged for 5 min at $1 \times 1{,}500 \times g$. Supernatant was aspirated and cell pellet was resuspended in 1 mL DMEM complete medium (*see* **Note** 7).
3. Cells were named 28-2 and were placed in a T-25 cell culture flask, allowed to propagate, and the colony was expanded with normal subculturing procedures (*see* **Note 8**).

3.2.2 IP Cell Line

1. At 90 days PTI in the IP model, a peritoneal flush was performed with warmed PBS and fluid was aspirated.
2. Abdominal aspirate was centrifuged for 5 min at $1 \times 1{,}500 \times g$. Supernatant was aspirated and cell pellet was resuspended in 1 mL DMEM complete medium.
3. Cells were named IP and were placed in a T-25 cell culture flask, allowed to propagate, and the colony was expanded with normal subculturing procedures (*see* **Note 9**).

3.2.3 Explant Cell Line

1. At 90 days PTI, a separate group of animals is used to generate a primary explant cell line.

2. Mice are euthanized with CO_2 asphyxiation and immediately the primary ovarian tumor is removed through a midline abdominal incision.
3. Tumor tissue is minced into 2–3 pieces and placed in a 10 cm culture dish in DMEM complete medium (*see* **Note 10**).
4. Cells are allowed to grow out from the primary tumor for 3 days at which time single cells were selected, replated, and allowed to propagate normally (*see* **Note 11**).

3.3 Assessment of the Effect of Epithelial–Stromal Interaction

To determine the effects of epithelial–stromal interaction, we evaluated the expression and localization of proliferative, apoptotic, and angiogenic proteins using immunofluorescence and immunoblotting. We also evaluated cell motility using the scratch assay. Immunofluorescence allows the determination of the proportion of cells that are expression a particular protein, as well as any changes in cellular localization. Immunoblotting can provide quantitative information on the amount of protein expressed by cells in vitro or by tissues extracted at euthanasia. Both of these techniques require a similar amount of time to complete and provide different but complementary information. The scratch assay provides information on the proliferative and migratory capacity of cells in vitro. Other complementary assays would be the transwell or Boyden chamber assays to study migration and bromodeoxyuridine (BrdU) incorporation or Ki67 immunostaining to evaluate cellular proliferation.

3.3.1 Immunofluorescence Staining of the Attached Cells

1. Place 22 × 22 mm glass coverslips in the bottom of 6-well culture vessels.
2. Seed 1×10^6 S/T-OSE, 28-2, IP, or explant cells in 2 mL DMEM complete medium to each well.
3. At 80 % confluence, DMEM media is aspirated, cells are rinsed with warmed PBS, and then fixed in 1 mL 10 % neutral buffered formalin for 1 h at room temperature.
4. Perform cell membranes permeabilization with 0.2 % Triton X-100 in PBS for 15 min at room temperature.
5. Place coverslips with adherent cells in blocking solution for 10 min at room temperature.
6. Dilute antibodies to their appropriate concentration in Antibody Diluting Solution and pipetted on top of the coverslip.
7. Place a cover of paraffin over the coverslip to prevent evaporative loss (*see* **Note 12**).
8. Incubate cells with primary antibody, anti-Ki67, overnight at 4 °C.
9. Rinse coverslips with adherent cells for 2 min twice with PBS.

10. Apply anti-rabbit secondary antibody conjugated to Alexa Fluor 488 to each coverslip for 2 h at room temperature.
11. Repeat **step 9**.
12. DAPI diluted in PBS is added to each coverslip for 2 min.
13. A drop of ProLong Gold antifade is added to a glass slide and each coverslip is mounted to a slide and allowed to cure overnight (*see* **Note 13**).
14. Coverslips are imaged with an inverted fluorescence microscope where Ki67- and DAPI-positive channels are collected and then overlayed using integrated morphometry software (*see* **Note 14**).
15. The results are expressed as a percentage of Ki67 positive cells.

3.3.2 Immunoblotting

1. Scrap and triturate the cells (S/T-OSE,28-2, IP, explant) in RIPA buffer. Incubate in RIPA buffer on ice for 5 min.
2. Quantify protein using a Protein Quantification Assay (Biorad or other suitable).
3. Prepare resolving gel (12 % acrylamide): mix 3.3 mL of ddH_2O, 4 mL of 30 % acrylamide, 2.5 mL of resolving gel buffer, 100 μL of 10 % SDS, 100 μL of 10 % ammonium persulfate and 4 μL of TEMED in a 50 mL conical flask and pour into 7.25 cm × 10 cm × 1.5 mm cassette. Overlay the resolving gel with water.
4. Prepare stacking gel (4 % acrylamide): mix 6 mL of ddH_2O, 1.3 mL of 30 % acrylamide, 2.5 mL of resolving gel buffer, 100 μL of 10 % SDS, 100 μL of 10 % ammonium persulfate and 4 μL of TEMED in a 50 mL conical flask and pour over the resolving gel.
5. Insert 10 well, 1.5 mm thick comb immediately.
6. Calculate the volume of sample needed to load 20 μg protein per lane (*see* **Note 15**).
7. Vortex cell lysate samples, pulse spin (5,000 × *g* for 20 s) and heat at 95 °C or 5 min in heating block.
8. After heating, pulse spin (5,000 × *g* for 20 s).
9. Load molecular weight marker and 20 μg each of S/T-OSE, 28-2, IP, and explant cell lysate per lane.
10. Electrophorese at 100 mV until dye front has reached the bottom of the gel.
11. Approximately 20 min before samples are ready to transfer, presoak the following in transfer buffer: sponge pads, Whatmann paper, PVDF membrane.
12. Pry glass plates apart with spatula and transfer the plate with the gel remaining to a dish with transfer buffer.

13. Remove the stacking gel and slide the resolving gel onto PVDF membrane.
14. Gently remove air bubbles from between the gel and membrane.
15. Sandwich gel/membrane between 2 pieces of Whatmann paper and then 2 sponges and assemble in the transfer apparatus and insert into transfer chamber.
16. Fill transfer chamber with transfer buffer until the sponge pads are covered.
17. Transfer at 300 mA for 2 h.
18. After transfer, disassemble and wash membranes for10 min twice in TBS-T to remove methanol.
19. Place membrane in 25 mL of blocking solution and agitate for 1 h. at room temperature.
20. After blocking, incubate membrane with the primary antibody at the appropriate dilution (*see* **Note 16**).
21. The membrane is washed 3 × 10 min with 10 mL TBS-T and the secondary antibody applied at concentration of 1:1,000 for 1 h on a rocker at room temperature.
22. Membrane is washed 3 × 10 min with 10 mL TBS-T.
23. Place membrane on a piece of overhead transparency film, and add 1.0 mL of chemiluminescence substrate, cover with second piece of transparency film and incubate for 1 min.
24. Protein signal is transferred to x-ray film and imaged using an optical imaging system.
25. Epithelial–stromal interaction resulted in increased expression of angiogenic (VEGF, pVEGFR-2), survival (pAKT, bcl-2) and proliferative (PCNA) markers and a decreased expression of apoptotic proteins (Bax) (Fig. 2).

3.4 Scratch Assay

1. Add 1×10^6 S/T-OSE, 28-2, or explant cells to each well of a 6-well culture dish in 2 mL DMEM complete medium.
2. Allow cells to reach approximately 80 % confluence.
3. Make a scratch across the bottom of the 6-well plate with a plastic pipette (*see* **Note 17**).
4. At 12 and 24 h post scratch, image the bottom of the 6-well dish with brightfield microscopy and quantify the area of the scratch filled in by proliferating/migrating tumor cells (*see* **Note 18**).
5. Epithelial–stromal interaction results in a more rapid cellular proliferation and increased rate of scratch wound closure (Fig. 3).

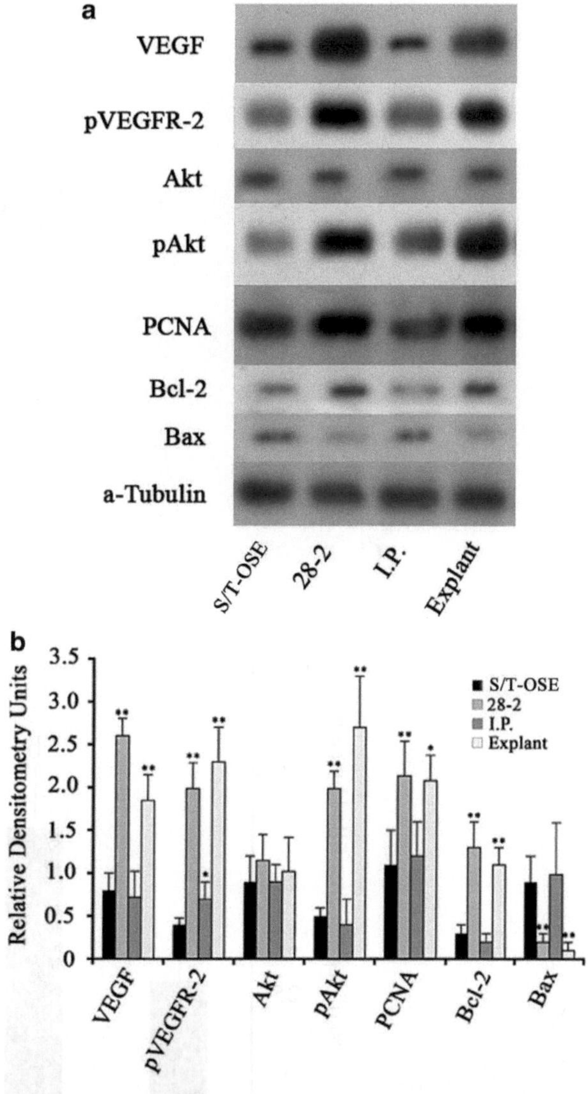

Fig. 2 Following stromal interaction, tumor cells have increased expression of angiogenic, proliferative, and survival factors. (**a**) Immunoblot analysis was performed on protein lysates from S/T-OSE, 28-2, I.P., and explant cells. (**b**) Densitometry was performed on a minimum of three different immunoblot experiments and results are expressed relative to α-tubulin. The graph represents the mean ± SEM expression of the different factors for each cell type. $*p<0.05$; $**p<0.001$ compared to S/T-OSE cells

4 Notes

1. C57BL-6 mice are syngeneic for the S/T-OSE cells generously donated by Drs. Roby and Terranova (Kansas State University). Mice are housed in accordance with the Canadian Council on Animal Care, on a 12 h light/dark schedule and allowed water and food ad libitum.

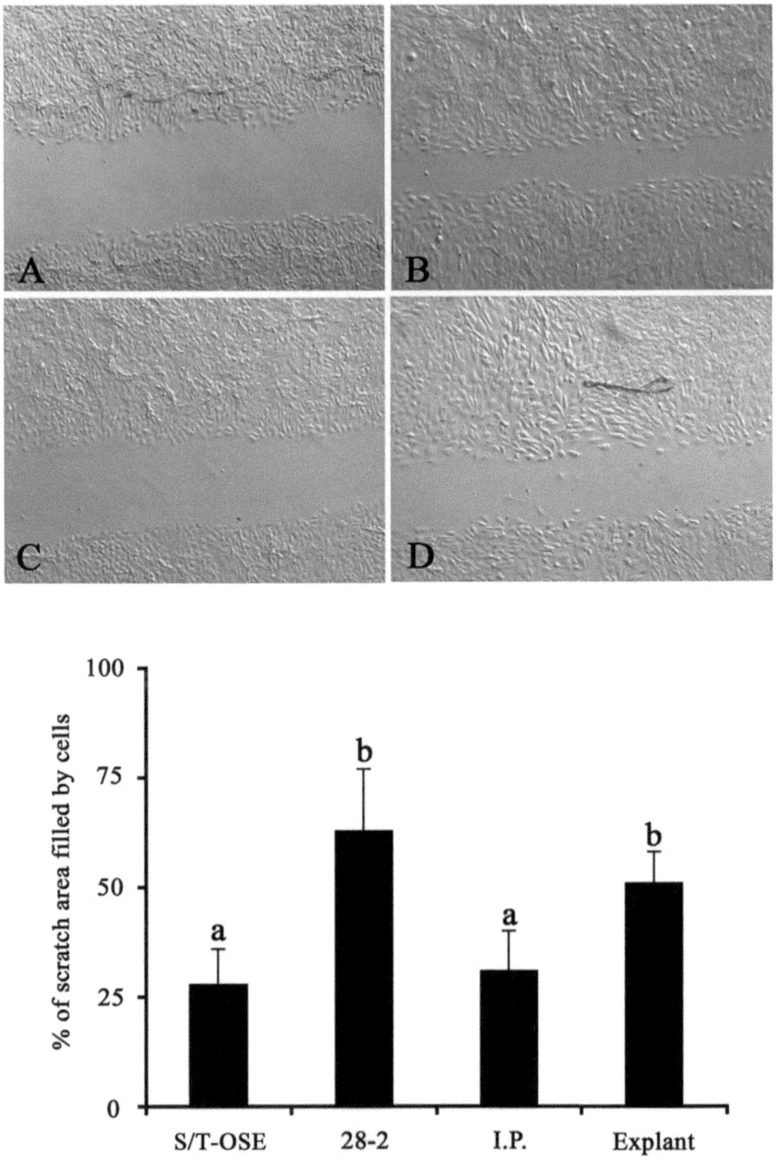

Fig. 3 The cell migration of S/T-OSE (**a**), 28-2 (**b**), I.P. (**c**), and explant (**d**) cell lines in the in vitro scratch wound healing assay. The graph represents the mean ± SEM percentage of the scratch area filled by the cells after 24 h post-scratch culture. Bars with *different letters* are statistically different ($p < 0.05$)

2. If performing surgeries on a number of mice, it is important to generate a fresh supply of cells hourly, as prolonged periods in PBS during the surgical procedure can reduce viability.
3. Once the skin is incised, it is still necessary to go through the epaxial muscle group and the dorsal peritoneal fascia in order to access the peritoneal space which contains the abdominal organs, including the ovaries.

4. It is important to express the cell solution slowly. The bursa will expand like a balloon and rupture is possible if inflation occurs too quickly.
5. The use of a PBS (vehicle) control will allow us to monitor any changes in the ovary that may be due to bursal disruption or irritation of the epithelial surface of the ovary due to the injection procedure or presence of 5 μL PBS. To date, we have not seen any reactive changes in the PBS-injected group.
6. It is important to keep mice on a warming pad during the surgery and recovery. This prevents excessive heat loss and greatly reduces recovery time.
7. Typically, there are enough cells from the ascites aspirate from a single mouse to initiate a culture. However, pooling cells from additional mice within the same group is an option to increase yield.
8. For in vitro experiments, this cell line represented the tumorigenic murine ovarian surface epithelial cells that had interacted with the ovarian stroma. We know that following bursal injection, the cells invade through the basement membrane and are exposed to the hormone- and growth factor-rich stromal environment. This approach facilitates the epithelial–stromal interaction that we hypothesize is important in development of the etiology of EOC.
9. This cell line represents the tumorigenic epithelial cell line that did not interact with the ovarian stroma, but were still allowed access to the peritoneal space, as were the 28-2 cells following dissemination from the tumor.
10. As with the ascites cells, a tumor explant from an individual mouse will provide sufficient cells, but pooling different tumor tissues to increase yield is an option.
11. From the explants, there could be a heterogeneous population of cells that grow out initially. However, the cells that grew out from the tumor explant appeared morphologically to be epithelial. In a subset of colonies selected, we performed immunohistochemical analysis for cytokeratin 8 and 18 and confirmed that the explant cell culture consisted of epithelial cells. These cells, when compared to the IP cell line, allowed us to determine the role of the epithelial–stromal interaction in EOC progression.
12. It is important not to press down on the paraffin cover when applying as this may disperse the antibody solution underneath and result in variable binding.
13. Getting the glass coverslip out of the 6-well plate can be difficult. We find that using a scalpel blade to gently raise one side of the coverslip and then grasping with forceps gives the best results.

14. Although DAPI is collected at 461 nm (blue), we pseudocolored the fluorochrome red with the software as this gave us the best indication of co-localization. Suitable software for this type of image analysis includes Metamorph or ImagePro Plus.
15. Higher concentration proteins that require lower volume should be made isovolumetric with the sample with the lowest concentration with the addition of an appropriate amount of water.
16. Antibodies used detect proteins associated with angiogenesis (VEGF, VEGFR2), cell survival (Akt, pAkt), proliferation (PCNA), and cell death (Bcl-2, Bax).
17. Following the scratch, it helps to swirl the dish a few times. This will dislodge the cells dispersed by the pipette and eliminate frayed edges that otherwise may occur.
18. It is important to image the same area of the dish every time as the width of the scratch typically varies somewhat down its length.

Acknowledgments

This work was supported by grants from the Canadian Institutes for Health Research and the Natural Sciences and Engineering Research Council of Canada. We would like to thank Michelle Ross for technical support and assistance.

References

1. Vanderhyden BC, Shaw TJ, Ethier JF (2003) Animal models of ovarian cancer. Reprod Biol Endocrinol 1:67–78
2. Nitta M, Katabuchi H, Ohtake H, Tashiro H, Yamaizumi M, Okamura H (2001) Characterization and tumorigenicity of human ovarian surface epithelial cells immortalized by SV40 large T antigen. Gynecol Oncol 81:10–17
3. Su G, Kozak KR, Imaizumi S, Gao F, Amneus MW, Grijalva V, Ng C, Wagner A, Hough G, Farias-Eisner G, Anantharamaiah GM, Van Lenten BJ, Navab M, Fogelman AM, Reddy ST, Farias-Eisner R (2010) Apolipoprotein A-I (apoA-I) and apoA-I mimetic peptides inhibit tumor development in a mouse model of ovarian cancer. Proc Natl Acad Sci USA 107:1997–20002
4. Zheng J, Mercado-Uribe I, Rosen DG, Chang B, Liu P, Yang G, Malpica A, Noara H, Auersperg N, Mills GB, Bast RC, Liu J (2010) Induction of papillary carcinoma in human ovarian surface epithelial cells using combined genetic elements and peritoneal microenvironment. Cell Cycle 9:140–146
5. Greenaway JB, Koehler A, McCulloch CA, Petrik J, Brown TJ, Ringuette MJ (2012) The impact of the ovarian microenvironment on the anti-tumor effect of SPARC on ovarian cancer. Biochem Cell Biol 90:96–107. PMID: 22003835
6. Quinn BA, Xiao F, Bickel L, Martin L, Hua X, Klein-Szanto A, Connolly DC (2010) Development of a syngeneic mouse model of epithelial ovarian cancer. J Ovarian Res 3:24–42
7. Wertel I, Nowicka A, Rogala E, Kotarski J (2011) Peritoneal immune system in patients with advanced epithelial ovarian cancer. Int Rev Immunol 30:87–101
8. Preston CC, Goode EL, Hartmann LC, Kalli KR, Knutson KL (2011) Immunity and immune suppression in human ovarian cancer. Immunotherapy 3:539–556

9. Berezhnaya NM (2010) Interaction between tumor and immune system: the role of tumor cell biology. Exp Oncol 32:159–166
10. Roby KF, Taylor CC, Sweetwood JP, Cheng Y, Pace JL, Tawfik O, Persons DL, Smith PG, Terranova PF (2000) Development of a syngeneic mouse model for events related to ovarian cancer. Carcinogenesis 21:585–591
11. Yang WL, Godwin AK, Xu XX (2004) Tumor necrosis factor-alpha-induced matrix proteolytic enzyme production and basement membrane remodeling by human ovarian surface epithelial cells: molecular basis linking ovulation and cancer risk. Cancer Res 64: 1534–1540
12. Purdie DM, Bain CJ, Siskind V, Webb PM, Green AC (2003) Ovulation and risk of epithelial ovarian cancer. Int J Cancer 104:228–232
13. Shaw TJ, Senterman MK, Dawson K, Crane CA, Vanderhyden BC (2004) Characterization of intraperitoneal, orthotopic, and metastatic xenograft models of human ovarian cancer. Mol Ther 10:1032–1042
14. Martinez-Poveda B, Gomez V, Alcaide-German M, Perruca S, Vazquez S, Alba LE, Casanovas O, Garcia-Bermejo ML, Peso L, Jimenez B (2011) Non-invasive monitoring of hypoxia-inducible factor activation by optical imaging during antiangiogenic treatment in a xenograft model of ovarian carcinoma. Int J Oncol 39:543–552
15. Greenaway J, Moorehead R, Shaw P, Petrik J (2008) Epithelial stromal interaction increases cell proliferation, survival and tumorigenicity in a mouse model of epithelial ovarian cancer. Gynecol Oncol 108:385–394
16. Woolery KT, Kruk PA (2011) Ovarian epithelial-stromal interactions: role of interleukins 1 and 6. Obstet Gynecol Int. Article ID. 358493 Epub ahead of print. PMID: 21765834.

Chapter 32

Immunocompetent Mouse Model of Ovarian Cancer for In Vivo Imaging

Selene Nunez-Cruz and Nathalie Scholler

Abstract

Syngeneic and transgenic mouse models are important tools for the study of the biology of cancer. While syngeneic mouse models are generated through the implantation in host animals of tumor cells from genetically and immunologically compatible donors, transgenic mouse models are engineered to express genetic material with oncogenic properties in predetermined location. We have developed a syngeneic mouse model of ovarian cancer permitting in vivo imaging in immunocompetent recipients by implanting ovaries with fluorescently labeled cancer cells that derived from a spontaneous ovarian tumor developing in a transgenic mouse model. Tumor cells were retrovirally transduced with a far-red fluorescent protein. This animal model combines the advantages of syngeneic and transgenic mouse models as it permits to both monitor tumor growth by in vivo imaging and to analyze the tumor microenvironment of an immunocompetent host.

Key words Transgene, Syngeneic, Katushka, Orthotopic, In vivo imaging, Ovarian cancer

1 Introduction

In vivo models of ovarian cancer are required to study cancer progression and to evaluate anticancer therapies. As mice do not spontaneously develop epithelial ovarian cancer (EOC), two main types of EOC mouse models have been developed, syngeneic by implantation of mouse ovarian cells immortalized in vitro [1] and transgenic through genetic engineering. EOC syngeneic mouse models were first established by implanting the ID8 mouse ovarian surface epithelial cell line (MOSEC) in various localizations, including subcutaneous, intraperitoneal [1], or orthotopic [2]. Recipient animals can be immune competent or immune compromised but must be of the same genetic background that of the implanted tumor cell line. Alternatively, transgenic mouse models of ovarian cancer are engineered to spontaneously develop tumor. The model developed by Connolly and colleagues permits the expression of the simian virus 40 tumor antigen (SV40 TAg) by the reproductive

Anastasia Malek and Oleg Tchernitsa (eds.), *Ovarian Cancer: Methods and Protocols*, Methods in Molecular Biology, vol. 1049, DOI 10.1007/978-1-62703-547-7_32, © Springer Science+Business Media New York 2013

tract, under the control of the Müllerian-inhibiting substance type II receptor (MISIIR) promoter [3]. Consequently, female mice transgenic for MISIIR (Tg *MISIIR*-TAg *DR26*) develop bilateral ovarian tumors with 100 % penetrance by 5–6 months of age [3]; transgenic mice are tolerant to SV40 tumor antigen but their immune response is otherwise normal and thus permits the study of the tumor microenvironment. However, monitoring ovarian tumor progression in this model is challenging due to the location of ovarian tumors deep inside the peritoneal cavity.

In vivo imaging technologies available for detection of ovarian cancer in live mice include ultrasonography, magnetic resonance imaging (MRI), micro-positron emission tomography (micro-PET) and computed tomography (CT) for spontaneous tumors, and, for tumors engineered with light-emitting reporter such as firefly luciferase or green fluorescent protein (GFP), bioluminescent imaging (BLI) or fluorescent imaging (FLI) [4]. Efficient visualization for internal tumor growth can be further improved by the use of dyes or proteins with emission spectra in the far-red wavelengths.

The present protocol describes the use of a model of ovarian cancer combining transgenic and syngeneic mice to follow ovarian cancer development by in vivo imaging in the context of an immune competent tumor microenvironment. This model utilizes the ovarian cancer cell line (MOV1) isolated from an ovarian tumor of a 26-week-old Tg *MISIIR*-TAg *DR26* mouse. MOV1 cells were retrovirally transduced with TurboFP635 Lentivirus mammalian vector that encodes the far-red fluorescent protein Katushka ($MOV1^{KAT}$) [5]. Katushka is a far-red fluorescent protein from the sea anemone *Entacmaea quadricolor* with emission spectra in the far-red wavelengths (excitation/emission maxima at 588/635 nm). Katushka's optical property, fast maturation, high pH stability, and photostability are favorable for deep imaging of animal tissues [6]. To further mimic ovarian cancer process, $MOV1^{KAT}$ cells were orthotopically implanted in the ovaries of mice also transgenic for *MISIIR*-TAg but issued from a strain that is not susceptible to cancer development [7]. Within 3 weeks following implantation, non-tumor-prone transgenic mice developed fluorescently labeled ovarian tumors that could be visualized by in vivo imaging and that were infiltrated with leukocytes. This novel syngeneic mouse model for ovarian cancer thus permits in vivo imaging and enables preclinical studies of the tumor microenvironment and tumor immune responses [5].

Similar systems can be created using different mouse strains. While it is likely that $MOV1^{KAT}$ cells will be rejected from mice of different background and/or non-transgenic for MISIIR, the model system described here can be implemented in other mouse strains. In fact, most mouse ovarian surface epithelial cells (MOSEC) can be immortalized in vitro by repeated passages and then selected in vivo for their tumor forming potential as first described by Roby et al. [1]. Thus, the system described here can be reproduced following these four steps: (1) in vitro and in vivo selections of an immortalized mouse ovarian cell line with tumorigenic properties, (2) transfection of the immortalized cell line with a marker for in vivo imaging, (3) orthotopic implantation into syngeneic mice (Subheadings 3.1–3.3), and (4) in vivo imaging (Subheading 3.4).

2 Materials

2.1 Cell Culture

Prepare all solutions in sterile conditions under a laminar/vertical hood, using deionized, ultrapure water dH2O2 (18 MΩ cm at 25 °C) and tissue culture grade reagents. All reagents and solutions must be sterile. Unless otherwise indicated, store reagents at room temperature.

1. MOV1^{KAT} cells (*see* **Note 1**).
2. Dulbecco's Modified Eagles Media (DMEM).
3. DMEM complete medium. Supplement Dulbecco's Modified Eagles Media (DMEM) with 10 % fetal bovine serum (FBS) and 1 % antibiotic/antimycotic. Store at 4 °C.
4. Phosphate-buffered saline buffer (PBS), ×1, sterile, Ca/Mg free.
5. PBS buffer with 0.002 M EDTA.
6. Trypsin–EDTA solutions: 0.05 % trypsin/0.53 mM EDTA. Store at 4 °C.
7. Baked Pasteur pipettes.
8. Tissue culture flasks T175.

2.2 Mouse Model

1. Tumor recipient: non-tumor prone mice of same background as the implanted tumor cells. Here we use non-tumor prone Tg MISIIR-TAg mice (*see* **Note 2**).

2.3 Material for Survival Surgery and In Vivo Imaging

1. Heating pad.
2. Isoflurane vaporizer.
3. Oxygen gas tank.
4. F/air carbon filters.
5. Nose cone-tubing system.
6. Hair removal cream.
7. Eye ointment.
8. Rodent clippers.
9. Insulin syringe 3/10, 5/10, and 1 cc U-100.

10. Sterile surgical instruments.
11. Plain Gut Absorbable suture.
12. Tissue adhesive.
13. Cotton-tipped applicators.
14. Cotton swabs (alcohol, povidone–iodine).
15. Isoflurane.
16. Ketoprofen.
17. Enrofloxacin (Baytril).
18. Trimethoprim–sulfamethoxazole (Bactrim) (*see* **Note 3**).
19. IVIS Spectrum Instrument.
20. Fisher Scientific 500 g scale.
21. 70 % ethanol.
22. Clidox.
23. KimWipes.
24. Paper towels.

3 Methods

3.1 Cell Culture

1. Culture MOV1^{KAT} cells in a T175 flask with DMEM complete medium until they reach 90 % confluence (*see* **Note 4**).
2. Bring PBS, trypsin–EDTA, and DMEM medium at room temperature before preparing the cells for injection (*see* **Note 5**).
3. Aspirate medium from the flasks containing the growing MOV1^{KAT} cells with a Pasteur pipette without disturbing the monolayer of MOV1^{KAT} cells.
4. Add 10 ml of PBS per flask.
5. Swirl PBS over the MOV1^{KAT} cells and aspirate with a Pasteur pipette without disturbing the cell monolayer.
6. Add 4 ml of trypsin–EDTA solution per flask.
7. Incubate the flask in a horizontal position for 3 min at 37 °C.
8. Add 10 ml of DMEM per flask (*see* **Note 6**).
9. Determine the cell number using a hemocytometer.
10. Once the cell concentration has been determined, pellet the cells by centrifugation for 5 min at $300 \times g$ at room temperature.
11. Gently resuspend the cells in an eppendorf tube with sterile PBS supplemented with 0.002 M EDTA to the concentration of 1×10^6 cells in 10 μl (*see* **Note 7**).

3.2 Presurgery

Appropriate preoperative and postoperative care of animals in accordance with established veterinary medical and nursing practices is required.

1. Place the mice in an isoflurane chamber connected to an isoflurane vaporizer. Turn ON the oxygen and the isoflurane level to 2 %.
2. Wait for 2 min before transferring the animal to the heating pad.
3. Add eye ointment to prevent eye dehydration.
4. Transfer an isoflurane-anesthetized mouse to a heating pad previously placed in a biosafety cabinet. Position the animal with the dorsolateral side to operate towards the operator.
5. Immediately insert the animal head into a nose cone system connected to the isoflurane vaporizer to deliver anesthesia throughout the surgery.
6. Disinfect the injection site with alcohol swabs.
7. Subcutaneously inject 5 mg/kg of Ketoprofen analgesic.
8. Shave the left caudal portion of the dorsum from the thoracolumbar junction to the base of the animal tail with rodent clippers.
9. Dab the clipped area with a piece of adhesive tape or moistened gauze to pick up loose hair that could otherwise migrate into the incision.
10. Apply hair removal cream for 1 min to completely remove hair (*see* **Note 8**).
11. Remove excess of hair and cream with a moistened gauze.
12. Sterilize the shaved area with povidone–iodine and alcohol swabs.
13. Place a sterile surgical drape to cover the animal body and expose the area of incision only.
14. Prior to surgery, fill up a 3/10 cc G31 insulin syringe with $MOV1^{KAT}$ cells at a concentration of 1×10^6 in 10 μl of PBS supplemented with 0.002 M EDTA.
15. Fill up a 5/10 cc insulin syringe with PBS.
16. Place all sterile surgical instruments and cotton swabs near the surgical site.

3.3 Surgery

Knowledge in mouse anatomy and experience in mouse surgery are required before performing any survival surgery. All survival surgery must be performed with aseptic procedures, including sterile gloves, masks, sterile instruments, and aseptic techniques. A dedicated surgical facility is not required for housing rodents, but surgery must be performed using aseptic techniques. Research personnel must be appropriately qualified and trained in all procedures to ensure correct surgical technique [8] (*see* **Note 9**).

1. Just before surgery, adjust the isoflurane vaporizer levels to 1.5 %.
2. Verify that the animal is completely anesthetized by pinching the foot pad (*see* **Note 10**).
3. Locate the spleen under the skin (*see* **Note 11**) and using surgical scissors make a dorsolateral incision of 1–2 cm long on the top right of the spleen.
4. Dissect the retroperitoneum with the surgical scissors. The fat pad surrounding mouse ovary will be observed (*see* **Note 12**).
5. Use curved forceps to grasp and expose the fat pad surrounding the mouse ovary.
6. Hydrate the organ with 2–4 drops of sterile PBS. Clean the excess of PBS dropped on the skin with a sterile cotton-tipped applicator.
7. Use curved forceps to grasp, retract, and position the ovary for injection.
8. While firmly grasping the ovary with the forceps, slowly inject 10 μl of $MOV1^{KAT}$ tumor cell suspension in the ovary (*see* **Note 13**).
9. A firm grasp will prevent fluid regurgitation or leakage.
10. Immediately following injection, release the tension exerted by the forceps. The perforation in the ovary should spontaneously retract and close.
11. Using a Plain Gut Absorbable suture attached to a needle, close the retroperitoneum wound.
12. Release the animal from the nose cone.
13. Stretch the skin and seal the dorsolateral wound edges with few drops of tissue adhesive.
14. The animal should wake up from anesthesia within 2–5 min.
15. To prevent infection, administer antibiotics (Bactrim) at 200 mg/kg. Supplement the drinking water with enrofloxacin (Baytril) at 200 mg/ml (*see* **Note 14**).
16. Place back the mouse in its cage and monitor for recovery (*see* **Note 15**).

3.4 In Vivo Imaging

This procedure can be performed at least 1 week after the orthotopic injection of tumor cells. The protocol is adopted to use the IVIS Lumina system (Xenogen). However, any similar equipment with appropriate software can be applied as well.

1. Transfer the mice in an isoflurane chamber connected to the isoflurane vaporizer and the IVIS Spectrum Instrument as described in presurgical section.
2. Turn ON the oxygen and the isoflurane level to 2 %. Monitor the mice for anesthesia.

3. Once mice are anesthetized, turn isoflurane chamber flow OFF and imaging chamber flow ON.
4. Transfer mice to imaging chamber.
5. Perform in vivo imaging according to the imaging system manufacturer's instructions. We routinely used the IVIS Lumina system (Xenogen).
6. To image, click the Living Image software desktop icon. Select "Initialize" on the IVIS Acquisition Control Panel. The instrument settings are analogous to camera settings.
7. On the Acquisition Control Panel, set up the instrument's acquisition parameters. For fluorescence, check "Fluorescent."
8. Click the Photograph box to acquire a photograph with each image.
9. Set the exposure time as Auto.
10. Under "Pixel binning or CCD resolution," check "Medium."
11. Under F/stop or aperture, check the value of 2.
12. Select the 535 excitation filter and the DsRed emission filter.
13. Under field of view, click on View B to image a single mouse.
14. Click on acquire to begin the image acquisition.
15. Once the image acquisition is complete, use the Region of Interest (ROI) tool to measure the signal. Click on the measurement icon to release the signal values and area.
16. Click on "save" to save the image in the user folder.
17. Turn imaging chamber flow OFF. Stop the administration of isoflurane and return the mouse to its cage.
18. The mouse should wake up immediately.
19. Using this protocol, the growth of an orthotopic ovarian cancer can be monitored in vivo for at least 3 weeks (*see* **Note 16** and Fig. 1).

4 Notes

1. MOV1^{KAT} is ovarian cancer cell line isolated from an ovarian tumor of Tg *MISIIR*-TAg *DR26* mouse and stably transduced with TurboFP635 Lentivirus mammalian vector that encodes Katushka, a far-red mutant of the red fluorescent protein from sea anemone Entacmaea quadricolor with excitation/emission maxima at 588/635 nm.
2. Non-tumor-prone Tg *MISIIR*-TAg mice were produced by the introduction of *MISIIR*-TAg construct into pronuclei of the first generation of a hybrid genetic background of C57BL/6 and C3H mice [7].

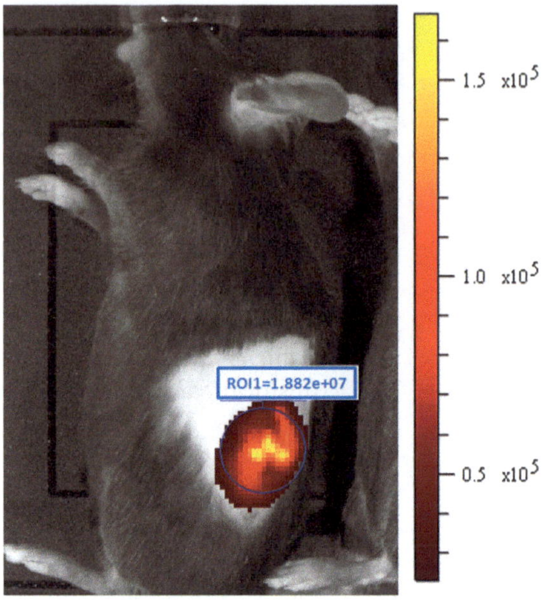

Fig. 1 In vivo imaging of orthotopic MOV1^{KAT} tumor. MOV1^{KAT} cells were orthotopically implanted into the ovary of a non-tumor-prone MISIIR-TAg mouse. In vivo imaging was performed 2 weeks later. The fluorescence emission generated by MOV1^{KAT} cells engrafted in the ovary produced a total signal of 1.882×10^7 over an area of 19 mm^2. Radian efficiency = (p/s/cm^2/sr)/(μW/cm^2). Color scale Min = 2.28e4, Max + 1.67e5

3. Antibiotic (Bactrim) administration in the drinking water is continued for 1 week.
4. MOV1^{KAT} cells are adherent and grow in monolayer. A T175 flask of MOV1^{KAT} cells at 90 % confluence yields 0.5–0.7 million cells.
5. Use one million cells per orthotopic implantation, which will require 1–2 T175 flasks at 90 % confluence.
6. The use of DMEM supplemented with 10 % (v/v) FBS and penicillin/streptomycin 1 % after trypsin–EDTA step increases cell viability before injection.
7. Keep the cells at 4 °C or in ice before injection to reduce clumps formation and cell mortality.
8. Rodent skin is very fragile. Add the hair removal cream for less than 4 min to avoid skin burn.
9. All animal procedures must to be in accordance with the Institutional Animal Care and Use Committee and conducted according to guidelines of the National Institutes of Health.
10. Anesthetized animals must be monitored through the procedure to insure they stay in the proper anesthetic plane. Frequently monitor respiratory pattern and frequency, mucous

membranes, and exposed tissues to keep track of anesthetic depth and potential complications.

11. Spleen is located on the left flank of the animal and can be easily visualized after cleaning the skin area with alcohol. The ovary is located next to the spleen. Make an incision on top right of the spleen to visualize the ovarian fat pad surrounding the ovary.
12. The mouse ovary is surrounded by a white fat pad. Due to its pale color, it could be confounded with the intestines but its texture is softer. In some cases, the ovary can be found embedded in the fat pad and thus may be difficult to observe. The pink–yellow color of the ovary should help its localization.
13. Ovaries are extremely small (2 mm) and no more than 20 μl can be injected to the organ. To inject the cancer cells, the syringe should be grabbed with the needle bevel faced up and the liquid should be pushed out slowly. Practice is required to successfully perform this procedure.
14. Keep the animal on antibiotics in the drinking water for 1 week.
15. Postoperative care includes monitoring the animal for several days after the surgical procedure to prevent development of postsurgical complications and provide analgesics if needed.
16. Katushka fluorescence can be visualized up to 5 weeks post injection of $MOV1^{KAT}$ cells. However, in our experience Katushka fluorescence is reduced after 6 weeks even when the tumor continues to grow. This method is thus most effective to visualize proper injection of tumor cells at the organ site and tumor growth at early stages.

References

1. Roby KF, Taylor CC, Sweetwood JP, Cheng Y, Pace JL, Tawfik O, Persons DL, Smith PG, Terranova PF (2000) Development of a syngeneic mouse model for events related to ovarian cancer. Carcinogenesis 21(4):585–591
2. Greenaway J, Moorehead R, Shaw P, Petrik J (2008) Epithelial-stromal interaction increases cell proliferation, survival and tumorigenicity in a mouse model of human epithelial ovarian cancer. Gynecol Oncol 108(2):385–394
3. Connolly DC, Bao R, Nikitin AY, Stephens KC, Poole TW, Hua X, Harris SS, Vanderhyden BC, Hamilton TC (2003) Female mice chimeric for expression of the simian virus 40 TAg under control of the MISIIR promoter develop epithelial ovarian cancer. Cancer Res 63(6): 1389–1397
4. Connolly DC, Hensley HH (2009) Xenograft and transgenic mouse models of epithelial ovarian cancer and non invasive imaging modalities to monitor ovarian tumor growth in situ – applications in evaluating novel therapeutic agents. Curr Protoc Pharmacol 45:14.12.11–14.12.26
5. NunezCruz S, Connolly DC, Scholler N (2010) An orthotopic model of serous ovarian cancer in immunocompetent mice for in vivo tumor imaging and monitoring of tumor immune responses. J Vis Exp 45:pii 2146
6. Shcherbo D, Merzlyak EM, Chepurnykh TV, Fradkov AF, Ermakova GV, Solovieva EA, Lukyanov KA, Bogdanova EA, Zaraisky AG, Lukyanov S, Chudakov DM (2007) Bright far-red fluorescent protein for whole-body imaging. Nat Methods 4(9):741–746
7. Quinn BA, Xiao F, Bickel L, Martin L, Hua X, Klein-Szanto A, Connolly DC (2010) Development of a syngeneic mouse model of epithelial ovarian cancer. J Ovarian Res 3:24
8. Gonder JC, Laber K (2007) A renewed look at laboratory rodent housing and management. ILAR J 48(1):29–36

Part VII

Non-Viral Drug Delivery System for Ovarian Cancer Therapy

Chapter 33

Drug Delivery Approaches for Ovarian Cancer Therapy

Anastasia Malek

Abstract

Tumor-specific drug delivery represents a challenging issue that restricts the clinical applications of many advanced anticancer therapeutics. Ovarian cancer exhibits a quite specific pattern of dissemination: it spreads primarily within the peritoneal cavity, providing a possibility of locoregional, intraperitoneal drug administration. Considering this unique aspect of ovarian cancer biology, this chapter provides a short review of most promising approaches for therapeutic delivery of genetic drugs.

Key words Ovarian cancer, Intraperitoneal therapy, Ovarian cancer-specific ligand, Polymers, Liposomes, Exosomes

1 Drug Delivery Approaches for Cancer Therapy

Cancer could become a treatable disease if a method for tumor-specific delivery of cytostatic agents is discovered. Research in the field of controlled directed drug delivery is essential for improving therapeutic outcomes for patients with solid tumors and has become more intensive in recent years. Due to recent advantages in conjugation chemistry and nanotechnology, simply understanding the classification of emerging drug delivery approaches has became a challenge. Drugs can be structurally organized into drug-carrier complexes as follows: (1) coupled/conjugated with carrier molecules, such as peptides, lipids, aptamers, or antibodies at specific molecular ratios; (2) mixed with lipids or polymers to form self-assembling multimolecular complexes at a nanoscale size; (3) attached/absorbed to the surface of synthetic nanomaterials, such as carbon nanotubes, quantum dots, or dendrimers; and (4) entrapped in complex formulations with meso-porous materials, such as metal-organic frameworks or silica-based substances. Passive and active targeting strategies can be distinguished in tumor-tissue achievement. Passive tumor targeting is based on hyperpermeability of the vasculature and immature lymph drainage systems in tumors (the enhanced permeation and retention

Anastasia Malek and Oleg Tchernitsa (eds.), *Ovarian Cancer: Methods and Protocols*, Methods in Molecular Biology, vol. 1049,
DOI 10.1007/978-1-62703-547-7_33, © Springer Science+Business Media New York 2013

effect or EPR) and assumes prolonged blood circulation of the drug. Tumor-specific antibodies and various types of ligands to tumor-specific surface molecules are being explored for active tumor-targeting drug delivery. Particular classes contain stimuli-sensitive carriers that release their cargo upon exposure to appropriate external impacts, such as high temperatures, low pH, or magnetic fields. Other factors, including biocompatibility, mode of biodegradation, clearance, and immune system involvement, are being considered in the development of new drug delivery approaches. There are several recent systematic reviews that describe state-of-the-art drug delivery research [1–3].

2 Intraperitoneal Drug Administration

We have highlighted methods that can be efficiently applied to treat ovarian cancer with a primarily peritoneal route of dissemination. The mechanisms involved in peritoneal metastasis and metastases morphology are distinct from the mechanisms involved in hematological routes of tumor spread [4]. The specificity of local therapeutic intervention can be defined in terms of particular pharmacokinetics, toxicity issues, dosage, and regime [5]. There is evidence that intraperitoneal drug administration is advantageous in patients with tumors that are confined to the peritoneal cavity. Several large randomized trials of conventional cytostatic agents in patients with stage III ovarian cancer who underwent optimal cytoreduction demonstrated a significant survival benefit when intraperitoneal chemotherapy was added to systemic therapy [6]. The efficacy of intraperitoneal therapy in ovarian cancer may be further improved through development of new drug delivery systems that explore the anatomical features of the peritoneal cavity, functional properties of the peritoneal-plasma barrier, cellular and subcellular ascitic fluids, molecular composition of the surface of peritoneal metastases, characteristics of multicellular conglomerates (spheroids) suspended in ascitic fluid, and many other site-specific factors [7].

3 Polymer- and Lipid-Based Delivery Systems

Regarding gene therapeutic approaches, the two main carrier systems include viral vectors and nonviral delivery systems. Viral vectors, including retroviruses, adenoviruses, and adeno-associated viruses, have a high efficiency of gene delivery [8]. Although laborious production and serious safety risks of viral vectors have become apparent in recent years, their utility is being reappraised. Nonviral delivery systems are generally less effective compared to viruses, although their preparation and application are more reproducible and better controlled. Various types of lipids and polymers (natural or synthetic) are utilized as vehicles for genetic drugs. The nanoscale complexes that form with nucleic acids (NA) are defined as "lipoplexes" or "polyplexes" and constitute promising alternatives to viral vectors in gene therapy. Interactions between the vectors and NA leading to nano-complex formation, the supramolecular structures of lipoplexes and polyplexes, and mechanisms of NA transfer are reviewed in the literature [9]. Properties including range of NA condensation and protection, size, shape regularity, surface charge, stability of the complexes, and efficiency of intracellular NA release define the efficiency and safety of nonviral vectors. Advanced strategies to employ both lipids and polymers to achieve optimal characteristics have been explored in recent studies [10]. The efficiency of nano-complexes as NA carriers is defined by the ability to penetrate the cellular membrane, although this property is associated with cytotoxicity. The cytotoxicity of polymer- and lipid-based delivery systems appears to be a major limiting factor to systemic intravenous application [11]. In the context of ovarian cancer therapy, a considerable reduction in the dose of nano-complexes in the bloodstream while maintaining a high local drug concentration may be achieved through intraperitoneal administration. Different doses of siRNA complexed with the cationic polymer PEI (polyethylenimine) applicable for i.p. and i.v. are described in Chapter 34, while relevant toxicological data have been previously published [12]. Intraperitoneal application of siRNA formulated with the neutral lipid DOPC (1,2-dioleoyl-*sn-glycero*-3-phosphatidylcholine) was explored in another study and resulted in significant modulation of the target gene and antitumor effects in preclinical models of peritoneally distributed ovarian cancer [13].

4 Multistage Nano-vectors

The transfection efficacy of polymer- and lipid-based NA complexes is defined by the ability to attach and penetrate the cell surface membrane as a result of their nanoscale size and positive surface charge. The same property mediates toxicity and rapid clearance from physiological fluids. The "therapeutic window" for this type of drug is between a dose that is high enough to provide a sufficient range of NA transfection and low enough to result in acceptable toxic effects. Because this therapeutic window is quite narrow, sustained drug administration appears to play a critical role.

The concept of multistage nano-vectors introduced in 2008 [14] was aimed to achieve both efficient drug transfection and sustained release of transfection complexes close to the target lesion. These vectors are comprised of two distinct nano-elements or "stages." First-stage meso-porous silicon particles are designed to protect, safely deliver, and optimally distribute drug cargo within the body, and second-stage nanoparticles are embedded within the porous structure and can penetrate the tissues and introduce drug cargo in the target cells after release. To yield precise control of the characteristics of first-stage particles (e.g., size, shape, morphology, and surface charge), they are produced using semiconductor fabrication techniques, including photolithography and electrochemical etching [15]. The kinetics of second-stage nanoparticle release is defined by morphology and the degradation rate of the first-stage vehicles. Multistage nano-vector systems can be adjusted to deliver various types of agents, including cytostatics, metal nanoparticles, imaging agents, and NA-containing transfection complexes [16]. The efficacy of meso-porous silicon particles loaded with siRNA-DOPC (dioleoyl phosphatidylcholine) nano-liposomes was evaluated in orthotopic models of ovarian cancer following 3 weeks of sustained target gene silencing after a single i.v. injection [17]. The methods used to prepare the multistage vectors used in this study are included in Chapter 36. However, further investigation is required to estimate whether multistage vectors can be efficiently applied in intraperitoneal therapy and whether this route of administration improves the therapeutic effect.

5 Natural Transport Pathways as Drug Delivery Systems

In parallel to developing comprehensive and highly technological drug delivery systems, analysis of natural transport pathways implicated in molecular turnover across body compartments may provide promising solutions. For example, high-density lipoproteins are a class of native multimolecular complexes that enable lipids, such as cholesterol and triglycerides, to be transported within the bloodstream. In addition to lipid cargo, HDLs contain multiple specific proteins with structural, receptor, and transmembrane transport functions and signalling lipids and microRNA that maintain complex and highly regulated lipid turnover. The function of HDL is mediated by enzymes that alter its structure and composition and cellular receptors that guide transport and facilitate loading of the lipid cargo. Various advanced strategies to utilize HDL are discussed in literature [18]. One of these approaches is to modulate the natural homing of HDL nanoparticles to cholesterol-recipient cells and redirect to target tissues. Scavenger receptor class B member 1 (SR-BI) expressed on the surface of numerous tissues normally mediates the homing of HDL particles and facilitates uptake of cholesterol via interaction with apolipoprotein A-I, the major protein component in HDL complexes. Conjugation of cancer-specific ligands with the ApoA-I protein can abolish its natural binding capacity and redirect modified HDLs to cancer cells. Rerouting HDL particles from SR-BI receptors to folic acid receptors that are frequently overexpressed in ovarian cancer cells provides a biomimetic system that enables ovarian cancer-directed drug delivery (Chapter 35). Therapeutic siRNA delivery by conjugation with native lipids circulating in the bloodstream has been explored in other studies [19–21]. Considering the list of ovarian cancer-specific surface molecules and opportunities for intraperitoneal administration of HDL-based siRNA-loaded nanoparticles, the described approach appears to be very attractive.

Membranous microvesicles, or "exosomes," are another native system of intercellular communication [22] that have emerged as promising drug delivery vehicles in recent years. These secreted particles are 30–200 nm in diameter, are delimited by a lipid bilayer, and contain a wide range of membrane-bound or free proteins and nucleic acids (mRNA and miRNA, in particular). The exact biological functions of exosomes are still being investigated, although their role in intercellular signalling and exchange of regulatory miRNA has been established [23]. Implication of exosomes in the development of various diseases and cancer progression has been discussed in the literature [24, 25]. Recent studies have successfully shown that exosomes isolated from cultured cells can be loaded with siRNA and applied in experimental gene silencing therapy in vitro and in vivo [26, 27]. In the context of ovarian cancer, extracting exosomes from the ascitic fluid of patients is a possibility [28]. Moreover, the release and uptake of exosomes by cultured SKOV3 cells was recently observed [29], confirming the role of micro-vesicular communication in ovarian cancer. These data suggest the theoretic possibility of obtaining exosomes from the ascitic fluid of patients for use as auto-vehicles for drug administration with minimal toxic or immune side effects. Chapter 37 presents methods of exosome isolation, labelling, and purification followed by in vitro exosome internalization assays that provide a basis for further exploration as a drug delivery approach.

References

1. Sultana S, Khan MR, Kumar M, Kumar S, Ali M (2013) Nanoparticles-mediated drug delivery approaches for cancer targeting: a review. J Drug Target 21(2):107–125. doi:10.3109/1061186X.2012.712130
2. Diou O, Tsapis N, Fattal E (2012) Targeted nanotheranostics for personalized cancer therapy. Expert Opin Drug Deliv 9:1475–1487
3. Hirsjarvi S, Passirani C, Benoit JP (2011) Passive and active tumour targeting with nanocarriers. Curr Drug Discov Technol 8:188–196
4. Sodek KL, Murphy KJ, Brown TJ, Ringuette MJ (2012) Cell–cell and cell-matrix dynamics in intraperitoneal cancer metastasis. Cancer Metastasis Rev 31:397–414
5. Hasovits C, Clarke S (2012) Pharmacokinetics and pharmacodynamics of intraperitoneal cancer chemotherapeutics. Clin Pharmacokinet 51:203–224
6. Ceelen WP, Flessner MF (2010) Intraperitoneal therapy for peritoneal tumors: biophysics and clinical evidence. Nat Rev Clin Oncol 7:108–115
7. Zahedi P, Yoganathan R, Piquette-Miller M, Allen C (2012) Recent advances in drug delivery strategies for treatment of ovarian cancer. Expert Opin Drug Deliv 9:567–583

8. Kanerva A, Raki M, Hemminki A (2007) Gene therapy of gynaecological diseases. Expert Opin Biol Ther 7:1347–1361
9. Tros de Ilarduya C, Sun Y, Duzgunes N (2010) Gene delivery by lipoplexes and polyplexes. Eur J Pharm Sci 40:159–170
10. Garcia L, Urbiola K, Duzgunes N, Tros de Ilarduya C (2012) Lipopolyplexes as nanomedicines for therapeutic gene delivery. Methods Enzymol 509:327–338
11. Malek A, Merkel O, Fink L, Czubayko F, Kissel T et al (2009) In vivo pharmacokinetics, tissue distribution and underlying mechanisms of various PEI(-PEG)/siRNA complexes. Toxicol Appl Pharmacol 236:97–108
12. Hobel S, Koburger I, John M, Czubayko F, Hadwiger P et al (2010) Polyethylenimine/small interfering RNA-mediated knockdown of vascular endothelial growth factor in vivo exerts anti-tumor effects synergistically with Bevacizumab. J Gene Med 12:287–300
13. Mangala LS, Han HD, Lopez-Berestein G, Sood AK (2009) Liposomal siRNA for ovarian cancer. Methods Mol Biol 555:29–42
14. Tasciotti E, Liu X, Bhavane R, Plant K, Leonard AD et al (2008) Mesoporous silicon particles as a multistage delivery system for imaging and therapeutic applications. Nat Nanotechnol 3:151–157
15. Chiappini C, Tasciotti E, Fakhoury JR, Fine D, Pullan L et al (2010) Tailored porous silicon microparticles: fabrication and properties. Chemphyschem 11:1029–1035
16. Godin B, Tasciotti E, Liu X, Serda RE, Ferrari M (2011) Multistage nanovectors: from concept to novel imaging contrast agents and therapeutics. Acc Chem Res 44:979–989
17. Tanaka T, Mangala LS, Vivas-Mejia PE, Nieves-Alicea R, Mann AP et al (2010) Sustained small interfering RNA delivery by mesoporous silicon particles. Cancer Res 70:3687–3696
18. Liu X, Suo R, Xiong SL, Zhang QH, Yi GH (2012) HDL drug carriers for targeted therapy. Clin Chim Acta 415C:94–100
19. Shahzad MM, Mangala LS, Han HD, Lu C, Bottsford-Miller J et al (2011) Targeted delivery of small interfering RNA using reconstituted high-density lipoprotein nanoparticles. Neoplasia 13:309–319
20. Nakayama T, Butler JS, Sehgal A, Severgnini M, Racie T et al (2012) Harnessing a physiologic mechanism for siRNA delivery with mimetic lipoprotein particles. Mol Ther 20:1582–1589
21. Ding Y, Wang W, Feng M, Wang Y, Zhou J et al (2012) A biomimetic nanovector-mediated targeted cholesterol-conjugated siRNA delivery for tumor gene therapy. Biomaterials 33:8893–8905
22. Bang C, Thum T (2012) Exosomes: new players in cell–cell communication. Int J Biochem Cell Biol 44:2060–2064
23. Vickers KC, Remaley AT (2012) Lipid-based carriers of microRNAs and intercellular communication. Curr Opin Lipidol 23:91–97
24. Ohno S, Ishikawa A, Kuroda M (2013) Roles of exosomes and microvesicles in disease pathogenesis. Adv Drug Deliv Rev 65(3):398–401. doi:10.1016/j.addr.2012.07.019
25. Martins VR, Dias MS, Hainaut P (2013) Tumor-cell-derived microvesicles as carriers of molecular information in cancer. Curr Opin Oncol 25(1):66–75. doi:10.1097/CCO.0b013e32835b7c81
26. El-Andaloussi S, Lee Y, Lakhal-Littleton S, Li J, Seow Y et al (2012) Exosome-mediated delivery of siRNA in vitro and in vivo. Nat Protoc 7:2112–2126
27. El Andaloussi S, Lakhal S, Mager I, Wood MJ (2013) Exosomes for targeted siRNA delivery across biological barriers. Adv Drug Deliv Rev 65(3):391–397. doi: 10.1016/j.addr.2012.08.008
28. Peng P, Yan Y, Keng S (2011) Exosomes in the ascites of ovarian cancer patients: origin and effects on anti-tumor immunity. Oncol Rep 25:749–762
29. Escrevente C, Keller S, Altevogt P, Costa J (2011) Interaction and uptake of exosomes by ovarian cancer cells. BMC Cancer 11:108

Chapter 34

Polymer-Based Delivery of RNA-Based Therapeutics in Ovarian Cancer

Ulrike Weirauch, Daniela Gutsch, Sabrina Höbel, and Achim Aigner

Abstract

RNA interference (RNAi) is a naturally occurring, powerful mechanism for gene silencing, based on the cleavage of a given target mRNA. It relies on small interfering RNAs (siRNAs) in the cell. Being similar in structure, microRNAs (miRNAs) are important regulators of gene expression which mainly act by blocking mRNA translation. In cancer, certain miRNAs have been found to be pathologically downregulated. The therapeutic application of siRNAs or miRNAs for the induction of RNAi or miRNA replacement, respectively, relies on their efficient delivery through a non-viral formulation. Complexation of siRNAs/miRNAs in polymeric nanoparticles based on polyethylenimines (PEIs) offers protection against degradation, delivery to the target site, cellular uptake, and intracellular release. This chapter provides protocols for therapeutic gene silencing and miRNA replacement therapy, based on PEI complexes for in vitro and in vivo use.

Key words RNAi, miRNA, siRNA, Polyethylenimine, PEI, Gene knockdown, miRNA replacement therapy, Nanoparticles

1 Introduction

RNA interference (RNAi) relies on the action of small interfering RNAs, siRNAs, which are incorporated into the so-called RNA-induced silencing complex (RISC). The specific binding of the siRNA to its target mRNA, based on Watson–Crick base pairing, leads to target mRNA cleavage due to the nuclease activity of RISC. The mRNA is then rapidly degraded and thus unavailable for translation [1]. To explore RNAi for the knockdown of a given target gene, however, siRNAs can be directly delivered into the cell. An alternative is the transfection of expression vectors which encode for longer double-stranded RNAs (small hairpin RNAs, shRNA), serving as Dicer substrate for cellular siRNA production [2]. Importantly, all other components of the RNAi machinery are provided by the cell, and thus the delivery of siRNAs or shRNA-encoding vectors is necessary and sufficient for the induction of

Anastasia Malek and Oleg Tchernitsa (eds.), *Ovarian Cancer: Methods and Protocols*, Methods in Molecular Biology, vol. 1049, DOI 10.1007/978-1-62703-547-7_34, © Springer Science+Business Media New York 2013

RNAi. However, due to poor pharmacokinetic properties, this represents a major bottleneck in the use of RNAi, especially in vivo with regard to therapeutic applications [3–5].

More recently, microRNAs (miRNAs) have been recognized as important regulators of gene expression [6]. Comparable to siRNAs, they are incorporated into RISC but act based on an imperfect base pairing with their target mRNA(s). This leads to blocking of mRNA translation or to mRNA cleavage. While miRNAs may exert milder effects with regard to the inhibition of a single target gene, a given miRNA may well inhibit multiple target genes. Several miRNAs have been recognized as up- or downregulated in tumors including ovarian carcinoma and have been identified as disease relevant [7, 8]. While miRNA overexpression can be addressed by the introduction of miRNA inhibitors like antimiRs, a very promising approach for restoring aberrantly low levels of a given miRNA is its reintroduction [9]. Thus, this so-called miRNA replacement therapy aims at restoring the physiological state of a diseased cell, making this approach a very promising strategy for therapeutic intervention.

The delivery of nucleic acids represents a major challenge for their application, particularly in the in vivo situation. Due to their marked instability, this is especially true for RNA molecules. Gene delivery can be achieved by viral or by non-viral vectors. Viruses come with certain issues including potential safety problems due to the induction of toxic immune responses, the application of recombinant DNA, the risk of its random integration in the host genome, and a possible oversaturation of the RISC machinery in the case of shRNA expression vectors [10]. Consequently, despite lower efficacies, non-viral approaches offer advantages. The delivery of RNA molecules like siRNAs or miRNAs exclusively relies on non-viral systems [4, 11].

Strategies for the non-viral delivery of nucleic acids include their chemical modification and/or coupling to peptides, lipids, aptamers or antibodies, their encapsulation in lipids, or the formation of liposomal or polymeric nanoparticles for protection and cellular uptake [5, 12].

Regarding their physicochemical properties, positively charged nanoscale particles are optimal for cellular uptake. Thus, cationic lipids and polymers are the most abundantly used substances for non-viral delivery of nucleic acids. Several different natural and synthetic cationic polymers are available for nucleic acid complexation and condensation. While atelocollagen and chitosan are the most often used natural polymers, examples for synthethic polymers include poly-l-lysin, cyclodextrin, polylactic acid (PLA), poly(lactic-co-glycolic acid) (PLGA), and poly-β-aminoesters. The various cationic polymers differ greatly in their transfection efficiencies. Reasons are differences in cellular uptake, complex stability, and lysosomal escape [13]. Furthermore, different cationic polymers show a correlation between toxicity and transfection efficiency. This can be explained by the need of a positive charge for efficient cellular uptake which is also responsible for cytotoxicity [14]. In vivo, charged nanoparticles cause nonspecific interactions with proteins and blood components mediating aggregation and opsonization by the reticuloendothelial system (RES) [15, 16]. Therefore, strategies to improve the nanoparticles biocompatibility and target specificity are investigated in terms of surface shielding modifications and coupling of tissue-specific ligands, and the selection of optimal polymers is critical for successful intervention.

Polyethylenimines (PEIs) are synthetic linear or branched polymers of various molecular weights [17, 18]. The partial protonation of their amino groups results in a high cationic charge density, which allows them to form non-covalent complexes with negatively charged nucleic acids. This leads to full siRNA/miRNA protection against degradation, their cellular uptake, and, due to the so-called proton sponge effect, their intracellular escape from endosomes/lysosomes into the cytoplasm [19]. Although the ability of nucleic acid complexation is a general feature of polyethylenimines, only certain PEIs are suitable in terms of biological efficacy, optimal complex stability, and absence of cytotoxic effects [20, 21]. These include the branched ~10 kDa PEI F25-LMW, purified from a 25 kDa PEI by gel permeation chromatography [22], and the commercially available linear ~22 kDa jetPEI™ [23, 24]. Notably, these PEIs can also be used as DNA transfection reagents [25]. Since physicochemical and biological properties of the complexes are dependent on the complexation conditions, optimal protocols for complex preparation are critical for biological activity [26, 27].

The application of PEI/siRNA as well as PEI/miRNA complexes resulted in significant antitumor effects in vivo in various xenograft models [9, 23, 24, 28–33]. Thus, the PEI-mediated delivery of small RNA molecules is a powerful system for the investigation of therapeutic effects of a given siRNA or miRNA in vivo.

In this chapter, two approaches for gene knockdown in ovarian carcinoma are described, based either on the direct delivery of siRNAs or on the transfection of shRNA-encoding plasmids. Furthermore, the delivery of small RNAs is extended towards miRNAs, aiming at miRNA replacement therapy. While initial experiments will rely on in vitro systems (tissue culture) for analysis, the in vivo application of PEI-based complexes, performed in preclinical mouse tumor models, is the major focus. Since the in vivo biodistribution of the complexes is dependent on their mode of administration [28], different routes of injection are described, depending on the target organ/target tissue. Because the various siRNAs or miRNAs will only differ with regard to their sequence, and the size of the nucleic acid is not critical over a wide range, the PEI complexation can be considered as a general platform for nucleic acid delivery including small RNAs for knockdown approaches. Several oncogenes have been described as upregulated and functionally relevant in ovarian cancer, and consequently these knockdown strategies offer novel approaches in ovarian carcinoma treatment.

2 Materials

2.1 Preparation of PEI Complexes

1. Complexation Buffer: 0.15 M NaCl, 0.01 M HEPES, pH 7.4. Prepare with nuclease-free water (*see* **Note 1**) and adjust the pH with HCl. Store sterile filtered 50 mL aliquots at −20 °C or, once thawed, at 4 °C.
2. Glucose Solution: 5 % (w/v) glucose in nuclease-free water. Store sterile filtered 50 mL aliquots at −20 °C or, once thawed, at 4 °C.
3. Nucleic acids, i.e., siRNAs, miRNAs, or shRNA plasmids (*see* **Note 2**).

   Dissolve custom made siRNAs or miRNAs according to the manufacturer's instructions in buffer or nuclease-free water. Store aliquots of a 100 μM stock solution at −80 °C. Use a 20 μM dilution as working solution, which is stored at −20 to −80 °C. Clone shRNA-encoding sequences into appropriate RNAi vectors according to standard procedures.

   Luciferase encoding plasmid (e.g., pGL3-Control, Promega, Madison, WI).

   siRNA GL3, a luciferase siRNA specific for pGL3-Control plasmid: passenger strand sequence 5′-CUUACGCUGAGUACUUCGATT-3′ and guide strand sequence 5′-UCGAAGUACUCAGCGUAAGTT-3′.

   siRNA GL2, a luciferase siRNA nonspecific for pGL3-Control plasmid, serving as negative control: passenger strand sequence 5′-CGUACGCGGAAUACUUCGATT-3′ and guide strand sequence 5′-UCGAAGUAUUCCGCGUACGTT-3′.
4. jetPEI™ and in vivo-jetPEI™ (Polyplus, Illkirch, France).
5. PEI F25-LMW.

   Prepare from the commercially available branched 25 kDa polyethylenimine by gel filtration as described [22]. PEI F25-LMW is filter sterilized through a 0.2 μm filter and stored at 4 °C (*see* **Note 3**).

2.2 Tissue Culture

1. Dulbecco's PBS without Ca and Mg. Store at 4 °C.
2. Trypsin–EDTA solution: 0.05 %-trypsin/0.53 mM EDTA. Store at −20 °C or, for shorter time periods, at 4 °C.

3. Fetal calf serum (FCS). Dispense into 50 mL aliquots and store at −20 °C. Thaw before adding to culture medium.
4. Iscove's Modified DMEM (IMDM) supplemented with 10 % fetal calf serum (FCS) and 10× DMEM are stored at 4 °C. Normocin 50 mg/mL. Store at −20 °C.

   Dilute 1 mL Normocin in 500 mL cell culture medium to achieve antibacterial and fungicide effect (*see* **Note 4**).
5. Cell proliferation reagent WST-1. Store at −20 °C.
6. Agar solution: 2.4 % in water. Autoclave and store at RT.
7. Agar mixture:

   72.5 % medium, supplemented with 10 % FCS, 25 % agar solution (2.4 %), 2.5 % 10× medium. Heat solidified agar solution in the microwave and cool down in a 42 °C water bath. Preheat other ingredients to 37 °C and add to the agar solution. Keep the mixture fluid at 42 °C until use.

2.3 Quantitative RT-PCR (qRT-PCR)

1. RNA extraction solution containing guanidinium thiocyanate, phenol, and chloroform (TRI, e.g., peqGOLD TriFast™, PEQLAB, Erlangen, Germany). Store at 4 °C and protect from the light. Work under a hood and avoid skin contact.
2. Reverse Transcriptase (e.g., Revert Aid™ H Minus M-MuLV Reverse Transcriptase), 200 U/μL supplied with 5× Reaction Buffer. Store at −20 °C.
3. Random Hexamer Primer 20×: 100 μM mixture of single-stranded random hexanucleotides with 5′- and 3′-hydroxyl ends. Store at −20 °C.
4. dNTP Mix 10 mM. Store at −20 °C.
5. RiboLock™ RNase Inhibitor, 40 U/μL (e.g., Fermentas, St. Leon-Rot, Germany). Store at −20 °C.
6. QuantiTect™ SYBR® Green PCR Kit (Qiagen, Hilden, Germany) or equivalent.
7. qRT-PCR primers specific for the gene of interest dissolved in nuclease-free water. Store a 100 μM stock solution and 5 μM aliquots of a mix of forward and reverse primers at −20 °C.
8. Primers for a housekeeping gene, e.g., actin (forward: 5′-CCA ACC GCG AGA AGA TGA-3′ and reverse: 5′-CCA GAG GCG TAC AGG GAT AG-3′). Prepare stock and work solutions and store as indicated above.
9. 6× DNA loading dye and GeneRuler™ 1 kbp DNA Ladder (or similar). Store at 4 °C.

2.4 Luciferase Assay

1. Luciferase Assay System (e.g., Promega, Madison, WI). Store substrates in aliquots at −20 °C for up to 1 month or at −70 °C for up to 1 year. Protect from light (*see* **Note 5**).

2.5 Mouse Tumor Xenograft Models

1. Athymic nude mice for experiments with tumor xenografts, for other applications use immunocompetent mice or other transgenic/mutant mice (*see* **Note 6**).
2. Isoflurane. Store at 4 °C and avoid exposure.
3. Sterile single-use syringes and needles (26 G × ½″ for subcutaneous cell injection and i.p. complex injection, 30 G × ½″ for i.v. complex injection).
4. Microvette® CB 300, system for capillary blood collection.

2.6 [^{32}P]-Labeling of siRNA/miRNA

1. [^{32}P]-ATP (6,000 Ci/mmol, 20 mCi/mL EasyTide Lead; PerkinElmer, Waltham, MA, USA). Store at 4 °C.
2. T4 Polynucleotide Kinase. Store at −20 °C.
3. 0.5 M EDTA, pH 8.0. Store at room temperature.
4. Micro Bio-Spin® 6 Chromatography Columns (Bio-Rad, Hercules, CA, USA). Store at 4 °C.

2.7 RNA Preparation, Agarose Gel Electrophoresis, Blotting, and Autoradiography

1. Agarose NEEO.
2. MOPS buffer (10×): 0.4 M MOPS (3-(*N*-morpholino) propanesulfonic acid), pH 7.0, 0.1 M Na-acetate, 0.01 M EDTA. Dissolve in DEPC-treated, autoclaved water. Filter buffer and store at room temperature. Protect from light.
3. SSC buffer (20×): 3 M NaCl and 0.3 M Na_3-citrate × $2H_2O$. Dissolve in ddH_2O and autoclave. Store at room temperature.
4. RNA Loading Buffer (10×): 0.1 % (w/v) xylenecyanol, 0.1 % (w/v) bromophenol blue, 50 % (v/v) glycerol, 50 % (v/v) ddH_2O. Store at room temperature or at 4 °C.
5. Nylon membrane.
6. Chromatography paper.

2.8 Equipment and Supplies

1. Laminar flow bench and cell culture incubator.
2. Multi-well microtiter plate reader equipped with a 450 nm filter (for WST).
3. Luminometer.
4. Fume hood.
5. UV/Vis spectrophotometer.
6. PCR thermal cycle system.
7. Real-time PCR thermal cycle system.
8. Agarose Electrophoresis Equipment.
9. Ocular lens with grid.
10. Experimental animal facilities.

3 Methods

The PEI-mediated delivery of nucleic acids, like other non-viral delivery approaches, relies on several critical parameters including size, surface charge, and stability of the complexes as well as complexation efficacy and biocompatibility/toxicity. These properties are influenced by the PEI's molecular weight and degree of branching, the ratio between PEI and nucleic acids (the so-called N/P ratio referring to the nitrogen atoms of PEI and the nucleic acid phosphates), the buffer conditions employed during complexation, and, to a lesser extent, the molecular weight of the nucleic acid. Additionally, covalent coupling of the PEI to other polymers like polyethyleneglycol (= PEGylated PEIs, PEG-PEIs) can lead to markedly altered complex properties due to shielding of the net complex charge [34–36].

For the in vitro delivery of nucleic acids, several transfection reagents are commercially available, with PEI being one example. However, many transfection agents rely on certain conditions for their application and cannot be used in vivo, and small nucleic acid molecules like siRNA and miRNA are less easily complexed than larger nucleic acids. Thus, in particular for the direct application of siRNAs or miRNAs for the induction of RNAi or gene replacement for therapeutic purposes, only a very limited set of reagents or strategies exist. The two low molecular weight PEIs described here have been shown to efficiently deliver siRNAs, miRNAs, and shRNA-encoding plasmids while displaying low cytotoxicity (Fig. 1).

3.1 Preparation of PEI Complexes

Among cationic polymers, some polyethylenimines display excellent properties with regard to nucleic acid complexation and cellular delivery. However, high molecular weight PEIs cannot be used due to their cytotoxicity, and only certain low molecular weight PEIs display sufficient bioactivity. These include the linear jetPEI and the branched PEI F25-LMW. The N/P ratio is critical for efficient formation and cellular uptake of the complexes and depends on the PEI rather than on the nucleic acid. While optimal PEI/nucleic acid ratios are given in this protocol, the reader is also referred to **Note 7**.

To control for nonspecific effects of the transfection or the carrier influencing gene expression, the PEI complexation of a nonspecific or scrambled siRNA/miRNA/shRNA needs to be performed in parallel. Upon transfection, these cells or mice treated with nonspecific nucleic acids will serve as a negative control in addition to nontransfected cells or untreated mice, respectively. This includes control for the absence of vector and/or nucleic acid-mediated off-target effects, immunostimulation by the nucleic acid, and nonspecific cytotoxicity.

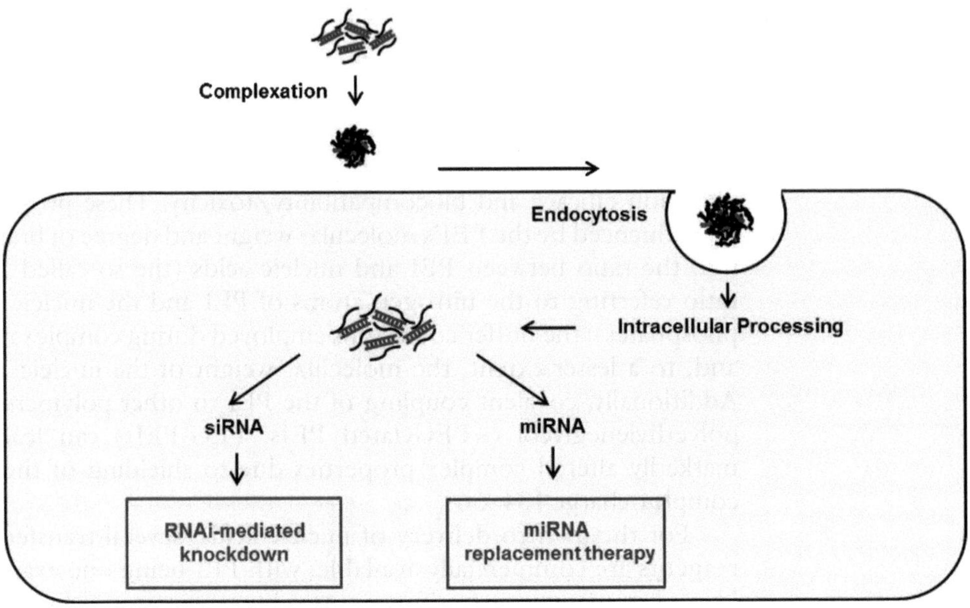

Fig. 1 Complexation of siRNA or miRNA molecules by polyethylenimine. Ionic interactions between small RNAs and PEI result in formation of nanoscale polyplexes, which can enter the cell via endocytosis. Upon intracellular processing (release from the endosomal/lysosomal system, decomposition of the polyplexes), released siRNAs/miRNAs allow RNAi-mediated gene knockdown (PEI/siRNA complexes) or miRNA replacement therapy (PEI/miRNA complexes)

For the optimization of complexation conditions, the knockdown of a reporter gene like luciferase (*see* below) can be performed. In this case, stably luciferase expressing cells can be employed, or cells can be transiently transfected with a luciferase expression vector 24 h prior to siRNA or shRNA–plasmid transfection, using any commercially available transfection reagent.

The following protocols for in vitro transfection refer to 24-well plates. Smaller or larger complex amounts can be prepared at the same mixing ratios. The presence of serum in the medium may influence transfection efficacy (*see* **Note 8**).

3.1.1 Complexation for In Vitro Transfection with PEI/DNA-Complexes (Including shRNA Constructs) in 24-Well Plates

1. Dilute 0.5 μg of DNA in 40 μL Complexation Buffer.
2. Mix and incubate for 5–10 min (Vial 1).
3. In parallel, prepare 40 μL PEI F25-LMW or jetPEI solution: Add 2.5 μL 1 mg/mL PEI F25-LMW solution to 37.5 μL Complexation Buffer or 1 μL 7.5 mM jetPEI solution to 39 μL Complexation Buffer. Mix and incubate at room temperature for 10 min (Vial 2).
4. For complex preparation, add the PEI solution (Vial 2) to the nucleic acid solution (Vial 1).
5. Mix by vortexing for 5 s.

6. Incubate the complexes for 30–60 min at room temperature and briefly vortex again prior to transfection.
7. Add 80 μL of complex solution directly into to the well containing 0.5–1.0 mL of medium.

3.1.2 Complexation for In Vitro Transfection with PEI/RNA-Complexes (siRNA or miRNA) in 24-Well Plates

1. Dilute 0.8 μg siRNA or miRNA in 40 μL Complexation Buffer.
2. Mix and incubate for 5–10 min (Vial 1).
3. In parallel, prepare 40 μL PEI F25-LMW or jetPEI solution: Add 4 μL 1 mg/mL PEI F25-LMW solution to 36 μL Complexation Buffer or 1.6 μL 7.5 mM jetPEI solution to 38.4 μL Complexation Buffer. Mix and incubate at room temperature for 10 min (Vial 2).
4. Refer to **steps 4–7** of the previous protocol (Subheading 3.1.1).

3.1.3 Complexation for a Single Standard Injection of PEI F25-LMW/Nucleic Acid Complexes (10 μg Nucleic Acid) into a Mouse

The following protocols are for in vivo application and refer to single injections for one mouse with a body weight of about 30 g. For the preparation of larger amounts up to 100 μg nucleic acid, the protocol can be upscaled accordingly. For amounts >100 μg nucleic acid, however, multiple complexation reactions should be run in parallel. Upon completion of complex formation, combine the contents of the different vials (each containing 1.5 mL complex solution) and briefly vortex again. PEI F25-LMW-based complexes can be stored frozen (*see* **Note 9**).

1. Dilute 10 μg nucleic acid in 75 μL Complexation Buffer.
2. Mix and incubate for 5–10 min (Vial 1).
3. In parallel, prepare 75 μL PEI F25-LMW solution. Add 10 μL of a 5 mg/mL PEI F25-LMW solution to 65 μL Complexation Buffer, mix, and incubate at room temperature for 5–10 min (Vial 2).
4. For complex preparation, add the polymer solution (Vial 2) to the nucleic acid solution (Vial 1).
5. Mix by vortexing for 5 s.
6. Incubate the complexes for 30–60 min at room temperature and briefly vortex again prior to injection.

3.1.4 Complexation Protocol for a Single Standard Injection of jetPEI/Nucleic Acid Complexes (10 μg Nucleic Acid) into a Mouse

1. Dilute 10 μg nucleic acid in 75 μL Complexation Buffer.
2. Mix and incubate for 5–10 min (Vial 1).
3. In parallel, prepare 75 μL jetPEI solution. Dilute 20 μL of a 7.5 mM jetPEI solution or 5 μL of a 4× jetPEI solution in Complexation Buffer, mix, and incubate at room temperature for 5–10 min (Vial 2).
4. Refer to **steps 4–6** of the previous protocol (Subheading 3.1.3).

3.1.5 Complexation Protocol for a Single Standard Injection of In Vivo-jetPEI/Nucleic Acid Complexes (10 μg Nucleic Acid) into a Mouse

Dilute 10 μg nucleic acid in 75 μL 5 % (w/v) glucose.

1. Mix and incubate for 5–10 min (Vial 1).
2. In parallel, prepare 75 μL in vivo-jetPEI solution. Add 1 μL of a 150 mM in vivo-jetPEI solution to 74 μL 5 % (w/v) glucose, mix, and incubate at room temperature for 5–10 min (Vial 2).
3. Refer to **steps 4–6** of the previous protocol (Subheading 3.1.3).

3.2 Determination of In Vitro Transfection Efficacy Using the Luciferase System

For the simple and accurate analysis of gene-targeting efficacies, the determination of luciferase activity can be performed either in stably luciferase expressing cells (if available), e.g., SKOV-3-Luc [23], or in wild-type cells upon their prior transient transfection with a luciferase expression vector. Luciferase knockdown after siRNA transfection usually reaches maximum values at 48–96 h after siRNA transfection. In the case of shRNA expression plasmids, the effect may take a bit longer due to the requirement of DNA transcription and shRNA processing prior to RISC loading. However, in both cases, optimal time ranges will mainly depend on the target gene and the cell line and may require optimization. The activity of the luciferase enzyme is measured in a luminometer and expressed in relative light units (RLU).

Using the luciferase quantitation kit from Promega, we employed the following, slightly modified, protocol, which refers to experiments in the 24-well plate format:

1. Prepare the 1× Lysis buffer by adding 4 volumes of water to 1 volume of 5× lysis buffer.
2. Remove the growth medium from adherent cells (or, in the case of cells in suspension, after spinning them down at 800 rpm and aspirating the medium).
3. Add 100 μL/well Lysis Buffer to the cells and incubate on a rocking platform for 10 min at room temperature.
4. Check complete cell lysis under the microscope.
5. For the measurement of the luciferase activity in the luminometer, dispense 25 μL of the Luciferase Assay Reagent into a luminometer tube, add 10 μL of the cell lysate, mix both components by carefully tapping against the tube, and measure immediately.
6. To avoid background signals, no gloves should be worn when handling the luminometer tubes.

3.3 Determination of Target Gene Knockdown (mRNA Knockdown Efficacies)

The ultimate goal is the knockdown of a given target gene of interest. For the identification of the best siRNA or shRNA from a set of candidates, other transfection reagents can be used besides PEI (*see* **Note 10**). Knockdown efficacies can be determined on mRNA level by Northern blotting or, being more accurate and relying on smaller RNA amounts, by quantitative RT-PCR (qRT-PCR). For the correct estimation of the target gene knockdown efficacy, control transfections with PEI/nonspecific siRNA complexes should be done in parallel. Knockdown efficacies are determined by the comparison of expression levels of the target gene in cells treated with the specific PEI/siRNA complexes versus control transfected cells and are expressed in "% remaining expression over control" or in "% knockdown compared to control".

3.3.1 Total RNA Isolation

1. Grow cells in 6-well plate to achieve 60–70 % of confluence.
2. Transfect the cells as described above and wait for 72–120 h after transfection.
3. Add 1 mL TriFast™ reagent per well.
4. Incubate for 5 min at room temperature.
5. Mix cell lysate by pipetting up and down several times prior to its transfer into a 1.5 mL vial.
6. Add 0.2 mL chloroform to each mL of TriFast™ and shake vigorously for 15 s.
7. Incubate at room temperature for 3–10 min.
8. Centrifuge at 12,000 × *g* for 10 min at 4 °C.
9. Transfer the aqueous upper phase containing the RNA into a new tube.
10. Add 0.5 mL isopropanol per 1 mL of TriFast™ and incubate 5–15 min on ice for RNA precipitation.
11. Centrifuge at 12,000 × *g* for 10 min at 4 °C.
12. Remove the supernatant and wash the RNA pellet with 75 % ethanol.
13. Centrifuge again at 7,500 × *g* for 5–10 min at 4 °C.
14. Air-dry the RNA pellet until all excess ethanol is evaporated completely and then resuspend the RNA in 10–50 μL nuclease-free water. Freezing and incubating the solution for 5 min at 65 °C will aid the resolubilization of the RNA.
15. Determination of quality/quantity of isolated RNA.

Target mRNA levels can now be determined either by Northern blotting or qRT-PCR. For Northern blotting, RNA pellets can be directly dissolved in RNA Loading Buffer and further processed according to standard Northern blot protocols. For qRT-PCR, cDNA can be generated using the RevertAid™ H Minus M-MuLV Reverse Transcriptase in accordance with the following protocol.

3.3.2 Reverse Transcription

1. Mix 1 μg of total RNA, 1 μL Random Hexamer Primer, and DEPC-treated water, added to a final volume of 12.5 μL in a PCR tube.
2. Incubate for 5 min at 65 °C and chill on ice.

3. After spinning down the solution by short centrifugation, 4 μL 5× reaction buffer, 0.5 μL RiboLock™ RNase Inhibitor, 2 μL 10 mM dNTP Mix, and 1 μL RevertAid™ H Minus M-MuLV Reverse Transcriptase are added.
4. All components are mixed, the solution is spun down by brief centrifugation, and the tubes are placed into a Thermo Cycler.
5. The initial incubation is at 25 °C for 10 min, followed by the elongation step at 42 °C for 60 min and an enzyme inactivating step at 70 °C for 10 min.
6. The cDNA is cooled down to 4 °C and used directly for PCR, or stored at −20 °C.

3.3.3 Quantitative PCR

1. Dilute cDNA 1:10 in DEPC-treated water.
2. For duplicates, add 2.2 μL 5 μM Primer-Mix (containing appropriate primers to amplify the gene of interest or, as a loading control, a housekeeping gene) and 10 μL SYBR Green mix (prepared according to the manufacturer's instructions) to 8.8 μL cDNA.
3. Mix the components thoroughly by pipetting the solution up and down for at least ten times, and transfer 10 μL of the reaction mixture into a LightCycler capillary.
4. In the LightCycler, preincubate the reaction at 95 °C for 15 min to activate the HotStarTaq® DNA Polymerase.
5. Parameters for PCR are the following: denaturation step 10′/95 °C, annealing step 10′/55 °C, extension step 10′/72 °C—for 55 cycles—and then cooling down to 4 °C. The annealing temperature may vary dependent on the primers used and may require optimization.
6. Run PCR reactions with target gene-specific and, for normalization, with housekeeping gene-specific primer sets (e.g., actin) in parallel for each sample, and determine expression levels of the gene of interest by the formula $2^{\Delta CP(\text{target gene})}/2^{\Delta CP(\text{actin})}$ with CP = cycle number at the crossing point (0.3).

The most reliable documentation of gene knockdown relies on the parallel determination of targeting efficacies on both mRNA and protein levels (*see* **Note 11**) and is often required by referees when submitting articles to peer-reviewed journals. Dependent on the target gene, the quantitation of protein levels may rely on Western blotting, ELISA, FACS, or assays for enzyme activity, substrate binding, or downstream effects of the target protein.

3.4 Determination of miRNA Target Molecule Levels

To determine the molecular effects of a given miRNA of interest, its inhibitory activity on potential (predicted in silico, as available in databases like www.mirdb.org) or already established target genes can be measured. Except for the conserved seed region, miRNAs, unlike siRNAs, show incomplete sequence complementarity with their target mRNA and thus exert their effects of preventing protein biosynthesis mainly by the inhibition of protein translation rather than mRNA cleavage. Consequently, miRNA effects may not be seen on mRNA level, and it is necessary to determine the levels of protein expression of the target molecule.

The method of choice for the quantitation of protein levels will strongly depend on the protein of interest and the assays or reagents available (antibodies, substrates, distinct signal transduction pathways). As stated above, this includes Western blotting, ELISA, FACS, and assays for enzyme activity, substrate binding, or downstream effects of the target protein.

To confirm the enrichment of the transfected miRNA in the cells, a quantification of this miRNA may be performed by PCR using stem-loop primers [37]. The cell or tissue lysate is subjected to RNA extraction with enriching small RNAs. For reverse transcription, stem-loop primers are employed due to the shortness of the miRNA sequence. These primers are ~50 nt in length and have an overhang on one side of the stem that is complementary to the miRNA sequence, thus forming a cDNA hybrid of miRNA and primer. For the quantitative PCR reaction, one primer specific for the miRNA and one recognizing the loop sequence are used.

3.5 Analysis of Biological Effects in Ovarian Cancer Cells In Vitro

An important biological effect on cancer cells upon siRNA, miRNA, or shRNA transfection is their often impaired capacity to proliferate (*see* **Note 12**). To study anchorage-dependent proliferation, a colorimetric assay based on the time-dependent measurement of cell viability is carried out in a 96-well format. For the assessment of anchorage-independent proliferation, a soft agar assay for monitoring the three-dimensional colony formation in an agar matrix is employed. For both assays, triplicates should be carried out for each treatment group.

3.5.1 Assessment of Anchorage-Dependent Proliferation

1. Seed ~1,000 cells in 100 μL medium/well.
2. Transfect on the same day, or 1 day later, with 0.08 μg DNA or 1.3 μg siRNA, respectively, complexed as described above (*see* **Note 13**).
3. For the determination of the number of viable cells, mix 5 μL of WST-1 Reagent with 50 μL serum-free medium.
4. Aspirate medium in the wells and add 50 μL of the WST-1 mixture. Incubate for 1 h at 37 °C.
5. Measure absorption at 450 nm in a microplate reader.
6. Depending on the cell line and the target gene, the establishment of antiproliferative effects will take several days and can be accurately monitored by measuring the number of viable cells over 3–6 days.

3.5.2 Assessment of Anchorage-Independent Proliferation (Soft Agar Assay)

1. Seed cells into 24-, 12- or 6-well plates at ~30,000, ~60,000 or ~150,000 cells per well.
2. Transfect cells on the same day or 1 day later as described above.
3. Trypsinize cells 1 day after transfection.
4. Count cells and adjust concentration to 60,000 cells/mL.
5. Add 1 mL prewarmed agar mixture per well of a 6-well plate and distribute evenly. Let solidify.
6. Mix 1.5 mL prewarmed agar mixture quickly with 1 mL cell suspension in the water bath and pipette 0.8 mL/well on top of the bottom agar.
7. Incubate at 37 °C under standard cell culture conditions.
8. Count single cells in ten fields of each well 1 day after plating to normalize for differences in initial cell numbers.
9. Monitor colony growth by counting colonies above a certain cutoff in 10 fields/well (*see* **Note 14**).

3.6 Intraperitoneal Delivery of PEI Complexes In Vivo

While several transfection reagents suitable for delivery of siRNAs and miRNAs have been introduced for in vitro use, the in vivo situation is considerably more complex. Among others, the following additional requirements have to be met: protection of siRNA molecules against degradation; transfer through several biological membranes; favorable pharmacokinetic properties, for example, with regard to serum half-life and biodistribution; efficient delivery to and uptake into the target organ as well as high biocompatibility; and the absence of other unwanted effects. PEI/siRNA and PEI/miRNA complexes based on jetPEI and PEI F25-LMW have been successfully used for systemic or local application. Systemic administration of PEI F25-LMW/siRNA and PEI F25-LMW/miRNA complexes can be performed through intraperitoneal or intravenous injection (*see* **Notes 15** and **16**).

3.6.1 Intraperitoneal Administration of PEI F25-LMW/siRNA and PEI F25-LMW/miRNA Complexes

1. For i.p. injections in mice, a rather broad range of injection volumes has been described; however, the maximum volume is ~50 mL/kg, i.e., 1.5 mL for a mouse with 30 g body weight. For i.v. injections, a maximum volume of 150 μL for a 30 g mouse should not be exceeded and the injection should be performed slowly. Typically, we use 150 μL for i.p. and 100 μL for i.v. injections in our experiments.
2. Prior to in vivo applications, toxicity studies may be performed to determine maximum amounts of PEI/siRNA or PEI/miRNA complexes that allow repeated application without adverse effects (*see* **Note 17**). In mice, repeated injection of 10–30 μg (i.p.) or 10 μg (i.v.) PEI-complexed siRNA was well tolerated.

3.6.2 Local Application of PEI F25-LMW/siRNA and PEI F25-LMW/miRNA Complexes

Local applications of PEI/siRNA or PEI/miRNA complexes can be performed as well. Among others, these include intrathecal injections into the brain or instillation into the lung. Special care needs to be taken not to exceed maximum volumes for these modes of administration (~2 or ~50 μL, respectively, in mice). If the volume is a limiting factor, complexation conditions (*see* Subheading 3.1.) can be modified by reducing volumes of the Complexation Buffers (HEPES/NaCl and Glucose Solution) in order to achieve higher complex concentrations.

3.7 Determination of siRNA/miRNA Biodistribution Through [^{32}P]-Labeling of siRNA/miRNA

For the induction of RNAi in vivo, the delivery of intact nucleic acids is of critical importance. Thus, prior to a large therapeutic experiment involving several treatment groups, it may be advantageous to test for siRNA/miRNA delivery into the target tissue/organ of interest. Likewise, when observing therapeutic effects, the method described below allows to demonstrate that those are indeed based on the in vivo delivery of intact siRNA/miRNA molecules, thus validating the results with regard to specificity. In contrast to other methods relying on the in situ detection of labeled nucleic acids, this protocol tests exclusively for intact siRNA/miRNA molecules since degradation products will not contribute to the signal. Please note, however, that this method relies on radioactive labeling (*see* **Note 18**).

3.7.1 Nucleic Acid Labeling and siRNA/miRNA Biodistribution

1. 5′-Labeling of siRNAs/miRNAs: In a 1.5 mL reaction tube, mix 7.5 μg siRNA/miRNA with 10 μL [γ-^{32}P]ATP, 5 μL 10× reaction buffer A (Fermentas), 2 μL T4 Polynucleotide Kinase, and add water to 50 μL.
2. Incubate the mixture for 30 min at 37 °C.
3. Stop the reaction by adding 2 μL 0.5 M EDTA, pH 8.0, and purify labeled nucleic acid molecules from free nucleotides by gel filtration. For example, use Micro Bio-Spin® 6 Chromatography Columns according to the manufacturer's DNA purification protocol: Resuspend the resin, place the column into a 2.0 mL tube, and remove the cap of the tube. Wait until the packing buffer has drained and empty the 2.0 mL tube. Centrifuge the column for 2 min at 1,000 ×*g* and place it into a new 1.5 mL tube. Apply the labeling reaction mix onto the resin and centrifuge the column for 4 min at 1,000 ×*g*. The flow-through contains the labeled, purified nucleic acids.
4. Prepare PEI/siRNA complexes or PEI/miRNA complexes as described in Subheading 3.1 with a maximum of 3 μg radioactively labeled nucleic acids/injection per mouse (fill up with nonlabeled siRNAs/miRNAs to reach desired nucleic acid amounts, if applicable).
5. Inject the complex solution into the mouse and wait 1–3 min prior to collecting blood from the tail artery using a capillary tube like Microvette® CB 300.

6. At the time point(s) of interest, typically between 30 min and 8 h, sacrifice the mice, e.g., by exposing to an overdose of isoflurane and cervical dislocation, immediately take blood by puncturing the heart, and remove organs to be analyzed, e.g., lung, liver, kidney, spleen, skeletal muscle, tumor xenografts, and brain. For most accurate results, analyze the whole organ/tissue if possible (*see* **Note 19**).
7. Rinse tissues in PBS to remove excess blood and determine the exact weight. Freeze the tissues in liquid nitrogen or proceed immediately with the homogenization of the tissue.

3.7.2 RNA Preparation and Autoradiography

1. Put the tissue sample into a mortar and, if frozen, wait until the tissue starts to thaw. Using a pistil, press the sample flat and add some liquid nitrogen. Grind the tissue with the pistil while adding more liquid nitrogen, if necessary, until a fine powder is obtained.
2. Add 0.75 mL TriFast™ and transfer the suspension into a 2.0 mL reaction tube. Rinse the mortar with 0.75 mL fresh TriFast™ to collect residual tissue material, and combine with the first suspension.
3. Proceed with the preparation of RNA as described in Subheading 3.3.
4. Resuspend the RNA pellet in 50 μL 1× RNA Loading Buffer.
5. Gel electrophoresis: Prepare a 1 % agarose gel by dissolving 2 g agarose in 175 mL boiling water. Let the solution cool down to 55–60 °C prior to adding 20 mL 10× MOPS buffer and 5 mL 37 % formaldehyde (work under a chemical hood!) and pouring the gel in an appropriate gel electrophoresis device.
6. Load equal amounts of the samples and run the gel until the loading dye reaches the lower end (e.g., 80 V for ~90 min).
7. Capillary transfer: Fill a wide container with 20× SSC buffer and place a glass plate on its top. Place a sheet of Whatman 3 MM chromatography paper on the glass plate with its ends reaching into the buffer. Soak the whole paper in buffer prior to placing the gel upside down onto the paper. Presoak a gel-size nylon membrane and four gel-size chromatography sheets in 20× SSC buffer and place them, nylon membrane first, onto the gel. Carefully remove any bubbles from the sandwich, overlay with a ~10 cm layer of dry paper towels, put a ~1 kg weight on top, and allow the capillary transfer to proceed overnight.
8. Autoradiography: Expose the nylon membrane (wrapped in plastic) to an X-ray film or a phosphoimager screen. Scan the film or screen and determine signal intensities using any appropriate software (Fig. 2).

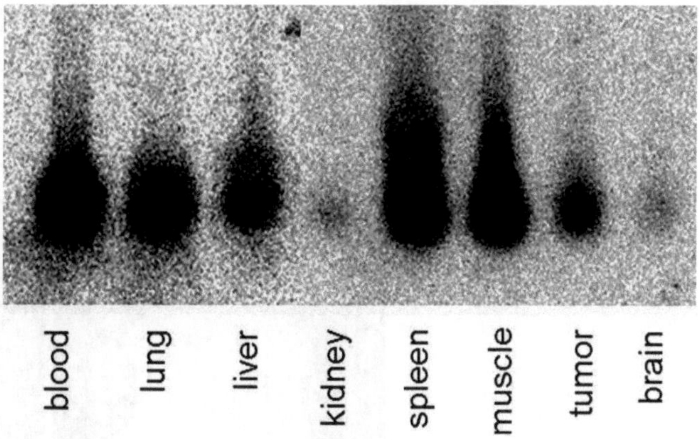

Fig. 2 Biodistribution of PEI/siRNA complexes. PEI F25-LMW/siRNA complexes were injected via i.p.-injection into a mouse bearing s.c. tumor xenografts. The mouse was sacrificed after 60 min and tissues analyzed as described above. Autoradiographic signals represent intact ^{32}P-labeled siRNA molecules in the different tissues

3.8 Therapeutic Treatment and Analysis of Antitumor Effects in a Subcutaneous Ovarian Carcinoma Xenograft Model (Example: PEI/siHER2) [23]

1. Establishment of s.c. ovarian carcinoma xenografts: Inject 2.5×10^6 SKOV-3 cells in 150 μL PBS subcutaneously in both flanks of 6- to 8-week old nude mice.
2. After reabsorption of the fluid, i.e., 3–5 days after injection, measure tumor sizes regularly every 2–3 days and estimate tumor volumes from the product of its perpendicular diameters.
3. When tumors are well established, randomize mice into groups. In addition to the treatment group(s) that receive PEI-complexed specific siRNAs (e.g., siHER2), two control groups are necessary to monitor nonspecific effects, one being left untreated and the other receiving a nonspecific PEI-complexed siRNA.
4. Treat mice systemically by i.p. injection of PEI/siRNA complexes containing 8 μg siRNA every 2–3 days (*see* **Note 20**). Note that dosages can also be increased, with up to 30 μg siRNA/injection being well tolerated in mice. Using the same protocol, PEI-complexed miRNAs can be applied as well.
5. After 2–4 weeks, dependent on the tumor size and the observed effects, terminate the experiment and sacrifice mice by exposure to an overdose of isoflurane and cervical dislocation (*see* **Note 21**).
6. Remove the tumors and divide the tissue into several samples: Use one sample for RNA preparation and Northern blotting/qRT-PCR to determine mRNA levels of the target gene

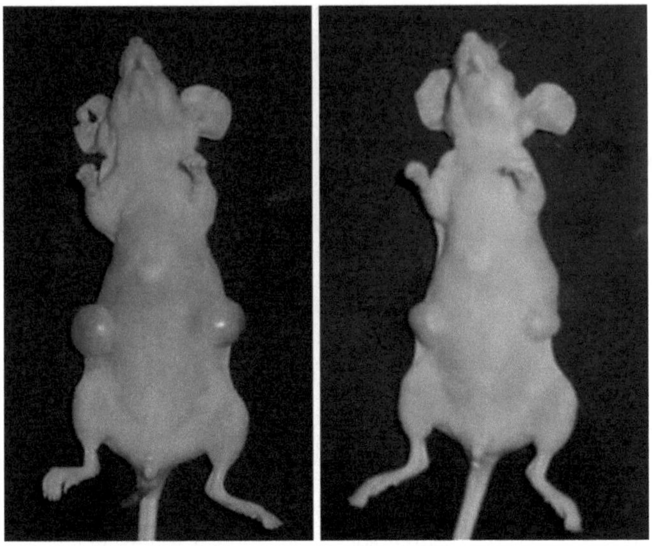

Fig. 3 Tumor xenografts in athymic nude mice. Subcutaneously injected SKOV-3 ovarian carcinoma cells formed tumor xenografts in immunocompromised animals

(e.g., HER2). Take a second part of the tumor and fix immediately by transferring into 10 % formalin, prior to paraffin embedding and immunohistochemical staining of tissue sections (e.g., for HER2 protein). If applicable, determine protein levels of the target gene from tumor lysates by Western blotting, ELISA, or other assays available (Fig. 3).

3.9 Therapeutic Treatment and Analysis of Antitumor Effects in an i.p. Ovarian Carcinoma Xenograft Model (Example: PEI/shHMGA2) [38]

1. Inject 1×10^7 Ovcar-3 cells in 500 μL PBS into the peritoneum of athymic nude mice to establish i.p. ovarian carcinoma xenografts.
2. Randomize mice into treatment groups 2 weeks after injection of the tumor cells. In this example, mice received PEI-complexed vector encoding either a HMGA2 specific or a corresponding scrambled sequence as nonspecific control or remained untreated.
3. Administer complexes once a week by i.p. injection with 35 μg shRNA-encoding vector complexed with PEI for a total period of time of 4 weeks (*see* **Notes 20** and **21**).
4. Sacrifice mice 1 week after the last injection by exposure to an overdose of isoflurane and cervical dislocation.
5. Remove intraperitoneal tumors surgically and measure their weight.

Dependent on the available analytical tools, samples of the tumor tissues are collected for RNA preparation and subsequent qRT-PCR, immunohistochemical staining, and/or determination of protein levels from lysates.

3.10 miRNA Replacement Therapy and Analysis of Antitumor Effects in an s.c. Ovarian Carcinoma Xenograft Model (Example: PEI/miRNA, Intratumoral Injection)

1. Establish and monitor subcutaneous tumors as described above (*see* Subheading 3.7.).
2. Randomize mice into treatment and negative control groups.
3. Inject PEI/miRNA complexes directly into the tumor mass upon establishment of the tumors (*see* **Note 22**).

4 Notes

1. To avoid nuclease degradation, resuspension and dilution of nucleic acids should be performed with solutions free of DNases and RNases. For the preparation of Complexation Buffer and Glucose Solution, DEPC-treated bidestilled water should be used.
2. Predesigned siRNAs against reporter genes like luciferase (e.g., luciferase siRNAs GL2 and GL3 from MWG, Ebersberg, Germany) or constructs encoding shRNAs against luciferase can be used for the optimization of gene knockdown conditions in a given stably or transiently luciferase expressing cell line.
3. If not protected from light, PEI F25-LMW solutions may change over a longer time period to a yellow or light-brown color. To our knowledge, this does not impair its transfection performance.
4. Since seemingly poor transfection efficacies in tissue culture and poor formation of xenografts in animal experiments may be due to mycoplasma contamination of the cells, we recommend regular testing and/or treatment of cells with an antibiotic against mycoplasma infection.
5. Oxidative processes in Luciferase Assay Reagent might result in detection of low levels of light units. Thus, adjusting reductive conditions by adding 2-mercaptoethanol to the Luciferase Assay Reagent can recover optimal conditions for the luciferase reaction.
6. Mice need to be kept and handled according to the appropriate laboratory animal guidelines. For the successful establishment of s.c. tumors and for the accurate determination of three-dimensional sizes of xenografts, cells should be injected directly under the skin while avoiding injection into deeper regions. The genetic background (strain/gender) of athymic nude mice with the nu/nu mutation might also influence the establishment and growth of xenografts. Thus, in some cases,

a comparison of different nude mice can be helpful to determine the optimal strain for an experiment.

7. The transfection efficiency is strongly related to the optimal PEI/nucleic acid mass ratio or N/P ratio. For the branched PEI F25-LMW, optimal N/P ratios are usually between 38.5 and 77. According to the manufacturer's protocol, optimal N/P ratios for jetPEI and in vivo-jetPEI are between 5 and 10. Nevertheless, it can be useful to determine optimal N/P ratios for different applications and cell lines. Unless stated otherwise, the N/P ratios employed in the complexation protocols in this chapter are 38.5 for PEI F25-LMW and 5 for jetPEI or in vivo-jetPEI, respectively.
8. FCS in the transfection medium may impair transfection efficacy when using certain transfection reagents. For PEI F25-LMW, however, we did not notice a significant serum dependence in vitro, while jetPEI performed better at lower FCS concentrations under the conditions investigated by our group. It is usually not necessary to change the medium after transfection. However, a medium change after 6–8 h will not decrease the transfection efficacy.
9. Polyplexes with PEI F25-LMW and nucleic acids allow freezing. To this end, prepare appropriate ready-to-use aliquots and store at −20 or −80 °C until use. This procedure does not impair the biological activity of the complexes. Repeated freeze/thawing cycles should be avoided. Upon re-thawing, briefly vortex and incubate complexes for 30 min prior to use.
10. Depending on the cell line used, the PEI-mediated delivery of nucleic acids in vitro may be less efficient compared to other transfection reagents and methods. In this case, the in vitro identification of the best siRNA or shRNA from various predesigned candidates against a given target gene can also be done using other transfection reagents that may be more efficient in the cell line studied.
11. In addition to the determination of mRNA levels by Northern blotting or qRT-PCR, other methods for the measurement of expression levels can be employed. These include, but are not limited to, protein quantitation by ELISA, FACS, or Western blotting as well as various tests for protein or enzyme activity and will strongly depend on the protein of interest.
12. Dependent on the cell line, cytotoxic effects may be observed in vitro upon treatment with PEI complexes. To accurately determine threshold concentrations of PEI, commercially available tests for the assessment of viable cells (MTT assay, WST-1 assay) or cell death (LDH release assay) can be performed. The same tests may be used for monitoring specific effects upon gene targeting, i.e., if antiproliferative or apoptotic effects are anticipated after knockdown of the gene of interest.

13. The WST-1 assay is an endpoint measurement. For every time point, at least triplicate wells are needed. Avoid using the wells located next to the borders of the plate since the medium evaporates faster here, leading to artifacts. Fill border wells with PBS or medium instead. Cells should not reach confluency or the lag phase of proliferation.
14. Colony formation may take several days or weeks. Colonies should be counted by at least two independent and blinded investigators. To define a cutoff for colony counting, an ocular lens with grid may be used.
15. In mice, the tail veins are located on the left and right side of the tail, whereas the arteries are located on the dorsal and ventral side of the tail. For i.v. injection, the mice should be transferred to a restraining device to avoid movement. Warming the tail with an infrared lamp or warm water will enlarge the veins. Alternatively, a disinfectant solution can be sprayed onto the skin of the tail for vein enlargement. For injection in mice, we suggest to use a 30 Gauge needle.
16. To facilitate the penetration of the needle during i.p. injection, hold the mouse tightly. It may happen that organs in the abdomen and pelvis, e.g., colon or bladder, are accidentally punctured. To avoid this, the lower left part of the abdomen is proposed as site of injection.
17. Despite careful design of siRNA and shRNA molecules, the absence of off-target effects and immunostimulation in vivo as well as adverse effects of the delivery system should be excluded by performing tests like ELISA for cytokines or determination of the activity of liver enzymes.
18. Special care needs to be taken when working with [^{32}P]-labeled material. Consult your lab safety manuals and radiation safety personnel.
19. Since the distribution in a tissue or organ can be quite heterogeneous, it is necessary to homogenize the whole organ (e.g., liver or kidney).
20. Based on biodistribution experiments in our lab, we propose the i.p. injection of PEI/nucleic acid complexes for the therapeutic treatment of s.c. xenografts. Depending on the target tissue, other modes of administration may be used.
21. Tumor growth rate and appearance as well as animal welfare determine the duration of an experiment.
22. Injection volumes are dependent on the tumor size and are generally in the range of 50 μL. While, for comparability, it is crucial that equal complex amounts are used in all groups at a given time point, injection volumes may be increased during

the experiment when the tumors get larger. Typically, ~4 μg miRNA per injection is employed.

23. Experiments described here may include the work with potentially hazardous or genetically modified material. Please consult the safety guidelines in your lab for proper handling.

Acknowledgments

This work was supported by grants from the Deutsche Forschungsgemeinschaft (Forschergruppe "Nanohale" (AI 24/6-1) and AI 24/9-1), the German Cancer Aid (Deutsche Krebshilfe, grants 106992 and 109128), and the VfK Verein für Krebsforschung.

References

1. Meister G, Tuschl T (2004) Mechanisms of gene silencing by double-stranded RNA. Nature 431:343–349
2. Siolas D, Lerner C, Burchard J et al (2005) Synthetic shRNAs as potent RNAi triggers. Nat Biotechnol 23:227–231
3. de Fougerolles A, Vornlocher HP, Maraganore J et al (2007) Interfering with disease: a progress report on siRNA-based therapeutics. Nat Rev Drug Discov 6:443–453
4. Aigner A (2007) Applications of RNA interference: current state and prospects for siRNA-based strategies in vivo. Appl Microbiol Biotechnol 76:9–21
5. Rettig GR, Behlke MA (2011) Progress toward in vivo use of siRNAs-II. Mol Ther 20(3):483–512
6. Bartel DP (2004) MicroRNAs: genomics, biogenesis, mechanism, and function. Cell 116:281–297
7. Lovat F, Valeri N, Croce CM (2011) MicroRNAs in the pathogenesis of cancer. Semin Oncol 38:724–733
8. Aigner A (2011) MicroRNAs (miRNAs) in cancer invasion and metastasis: therapeutic approaches based on metastasis-related miRNAs. J Mol Med 89:445–457
9. Ibrahim AF, Weirauch U, Thomas M et al (2011) MicroRNA replacement therapy for miR-145 and miR-33a is efficacious in a model of colon carcinoma. Cancer Res 71(15):5214–5224
10. Grimm D, Streetz KL, Jopling CL et al (2006) Fatality in mice due to oversaturation of cellular microRNA/short hairpin RNA pathways. Nature 441:537–541
11. Merdan T, Kopecek J, Kissel T (2002) Prospects for cationic polymers in gene and oligonucleotide therapy against cancer. Adv Drug Deliv Rev 54:715–758
12. Aigner A (2008) Cellular delivery in vivo of siRNA-based therapeutics. Curr Pharm Des 14:3603–3619
13. Tang MX, Szoka FC (1997) The influence of polymer structure on the interactions of cationic polymers with DNA and morphology of the resulting complexes. Gene Ther 4:823–832
14. Eliyahu H, Barenholz Y, Domb AJ (2005) Polymers for DNA delivery. Molecules 10:34–64
15. Liu F, Huang L (2002) Development of non-viral vectors for systemic gene delivery. J Control Release 78:259–266
16. Basarkar A, Singh J (2007) Nanoparticulate systems for polynucleotide delivery. Int J Nanomedicine 2:353–360
17. Boussif O, Lezoualc'h F, Zanta MA et al (1995) A versatile vector for gene and oligonucleotide transfer into cells in culture and in vivo: polyethylenimine. Proc Natl Acad Sci USA 92:7297–7301
18. Lungwitz U, Breunig M, Blunk T et al (2005) Polyethylenimine-based non-viral gene delivery systems. Eur J Pharm Biopharm 60:247–266
19. Behr JP (1997) The proton sponge: a trick to enter cells the viruses did not exploit. Chimia 51:34–36
20. Godbey WT, Wu KK, Mikos AG (1999) Size matters: molecular weight affects the efficiency of poly(ethylenimine) as a gene delivery vehicle. J Biomed Mater Res 45:268–275
21. Breunig M, Lungwitz U, Liebl R et al (2007) Breaking up the correlation between efficacy and toxicity for nonviral gene delivery. Proc Natl Acad Sci USA 104:14454–14459

22. Werth S, Urban-Klein B, Dai L et al (2006) A low molecular weight fraction of polyethylenimine (PEI) displays increased transfection efficiency of DNA and siRNA in fresh or lyophilized complexes. J Control Release 112:257–270
23. Urban-Klein B, Werth S, Abuharbeid S et al (2005) RNAi-mediated gene-targeting through systemic application of polyethylenimine (PEI)-complexed siRNA in vivo. Gene Ther 12:461–466
24. Grzelinski M, Urban-Klein B, Martens T et al (2006) RNA interference-mediated gene silencing of pleiotrophin through polyethylenimine-complexed small interfering RNAs in vivo exerts antitumoral effects in glioblastoma xenografts. Hum Gene Ther 17:751–766
25. Zou SM, Erbacher P, Remy JS et al (2000) Systemic linear polyethylenimine (L-PEI)-mediated gene delivery in the mouse. J Gene Med 2:128–134
26. Boussif O, Zanta MA, Behr JP (1996) Optimized galenics improve in vitro gene transfer with cationic molecules up to 1000-fold. Gene Ther 3:1074–1080
27. Hobel S, Prinz R, Malek A et al (2008) Polyethylenimine PEI F25-LMW allows the long-term storage of frozen complexes as fully active reagents in siRNA-mediated gene targeting and DNA delivery. Eur J Pharm Biopharm 70(1):29–41
28. Hobel S, Koburger I, John M et al (2010) Polyethylenimine/small interfering RNA-mediated knockdown of vascular endothelial growth factor in vivo exerts anti-tumor effects synergistically with Bevacizumab. J Gene Med 12:287–300
29. Kaestner P, Aigner A, Bastians H (2011) Therapeutic targeting of the mitotic spindle checkpoint through nanoparticle-mediated siRNA delivery inhibits tumor growth in vivo. Cancer Lett 304:128–136
30. Hendruschk S, Wiedemuth R, Aigner A et al (2011) RNA interference targeting survivin exerts antitumoral effects in vitro and in established glioma xenografts in vivo. Neuro Oncol 13:1074–1089
31. Gunther M, Lipka J, Malek A et al (2011) Polyethylenimines for RNAi-mediated gene targeting in vivo and siRNA delivery to the lung. Eur J Pharm Biopharm 77(3):438–449
32. Ripka S, Neesse A, Riedel J et al (2010) CUX1: target of Akt signalling and mediator of resistance to apoptosis in pancreatic cancer. Gut 59(8):1101–1110
33. Schulze D, Plohmann P, Hobel S et al (2011) Anti-tumor effects of fibroblast growth factor-binding protein (FGF-BP) knockdown in colon carcinoma. Mol Cancer 10:144
34. Harris JM, Martin NE, Modi M (2001) Pegylation: a novel process for modifying pharmacokinetics. Clin Pharmacokinet 40:539–551
35. Malek A, Czubayko F, Aigner A (2008) PEG grafting of polyethylenimine (PEI) exerts different effects on DNA transfection and siRNA-induced gene targeting efficacy. J Drug Target 16:124–139
36. Malek A, Merkel O, Fink L et al (2009) In vivo pharmacokinetics, tissue distribution and underlying mechanisms of various PEI(-PEG)/siRNA complexes. Toxicol Appl Pharmacol 236:97–108
37. Chen C, Ridzon DA, Broomer AJ et al (2005) Real-time quantification of microRNAs by stem-loop RT-PCR. Nucleic Acids Res 33:e179
38. Malek A, Bakhidze E, Noske A et al (2008) HMGA2 gene is a promising target for ovarian cancer silencing therapy. Int J Cancer 123:348–356

Chapter 35

Ligand-Coupled Lipoprotein for Ovarian Cancer-Specific Drug Delivery

Ian R. Corbin

Abstract

Lipoproteins are natural nanosized delivery vehicles within the circulatory system of all mammals. Scientists have long been interested in utilizing these endogenous macromolecules to transport exogenous imaging or therapeutic agents to specific cells or tissues in the body. The broad distribution of lipoprotein receptors throughout the body however has limited the utility of this approach for targeted delivery of medicinal agents. In recent years lipoprotein rerouting strategies have been developed wherein lipoproteins can be redirected from their natural lipoprotein receptors to an alternate receptor of choice. In this chapter we describe the basic methods of preparing folic acid-conjugated high-density lipoprotein nanoparticles for targeted delivery of imaging or chemotherapeutic agents to ovarian cancer cells.

Key words Nanoparticles, High-density lipoprotein, Folic acid, Folate receptor

1 Introduction

Plasma lipoproteins are a family of endogenous macromolecules which serve to transport fat and cholesterol from one cell type to another in a highly organized and coordinated manner. The core-shell structure of lipoproteins together with its receptor-targeting apoprotein moieties resembles many of the synthetic nanoparticles engineered today. In fact many research groups over the years have tried to utilize lipoproteins for drug delivery against cancer. While most cancer cells do express lipoprotein receptors (Particularly for HDL and LDL), many normal tissues also express these receptors at high levels. The poor discrimination of lipoprotein receptor targeting, unfortunately, limits the utility of this strategy. The work of Zheng et al. recently developed and validated a general strategy for rerouting LDL particles to alternate receptors [1]. This approach not only provides a method for targeting lipoproteins to cancer cells with greater specificity but also expands the utility of lipoprotein-based drug delivery systems to cancer cells not expressing LDLR.

Anastasia Malek and Oleg Tchernitsa (eds.), *Ovarian Cancer: Methods and Protocols*, Methods in Molecular Biology, vol. 1049,
DOI 10.1007/978-1-62703-547-7_35, © Springer Science+Business Media New York 2013

The rerouting strategy involves alkylating cancer homing molecules to lysine (Lys) residues in the receptor-targeting moiety of apoB-100 apoprotein. This chemical modification will essentially abolish the binding capability of apoB-100 for the LDLR [2] and simultaneously enable the lipoprotein particle with recognition and affinity for a new receptor dictated by the alkylating ligand. Proof of this rerouting strategy was demonstrated both in vitro and in vivo with folic acid (FA)-conjugated fluorescent LDL nanoparticles [1, 3]. Several years later, this technology was applied to high-density lipoproteins (HDL) [4], the smallest member of the lipoprotein family which in many respects is an ideal candidate as a nanocarrier. The small size (7–12 nm) and endogenous nature of HDL allows it to escape reticular endothelial system (RES) surveillance and circulate for long periods granting it access to most tissues in the body. Furthermore, reconstituted HDL ($_r$HDL) can be self-assembled from individual components (apoA-I and commercial lipids) [5]; this makes it suitable for large-scale production and provides opportunities to introduce alternate components to the nanoparticle formulation. The FA-conjugated HDL prototype was recently reported to be highly efficacious in an orthotopic murine model of ovarian cancer [12]. The high prevalence of FR overexpression in ovarian cancer [6] and the fully biocompatible nature of the HDL nanoparticle make this a rather attractive drug delivery system for ovarian malignancies. Herein we describe the basic methods of preparing FA-conjugated HDL nanoparticles for targeted delivery of diagnostic or therapeutic agents to ovarian cancer cells.

2 Materials

2.1 Apoprotein A-I Isolation

1. HDL isolated from fresh or frozen human plasma (*see* **Note 1**).
2. Diethyl ether and ethanol.
3. Concentrated urea solution: 4 M urea in water.
4. 0.9 % NaCl saline.

2.2 Preparation of $_r$HDL Particles

1. Sonication buffer: 10-mM Tris–HCl, containing 0.1-M KCl, 1-mM EDTA, pH 8.0. Store at room temperature.
2. Egg yolk phosphatidylcholine and cholesteryl oleate.
3. Chloroform.
4. Millipore 0.1-μm syringe filters.
5. Tris buffer saline: 10-mM Tris–HCl, with 0.15-M NaCl, 1-mM EDTA, pH 7.5. Store at room temperature.

2.3 Purification of $_r$HDL Particles

1. KBr Buffer: 0.15-M NaCl, 2-mM EDTA, pH 7.4, KBr is added to produce a density of 1.066 g/ml.
2. Ultracentrifuge.
3. Amicon Centrifugation Filter Device, 10,000-MW cutoff (Millipore, Billerica, MA).
4. Akta FPLC system and a Superdex 200 column (60 × 16 cm) (GE Healthcare, Piscataway, NJ).

2.4 Folic Acid Conjugation of $_r$HDL Nanoparticles

1. Folic acid dehydrate, anhydrous dimethyl sulfoxide (DMSO), triethylamine, *N*-Hydroxysuccinimide (NHS), and dicyclohexylcarbodiimide (DCC).
2. Sodium phosphate/boric acid buffer (0.1 M NaH_2PO_4, 0.1 M H_3BO_3, 1 mM EDTA), pH 9.4, 10 and 10.9.

2.5 Nanoparticle Composition

1. Lowry protein assay kit (Sigma-Aldrich, St. Louis, MO).
2. Phospholipid and cholesteryl-oleate assay kits (Wako Diagnostics, Richmond, VA).
3. UV Spectrophotometer.

2.6 Nanoparticle Size and Morphology

1. Zetasizer Nano-ZS90 (Malvern Instruments, Malvern, UK).
2. Uranyl acetate solution: 2 % saturated aqueous uranyl acetate.
3. Transmission Electron Microscope.

2.7 Equipment and Supplies

1. Millipore 0.1-μm syringe filters.
2. Ultracentrifuge.
3. Amicon Centrifugation Filter Device, 10,000-MW cutoff (Millipore, Billerica, MA).
4. Akta FPLC system and a Superdex 200 column (60 × 16 cm) (GE Healthcare, Piscataway, NJ).
5. UV Spectrophotometer.
6. Zetasizer Nano-ZS90 (Malvern Instruments, Malvern, UK).
7. Uranyl acetate solution: 2 % saturated aqueous uranyl acetate.
8. Transmission Electron Microscope.

3 Methods

3.1 Apoprotein A-I

HDL can be purchased from commercial vendors or isolated from fresh or frozen plasma of healthy donors by sequential ultracentrifugation (*see* **Note 1**). A protocol for the isolation of lipoprotein from plasma will not be discussed in the present work; for a detailed description of this procedure, see Havel et al. [7]. Once the HDL fraction has been isolated from plasma, HDL apoproteins can subsequently be extracted using the delipidation procedure described by Scanu [8]. During this procedure the lipid components of the HDL are completely extracted from the particle with the ethanol–diethyl ether solvent. The remaining protein subsequently precipitates from this solution (due to its low solubility at the indicated temperatures). It is important to note that the protein precipitate occurs when HDL, prior to delipidation, is dialyzed against NaCl, 0.15 M, pH 7 (or buffers of similar pH) but not when the HDL is dialyzed against alkaline buffers (pH 8.6).

1. Mix 1 ml of HDL (approximately 5 mg/ml of protein in 0.9 % NaCl saline) with 50 ml of a prechilled ethanol–diethyl ether 3:2 (v/v). Place the mixture on a multipurpose rotator and rotate the solution for 6 h at −10 to −20 °C. Under these conditions the HDL apoproteins will precipitate from solution (*see* **Note 2**).
2. After the 6-h period, centrifuge (790 × *g*) the sample for 15 min at 1 °C and remove the supernatant. Add 50 ml of fresh prechilled diethyl ether to the protein pellet and return the sample to the rotator to allow further precipitation to proceed overnight at −10 to −20 °C.
3. The next morning centrifuge (790 × *g*) the sample for 15 min at 1 °C and remove the supernatant. Wash the protein pellet three times with diethyl ether to remove any residual lipids (*see* **Notes 3** and **4**).
4. Finally, dry the delipidated protein under a stream of nitrogen and stored as a dry residue at −20°C until use. When the apoprotein is ready to be used for HDL particle formation, resuspend the protein in 4 M urea (*see* **Note 5**).

3.2 Preparation of $_r$HDL Nanoparticles

Reconstituted HDL will be prepared in a two-step process. In the first step, the commercial lipids, egg yolk phosphatidylcholine and cholesteryl oleate or linoleate, will be subjected to sonication to formulate lipid emulsions similar in composition to natural HDL. In the second step, Apo A-I protein is introduced and allowed to react with the lipid emulsion sample to produce the $_r$HDL nanoparticles.

1. Reconstituted HDL particles can be prepared by a co-sonication method (Fig. 1) similar to that described by Pittman [5]. Gently mix chloroform solutions of egg yolk phosphatidylcholine (9 mg), cholesteryl oleate, or linoleate (6 mg) in a glass test tube. Remove the solvent by drying the lipid mixture under a gentle stream of nitrogen to form a thin film of lipids (Fig. 1a). Thereafter, place the sample under a high vacuum for at least 2 h and store the dried lipids in a desiccator overnight at 4°C (*see* **Notes 6–8**).

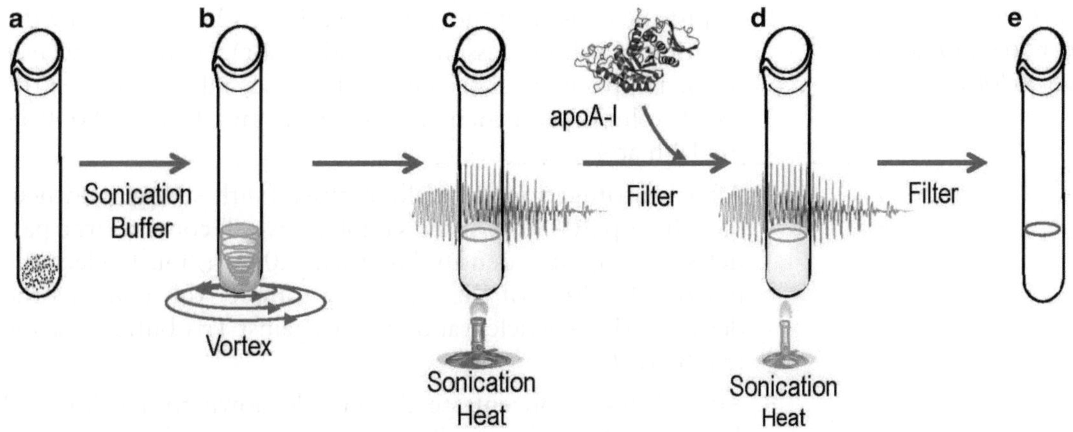

Fig. 1 Schematic depiction of the preparation of $_r$HDL nanoparticles. (**a**) Thin film of dried lipids. (**b**) Warm sonication buffer is added and sample is vortexed intermittently. (**c**) Lipid suspension is sonicated at 49–54 °C. (**d**) Sample is filtered and apoA-I is added dropwise as the sample is sonicated at 40–42 °C. (**e**) Filtered sample with $_r$HDL nanoparticles

2. The next day add 7 ml of warm (50 °C) degassed sonication buffer to the residue and vortex the sample intermittently for 5 min (Fig. 1b) (*see* **Note 9**).
3. After the vortexing step, sonicate the sample for 60 min at 49–54 °C under nitrogen (Fig. 1c) (*see* **Note 10**).
4. Following the first sonication step, filter the emulsion mixture using a 0.1-μm filter to remove large emulsion complexes from the sample (*see* **Note 11**).
5. Lower the temperature of the sonication bath to 40–42 °C and continue to sonicate the filtered sample. During this period, add 10 mg of apoA-I in 4-M urea dropwise to the emulsion mixture over 10-min period. Continue to sonicate the sample for an additional 20 min (Fig. 1d) (*see* **Note 12**).
6. Filter (0.1-μm filter) the heterogeneous mixture of $_r$HDL particles to remove large protein-free emulsion complexes (Fig. 1e) (*see* **Note 13**).

3.3 Purification of $_r$HDL Nanoparticles

In the section described above (Subheading 3.2), $_r$HDL nanoparticles are produced by self-assembly processes governed by the thermodynamics and stoichiometries of the associated apoA-I protein and lipids. As such a heterogenous population of $_r$HDL nanoparticles and emulsions (with and without small amounts of protein) are formed. Here purification of the sample is performed by density ultracentrifugation followed by gel filtration chromatography (*see* **Note 14**).

3.3.1 Removing of Large Low-Density Particles by Density Ultracentrifugation

1. Adjust the density of the $_r$HDL solution to 1.066 g/ml by the addition of solid potassium bromide (KBr). Next, slowly layer room temperature KBr buffer (1.066 g/ml) on top of the $_r$HDL solution and then centrifuge the sample at 160,000 × *g* for 18 h at 4 °C.
2. After centrifugation, carefully remove (with syringe and needle) the top 20–30 % of the sample; this will contain large particles floating at a density less than 1.066 g/ml. Collect the bottom 20–30 % of the remaining sample (this contains the desired $_r$HDL particles) and dialyze against Tris-buffered saline (*see* **Note 15**).
3. After dialysis, concentrate the sample down to a volume of 1 ml using the Amicon Ultra filter device.

3.3.2 Isolation of $_r$HDL Nanoparticles Using Gel Filtration Chromatography

1. The $_r$HDL sample can be further purified by gel filtration chromatography to remove any remaining large particles (void volume) and isolate population of particles resembling HDL_2 (1.063–1.125 g/ml, ~8.8–12 nm) or HDL_3 (1.125–1.21 g/ml, ~7.0–8.9 nm) species. Several gel filtration columns and systems are available; we found using the Superdex 200 column (60 × 16 cm) on the Akta FPLC system (GE Healthcare, Piscataway, NJ) produced very good results. Chromatography should be carried out according to manufacturer's instructions using Tris-buffered saline as a mobile phase at a flow rate of 1 ml/min (Fig. 2).
2. Transmission electron microscopy can be used to examine the size and morphology of the eluted particles of interest (Fig. 3) (*see* **Note 16**).

3.4 Folic Acid Conjugation of $_r$HDL Nanoparticles

To redirect $_r$HDL particles away from the HDL receptor (SR-BI) to FR, folic acid molecules will be attached to the lysine residues of apoA-I. In this procedure the gamma carboxyl of folic acid will be linked to the lysine epsilon amino group of apoA-I via a hydroxysuccinimide ester linker. In the subsections to follow, the folic acid derivative, folate-*N*-hydroxysuccinimide ester, will first be prepared. Thereafter, it will be reacted with $_r$HDL to produce folic acid-conjugated $_r$HDL particles.

3.4.1 Preparation of Folic Acid for Conjugation: Synthesis of Folate-N-Hydroxysuccinimide Ester (FA-NHS) (Fig. 4)

1. Dissolve 54-mg (113-μmol) folic acid dehydrate in a 20-ml reaction flask containing 1 mL of anhydrous dimethyl sulfoxide (DMSO) and 20 μL of triethylamine. Allow this mixture to stir for 1–2 h to dissolve most of the folic acid.
2. Next add 20-mg (170-μmol) *N*-Hydroxysuccinimide and 26-mg (226-μmol) dicyclohexylcarbodiimide to the mixture and allow the reaction to proceed under argon at room temperature for 24 h.
3. Following the reaction, purify the final product FA-NHS by removing by-product dicyclohexylurea by filtration (*see* **Note 17**).

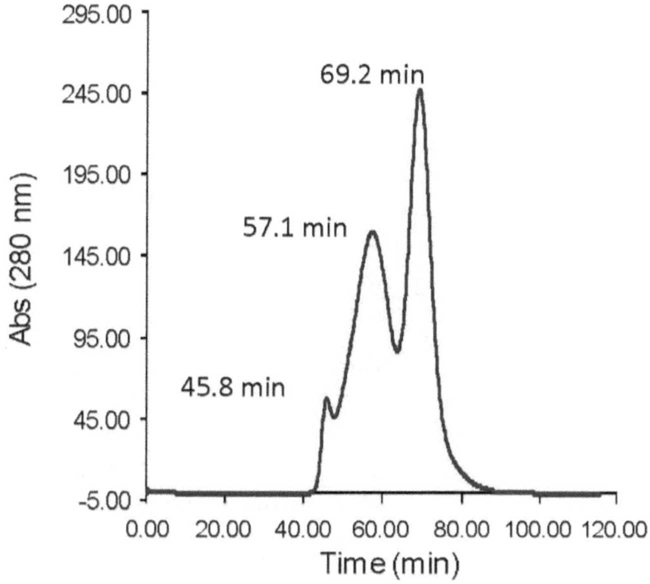

Fig. 2 FPLC profile of $_r$HDL particles. Large particles (>20 nm) from the void volume elute at 46 min. The particles eluting at 57 and 69 min are approximately 13 and 8 nm in size, respectively

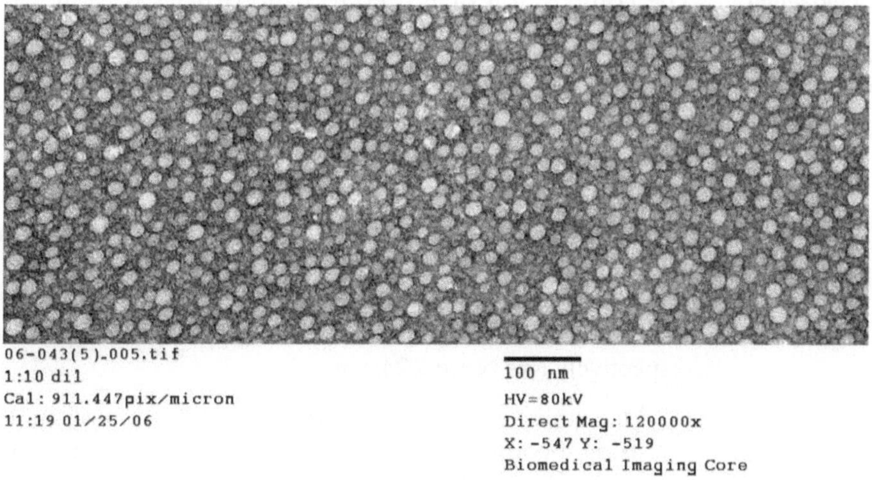

Fig. 3 Transmission electron micrograph of $_r$HDL particles following FPLC (69 min fraction)

3.4.2 Synthesis of FA-$_r$HDL Nanoparticle

1. Aliquot the equivalent of 1 mg of $_r$HDL protein into a separate tube. Raise the pH of the solution to 9.4 by exchanging the Tris-buffered saline with sodium phosphate/boric acid buffer pH 9.4 using the Amicon filter device. Wash the $_r$HDL particles with a total of 6 ml of sodium phosphate/boric acid buffer pH 9.4 and then concentrate the sample down to a volume of 500 μl.

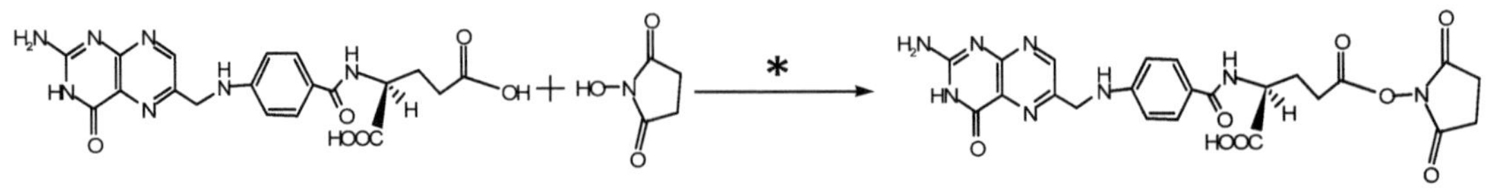

Fig. 4 Reaction scheme for synthesis of FA-NHS

2. In a stepwise fashion, increase the pH of the solution to 10 and then 10.9 as described above (*see* **Note 18**).
3. After the final wash, resuspend the $_{r}$HDL particles in 3 ml of sodium phosphate/boric acid buffer pH 10.9 to give an approximate protein concentration of 0.33 mg/ml.
4. Slowly add the FA-NHS in anhydrous DMSO dropwise to the $_{r}$HDL solution at a molar ratio of 80:1 (FA-NHS–$_{r}$HDL protein). Allow the reaction to run at room temperature for 6–8 h (*see* **Note 19**).
5. Stop the reaction by extensively dialyzing the sample against repeated volumes of Tris-buffered saline overnight at 4 °C. Remove any precipitate that formed during dialysis by filtering sample through a 0.2-μm filter (*see* **Notes 20** and **21**).

3.5 Characterization

3.5.1 Nanoparticle Composition

The composition of FA-$_{r}$HDL nanoparticles is easily determined using a few standard biochemical assays. Typically the composition of these particles is expressed as molar ratios of components per particle. For the smaller (7–9 nm) $_{r}$HDL nanoparticles, usually two apoA-I molecules associate with the particle. The typical molar ratio of phospholipid–cholesteryl oleate–apoA-I–FA for these particles is 56:16:2:40, respectively. Conversely the larger (10–12 nm) $_{r}$HDL nanoparticles can have 3–5 apoA-I molecules per particle. If four molecules of apoA-I is identified with the large $_{r}$HDL (usually the case), the molar ratio of phospholipid–cholesteryl oleate–apoA-I–FA for these particles should be approximately 232:84:4:80, respectively (*see* **Note 22**).

1. Determine the apoA-1 protein concentration of the FA-$_{r}$HDL using a commercial Lowry protein assay kit using a molecular weight of 28,000 Da.
2. Similarly phospholipid and cholesteryl-oleate concentrations can be determined using assay kits from Wako Diagnostics.
3. The amount of FA molecules attached to $_{r}$HDL can be determined from the unique UV absorbance of FA at 280 nm (Fig. 5). Transfer 10 μl of the FA-$_{r}$HDL solution into 1 ml of saline and record the UV spectrum of the diluted sample over a wavelength range of 200–500 nm. The concentration of FA molecules conjugated to $_{r}$HDL can be calculated from a standard curve of free FA (*see* **Note 23**).

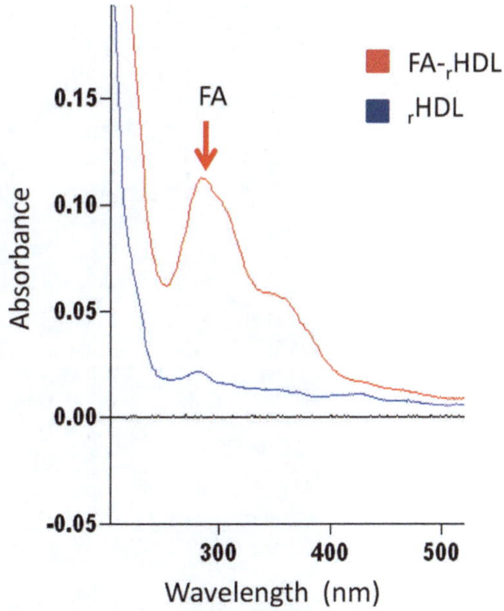

Fig. 5 UV spectra of $_r$HDL (*blue trace*) and FA-$_r$HDL (*red trace*). Characteristic peak belonging to FA is identified at 285 nm

3.5.2 Nanoparticles Size and Morphology

The size and morphology of the FA-$_r$HDL nanoparticles will resemble the quasi-spherical shape of $_r$HDL. The FA-$_r$HDL particles however may report a slightly larger diameter than its starting $_r$HDL nanoparticle due to the addition of folic acid residues to its surface.

1. Take about 20 μl of FA-$_r$HDL nanoparticles, dilute up to 1 ml with purified water, and place in a sample cell of a light-scattering device like Zetasizer Nano-ZS90. Measure the size of the particles following the directions of the instrument.
2. To examine the morphology of the FA-$_r$HDL nanoparticles, a diluted aliquot of the sample should be negatively stained with uranyl acetate solution and viewed using a Transmission Electron Microscope.

3.6 In Vitro FR Targeting with FA-$_r$HDL

To demonstrate the lipoprotein retargeting strategy, $_r$HDL nanoparticles were formulated with the near infrared dye, DiRBOA (1,1′-dioctadecyl-3,3,3′,3′-tetramethylindotricarbocyanine iodide bis-oleate). Thereafter, the folic acid-conjugated $_r$HDL-DiRBOA was prepared. FR-positive murine ovarian cancer cells, MOSEC clonal line IC5, were exposed to equal concentrations of $_r$HDL-DiRBOA and FA-$_r$HDL-DiRBOA (Fig. 6a, b). Figure 6a demonstrates that very little of the $_r$HDL was taken up by the ovarian cancer cells indicated by the low levels of fluorescence; conversely following FA-$_r$HDL-DiRBOA incubation, pronounced fluorescence can be

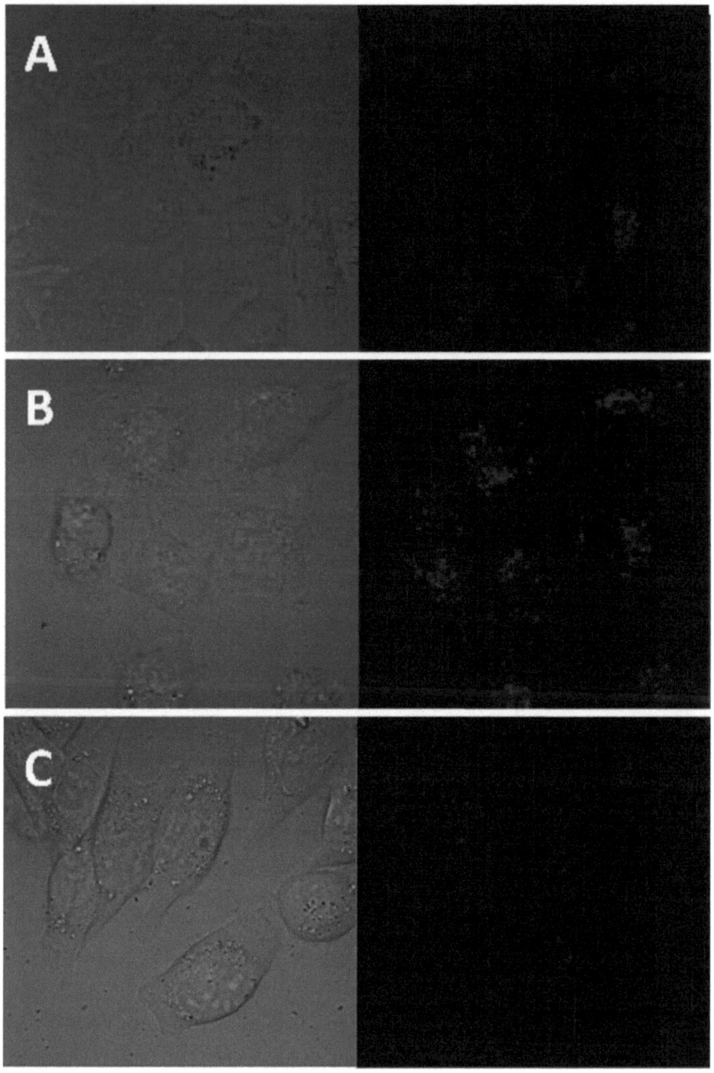

Fig. 6 Fluorescent (*right*) and corresponding bright field (*left*) confocal images of IC5 ovarian cancer cells incubated with (**a**) $_r$HDL-DiRBOA (1.2 μM) or (**b**) FA-$_r$HDL-DiRBOA (1.2 μM) for 3 h. Inhibition studies (**c**) were performed with FA-$_r$HDL-DiRBOA (1.2 μM) and 600-fold excess free folic acid

seen in the cells indicative of avid uptake of this nanoparticle. Additional studies later showed that excess free folic acid can block the uptake of FA-$_r$HDL-DiRBOA in IC5 ovarian cancer cells (Fig. 6c). Collectively these experiments demonstrate the enhanced efficacy of targeting ovarian cancer cells using FA-conjugated $_r$HDL nanoparticles.

4 Notes

1. A number of commercial vendors sell plasma lipoprotein products. However, these products are typically quite expensive at a cost $300–400 per 10-mg protein. Most investigators isolate their desired lipoproteins of interest from pathogen-free normal human plasma attained from a local blood bank or clinical laboratory.
2. A number of exchangeable apoproteins associate with plasma HDL; these include apoproteins A-I, A-II, CI, CII, CIII, D, and E. Of these proteins, apoprotein A-I (apoA-I) is the principle structural and functional protein of HDL, accounting for 70 % of the total HDL protein. Thus the major apoprotein extracted from the plasma HDL samples will be the apoA-I species.
3. The delipidation procedure will remove essentially all cholesterol and triglycerides and the majority of phospholipids from the sample. Only a residual amount of phospholipids are anticipated to remain after this procedure (~3 % by weight of the total isolated protein).
4. Supernatants collected from the 6 h and overnight incubations can be pooled to precipitate any residual protein remaining in these solutions.
5. The high ionic strength of the concentrated urea solutions maintains apoA-I in a denatured, unfolded monomeric state.
6. Phosphatidylcholine and cholesteryl oleate/linoleate were selected to make the $_{r}$HDL particles because they, respectively, make up 80 % and 25–60 % of the phospholipid and cholesterol ester species in plasma HDL [9, 10]. This two-component formulation simplifies the preparation $_{r}$HDL and accurately reproduces the basic composition of natural HDL.
7. Trace amounts of radio- (e.g., [1α, 2α(n)-^{3}H]cholesteryl oleate, L-3-Phosphatidylcholine, 1-palmitoyl-2-[1-^{14}C]oleoyl)—or fluorescent (e.g., NBD-12 cholesterol)—labeled lipids can be incorporated into the formulation of HDL. Such probes can be used to track the activity of the targeted HDL nanoparticle in subsequent functional and biodistribution studies.
8. Incorporating anticancer drugs into the $_{r}$HDL formulation is somewhat more challenging. First, the drug of choice must have a sufficient degree of hydrophobicity for it to strongly associate with the $_{r}$HDL particle. Second, a significant amount of drug must be incorporated into $_{r}$HDL in order for the particle to be therapeutically active. The incorporation of drugs or imaging probes into lipoprotein platforms is greatly facilitated if a long unsaturated hydrocarbon chain (e.g., oleic or linoleic acid)

or a branched side chain moiety (e.g., polyisoprenes such as phytol) is linked to the drug/probe. These fatty acyl groups help "anchor" the drug/probe into the lipoprotein particle. Paclitaxel oleate is an example of this [11].

9. Vortexing the sample prior to sonication aids in pulling the dried lipid residue off the test tube walls and into solution. As the lipids are pulled into solution, an opaque dispersion will be formed.
10. Sonication can be performed with either a needle tip or bath sonicator. For needle tip sonication, a Branson Sonifier 350 can be used. Samples are sonicated at a 5-min pulse followed by 1 min of cooling to prevent sample overheating. This cycle is repeated up to ten times until the sample becomes translucent. Alternately, a temperature-controlled Branson ultrasonic bath can be used; samples sealed under nitrogen can be sonicated continuously for 60 min. Regardless of which sonication method is selected, this procedure functions to mechanically disperse the emulsion particles and minimize the size and heterogeneity of particles in the sample.
11. Under these conditions the majority of emulsion particles formed should be approximately 35 nm in diameter. Filtration is performed to remove large emulsions that may later interfere with the apoA-I-mediated $_r$HDL formation in the subsequent steps.
12. ApoA-I, solubilized in 4 M urea, is slowly introduced into a tenfold greater volume of lipid dispersion during the second sonication step. This is performed to allow the urea concentration to fall below a critical concentration (0.4 M) needed for apoA-I protein renaturation. The renatured apoA-I preferentially and more efficiently associates with lipid dispersion than self-associate.
13. ApoA-I preferentially and more strongly associates with smaller emulsions (~35 nm). Upon binding and penetrating into the emulsions phospholipid surface entropic energetics favor the formation HDL like particles 7–12 nm in size. Conversely apoA-I binding to the larger emulsions are weaker, and thus the thermodynamics and stoichiometries are less likely to form particles similar in size to HDL.
14. For $_r$HDL nanoparticles labeled with a visible fluorophore/chromophore, the purification steps will be easier as you will be able to see the floating low-density particles and the pellet of $_r$HDL during ultracentrifugation and the eluted fractions of interest during gel filtration chromatography.
15. This density ultracentrifugation method will remove larger low-density particles and sediment particles with densities greater than 1.066 g/ml (native HDL density 1.063–1.21 g/ml).

16. Negative stain transmission electron microscopy (with uranyl acetate) is most typically used to observe lipoprotein particles. The $_r$HDL nanoparticles will display a quasi-spherical morphology, which is similar to that observed for natural HDL.
17. Due to stability issues, FA-NHS should be made fresh for each conjugation reaction.
18. The lysine residues in apoA-I on $_r$HDL have a pK_as ranging from 8.3 to 10.5. In order for the majority of the lysines to be able to react with FA-NHS, the $_r$HDL sample was titrated up to a pH of 10.9.
19. Each apoA-I protein contains 21 lysine residues. Given that each $_r$HDL nanoparticles has two apoA-I molecules, 42 lysine residues per particle are available for FA-NHS conjugation. Using the conditions described in Subheading 3.4.2 (molar ratio of FA-NHS–$_r$HDL protein = 80:1; fourfold excess), essentially all of the lysine residues (90–100 %) of apoA-I in $_r$HDL will be conjugated with FA.
20. Repeated dialysis should be performed after the FA-NHS–$_r$HDL conjugation to remove excess free FA-NHS.
21. In spite of the harsh conditions during FA-NHS conjugation, there is little degradation of the $_r$HDL nanoparticle. Typically no more than 10–20 % of the protein is lost during this procedure.
22. When an imaging probe or drug is added to the nanoparticle formulation, appropriate assays should be included to quantify the amount of these probes/drugs in the nanoparticle composition.
23. When quantifying the amount of FA-conjugated to $_r$HDL, a standard curve of HDL should also be performed to determine how much the $_r$HDL nanoparticles contribute to the absorbance reading at 280 nm.

Acknowledgement

This work was supported by the SW-SAIRP (U24 CA126608).

References

1. Zheng G, Chen J, Li H et al (2005) Rerouting lipoprotein nanoparticles to selected alternate receptors for the targeted delivery of cancer diagnostic and therapeutic agents. Proc Natl Acad Sci USA 102:17757–17762
2. Lund-Katz S, Ibdah JA, Letizia JY et al (1988) A 13C NMR characterization of lysine residues in apolipoprotein B and their role in binding to the low density lipoprotein receptor. J Biol Chem 263:13831–13838
3. Chen J, Corbin IR, Li H et al (2007) Ligand conjugated low-density lipoprotein nanoparticles for enhanced optical cancer imaging in vivo. J Am Chem Soc 129:5798–5799
4. Corbin IR, Chen J, Cao W et al (2007) Enhanced cancer-targeted delivery using engineered high-

density lipoprotein-based nanocarriers. J Biomed Nanotechnol 3:367–376

5. Pittman RC, Glass CK, Atkinson D et al (1987) Synthetic high density lipoprotein particles. Application to studies of the apoprotein specificity for selective uptake of cholesterol esters. J Biol Chem 262:2435–2442
6. Kalli KR, Oberg AL, Keeney GL et al (2008) Folate receptor alpha as a tumor target in epithelial ovarian cancer. Gynecol Oncol 108:619–626
7. Havel RJ, Eder HA, Bragdon JH (1955) The distribution and chemical composition of ultracentrifugally separated lipoproteins in human serum. J Clin Invest 34:1345–1353
8. Scanu A (1966) Forms of human serum high density lipoprotein protein. J Lipid Res 7:295–306
9. Lund-Katz S, Liu L, Thuahnai ST et al (2003) High density lipoprotein structure. Front Biosci 8:d1044–d1054
10. Wang ST, Andrusco R, Peter F (1987) A comparison of fatty acid composition of cholesteryl esters in subjects at various concentrations of serum lipid. Clin Biochem 20:31–35
11. Nikanjam M, Gibbs AR, Hunt CA et al (2007) Synthetic nano-LDL with paclitaxel oleate as a targeted drug delivery vehicle for glioblastoma multiforme. J Control Release 124: 163–171
12. Corbin IR, Ng KK, Ding L, Jurisicova A, Zheng G (2013) Near Infrared Fluorescent Imaging of Metastatic Ovarian Cancer using Folate Receptor Targeted High-density Lipoprotein Nanocarriers. Nanomedicine (Lond) 8(6):875–890

Chapter 36

Mesoporous Silicon Particles for Sustained Gene Silencing

Nafis Hasan, Aman Mann, Mauro Ferrari, and Takemi Tanaka

Abstract

RNA interference (RNAi) is a powerful approach for silencing oncogenes; however, in vivo RNAi delivery has remained a major challenge due to lack of safe, efficient, and sustained delivery. Here, we describe a novel approach to overcome these limitations using mesoporous silicon particles loaded with nanoparticles (i.e., liposomes) containing small interfering RNA (siRNA) targeted against oncoprotein that contributes to cancer cell survival. This delivery method resulted in sustained gene silencing for at least 3 weeks with substantial reduction of tumor growth with no overt toxicities in two independent orthotopic mouse models of ovarian cancer following a single intravenous administration of mesoporous silicon particles loaded with liposomal EphA2-siRNA.

Key words RNA interference, Small interfering RNA, Nanoparticle, Liposome, Multistage delivery, Ovarian cancer, Sustained gene silencing, Mesoporous silicon particle

1 Introduction

RNA interference (RNAi) has recently emerged as a new therapeutic option with exceptional promise because of its ability to silence any gene of known sequence. In the past 10 years, RNAi has evolved rapidly as a new therapeutic option for many types of diseases including cancer. For example, there are ongoing clinical trials to evaluate the efficacy of small interfering RNA (siRNA) for the treatment of cancer [1], age-related macular degeneration (AMD) [2, 3], and respiratory syncytial virus infection (RSV) [4].

While many new molecular targets have been identified [5], some are simply not druggable with conventional therapeutic strategies (i.e., small molecule inhibitors or monoclonal antibody). In fact, molecular targets for monoclonal antibodies are limited to extracellular components (i.e., ligands or surface receptors) [6, 7] and rational design information regarding three-dimensional structures. In this regard, RNAi is a particularly attractive approach and opens up a new window to modulate a wide variety of oncogenes, which have not been druggable. While RNAi offers a great promise for future

Anastasia Malek and Oleg Tchernitsa (eds.), *Ovarian Cancer: Methods and Protocols*, Methods in Molecular Biology, vol. 1049, DOI 10.1007/978-1-62703-547-7_36,

medicine, the challenges remain for RNAi to be clinically applicable, and these include the following: poor pharmacokinetics due to lack of serum stability and rapid clearance [8], poor cellular uptake due to the negative charge [9], and potential toxicities [10, 11].

To overcome these limitations, a number of delivery strategies have been developed. One such strategy is nanoparticle-mediated RNAi delivery which has achieved significant improvements in cellular uptake in both animal models [10, 12–14] and human clinical trials [2, 15]. Conversely, unfavorable pharmacokinetics of RNAi has not been improved yet and remains the major obstacle particularly for cancer treatment. Due to the fact that gene silencing requires continuous downregulation of a target gene, most of the current RNAi delivery approaches require frequent intravenous injection [16, 17]. For example, twice weekly intravenous or intraperitoneal administration of liposomes containing siRNA against oncogenes was essential to achieve continuous in vivo gene silencing accompanied by tumor growth inhibition in orthotopic ovarian cancer mouse models. While promising, a requirement of multiple injections is a substantial impediment for clinical applications [18], and therefore, the development of a safe delivery system that allows for sustained gene silencing is crucial.

We have developed a novel multistage delivery strategy based on nanoporous silicon particles (PSP) that can be microfabricated with different sizes, shapes, and porosities [19]. Size and shape are regulated by the photolithographic masks, whereas the pore dimension and porosity are adjusted through the chemical composition and anodization conditions. Based on protocol we developed, the outer dimension of the particles can be altered at ranges from 500 nm to 20 μm in size with different shapes. The mean pore size ranges from 5 to 80 nm, and the porosity ranged from 40 to 80 %. The surface chemistry of the PSPs can be modified to negative (oxidized), positive [3-aminopropyltriethoxysilane (APTES)-modified], or neutral charges (counterion or PEGylated). In principle, PSPs are loaded with nanoparticles such as liposome, Qdot, and metal nanoparticles, and their porous structure will be filled with nanoparticles. The nanoparticles can be released over time as the PSPs degrade, the overall size diminishes, and the pore size enlarges, allowing the delivery of large amounts of payload for prolonged periods. In addition, unlike bulk silicon, PSPs are highly biocompatible and biodegradable. Intravenous injection of PSPs induced neither the cytokine productions nor elevation of blood chemistry in mouse in both acute and chronic settings [20]. The PSPs degrade into silicic acid under physiological condition, either eliminated renally or deposited into connective tissues. The degradation kinetics depends on the surface modification and porosity of the PSPs. For example, for sustained delivery of liposomal siRNA, less porosified PSPs have been used, while highly porosified PSPs are ideal choice for rapid release of nanoparticles from the porous structure. The biodistribution of the PSP may be influenced by the size and shape of the PSPs. Following the intravenous injection of PSP, silicon content analysis demonstrated that PSPs were primarily accumulated in the liver (48 %) and spleen (17 % of total injected dose) and there was no to minimal PSP accumulation in the kidney, lung, and heart [20, 21]. Transmission electron microscopic analyses of the liver and spleen sections confirmed that PSPs remained within sinusoidal spaces in the liver and red pulp in the spleen. However, based on our microscopic analysis, there is no evidence of embolization of PSP in the capillaries. Interestingly, biodegradation of intravenously injected PSPs is also affected by the organs. When PSPs were intravenously injected, silicon contents in the spleen were reduced by 80 % in the first 2 weeks and cleared by the third week. In contrast, only 55 % of PSP was cleared from the liver in the first 2 weeks, and approximately 25 % of the injected PSP remained in the liver 3 weeks after injection [21].

The approach described herein was developed to achieve sustained in vivo gene silencing. We deployed a two-stage delivery system (so-called multistage vector or MSV) that is comprised of biocompatible and biodegradable mesoporous silicon particles (PSPs) which serve as a carrier and DOPC liposomes containing the siRNA against EphA2 that overexpresses in ovarian cancer (EphA2-siRNA-lip) [20]. Our study demonstrated that a single intravenous administration of PSP loaded with EphA2-siRNA-lip resulted in sustained gene silencing for 3 weeks concomitant with significant tumor growth inhibition with minimal toxicity in two independent mouse models of orthotopic ovarian cancer.

2 Materials

2.1 PSP Preparation

1. Si (100) wafer, p^{2+} type, with a resistivity of 0.005 Ω/cm, was purchased from Silicon Quest (San Jose, CA, USA).
2. Hydrofluoric acid 49 %.
3. 100 % ethanol.
4. Isopropanol.
5. Potassium phosphate buffer 10 mM (pH 7.3).
6. Freshly prepared piranha solution (1 volume H_2O_2 and 2 volumes H_2SO_4).
7. 3-Aminopropyltriethoxysilane (APTES) was purchased from Sigma-Aldrich (St. Louis, MO, USA).

2.2 Multistage Delivery System

1. Control siRNAs (5′-AATTCTCCGAACGTGTCACGT-3′) and Alexa 555-tagged counterparts (5′-AATTCTCCGAA-CGTGTCACGT-3′) were purchased from Qiagen (Valencia, CA, USA).
2. siRNAs against EphA2 (5′-AATGACATGCCGATCTA-CATG-3′) were purchased from Sigma-Aldrich.
3. 1,2-Dioleoyl-*sn*-glycero-3-phosphatidylcholine (DOPC) was purchased from Avanti Polar Lipids (Alabaster, AL, USA).
4. Porous silicon particles were fabricated as described.
5. Tertiary butanol (*t*-butanol) was purchased from Sigma Chemical.
6. Nominal molecular weight limit filter units were purchased from Millipore (Billerica, MA, USA).

2.3 Cell Culture

1. SKOV3ip1-Lc and HeyA8-Lc (obtained from Anil K. Sood laboratory, MD Anderson Cancer Center, Texas, USA).
2. Fetal bovine serum (FBS) was purchased from Gemini Bio Products (Calabasas, CA, USA). Dispense into 50 mL aliquots and store at −20°C. Thaw before adding to culture medium.
3. Serum-free Hank's buffered salt solution (HBSS) was purchased from Life Technologies (Carlsbad, CA, USA).
4. Roswell Park Memorial Institute, Formula 1640 (RPMI 1640) supplemented with 15 % fetal bovine serum (FBS) and 0.1 % gentamicin sulfate was purchased from Gemini Bio Products.

2.4 Animals

1. Female athymic nude mice (NCr-nu; 4–5 weeks old) were purchased from Taconic Farms (Hudson, NY, USA).

2.5 Western Blotting

1. Modified radioimmunoprecipitation assay (RIPA) buffer—50 mM Tris–HCl, 150 mM NaCl, 1 % Triton, 0.5 % deoxycholate plus 25 μg/mL leupeptin, 10 μg/mL aprotinin, 2 mM EDTA, and 1 m sodium orthovanadate (Sigma-Aldrich).
2. BCA Protein Assay Reagent Kit purchased from Pierce Biotechnology (Rockford, IL, USA).
3. 10 % SDS-PAGE.
4. Tris-buffered saline (TBS). 10× TBS: 0.5 M Tris base, 9 % NaCl, pH 8.4.
5. 5 % nonfat milk in TBS.
6. Horseradish peroxidase-conjugated IgG for EphA2 detection purchased from Amersham Biosciences (Piscataway, NJ, USA).
7. Chemiluminescence detection kit purchased from Pierce Biotechnology.
8. Semidry electrophoresis kit purchased from Bio-Rad Laboratories (Hercules, CA, USA).

9. Purified, monoclonal mouse anti-EphA2 antibody purchased from Upstate (Millipore, Billerica, MA, USA).
10. Horseradish peroxidase (HRP)-conjugated anti-mouse IgG was purchased from Amersham Biosciences.
11. Anti-β-actin primary antibody was purchased from Sigma Chemical.

2.6 Immunohistochemistry

1. Xylene.
2. Ethanol—100, 95, and 80 %.
3. Phosphate-buffered saline buffer (PBS), 10×: 137 mM NaCl, 2.7 mM KCl, 10 mM $Na_2HPO_4{\cdot}2H_2O$, 2 mM KH_2PO_4, pH 7.4.
4. 0.2 mol/L Tris–HCl (pH 9.0).
5. Hydrogen peroxide (H_2O_2), 30 %. Prepare 3 % H_2O_2 fresh.
6. Pap pen for hydrophobic barrier.
7. Mouse IgG Fc blocker was purchased from The Jackson Laboratory (Bar Harbor, ME, USA).
8. TSA Biotin System Kit for blocking agent purchased from PerkinElmer (Boston, MA, USA).
9. Primary antibody, mouse anti-EphA2 clone EA5, was a kind gift from Dr. Michael Kinch, MedImmune Inc. (Gaithersburg, MD, USA).
10. Secondary antibody, biotinylated horse anti-mouse, purchased from Vector Labs (Burlingame, CA, USA).
11. Secondary Ab signal enhancer, streptavidin-HRP, purchased from DakoCytomation (Carpinteria, CA, USA).
12. Signal detection with 3,3′-diaminobenzidine (DAB) purchased from Phoenix Biotechnologies (Huntsville, AL, USA).
13. Hematoxylin solution, Gill no. 3, from Sigma Chemical.

2.7 Equipment and Supplies

1. Electrochemical etching (Model 790+® RIE Plasma-Therm, USA).
2. Sputtering system (Varian sputter, San Jose, USA).
3. Sonicator (Model 2510, Branson, USA).
4. ZetaPALS analyzer (Brookhaven Instruments, Holtsville, NY, USA).
5. Multisizer (Beckman Coulter, Brea, CA, USA).
6. Quantachrome Autosorb-3B surface analyzer (Quantachrome Instruments, Boynton Beach, FL, USA).

3 Methods

3.1 Preparation and Assembly of Multistage Delivery System

The multistage delivery system devised for sustained siRNA delivery is comprised of two delivery systems—mesoporous silicon particles (PSP) and the DOPC liposomes containing the siRNA (Fig. 1).

3.1.1 Preparation of Mesoporous Silicon Particles

The microfabrication of mesoporous silicon particles requires access to a cleanroom facility.

1. To fabricate the mesoporous silicon particles of a desired porosity, pore size, and thickness, apply electrochemical etching of a heavily doped p^{2+} type Si (100 mm) wafer with a resistivity of 0.005 Ω/cm, as previously described [19]. Apply a current density of 320 mA/cm^2 for 6 s in a 49 % hydrofluoric acid (HF): ethanol mixture with a ratio of 2:5 (v/v) to adjust the density of porous silicon particles (1.6 μm diameter) with

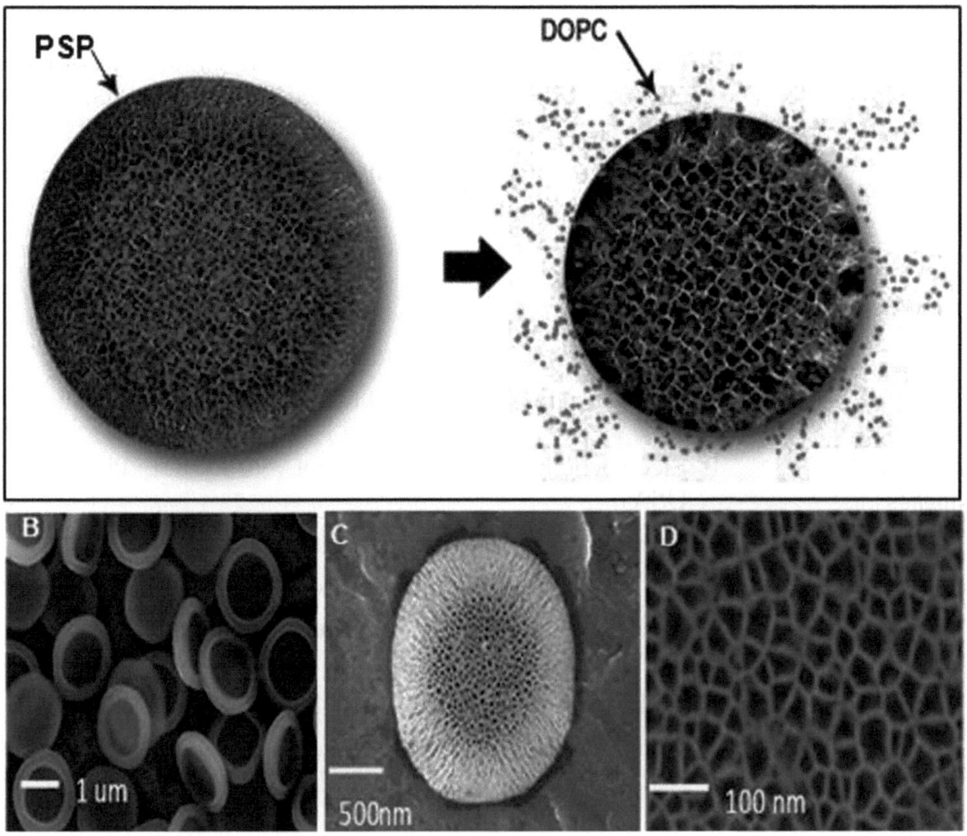

Fig. 1 Assembly of PSP-siRNA-lip. (**a**) Concept of multistage delivery system. (**b–d**) Scanning electron microscopic images of PSP at different magnifications

pore size (40–60 nm). After removing the nitride layer by HF, rinse and spin-dry the wafer, then place in a glass crystallization dish filled with isopropanol (IPA) (40 mL), and sonicate for 1 min to detach the particles from the bulk wafer. Finally, transfer the release suspension to a 50 mL low-retention tube and store in a controlled-temperature environment at 20 °C.

2. Analyze the surface charge of the particles using a ZetaPALS instrument and the size and the number of PSP using a Multisizer. For charge measurement, add 2 μL of PSPs to 1.4 mL of 10 mM phosphate buffer (pH 7.3) and conduct the analysis at room temperature (23 °C) in triplicates. To measure the surface area and pore size of the PSPs, use N_2 adsorption–desorption isotherms on a Quantachrome Autosorb-3B surface analyzer [19]. Quality control techniques such as scanning electron microscopy and transmission electron microscopy can also be employed to determine the pore shape and structure as previously described [19].
3. Modify the surface of PSP by transferring the suspension containing PSP to a glass beaker and evaporate the IPA overnight using a hot-plate set at 110 °C. Treat the dried PSP with piranha solution (1 volume H_2O_2 and 2 volumes H_2SO_4) with heating to 110–120 °C for 2 h with intermittent sonication to disperse the PSP. Wash the oxidized PSP in IPA, and then suspend in IPA containing 9 % (v/v) 3-aminopropyltriethoxysilane (APTES) for 16 h at 35 °C and 340×*g*. Wash the APTES-modified PSP in 100 % IPA for five times and store in IPA at 4 °C. Measure the surface charge of PSP by ZetaPALS to confirm modification. PSP is amino functionalized.

3.1.2 Liposome Preparation and Multistage Delivery System Assembly

1. Mix 1,2-dioleoyl-*sn*-glycero-3-phosphocholine (DOPC) with siRNA (20:1, mol/mol) in the presence of excess *t-butanol* to self-assemble the liposomes containing the EphA2-siRNA.
2. Add Tween 20 to the mixture in a ratio of 1:19 Tween 20:siRNA/DOPC.
3. Vortex, freeze the mixture in an acetone/dry ice bath, and lyophilize overnight (*see* **Note 1**).
4. Mix the amino-functionalized PSP (1×10^7 particles) with 100 μL of *t*-butanol and sonicate briefly. Spin down at 785×*g* at room temperature and repeat this process three times (*see* **Note 2**).
5. Resuspend silicon particles in 50 μL *t*-butanol and dry using SpeedVac at room temperature. The dried particles can be stored in either −20° or 4 °C for up to 5 months (*see* **Note 3**).
6. Reconstitute DOPC liposomes containing siRNA (5 μg siRNA) in 15 μL water followed by brief sonication in water bath (*see* **Note 4**).

7. Mix dry silicon particles pellet with 15 μL liposomes containing siRNA (siRNA-lip).
8. Briefly sonicate the mixture in water bath sonicator for 1 min (*see* **Note 5**).
9. Centrifuge at 1,400 × *g* to remove supernatant containing unincorporated free siRNA-lip (*see* **Note 6**).
10. Wash the pellet with 100 μL of DI water (*see* **Note** 7).
11. Centrifuge at 1,400 × *g* for 1 min at room temperature.
12. Resuspend the pellet in 100 μL saline and sonicate briefly before injection to mice (*see* **Note 8** and Fig. 1).

3.2 Orthotopic Ovarian Tumor Mouse Model and MSV Application

1. Acclimate mice to their surroundings for 7–10 days before initiation of any experimental procedures.
2. Two different ovarian cancer cell lines were used for the study—SKOV3ip1-Lc and HeyA8-Lc. Maintain both cultures in complete RPMI 1640 medium. All experiments should be performed at 70–80 % confluency of the cells (*see* **Note 9**).
3. For in vivo injection, trypsinize and centrifuge cells at 87 × *g* for 7 min at 4 °C, wash twice, and reconstitute in serum-free HBSS at a concentration of 1×10^6 cells/mL for 200 μL i.p. injections.
4. Inject the cells (1×10^6 cells in 0.2 mL HBSS) into female nude mice intraperitoneally using a 21–23 gauge needle (*see* **Note 10**).
5. Intravenously inject PSP loaded with triple-dose EphA2-siRNA-lip (15 μg EphA2-siRNA/2×10^6 PSP in 100 μL saline) via the tail vein ($n = 5$) (*see* **Notes 11** and **12**).
6. Approximately 2 to 3 weeks after the injection of PSP, tumor should be collected for sustained gene silencing. Alternatively, tumors can be collected weekly after PSP injection to ensure the sustained gene silencing.
7. For sample collection, euthanize mice using CO_2 chamber. Harvest tumors from peritoneal cavity and measure the weight and number of tumor nodules.
8. Snap freeze tumors in liquid nitrogen for Western blotting and fix in buffered formalin for immunohistochemistry.
9. A single intravenous administration of PSP loaded with triple-dose EphA2-siRNA-lip resulted in a significant reduction of tumor growth (tumor weight) in both SKOV3 and HeyA8 ovarian cancer mouse models (Fig. 2).

3.3 Evaluation of Gene Silencing

Tumor samples were analyzed post-treatment with the PSP-siRNA-lip constructs using Western blotting and immunohistochemistry.

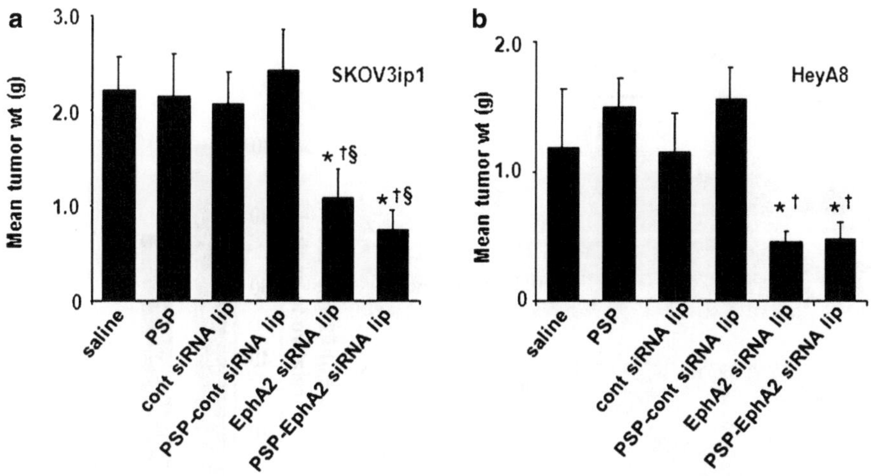

Fig. 2 Therapeutic efficacy of sustained EphA2-siRNA-liposome (EphA2-siRNA-lip) delivery by PSP. Nude mice were injected i.p. with SKOV3ip1 or HeyA8 cells and randomly allocated to one of six treatment groups ($n = 10$): (a) saline, (b) PSP, (c) nonsilencing control siRNA-lip, (d) PSP-nonsilencing control siRNA-lip, (e) EphA2-siRNA-lip, and (f) PSP-EphA2-siRNA-lip. siRNA-lip was i.v. injected biweekly at a dose of 5 μg siRNA. PSP-EphA2-siRNA-lip was injected in a single administration in 3 weeks at a dose of 15 μg siRNA. The mice were injected with saline biweekly in the rest of treatment period. When control animals (saline- and nonsilencing siRNA-treated mice) began to appear moribund (4–5 weeks after cell injection), all animals in an experiment were sacrificed, and mouse weight, tumor weight (wt), tumor number, ascites volume, and tumor location were recorded. Columns, mean tumor weight from SKOV3ip1 (**a**) or HeyA8 cells (**b**); bars, SD (*$p < 0.05$ compared to PSP, §$p < 0.05$ compared to saline, †$p < 0.05$ compared to PSP-cont siRNA-lip)

3.3.1 Western Blotting

1. Prepare lysate from snap-frozen tissues with the following steps—incubate approximately 30-mm³ sections of tissue on ice in RIPA buffer for 30 min and disrupt with a potter homogenizer (10–15 strokes) (*see* **Note 13**).
2. Centrifuge at 17,100 × *g* for 10 min at 4 °C to collect supernatants. Store the supernatant at −80 °C until used.
3. Determine protein concentrations using a BCA Protein Assay Reagent Kit and use 30 μg of total proteins for 10 % SDS-PAGE (*see* **Note 14**).
4. Transfer samples to a polyvinylidene difluoride membrane, block with 5 % nonfat milk, and incubate with primary antibody overnight at 4 °C.
5. Detect primary antibody against EphA2 with horseradish peroxidase-conjugated IgG.
6. Visualize the target gene expression using an enhanced chemiluminescence detection kit. Test membranes for β-actin to confirm equal loading.
7. Western blot data demonstrated that a single intravenous administration of PSP loaded with triple-dose EphA2-siRNA-lip resulted in reduced protein expression of EphA2 in the ovarian tumors at least for 21 days (Fig. 3a, b) (*see* **Note 15**).

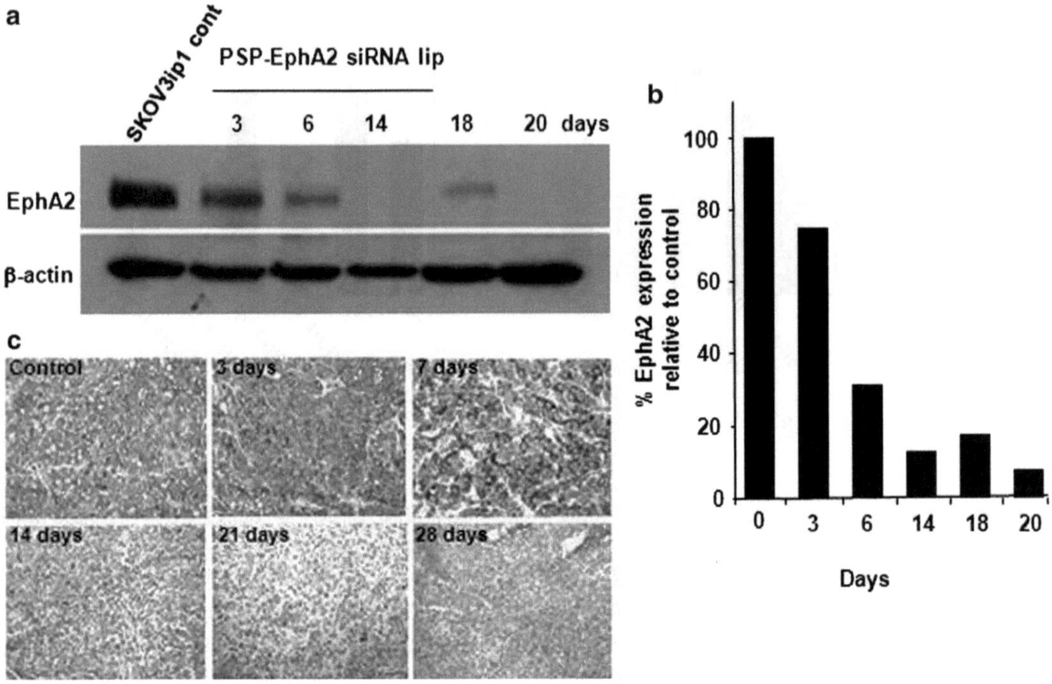

Fig. 3 Systemic delivery of siRNA-liposome (siRNA-lip) using PSP results in long-lasting in vivo gene silencing. The mice (three mice per time point) bearing SKOV3ip1 orthotopic ovarian tumors were injected with PSP-EphA2-siRNA-lip or left nontreated. (**a**) The tumors were harvested at the indicated time points for Western blot to measure EphA2 expression levels. (**b**) Densitometric analysis was performed to normalize EphA2 expression by β-actin. Data were expressed as % of normalized value to the nontreated. (**c**) Immunohistochemical analysis of EphA2 expression in the SKOV1ip3 tumor. Images were taken at original magnification of ×400

3.3.2 Immunohistochemistry

1. Use formalin-fixed, paraffin-embedded tumor sections of 8 μm thickness for EphA2 staining.
2. Bake the slides in 60 °C oven overnight.
3. Deparaffinize sections by sequential washing with xylene, 100 % ethanol, 95 % ethanol, 80 % ethanol, and 100 % DI water and PBS.
4. Perform antigen retrieval by heating in a steam cooker in 0.2 mol/L Tris–HCl (pH 9.0) for 20 min.
5. Draw a hydrophobic boundary around section using a pap pen.
6. Following cooling and PBS wash, block endogenous peroxide using 3 % H_2O_2 in methanol for 5 min.
7. Block nonspecific proteins and exposed endogenous mouse IgG antibodies with 0.13 μg/mL mouse IgG Fc blocker in 0.5 % blocking agent overnight at 4 °C.
8. Incubate slides with primary antibody, 5 μg/ml mouse anti-EphA2 clone EA5 for 4 h at 4 °C, and wash with PBS.

9. Incubate the slides for 1 h incubation at room temperature with 1.5 μg/mL biotinylated horse anti-mouse.
10. Wash the slides with PBS three times.
11. Add 0.75 μg/mL streptavidin-HRP for 30 min to enhance secondary antibody signal, and detect with 3,3′-diaminobenzidine (DAB) for 7 min.
12. Wash the slides three times with PBS.
13. Counterstain with Gill no. 3 hematoxylin for 20 s.
14. Wash with water and then PBS.
15. For image analysis, examine five randomly selected high-power (100×) fields exclusive of necrotic areas per slide and at least three individual tumors per group. Count positively stained cells and express as % of total number of cells in a particular field of view.
16. Immunohistochemistry of EphA2 demonstrated that a single intravenous administration of PSP loaded with triple-dose EphA2-siRNA-lip resulted in a reduced expression of EphA2 in the ovarian epithelium (Fig. 3c).

4 Notes

1. After lyophilization, liposome should form dry powder. If it looks wet, liposome may not be used for the loading to PSP.
2. Fixed-angle microcentrifuge can be used to pellet them down when PSP is resuspended in *t*-butanol. Sonication is needed to avoid aggregation.
3. Loading capacity of PSP remains intact for at least 5 months when stored in −20 °C.
4. Amount of liposome/siRNA was determined to achieve >50 % of downregulation of EphA2 protein expression. A brief sonication is recommended to avoid the aggregation and formation of large liposomes.
5. Probe sonication is not recommended for this procedure.
6. To evaluate the loading efficiency, fluorescently labeled siRNA with Alexa 555 can be used, and fluorescence intensity of the supernatant can be measured at Ex 555/Em 592. Successful loaded should yield approximately 80 % of loading (i.e., 1 μg siRNA remains in the supernatant and 4 μg of siRNA loading into 1×10^6 particles).
7. Washing the PSP/liposome pellet with DI water does not cause release of liposome from the silicon particles. However, if necessary, PBS wash results in release of liposomes that attach to the surface of the PSP.

8. PSP/liposome pellet may be aggregated, and therefore, brief sonication prior to injection is necessary, especially for intravenous injection. Intravenous injection of aggregated microparticles will cause embolization.
9. These cells are stably transfected with firefly luciferase to detect tumor growth. Generally, tumor take rates are approximately 60–80 %.
10. Tumors are palpable in the peritoneal cavity within 2 weeks.
11. Amount of siRNA to achieve sufficient gene silencing with biological effects should be determined for each target. When the PSP is washed with DI water, two phases of release (approx. 30 % of burst release and 70 % of sustained release) can be expected (*see* **Note** 7). Delivery of 15 μg siRNA (triple dose) was necessary to achieve the initial gene silencing via burst release (approx. 5 μg of siRNA was released in the serum right after the i.v. injection). Alternatively, instead of burst release, PBS washed PSP loaded with liposomal siRNA can be co-injected with necessary amounts of liposomal siRNA for the initial gene silencing. While triple dose is used, this will not cause toxicity because release rate is slow over a few weeks.
12. Intraperitoneal injection of PSP/liposome did not result in sustained gene silencing.
13. Alternatively, this procedure can be carried out using a probe sonicator.
14. The amounts of proteins loaded onto the gel should be optimized based on the abundance of the target protein.
15. A single injection of PSP-loaded liposomal siRNA will achieve equivalent gene silencing to twice weekly injections of liposomal siRNA

References

1. Davis ME, Zuckerman JE, Choi CH, Seligson D, Tolcher A, Alabi CA, Yen Y, Heidel JD, Ribas A (2010) Evidence of RNAi in humans from systemically administered siRNA via targeted nanoparticles. Nature 464(7291):173–184
2. Kim DH, Rossi JJ (2007) Strategies for silencing human disease using RNA interference. Nat Rev Genet 8(3):173–184
3. Check E (2005) A crucial test. Nat Med 11(3):243–244
4. DeVincenzo JP (2008) RNA interference strategies as therapy for respiratory viral infections. Pediatr Infect Dis J 27(10 Suppl):S118–S122
5. Vogelstein B, Kinzler KW (2004) Cancer genes and the pathways they control. Nat Med 10(8):789–799
6. Rugo HS (2004) Bevacizumab in the treatment of breast cancer: rationale and current data. Oncologist 9(Suppl 1):43–49
7. Tripathy D (2005) Targeted therapies in breast cancer. Breast J 11(Suppl 1):S30–S35
8. Bumcrot D, Manoharan M, Koteliansky V, Sah DW (2006) RNAi therapeutics: a potential new class of pharmaceutical drugs. Nat Chem Biol 2(12):711–719
9. Aagaard L, Rossi JJ (2007) RNAi therapeutics: principles, prospects and challenges. Adv Drug Deliv Rev 59(2–3):75–86

10. Heidel JD, Yu Z, Liu JY, Rele SM, Liang Y, Zeidan RK, Kornbrust DJ, Davis ME (2007) Administration in non-human primates of escalating intravenous doses of targeted nanoparticles containing ribonucleotide reductase subunit M2 siRNA. Proc Natl Acad Sci USA 104(14):5715–5721
11. Desai AA, Schilsky RL, Young A, Janisch L, Stadler WM, Vogelzang NJ, Cadden S, Wright JA, Ratain MJ (2005) A phase I study of antisense oligonucleotide GTI-2040 given by continuous intravenous infusion in patients with advanced solid tumors. Ann Oncol 16(6):958–965
12. Frank-Kamenetsky M, Grefhorst A, Anderson NN, Racie TS, Bramlage B, Akinc A, Butler D, Charisse K, Dorkin R, Fan Y et al (2008) Therapeutic RNAi targeting PCSK9 acutely lowers plasma cholesterol in rodents and LDL cholesterol in nonhuman primates. Proc Natl Acad Sci USA 105(33):11915–11920
13. Morrissey DV, Lockridge JA, Shaw L, Blanchard K, Jensen K, Breen W, Hartsough K, Machemer L, Radka S, Jadhav V et al (2005) Potent and persistent in vivo anti-HBV activity of chemically modified siRNAs. Nat Biotechnol 23(8):1002–1007
14. Zimmermann TS, Lee AC, Akinc A, Bramlage B, Bumcrot D, Fedoruk MN, Harborth J, Heyes JA, Jeffs LB, John M et al (2006) RNAi-mediated gene silencing in non-human primates. Nature 441(7089):111–114
15. Davis ME (2009) The first targeted delivery of siRNA in humans via a self-assembling, cyclodextrin polymer-based nanoparticle: from concept to clinic. Mol Pharm 6(3):659–668
16. Merritt WM, Lin YG, Spannuth WA, Fletcher MS, Kamat AA, Han LY, Landen CN, Jennings N, De Geest K, Langley RR et al (2008) Effect of interleukin-8 gene silencing with liposome-encapsulated small interfering RNA on ovarian cancer cell growth. J Natl Cancer Inst 100(5):359–372
17. Landen CN Jr, Chavez-Reyes A, Bucana C, Schmandt R, Deavers MT, Lopez-Berestein G, Sood AK (2005) Therapeutic EphA2 gene targeting in vivo using neutral liposomal small interfering RNA delivery. Cancer Res 65(15):6910–6918
18. Lara PN Jr, Higdon R, Lim N, Kwan K, Tanaka M, Lau DH, Wun T, Welborn J, Meyers FJ, Christensen S et al (2001) Prospective evaluation of cancer clinical trial accrual patterns: identifying potential barriers to enrollment. J Clin Oncol 19(6):1728–1733
19. Tasciotti E, Liu X, Bhavane R, Plant K, Leonard AD, Price BK, Cheng MM, Decuzzi P, Tour JM, Robertson F et al (2008) Mesoporous silicon particles as a multistage delivery system for imaging and therapeutic applications. Nat Nanotechnol 3(3):151–157
20. Tanaka T, Godin B, Bhavane R, Nieves-Alicea R, Gu J, Liu X, Chiappini C, Fakhoury JR, Amra S, Ewing A, Li Q, Fidler IJ, Ferrari M (2010) In vivo evaluation of safety of nanoporous silicon carriers following single and multiple dose intravenous administrations in mice. Int J Pharm 402(1–2):190–197
21. Tanaka T, Mangala LS, Vivas-Mejia PE, Nieves-Alicea R, Mann AP, Mora E, Han HD, Shahzad MM, Liu X, Bhavane R et al (2010) Sustained small interfering RNA delivery by mesoporous silicon particles. Cancer Res 70(9):3687–3696

Chapter 37

Exosomes as a Potential Tool for a Specific Delivery of Functional Molecules

Irina Nazarenko, Anne-Kathleen Rupp, and Peter Altevogt

Abstract

Extracellular membrane vesicles derived from the endosomal compartments and released by the fusion of the multivesicular bodies with the cell membrane are referred as exosomes (Exo) [Van Niel et al., J Biochem 140:13–21, 2006]. They function as mediators of intercellular communication and are employed by the organism in the regulation of systemic and local processes. Meantime, Exo are recognized as an indispensable entity of physiological fluids [Caby et al., Int Immunol 17:879–887, 2005; Lasser et al., J Transl Med 9:9, 2011; Lasser et al., Am J Rhinol Allergy 25:89–93, 2011]. Exo and other types of extracellular vesicles, e.g., exosome-like vesicles [van Niel et al., Gastroenterology 121:337–349, 2001] and microvesicles (MV) [Daveloose et al., Thromb Res 22:195–201, 1981], contain multiple functional molecules including lipids [Vidal et al., J Cell Physiol 140:455–462, 1989]; proteins [Simpson et al., Expert Rev Proteomics 6:267–283, 2009]; mRNA [Valadi et al., Nat Cell Biol 9:654–659, 2007]; DNA [Waldenstrom et al., PLoS One 7:e34653, 2012]; noncoding RNA, e.g., miRNA [Simpson et al., Expert Rev Proteomics 6:267–283, 2009]; and retrotransposon elements [Balaj et al., Nat Commun 2:180, 2011]. Assessment of the biological functions of Exo showed that they deliver specifically their cargo from the donor to recipient cells. Albeit the molecular mechanisms of this process are not fully understood, approaches for the application of Exo and MV as a tool for a cell-specific delivery of signalling molecules were successfully tested in in vitro and in vivo models [Maguire et al., Mol Ther 20:960–971, 2012]. Ovarian cancer cells release Exo, which bind stroma cells as well as donor cancer cells [Escrevente et al., BMC Cancer 11:108, 2011].

Here we describe an experimental approach for the assessment of Exo interaction and uptake by target cells. Methods for the isolation and purification of Exo from cell culture supernatants are included. To allow visualization of vesicle uptake, labelling of Exo with different fluorescent dyes, such as CFSE, PKH, DHPE, and $DiOC_{18}$, is presented. Finally, we explain qualitative and quantitative analysis of Exo uptake by immunofluorescence and flow cytometry, respectively.

Key words Exosomes, Microvesicles, Exosome uptake, Exosome labelling, Ovarian cancer, Cell-specific delivery

1 Introduction

Cancer cells release into the extracellular environment multiple factors composed of soluble components, e.g., cytokines, growth factors, and different types of extracellular membrane vesicles,

Anastasia Malek and Oleg Tchernitsa (eds.), *Ovarian Cancer: Methods and Protocols*, Methods in Molecular Biology, vol. 1049, DOI 10.1007/978-1-62703-547-7_37, © Springer Science+Business Media New York 2013

e.g., microvesicles (MV) and exosomes (Exo), which altogether support cancer progression on multiple levels, inducing angiogenesis and vasculogenesis [14], immunosuppression [16], and recruitment of bone-marrow-derived progenitors to the primary tumor or to the sites of metastasis [15].

Exo are defined as a population of small extracellular membrane vesicles with a diameter of 30–100 nm, formed by the internalization of a portion of the limiting membrane in the late endosomes which then referred as multivesicular bodies (MVBs) [17]. Secretion of the Exo occurs upon fusion of MVBs with the cell membrane [18–20]. According to the recent findings, the formation of intraluminal vesicles of MVBs is likely being a lipid-driven process regulated by components of the ESCRT (endosomal sorting complex required for transport) machinery [21]. The subsequent event, the fusion of MVBs with the cell membrane leading to the Exo secretion, is controlled by the RAB family of small GTPases, e.g., Rab27, Rab11, Rab35, and SNARE proteins, recently reviewed by Bobrie et al. [22].

There is a profile of proteins, comprised of components of the recycling and vesicular transport machinery identified in Exo of different origins, suggesting a universal mechanism of their formation. Among them, several Exo markers are determined, such as tetraspanins CD63 and CD81, major histocompatibility complex I (MHCI), lysosomal-associated membrane proteins 1 and 2 (LAMP1, LAMP2), and tumor susceptibility gene 101 (TSG101) [22]. Additionally, Exo reveal a pattern of proteins and nucleic acids, which is specific for the cell of origin and can be defined as a "fingerprint" or a "signature" of a donor cell [3, 8, 9, 18, 19, 23–26]. Albeit the molecular mechanisms of this process are not clarified in all details, we and others demonstrated that some proteins, for instance, tetraspanins, contribute to the recruitment of certain components to the Exo [23, 27]. Also, glycosylphosphatidylinositol-anchored membrane proteins such as CD24 are preferentially recruited into Exo [28]. Further investigations are required to learn more about the regulation of the Exo content. However, based on the available data, we can conclude that cargo of Exo is tightly regulated by the donor cells and includes molecules, responsible for a targeting of Exo to recipient cells either in the same organ or on distant sites. Furthermore, Exo contain a specific set of proteins, mRNA, miRNA, and possibly other components, assuring for their biological effects.

Once being secreted into the extracellular environment, Exo are distributed through the whole body within the physiological fluids and can be delivered to their target cells/organs. In the tumor context, Exo released by the tumor cells are enriched in the blood of patients. Recent findings demonstrated that tumor Exo represent on the first line an easy accessible source for biological markers which possess a high potential to improve current diagnostic accuracy, as has been demonstrated for ovarian cancer [28–31]. Furthermore, Exo represent a specific transport mechanism between donor and recipient cells that can be applied for a specific delivery of certain molecules to a desired recipient.

Here, we describe an experimental setup allowing to assess interaction and uptake of Exo by the recipient cells. This chapter contains methods for the Exo isolation and labelling with different fluorescent dyes, followed by the setting of interaction assay and analysis of Exo uptake using immunofluorescence and flow cytometry. Furthermore, we emphasize that Exo released by ovarian cancer cells not only are able to target distant recipient cells, for instance, adipose tissue-derived mesenchymal stem cells [32], but might act in an autocrine manner, being internalized by tumor cells [13].

2 Materials

2.1 Isolation of Exo from the Cell Culture Supernatants

1. Human ovarian carcinoma cell line SKOV3ip.
2. DMEM (Dulbecco's Modified Eagle Medium) cell culture medium, supplemented with 10 % FCS (fetal calf serum), 2 mM glutamine, 4.5 g/l glucose (corresponds to high-glucose DMEM), and 1.5 g/l sodium pyruvate.
3. Serum-free supernatants of cells used as donor for Exo production (*see* **Note 1**).
4. 1× phosphate-buffered saline buffer (PBS): buffer prepared from the 10× PBS stock solution (137 mM NaCl, 8.1 mM Na_2HPO_4, 2.7 mM KCl, 1.5 mM KH_2PO_4, pH 7.2–7.4).
5. Proteinase inhibitor stock solution prepared, for instance, by dissolving commercially available tablets containing a mixture of proteases in bi-distilled (18.0 Ω) water. Standard-wise 25×–100× stock solution is used. The stock can be stored at −20 °C.
6. Optional, a fixed-angle ultracentrifuge rotor, such as 45Ti or 50.2 Ti (Beckman Coulter, Krefeld, Germany), should be used for sedimentation of Exo (*see* **Note 3**).

2.2 Labelling of Exo with a Fluorescent Dye

1. A kit for measurement of protein concentration routinely used in your laboratory.
2. Red fluorescent reagent, PKH26 (Sigma-Aldrich, Munich, Germany).
3. Green fluorescent reagent, PKH67 (Sigma-Aldrich, Munich, Germany).
4. Red fluorescent rhodamine-labelled phospholipid, rhodamine-DHPE(Lissamine-rhodamine-B-sulfonyl)-1,2-dihexadecanoyl-sn-glycero-3-phosphoethanolamine (Life Technologies, Darmstadt, Germany).

5. Green fluorescent pro-dye CFSE (carboxyfluorescein diacetate succinimidyl ester) (Sigma-Aldrich, Munich, Germany).
6. Green fluorescent, lipophilic carbocyanine $DiOC_{18}$ (3,3′ Dioctadecyloxacarbocyanine Perchlorate) (Life Technologies, Darmstadt, Germany).
7. 1 ml syringe and 27–31 G needle.
8. Chloroform.
9. Ethanol 95 %.
10. 1× PBS buffer.
11. BSA 0.5 % solution in 1× PBS.
12. SW40/SW41Ti ultracentrifugation rotor (Beckman Coulter, Krefeld, Germany).
13. Polyallomer or polycarbonate ultracentrifugation tubes appropriate for the rotor used.
14. For purification of exosomes through discontinuous sucrose gradient: 2.5 M sucrose solution in 20 mM HEPES/NaOH, pH 7.2; 0.25 M sucrose solution in 20 mM HEPES/NaOH, pH 7.2; gradient mixer, 10× HBS solution (78.8 g/l NaCl, 7.4 g/l KCl, 0.81 $MgCl_2$, 1.1 g/l $CaCl_2$, 23.6 g/l HEPES, pH 7.4 NaOH). Filter-sterilize all solutions by passing through 0.22 μm filter and store for up to 10 weeks at 4 °C.
15. For purification of Exo on sucrose cushion, prepare 30 % sucrose solution in D_2O and 200 mM Tris base, pH 7.4, filter-sterilized by passing through 0.22 μm filter. Store for up to 10 weeks at 4 °C.
16. Amicon Ultra-4 centrifugal filter units, PLKH Ultracel-PL Membrane 100 kDa.

2.3 Interaction Assay Between Exo and Recipient Cells

1. Lab-Tek chamber slides with removable media chamber.
2. BD Falcon 24-well multiwell plates.
3. 1× PBS buffer.
4. 4 % paraformaldehyde solution in 1× PBS.
5. 0.2 % Tween 20 solution in 1× PBS.
6. Primary antibody recognizing human alpha-tubulin, for instance, mouse monoclonal anti-alpha-tubulin antibody DM1.
7. WGA-Alexa 647 (wheat germ agglutinin).
8. Secondary antibody donkey anti-mouse IgG Alexa Fluor 594.
9. Blocking buffer: 0.2 % (w/v) cold-water fish gelatine (Sigma-Aldrich, Munich, Germany) + 0.5 % (w/v) BSA in 1× PBS.
10. Fluorescence mounting medium.
11. BD flow cytometer or an alternative.

12. Latex beads, aldehyde/sulfate, 4 % w/vol 4 μm (Life Technologies, Darmstadt, Germany).
13. Confocal microscope supplied with 63× objective.

3 Methods

3.1 Isolation of Exo from the Cell Culture Supernatants

According to our and others' experience, different cell types vary in the amount of Exo they produce. An average amount of Exo released by the tumor cells under conventional culture conditions results in 50–200 μg exosomal proteins/isolated from 1 l of cell culture supernatants. However, there are cell lines producing significantly lower amount of Exo; those functional analysis might be hindered because of low yields of Exo isolated.

Application of antibiotics should be avoided by cultivation of cells for Exo production. Only mycoplasma-free cells should be used for the Exo preparation:

1. Culture cells in FCS-containing standard growth medium in 14 cm cell culture plates dishes until they reach 70–80 % confluency.
2. For the Exo isolation, wash cells once with 1× PBS to remove traces of FCS and incubate cells for further 24–48 h in serum-free medium (15 ml/plate). Alternatively use cell culture medium supplemented with Exo-depleted FCS (*see* **Note 1**).
3. Control cell viability prior harvesting supernatants to minimize contamination of Exo fraction with apoptotic blebs and other types of vesicles. The portion of viable cells should be comparable with the cell culture growing in medium supplemented with FCS.
4. Harvest cell supernatants. It is advisable to start with approximately 200 ml.
5. To remove cells and cell debris, centrifuge 15 min at 2,000 × *g*, 4 °C and transfer supernatants carefully into fresh tubes. Discard pellets.
6. To remove larger vesicles (MVs), centrifuge 15 min at 5,000 × *g* and 30 min 12,000 × *g*, 4 °C. At that step, storage of supernatants prior proceeding with the isolation protocol is possible (*see* **Note 2**). Pellets can be discarded; alternatively, if examination of MVs is desired, pellets after centrifugation by 12,000 × *g* should be carefully resuspended in a small volume, e.g., 100 μl of 1× PBS supplemented with protease inhibitors and stored at −80 °C.
7. Filter supernatants through a 0.22 μm filter to assure that all larger particles are removed.
8. Sediment Exo by ultracentrifugation 120 min at 110,000 × *g*, 4 °C (*see* **Note 3**).

9. Finally, wash pellets with 1× PBS and centrifuge again at 110,000 ×*g*, at 4 °C for 90 min. According to our experience, Exo pelleted from the same supernatant can be pooled together for the washing step. For that purpose, resuspend all Exo in approximately 1 ml of cold PBS and transfer in one ultracentrifugation tube. Fill the tube with an appropriate volume of 1× PBS and proceed with ultracentrifugation.
10. Discard carefully supernatants immediately after centrifugation and resuspend exosome pellet in 1× PBS. We use 100 μl total volume of 1× PBS supplemented with protease inhibitors to resuspend Exo isolated from 200 to 300 ml of cell culture supernatant. Store Exo at −80 °C (*see* Fig. 1 and **Note 4**).
11. To estimate the amount of Exo isolated, frequently a measurement of exosomal proteins is performed. For that purpose, any standard approach established in your laboratory, such as Bio-Rad Protein Assay Kit or BCA Pierce Protein Assay Kit, can be applied. A protocol adjusted for the measurement of low protein concentrations is optional, considering that the average concentration of Exo proteins is between 0.05 and 1 μg/μl. Alternatively, several devices for a quantitative analysis of Exo, such as NanoSight, were developed during the recent years. However, their application is still not standardized and should be established if corresponding equipment is available. Therefore, these methods are not further considered in the protocol.

3.2 Labelling of Exo with Fluorescent Dye

Labelling of Exo can be performed using different dyes. Here we describe the preparation and application of three different types of dyes that can be chosen dependent on the aim of the experiment. First, there are lipophilic synthetic dyes able to incorporate into the cell membrane such as PKH26, PKH67, and $DiOC_{18}$ (dialkylcarbocyanine); second, there are phospholipids, e.g., DHPE (*N*-(Lissamine-rhodamine-B-sulfonyl)-1,2-dihexadecanoyl-sn-glycero-3-phosphoethanolamine), directly intercalating into the cell membrane; and the third type is represented by the intracellular membrane-permeable dyes, for instance, carboxyfluorescein diacetate succinimidyl ester (CFSE), that can be released within the Exo and consequently detected in the recipient cell after uptake.

The following features can be considered by the choice of the dye to apply:

1. Excitation and emission wavelength of the dyes: green fluorochromes, PKH67 Ex/Em (490/504 nm), CFSE Ex/Em (492/517 nm), and $DiOC_{18}$ Ex/Em (484/501), and red fluorochromes, PKH26 Ex/Em (551/567 nm) and DHPE Ex/Em (560/581 nm).

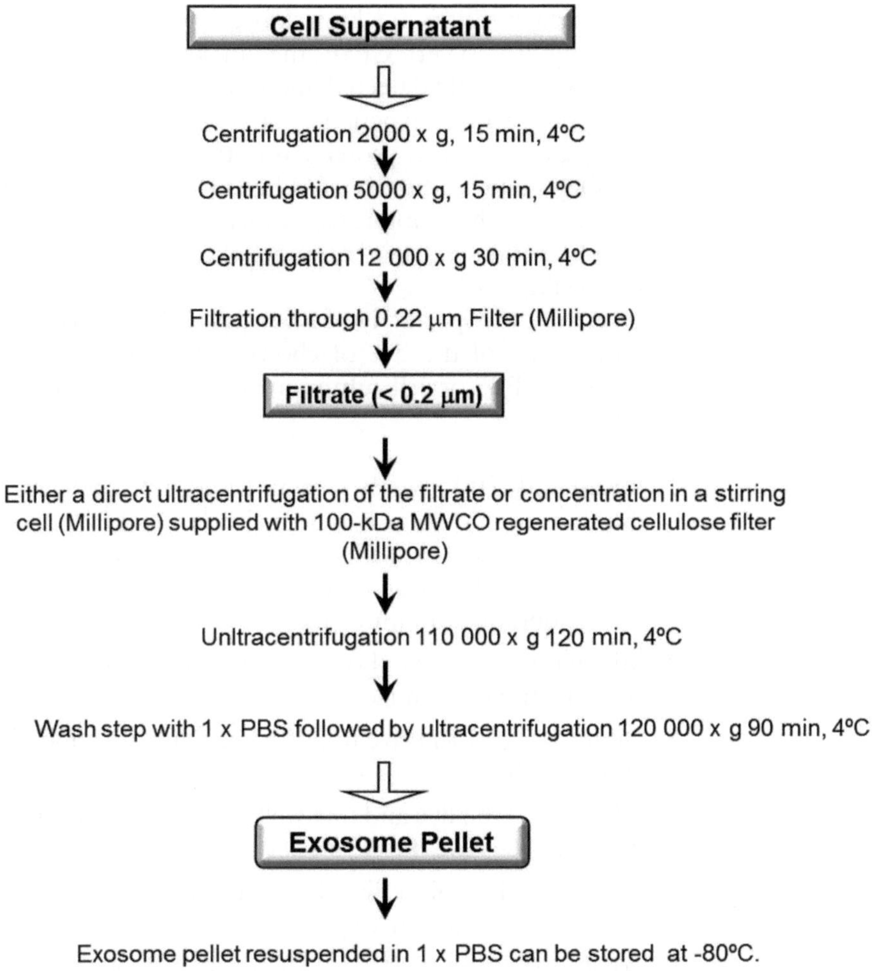

Fig. 1 Schema of Exo isolation from the cell culture supernatants

2. Mechanisms of function and potential application: PKH dyes are lipophilic fluorescent linkers, partitioning non-covalently into the cell membranes. They can be efficiently used by long-term visualization and Exo uptake studies.

DHPE is a phospholipid which doesn't transfer between lipid bilayers and therefore can be used for the investigation of fusion events based on fluorescence resonance energy transfer. Additionally, by labelling the cell membrane with this dye, endocytosis events, intracellular membrane traffic, and vesicle release can be visualized.

$DiOC_{18}$ is an analogue of long-chain dialkylcarbocyanine and is frequently used as a lipophilic tracer for *s* labelling of neuronal cells. The advantage of this tracer is that it does not affect cell viability and physiological properties.

CFSE is a colorless dye which passively diffuses through the cell membrane until the acetate group is cleaved by intracellular esterases, which results in a high fluorescence at 517 nm. Thus, by the labelling of Exo with CFSE, the uptake of Exo by the recipient cells can be efficiently detected and quantified as described below.

According to our experience, application of Exo corresponding 100 μg of exosomal proteins is optional for the establishment of the labelling procedure (*see* Subheading 3.1). Once established, adjust and keep the amount of Exo used constant, since the ratio between Exo and the dye is critical for the quality and the efficiency of the labelling.

To ensure the specificity of Exo uptake, it is advisable to use as a negative control the dye of choice diluted in a corresponding amount of 1× PBS or cell culture medium (use the same diluent as for the Exo).

3.2.1 Labelling of Exo with PKH Dyes

1. Resuspend 100 μg Exo sedimented by ultracentrifugation (Subheading 3.1; Fig. 1) in a final volume of 200 μl of ice-cold PBS supplemented with protease inhibitors. Approximately 300 ml of cell culture supernatant will be required to yield corresponding amount of Exo.
2. Mix gently with 500 μl of Diluent C provided by the supplier; keep the mixture on ice.
3. Dilute 1 μl of PKH dye in 500 μl of Diluent C and mix to disperse the dye.
4. Add Exo to the dye and mix well by pipetting. Total volume of the mixture is 1.2 ml.
5. Incubate for 5 min either by rotation at 4 °C or keeping the samples on ice and mixing periodically.
6. To stop staining, add 1 ml of the Exo-depleted FCS or 1 % BSA solution in 1× PBS, incubate for 1 min, and sediment Exo by ultracentrifugation at 110,000 × *g* for 2 h at 4 °C. Alternatively, Exo can be purified by sucrose gradient ultracentrifugation (Subheading 3.3.1; Fig. 2), sucrose cushion centrifugation (Subheading 3.3.2), or ultrafiltration (Subheading 3.3.3).
7. Resuspend pelleted Exo in a total volume of 50 μl 1× PBS.

3.2.2 Labelling of Exo with DHPE

1. Prepare 5 mg/ml DHPE stock solution in chloroform. The stock can be stored in darkness at −20 °C.
2. Resuspend 100 μg Exo sedimented by ultracentrifugation (Subheading 3.1; Fig. 1) in a final volume of 200 μl of ice-cold PBS supplemented with protease inhibitors. Approximately 300 ml of cell culture supernatant will be required to yield corresponding amount of Exo.
3. Dilute 1 μl of the DHPE stock solution in 50 μl of chloroform and vacuum-dry: the dye should form a thin film on the walls of the tube. Keep it protected from direct light.

Purification of labeled exosomes via continuous sucrose gradient

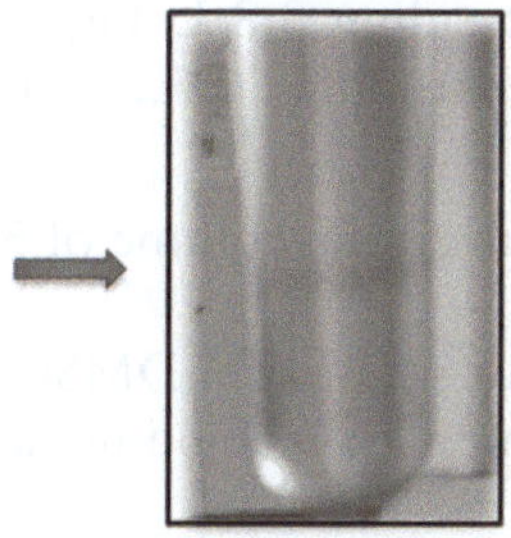

Fraction #	refractive index
1	1,3478
2	1,3565
3	1,3650
4	1,3720
5	1,3785
6	1,3860
7	1,3925
8	1,4005
9	1,4085
10	1,4160
11	1,4245
12	1,4250

Exosomes can be visualised in the layer between 1,11g/ml to 1,17g/ml sucrose, corresponding refraction index 1,39 to 1,41

Fig. 2 Purification of labelled Exo in continuous sucrose gradient. If labelling was performed with DHPE, the Exo layer is visible in light red (*red arrow*). Labelled Exo can be sedimented by ultracentrifugation and stored at −80 °C. However, higher uptake efficiency and biological activity are obtained if freshly prepared Exo are applied

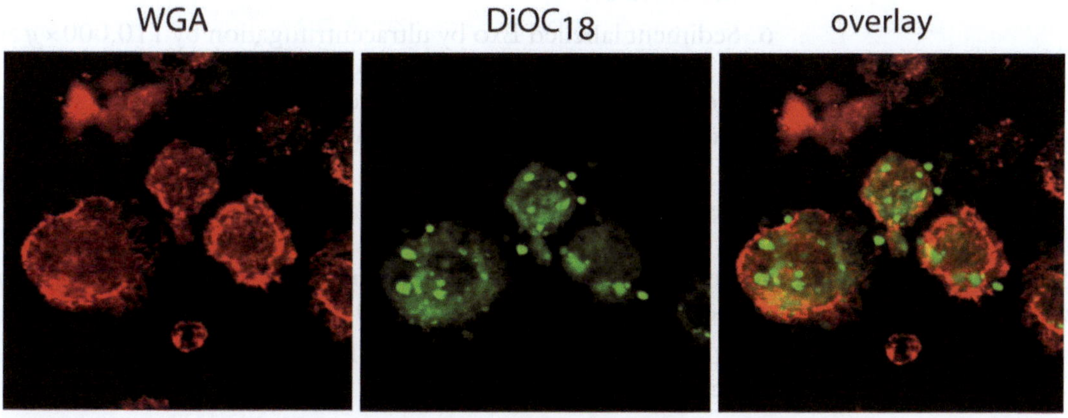

Fig. 3 Fluorescent staining of THP-1 cells after uptake of $DiOC_{18}$-labelled Exo from ovarian carcinoma ascites. Cellular membranes were visualized by staining with Alexa 647-WGA

4. Resuspend the dye in 50 μl of ice-cold 95 % ethanol by pipetting and vigorous vortexing.
5. Apply immediately into 500 μl of ice-cold 1× PBS using 1 ml syringe and a 31 G needle. Usage of a syringe allows more efficient distribution of the dye and consequently homogenous Exo labelling as compared with the application of a regular pipette tip.

6. Using the same syringe, inject the DHPE/1× PBS solution into the Exo suspension and incubate by gentle rotation for 1 h at 4 °C protected from light.
7. To remove unbound DHPE, purify Exo by sucrose gradient ultracentrifugation (Subheading 3.3.1; Fig. 2), sucrose cushion centrifugation (Subheading 3.3.2), or ultrafiltration (Subheading 3.3.3).
8. Resuspend pelleted Exo in a total volume of 50 μl 1× PBS.

3.2.3 Labelling of Exo with CFSE

1. Prepare 5 mM CFSE stock solution in DMSO. To avoid freezing-thawing cycles, prepare CFSE single-use aliquots and store at −20 °C or −80 °C.
2. Immediately prior Exo labelling, equilibrate an aliquot of CFSE solution to room temperature.
3. Resuspend 20–100 μg Exo sedimented by ultracentrifugation (Subheading 3.1; Fig. 1) in 1× PBS containing 0.5 % BSA in a final volume of 200 μl.
4. Add CFSE at final concentration of 5 μM to the Exo and incubate for 30 min at 37 °C by gentle rotation.
5. To stop labelling, dilute Exo approximately 65-fold with cell culture medium, supplemented with Exo-depleted FCS (*see* **Note 1**).
6. Sediment labelled Exo by ultracentrifugation by 110,000 ×*g* at 4 °C for 2 h. Alternatively, Exo can be purified by sucrose gradient ultracentrifugation (Subheading 3.3.1; Fig. 2), sucrose cushion centrifugation (Subheading 3.3.2), or ultrafiltration (Subheading 3.3.3).
7. Resuspend pelleted Exo in a total volume of 50 μl 1× PBS.

3.2.4 Labelling of Exo with $DiOC_{18}$

1. Resuspend 100 μg Exo sedimented by ultracentrifugation in 1× PBS in a final volume of 500 μl.
2. Add 5 μl of a 3 mM $DiOC_{18}$/DMSO solution to the resuspended Exo.
3. Incubate Exo for 2 h at 37 °C by gentle rotation.
4. Sediment labelled Exo by ultracentrifugation at 110,000 ×*g* for 2 h at 4 °C.
5. Resuspend the sample in 300 μl 1× PBS.
6. Repeat sedimentation of labelled Exo by ultracentrifugation at 110,000 ×*g*, at 4 °C for 2 h.
7. Resuspend pelleted Exo in a total volume of 60 μl 1× PBS.

3.3 Purification of Labelled Exo

To purify labelled Exo and to remove efficiently unbound dye, different methods can be applied. We describe here three approaches: sucrose gradient ultracentrifugation, sucrose cushion, and ultrafiltration. Albeit sucrose gradient-based techniques allow for a specific purification of intact Exo within a fraction of a given density, our and others' observations show that the Exo after purification exhibit a diminished biological activity. In contrast, application of ultrafiltration is a method of choice to remove unbound dye keeping Exo activity unchanged. However, bigger molecules, destroyed Exo, or other types of vesicles might remain in the preparation.

3.3.1 Purification of Exo by Sucrose Gradient Ultracentrifugation

1. Dilute labelled Exo in 1 ml 2.5 M sucrose dissolved in 20 mM HEPES/NaOH, pH 7.2, and load on the bottom of an ultracentrifugation tube for SW40/SW41 rotor (*see* **Note 5**).
2. Cover Exo with continues sucrose gradient (2.5 M sucrose—0.25 M sucrose prepared in 20 mM HEPES/NaOH, pH 7.2).
3. Centrifuge 15 h at 220,000 × *g*, 4 °C.
4. If the labelling was successful, a corresponding layer with Exo will be visible after ultracentrifugation (Fig. 2).
5. Carefully collect 12 fractions (1 ml/fraction) from the top. Don't disturb the gradient.
6. Dilute fractions containing Exo with 1× HBS and centrifuge 2 h at 110,000 × *g*, 4 °C to sediment Exo.
7. Resuspend pellet in 50 μl of 1× HBS.
8. Measure concentration of the exosomal proteins and dilute labelled Exo to the concentration of 10 μg/μl with cell culture medium for uptake assay.

3.3.2 Purification of Exo on a 30 % Sucrose Cushion

As an alternative to sucrose gradient, labelled Exo can be purified on 30 % sucrose cushion.

1. Load 1.5 ml of 30 % D2O/Tris solution on the bottom of SW40/SW41 centrifugation tube to make cushion.
2. Add Exo diluted in 10.5 ml PBS; don't disturb cushion.
3. Centrifuge 2 h at 110,000 × *g*, 4 °C.
4. Collect approximately 1 ml of cushion, which now contains Exo.
5. Transfer Exo into a fresh ultracentrifuge tube, dilute with PBS, and centrifuge 2 h, at 110,000 × *g*, 4 °C.
6. Resuspend Exo pellet in 50 μl 1× PBS.
7. Measure concentration of the exosomal proteins and dilute labelled Exo to the concentration of 10 μg/μl with cell culture medium for uptake assay.

3.3.3 Purification of Exo by Ultrafiltration

An alternative method for the purification of unbound dye is ultrafiltration. We describe here the application of Amicon Ultra-4 centrifugal filter units with 100 kDa molecular weight cutoff.

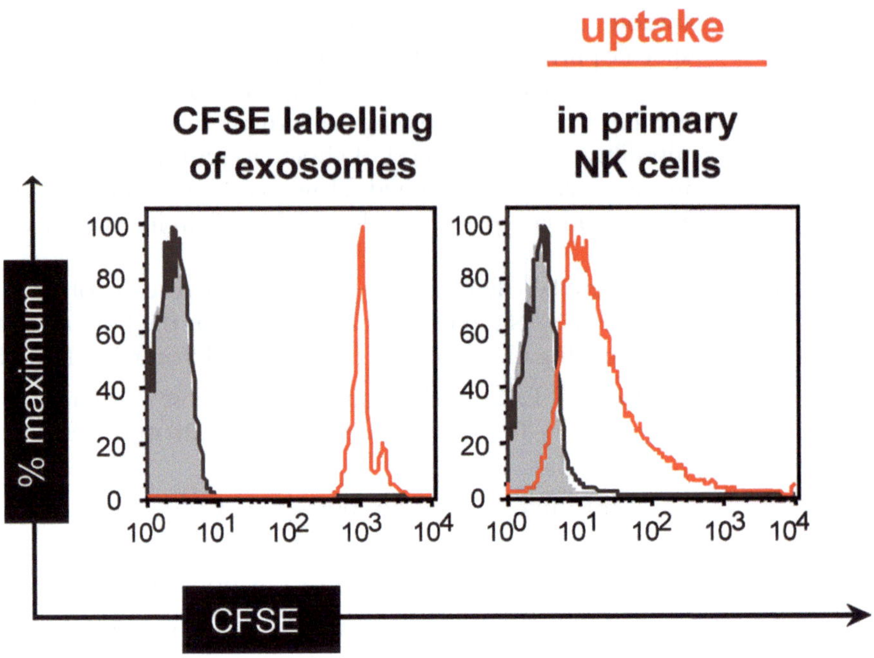

Fig. 4 Cytofluorographic analysis of primary NK cells following uptake of CSFE-labelled Exo from breast carcinoma ascites fluid (*right part* of the figure). The *left part* of the figure shows a control of Exo labelling: Exo adsorbed to aldehyde/sulfate latex beads

1. Dilute labelled Exo to 4 ml and fill an Ultra-4 centrifugal filter unit.
2. Centrifuge 20 min at 3,000 × *g*, 4 °C. Control volume, remained in the tube, centrifuge for additional 20 min if required.
3. Concentrate Exo to a final volume of 100 μl.
4. Measure concentration of the exosomal proteins and dilute labelled Exo to the concentration of 10 μg/μl with cell culture medium for uptake assay.

3.4 Flow Cytometry of Exo

As a control allowing estimation of the fluorescence of labelled Exo, flow cytometry can be performed (Fig. 4).

1. Dilute 5 μg of labelled Exo in 1× PBS to a final volume of 100 μl.
2. Add 3 μl of aldehyde/sulfate latex beads.
3. Incubate Exo with the beads for 15 min at room temperature (RT).
4. Add 800 μl 1× PBS to the Exo/bead mixture.
5. Incubate the Exo/bead mixture for 1 h at RT.
6. Block free aldehyde/sulfate binding groups by adding 100 μl of 1 M glycine/1× PBS and 100 μl of 10 % BSA/1× PBS to the mixture.
7. Incubate the Exo/bead mixture for 30 min at RT.

8. Pellet the beads by centrifugation 2 min at 10,000 × *g*, RT.
9. Wash the beads twice with 300 μl 3 % BSA/1× PBS.
10. Dilute the beads in 300 μl 3 % BSA/1× PBS and analyze them by flow cytometry.

3.5 Exo Uptake Assay

To study Exo uptake, different approaches can be applied dependent on the question addressed. Thus, for the assessment of intracellular localization of the Exo after uptake, immunofluorescence analysis allowing visualization of Exo and their colocalization with intracellular proteins could be a method of choice. In the protocol below, we use as an example staining with tubulin allowing colocalization of Exo with cytoskeleton. However, for a quantitative analysis, flow cytometry should be performed as described in Subheading 3.5.3.

3.5.1 Assessment of Exo Uptake by Adherently Growing Cells Using Immunofluorescence

1. To assess uptake of Exo, plate the cell in chamber slides for immunofluorescence analysis and in 24-well plates to examine uptake by flow cytometry.
2. Allow the cells to grow until they reach 60–80 % confluency.
3. Add Exo labelled with a fluorescent dye resuspended in cell culture medium at the final concentration 10–50 μg/ml as describe above.
4. Incubate Exo with the cells by 37 °C, 5 % CO_2, and 95 % humidity. Incubation time from 30 min up to 4 h should be tested to define optional duration of the procedure.
5. Remove Exo-containing medium from the single chamber slides.
6. Wash cells gently with 2× PBS to eliminate unbound Exo. This step is particularly important to avoid unspecific signal of Exo remaining on the cell surface.
7. Fix the cells in 4 % paraformaldehyde for 20 min, RT.
8. Wash three times with 1× PBS.
9. For staining of intracellular proteins, cells should be permeabilized. Use 0.2 % Tween 20 solution in 1× PBS and incubate cells for 5 min with the detergent, 4 °C. Longer application of Tween 20 or alternative harsh detergents, such as Triton X-100 or NP-40, might disrupt membrane proteins and lead to artificial results. Remove detergent and wash cells with 1× PBS three times.
10. To block unspecific bindings, incubate chamber slides with blocking for 30 min, RT.
11. Wash with 1× PBS three times.
12. To avoid drying of the cells, use a wet chamber for further steps.

13. Incubate with primary anti-tubulin antibody (1:2,000) diluted in the blocking buffer for 1 h; wash again with 1× PBS three times.
14. Incubate with the fluorescent secondary antibody (1:500) diluted in the blocking buffer for 45 min, RT; wash 1× PBS five times. Protect specimens from light during these steps.
15. Remove media chamber using forceps. Distribute mounting medium on a cover glass and mount the slide carefully avoiding building of air bubbles. Store mounted glass slides at 4 °C in the darkness until microscopy.
16. Proceed with immunofluorescence microscopy. To analyze colocalization of Exo with tubulin, laser confocal microscopy, allowing Z-stack analysis, should be used.

3.5.2 Assessment of Exo Uptake by Cells Growing in the Suspension Using Immunofluorescence

Since some ovarian tumor cell lines or primary tumor cells isolated from the ascites fluid might grow in the suspension, we include below a protocol for nonadherent cells:

1. Seed 2.5×10^5 cells grown in suspension in a 96-well cell culture plate.
2. Add labelled Exo in a concentration 50 μg/ml to the cells.
3. Incubate the cells with Exo for 3 h at 37 °C.
4. Pellet the nonadherent growing cells by centrifugation at $300 \times g$, RT.
5. Wash the pellet 2× with 1× PBS.
6. Add 200 μl of a 4 % paraformaldehyde/PBS solution to the cell pellet. Fix the cells for 20 min, RT.
7. Pellet the cells by centrifugation at $300 \times g$, RT, and wash with 1× PBS.
8. For labelling of the cell membrane, add 200 μl of a 5 μg/ml solution of WGA (wheat germ agglutinin) to the cells.
9. Incubate the cells for 15 min, RT, and wash with 1× PBS. Protect the samples from light.
10. Pellet the cells by centrifugation at $300 \times g$, RT.
11. Pipette the cells on poly-l-lysine-coated glass slides.
12. Incubate the cells on the slides for 1 h at RT in the dark.
13. Wash the slides by short dipping in H_2O and let them dry.
14. Mount the slides with a drop of Mowiol.
15. Proceed with immunofluorescence microscopy (Fig. 3).

3.5.3 Quantitative Analysis of Exo Uptake by Flow Cytometry

To quantify uptake of Exo, flow cytometry analysis should be performed. This method can be used for both adherent cells and cells growing in the suspension.

1. After incubation with Exo, detach cells using 0.05 % trypsin/10 mM EDTA solution (dependent on the cells used in the assay, higher percentage of trypsin, up to 0.5 % might be required. The optional trypsin concentration should be defined experimentally).
2. Wash cells twice with 1× PBS.
3. Resuspend cells with PBS supplemented with 2 % fetal calf serum; proceed with flow cytometry.
4. As a control apply untreated cells trypsinized as described above. Set forward/side scatter using as a minimum 2×10^3 events within the gated live population and calculate cell autofluorescence.
5. Measure PHP26- and DHPE-labelled Exo uptake by a shift of a peak fluorescence intensity in FL2 channel. If PHP67, CFSE, or $DiOC_{18}$ were applied, measure uptake by a shift of a peak fluorescence intensity in FL1 channel. For quantitative analysis use geometric mean of gated population.
6. Apply at least 3 biological and 2 technical replicates if statistical analysis should be performed. Use student's *t*-test; *p* values lower than 0.05 can be considered as significant.

4 Notes

1. Alternatively, medium for Exo production can be supplemented with the Exo-depleted fetal calf serum (FCS). For the depletion, FCS should be centrifuged overnight by 100,000 × *g*, 4 °C; the supernatants filter-sterilized and applied instead of FCS; the pellets containing FCS Exo can be discarded.
2. According to our experience, higher Exo yield can be enriched if fresh cell culture supernatants are used for the Exo isolation. If it is desired to store supernatants prior proceeding with the isolation protocol, cell debris should be removed (proceed until **step 6** of the protocol). Then protease inhibitors should be added to the supernatants to prevent Exo degradation. Supernatants can be stored for several weeks at −80 °C. However, according to our observations, amount and biological activity of Exo might be significantly decreased after storage.
3. If a fixed-angle rotor (45Ti or 50.2 Ti) for centrifugation of large volumes is not available, a concentration step can be included into the protocol after the cell culture supernatants were filtered through the 0.22 μm filter. For the concentration of supernatants to a desired volume, a stirred cell can be used, for instance, 8400 (Millipore) supplied with ultrafiltration disks made of regenerated cellulose (Ultracel Amicon Ultrafiltration Discs, 100 kDa).

Alternatively, one-way ultrafiltration units with 100 kDa molecular weight cutoff can be dependent on the rotor, different rmp correnspoding 110,00 × g will be applied, e.g. SW28 24,000 rpm; SW40 24.000 rpm; SW41 26,000 rpm; SW60 28.000 rpm used.

4. Integrity and quality of Exo preparation should be controlled by electron microscopy.
5. Dependent on the rotor applied for the sucrose gradient, loading on the bottom or on the top of the sucrose gradient can be performed. If the gradient is correctly equilibrated, both top and bottom loading should result in the same distribution of Exo in the gradient.

References

1. Van Niel G, Porto-Carreiro I, Simoes S, Raposo G (2006) Exosomes: a common pathway for a specialized function. J Biochem 140:13–21
2. Caby MP, Lankar D, Vincendeau-Scherrer C, Raposo G, Bonnerot C (2005) Exosomal-like vesicles are present in human blood plasma. Int Immunol 17:879–887
3. Lasser C et al (2011) Human saliva, plasma and breast milk exosomes contain RNA: uptake by macrophages. J Transl Med 9:9
4. Lasser C et al (2011) RNA-containing exosomes in human nasal secretions. Am J Rhinol Allergy 25:89–93
5. van Niel G et al (2001) Intestinal epithelial cells secrete exosome-like vesicles. Gastroenterology 121:337–349
6. Daveloose D et al (1981) Inhibitory effect of microvesicles collected from stored blood on platelet aggregation. Thromb Res 22:195–201
7. Vidal M, Sainte-Marie J, Philippot JR, Bienvenue A (1989) Asymmetric distribution of phospholipids in the membrane of vesicles released during in vitro maturation of guinea pig reticulocytes: evidence precluding a role for "aminophospholipid translocase". J Cell Physiol 140:455–462
8. Simpson RJ, Lim JW, Moritz RL, Mathivanan S (2009) Exosomes: proteomic insights and diagnostic potential. Expert Rev Proteomics 6:267–283
9. Valadi H et al (2007) Exosome-mediated transfer of mRNAs and microRNAs is a novel mechanism of genetic exchange between cells. Nat Cell Biol 9:654–659
10. Waldenstrom A, Genneback N, Hellman U, Ronquist G (2012) Cardiomyocyte microvesicles contain DNA/RNA and convey biological messages to target cells. PLoS One 7:e34653
11. Balaj L et al (2011) Tumour microvesicles contain retrotransposon elements and amplified oncogene sequences. Nat Commun 2:180
12. Maguire CA et al (2012) Microvesicle-associated AAV Vector as a Novel Gene Delivery System. Mol Ther 20:960–971
13. Escrevente C, Keller S, Altevogt P, Costa J (2011) Interaction and uptake of exosomes by ovarian cancer cells. BMC Cancer 11:108
14. Rak J, Yu JL, Klement G, Kerbel RS (2000) Oncogenes and angiogenesis: signaling three-dimensional tumor growth. J Investig Dermatol Symp Proc 5:24–33
15. Psaila B, Lyden D (2009) The metastatic niche: adapting the foreign soil. Nat Rev Cancer 9:285–293
16. Valenti R et al (2007) Tumor-released microvesicles as vehicles of immunosuppression. Cancer Res 67:2912–2915
17. Van Niel G, Porto-Carreiro I, Simoes S, Raposo G (2006) Exosomes: a common pathway for a specialized function. J Biochem 140:13–21
18. Stoorvogel W, Kleijmeer MJ, Geuze HJ, Raposo G (2002) The biogenesis and functions of exosomes. Traffic 3:321–330
19. Simons M, Raposo G (2009) Exosomes–vesicular carriers for intercellular communication. Curr Opin Cell Biol 21:575–581
20. van Niel G, Porto-Carreiro I, Simoes S, Raposo G (2006) Exosomes: a common pathway for a specialized function. J Biochem 140:13–21
21. Babst M (2011) MVB vesicle formation: ESCRT-dependent, ESCRT-independent

and everything in between. Curr Opin Cell Biol 23:6
22. Bobrie A, Colombo M, Raposo G, Thery C (2011) Exosome secretion: molecular mechanisms and roles in immune responses. Traffic 12:1659–1668
23. Nazarenko I et al (2010) Cell surface tetraspanin Tspan8 contributes to molecular pathways of exosome-induced endothelial cell activation. Cancer Res 70:1668–1678
24. Fevrier B, Raposo G (2004) Exosomes: endosomal-derived vesicles shipping extracellular messages. Curr Opin Cell Biol 16:415–421
25. Fevrier B, Vilette D, Laude H, Raposo G (2005) Exosomes: a bubble ride for prions? Traffic 6:10–17
26. Keller S, Sanderson MP, Stoeck A, Altevogt P (2006) Exosomes: from biogenesis and secretion to biological function. Immunol Lett 107:102–108
27. Rana S, Claas C, Kretz CC, Nazarenko I, Zoeller M (2011) Activation-induced internalization differs for the tetraspanins CD9 and Tspan8: Impact on tumor cell motility. Int J Biochem Cell Biol 43:106–119
28. Runz S et al (2007) Malignant ascites-derived exosomes of ovarian carcinoma patients contain CD24 and EpCAM. Gynecol Oncol 107:563–571
29. Taylor DD, Gercel-Taylor C, Parker LP (2009) Patient-derived tumor-reactive antibodies as diagnostic markers for ovarian cancer. Gynecol Oncol 115:112–120
30. Taylor DD, Gercel-Taylor C (2008) MicroRNA signatures of tumor-derived exosomes as diagnostic biomarkers of ovarian cancer. Gynecol Oncol 110:13–21
31. Li J et al (2009) Claudin-containing exosomes in the peripheral circulation of women with ovarian cancer. BMC Cancer 9:244
32. Cho JA et al (2011) Exosomes from ovarian cancer cells induce adipose tissue-derived mesenchymal stem cells to acquire the physical and functional characteristics of tumor-supporting myofibroblasts. Gynecol Oncol 123:379–386

INDEX

Anastasia Malek and Oleg Tchernitsa (eds.), *Ovarian Cancer: Methods and Protocols*, Methods in Molecular Biology, vol. 1049, DOI 10.1007/978-1-62703-547-7,

MIX
Papier aus verantwortungsvollen Quellen
Paper from responsible sources
FSC® C105338

If you have any concerns about our products,
you can contact us on
ProductSafety@springernature.com

In case Publisher is established outside the EU,
the EU authorized representative is:
Springer Nature Customer Service Center GmbH
Europaplatz 3, 69115 Heidelberg, Germany

Printed by Libri Plureos GmbH
in Hamburg, Germany